EMERGENCY MEDICINE

A COMPREHENSIVE STUDY GUIDE
FOURTH EDITION

Companion Handbook

EDITORS

David Cline, M.D.
Clinical Associate Professor, Assistant Residency Director, Department of Emergency Medicine, University of North Carolina School of Medicine, Chapel Hill, and Education Director, Wake Medical Center, Raleigh, North Carolina

O. John Ma, M.D.
Assistant Professor, Department of Emergency Medicine, University of North Carolina School of Medicine, Chapel Hill, North Carolina

Judith E. Tintinalli, M.D., M.S.
Steven J. Dresnick, M.D. Distinguished Professor and Chair in Emergency Medicine, Department of Emergency Medicine, University of North Carolina at Chapel Hill, Chapel Hill, North Carolina

Ernest Ruiz, M.D.
Professor of Clinical Emergency Medicine, University of Minnesota Medical School, and Head, Emergency Medicine Program, Minneapolis, Minnesota

Ronald L. Krome, M.D.
Professor of Emergency Medicine, Wayne State University, Detroit, Michigan

EMERGENCY MEDICINE

A COMPREHENSIVE STUDY GUIDE

FOURTH EDITION

Companion Handbook

American
College of
Emergency
Physicians

David Cline
O. John Ma
Judith E. Tintinalli
Ernest Ruiz
Ronald L. Krome

McGraw-Hill
Health Professions Division

*New York   St. Louis   San Francisco   Auckland
Bogotá   Caracas   Lisbon   London   Madrid
Mexico City   Milan   Montreal   New Delhi
San Juan   Singapore   Sydney   Tokyo   Toronto*

McGraw-Hill

*A Division of The **McGraw·Hill** Companies*

NOTICE

Medicine is an ever-changing science. As new research and clinical experience broaden our knowledge, changes in treatment and drug therapy are required. The editors and the publisher of this work have checked with sources believed to be reliable in their efforts to provide information that is complete and generally in accord with the standards accepted at the time of publication. However, in view of the possibility of human error or changes in medical sciences, neither the editors nor the publisher nor any other party who has been involved in the preparation or publication of this work warrants that the information contained herein is in every respect accurate or complete. Readers are encouraged to confirm the information contained herein with other sources. For example and in particular, readers are advised to check the product information sheet included in the package of each drug they plan to administer to be certain that the information contained in this book is accurate and that changes have not been made in the recommended dosages or in the contraindications for administration. This recommendation is of particular importance in connection with new or infrequently used drugs.

EMERGENCY MEDICINE, A Comprehensive Study Guide, 4/e
COMPANION HANDBOOK

Copyright © 1996 by The McGraw-Hill Companies, Inc. All rights reserved. Printed in the United States of America. Except as permitted under the United States Copyright Act of 1976, no part of this publication may be reproduced or distributed in any form or by any means, or stored in a data base or retrieval system, without the prior written permission of the publisher.

1 2 3 4 5 6 7 8 9   DOC DOC   9 8 7 6

ISBN 0-07-011402-1

This book was set in Times Roman by Monotype Composition Co., Inc. The editor was M.J. Wonsiewicz. The production supervisor was Rick Ruzycka; the cover designer was Grace Coughlan. The project coordination and management was performed by Monotype Editorial Services. R. R. Donnelley and Sons was printer and binder.

This book is printed on acid-free paper.

CONTENTS

Section 5 Cardiovascular Diseases   183

Section 6 Pulmonary Emergencies   229

Section 7 The Digestive System   251

Section 8 Renal and Genitourinary Disorders   313

Section 9 Gynecology and Obstetrics   333

Section 10 Pediatrics   365

Section 11 Infectious Diseases, Allergy, and Immunology   443

Section 12 Toxicology   499

Section 21 Muscular, Ligamentous, and Rheumatic Disorders   865

Section 22 Psychosocial Disorders, Abuse, and Assault   897

CONTRIBUTORS*

Stephanie Abbuhl, M.D. (26, 27), Medical Director, Emergency Department, Department of Emergency Medicine, University of Pennsylvania School of Medicine, Hospital of the University of Pennsylvania, Philadelphia, Pennsylvania

Amy J. Behrman, M.D. (39), Director, Occupational Health Services, Department of Emergency Medicine, University of Pennsylvania School of Medicine, Hospital of the University of Pennsylvania, Philadelphia, Pennsylvania

Burton Bentley II, M.D. (108, 137, 138, 139, 141, 171, 172), Attending Physician, Department of Emergency Medicine, Northwest Hospital, Tucson, Arizona

William J. Brady, M.D. (140, 142), Assistant Professor, Departments of Emergency Medicine and Internal Medicine, University of Virginia Health Sciences Center, Charlottesville, Virginia

David F. M. Brown, M.D. (38, 41), Attending Physician, Massachusetts General Hospital, and Instructor, Division of Emergency Medicine, Harvard Medical School, Boston, Massachusetts

Michael E. Chansky, M.D. (7, 55), Chief, Department of Emergency Medicine, Cooper Hospital/University Medical Center, Camden, New Jersey

David M. Cline, M.D. (1, 2, 25, 30, 31, 33, 60, 66, 67, 69, 70, 89), Clinical Associate Professor, Assistant Residency Director, Department of Emergency Medicine, University of North Carolina School of Medicine, Chapel Hill, and Education Director, Wake Medical Center, Raleigh, North Carolina

C. James Corrall, M.D., M.P.H. (73, 85), Adjunct Associate Professor of Clinical Pharmacology, Clinical Associate Professor of Pediatrics, Clinical Assistant Professor of Emergency Medicine, Department of Basic Sciences, University of Illinois College of Medicine–Peoria, Peoria, Illinois

David A. Dubow, M.D. (32, 34, 35, 36, 37), Clinical Instructor, Department of Emergency Medicine, University of North Carolina, Chapel Hill, and Attending Physician, Department of Emergency Medicine, Wake Medical Center, Raleigh, North Carolina

Angelique T. Fontenette, M.D. (48), Clinical Instructor, Department of Emergency Medicine, University of Arkansas for Medical Sciences, Little Rock, Arkansas

*The numbers in parentheses following the contributors' names indicate the chapters written by that contributor.

Sally S. Fuller, M.D. (64), Attending Physician, Department of Emergency Medicine, Wake Medical Center, Raleigh, North Carolina

Peggy E. Goodman, M.D. (13, 14, 44, 46), Assistant Professor, Department of Emergency Medicine, East Carolina University School of Medicine, Greenville, North Carolina

John E. Gough, M.D. (8, 9, 15), Assistant Professor, Assistant Medical Director, Division of Emergency Medical Services, Department of Emergency Medicine, East Carolina University School of Medicine, Greenville, North Carolina

Charles J. Graham, M.D. (3), Assistant Professor of Pediatrics, Associate Medical Director, Emergency Department, Arkansas Children's Hospital, Little Rock, Arkansas

Andrew Guertler, M.D. (143), Assistant Professor, Department of Emergency Medicine, University of Virginia Health Sciences Center, Charlottesville, Virginia

Gregory S. Hall, M.D. (53, 54, 88), Instructor, Department of Emergency Medicine, University of Arkansas for Medical Sciences, Little Rock, Arkansas

Kent N. Hall, M.D. (106, 128, 129, 150), Assistant Professor, Department of Emergency Medicine, University of Cincinnati Medical Center, Cincinnati, Ohio

Charles J. Havel, Jr., M.D. (103, 104, 144, 145, 148, 149, 162, 163), Pediatrics Emergency Medicine Fellow, Children's Hospital of Wisconsin, Milwaukee, Wisconsin

Marilyn P. Hicks, M.D. (71, 72, 74, 76), Clinical Assistant Professor, Department of Emergency Medicine, University of North Carolina School of Medicine, Chapel Hill, and Attending Physician, Department of Emergency Medicine, Wake Medical Center, Raleigh, North Carolina

Michael P. Kefer, M.D. (94, 117, 118, 119, 154, 155, 167, 168), Assistant Professor, Department of Emergency Medicine, Medical College of Wisconsin, Milwaukee, Wisconsin

David C. Kolb, M.D. (40), Assistant Professor, Department of Emergency Medicine, University of Arkansas for Medical Sciences, Little Rock, Arkansas

Judith Linden, M.D. (95, 101, 102, 158, 159, 164, 165), Attending Physician, Department of Emergency Medicine, Boston City Hospital, Boston, Massachusetts

O. John Ma, M.D. (100, 132, 133, 134, 135, 146, 147, 151), Assistant Professor, Department of Emergency Medicine, University of North Carolina School of Medicine, Chapel Hill, North Carolina

Juan A. March, M.D. (16, 17, 18, 19), Assistant Professor, Assistant Medical Director, Division of Emergency Medical Services, Department of Emergency Medicine, East Carolina University School of Medicine, Greenville, North Carolina

Cary C. McDonald, M.D. (43, 49, 50), Clinical Assistant Professor, Department of Emergency Medicine, University of North Carolina School of Medicine, Chapel Hill, and EMS Director, Department of Emergency Medicine, Wake Medical Center, Raleigh, North Carolina

Leslie C. McKinney, M.D. (79, 83), Medical Director of Urgent Care Operations, Cardinal Healthcare, P.A., Raleigh, North Carolina

Keith Mausner, M.D. (92, 98, 109, 110, 111, 115, 130, 131), EMS Fellow, Department of Emergency Medicine, Medical College of Wisconsin, Milwaukee, Wisconsin

Greg Mears, M.D. (97, 99, 136, 153, 160, 161, 166, 169), Assistant Professor, Department of Emergency Medicine, University of North Carolina School of Medicine, Chapel Hill, North Carolina

C. Crawford Mechem, M.D. (91, 93, 96, 116, 121, 122, 123, 124, 125, 174), Assistant Professor, Department of Emergency Medicine, University of Pennsylvania School of Medicine, Hospital of the University of Pennsylvania, Philadelphia, Pennsylvania

Stephen W. Meldon, M.D. (112, 113, 120, 152, 156, 157, 176, 177), Assistant Professor, Department of Emergency Medicine, Metrohealth Medical Center, Cleveland, Ohio

Frantz R. Melio, M.D. (5, 29, 42), Clinical Assistant Professor, Department of Emergency Medicine, University of North Carolina School of Medicine, Chapel Hill, and Chairman & Medical Director, Department of Emergency Medicine, Wake Medical Center, Raleigh, North Carolina

Dexter L. Morris, Ph.D., M.D. (90, 105, 107, 114, 170, 173), Assistant Professor and Vice Chair, Department of Emergency Medicine, University of North Carolina School of Medicine, Chapel Hill, North Carolina

Vincent Nacouzi, M.D. (4), Attending Physician, Department of Emergency Medicine, Wake Medical Center, Raleigh, North Carolina

Debra G. Perina, M.D. (20, 21, 68, 78), Associate Professor, Department of Emergency Medicine, University of Virginia Health Sciences Center, Charlottesville, Virginia

Michael C. Plewa, M.D. (77), Director of Research, Emergency Medicine Residency Program, St. Vincent Medical Center, Toledo, Ohio

N. Heramba Prasad, M.D. (47, 51, 56), Associate Professor and Chief, Division of Emergency Medical Services, Department of Emergency

Medicine, East Carolina University School of Medicine, Greenville, North Carolina

Rebecca S. Rich, M.D. (62, 63, 75, 80, 81, 82, 86, 87), Attending Physician, Emergency Department, Durham Regional Hospital, Durham, North Carolina

Elicia A. Sinor, M.D. (61), Assistant Professor, Residency Director, Department of Emergency Medicine, University of Arkansas for Medical Sciences, Little Rock, Arkansas

Eugenia B. Smith, M.D. (28), Clinical Instructor, Department of Emergency Medicine, University of North Carolina School of Medicine, Chapel Hill, and Attending Physician, Department of Emergency Medicine, Wake Medical Center, Raleigh, North Carolina

Marc D. Squillante, D.O. (57), Program Director, Emergency Medicine Residency, Saint Francis Medical Center, The University of Illinois College of Medicine—Peoria, Peoria, Illinois

Sarah A. Stahmer, M.D. (6), Assistant Professor, Associate Residency Program Director, Department of Emergency Medicine, University of Pennsylvania School of Medicine, Hospital of the University of Pennsylvania, Philadelphia, Pennsylvania

Arthur Tascone, M.D. (84), Attending Physician, Department of Emergency Medicine, Wake Medical Center, Raleigh, North Carolina

Stephen H. Thomas, M.D. (58, 59), Assistant Professor, Massachusetts General Hospital, Instructor, Division of Emergency Medicine, Harvard Medical School, and Associate Medical Director, Boston Med-Flight, Boston, Massachusetts

Judith E. Tintinalli, M.D., M.S. (126, 127), Steven J. Dresnick, M.D. Distinguished Professor and Chair in Emergency Medicine, Department of Emergency Medicine, University of North Carolina School of Medicine, Chapel Hill, North Carolina

Christian A. Tomaszewski, M.D. (10, 12, 45, 52), Medical Director, Hyperbaric Medicine, Carolinas Medical Center, Charlotte, North Carolina

Michael Utecht, M.D. (22, 23, 24), Clinical Instructor, Department of Emergency Medicine, University of North Carolina School of Medicine, Chapel Hill, North Carolina, and Attending Physician, Department of Emergency Medicine, Wake Medical Center, Raleigh, North Carolina

Gary D. Wright, M.D. (65), Assistant Professor, Department of Emergency Medicine, University of Arkansas for Medical Sciences, Little Rock, Arkansas

PREFACE

Since the book was first published in 1978, *Emergency Medicine: A Comprehensive Study Guide* has grown with the specialty of emergency medicine. The fourth edition, now hardback, is almost four hundred pages longer than the third edition. The growth of the parent text demanded that a *Companion Handbook* be published, and we are proud to be presenting it to you. We designed the handbook as a clinical tool to guide the diagnosis and management of patients presenting to the emergency department. Although based solely on the textbook, it is not intended to replace the original work. A complete discussion of pathophysiology that is essential to the clinician's understanding of the disease process and the logic behind treatment guidelines has not been included in this book. Instead, we hope that you will find the Handbook a helpful resource while seeing patients and as a supplement to the full text.

We would like to thank the original chapter authors for their hard work and the handbook authors for their practical insight into clinical management. Our goal, as editors, is to assist all physicians, residents, and students who practice in any emergency care setting to provide the best patient care possible.

Many people have contributed long hours to this project. In particular we would like to thank McGraw-Hill and Rosie Walsh for their invaluable assistance. Finally, without the love and support of our families, this book would not be possible. DMC thanks his family and his Father in Heaven; OJM thanks his parents, Simone and Mark; and JET thanks Anne, John, Fafa, and Burt.

David M. Cline, M.D.
O. John Ma, M.D.
Judith E. Tintinalli, M.D., M.S.

1 | RESUSCITATION AND INVASIVE MANAGEMENT

1 | Advanced Airway Support

David M. Cline

Control of the airway is the single most important task for emergency resuscitation. If the patient has inadequate oxygenation or ventilation, has inability to protect the airway due to altered sensorium from illness or drugs, or has external forces compromising the airway (i.e., trauma), he may need advanced airway techniques as described in this chapter.

INITIAL APPROACH

The initial approach to airway management is simultaneous assessment and management of the adequacy of airway patency (the A of ABCs) and oxygenation and ventilation (the B of ABCs).

1. Assess the patient's color and respiratory rate; marked hypoventilation with or without cyanosis may be an indication for immediate intubation.
2. Open the airway with head tilt–chin lift maneuver (use jaw thrust if C-spine injury is suspected). If needed, start bagging the patient with bag–valve–mask device, including an O_2 reservoir. Ensure properly sized mask for a good seal. This technique may require an oral or nasal airway or two rescuers to both seal the mask (two hands) and bag the patient.
3. Place the patient on a cardiac monitor, pulse oximetry, and, possibly, capnography (end–tidal CO_2), while collecting the remaining vitals, pulse, and blood pressure (temperature is important but can be delayed to assure the ABCs).
4. Determine the need for invasive airway management techniques, as described below. Do not wait for arterial blood gases (ABG) if your initial assessment declares the need for invasive airway management. If the patient does not require immediate airway or ventilation control, place the patient on oxygen by face mask, as necessary, to assure an O_2 saturation of 95% and draw laboratory studies as needed. Do not draw an ABG off oxygen unless deemed safe from your initial assessment.

OROTRACHEAL INTUBATION

The most reliable means to ensure a patent airway, provide oxygenation and ventilation, and prevent aspiration is endotracheal intubation. Many conscious patients require intubation (see Rapid Sequence Induction below). Selection of the blade should be considered in advance, if possible. The curved blade rests in the vallecula above the epiglottis and indirectly lifts it off the larynx because of traction on the frenulum. The straight blade is used to lift the epiglottis directly. The curved blade does a better job of clearing the tongue from view, and may be

3

less traumatic and reflex-stimulating. The straight blade is mechanically easier to insert in many patients.

Technique

1. Ensure adequate ventilation while preparing equipment. The patient should be preoxygenated, with or without a mask–valve–bag device, depending on the clinical need. Monitor vital signs and use pulse oximetry throughout the procedure.
2. Select your blade type and size (usually #3 or #4 curved blade, or #2 or #3 straight blade); test your blade light. Select your tube size (usually 7.5–8.0 in women, 8.0–8.5 in men); test the balloon cuff. Lubricate the end of the tube with lidocaine jelly or similar lubricant. Consider the use of a flexible stylet; bend the distal end up if the patient's anatomy requires it. Place your tube and tonsillar tip suction within easy reach. If you have an assistant, ask your assistant to hand you items when needed.
3. Position the patient with head extended and neck flexed, possibly with a rolled towel under the occiput. If C-spine injury is suspected, consider rapid sequence induction with in-line traction, nasotracheal intubation, or cricothyrotomy.
4. Insert the blade on the right, slowly advance the blade looking for the epiglottis, suction as necessary. If using the curved blade, slide the tip into the vallecula and lift (indirectly lifting the epiglottis); if using the straight blade, lift the epiglottis directly. Lift in the direction the handle points, that is, 90° to the blade. Do not rock the blade back on the teeth.
5. Once you visualize the vocal cords, do not take your eyes off them, ask your assistant to place the tube in your hand and pass the tube between the cords, avoiding force. Remove the stylet, inflate the balloon cuff, ventilate with a bag, and check for bilateral breath sounds. Confirm placement with an end-tidal CO_2 detector, if available (not reliable if the patient is in cardiac arrest). Check tube length; the usual distance (on the tube) from the corner of the mouth to 2 cm above the carina is 23 cm in men and 21 cm in women.
6. Tape the tube in place and insert a bite block. Verify correct intubation and tube placement with a portable chest X-ray.
7. If unsuccessful, reoxygenate with mask–valve–bag device. Consider changing the technique, possible using a smaller tube, different blade type or size, or repositioning the patient and reattempting intubation.

Short-term complications from orotracheal intubation (trauma to surrounding structures) are unusual, as long as correct position is confirmed. Failure to confirm position immediately can result in hypoxia and neurologic injury. Endobronchial intubation is usually on the right side and is corrected by withdrawing the tube 2 cm and listening for equal breath sounds.

NASOTRACHEAL INTUBATION

Indications and Contraindications

Nasotracheal intubation is indicated in situations where laryngoscopy is difficult, neuromuscular blockade is hazardous, or cricothyrotomy is unnecessary. Severely dyspneic, awake patients with congestive heart failure, chronic obstructive pulmonary disease (COPD), or asthma often cannot remain supine for other airway maneuvers but do tolerate nasotracheal intubation in the sitting position. Relative contraindications for this technique include complex nasal and massive midface fractures and bleeding disorders.

Technique

1. Spray both nares with a topical vasoconstrictor and anesthetic. Four percent to 10% cocaine solution is an appropriate single agent, but may cause unwanted systemic cardiovascular effects. Topical neosynephrine is an effective vasoconstrictor, and tetracaine is a safe, effective topical anesthetic.
2. Choose the tube size, usually 7.0 to 7.5 in women, and 7.5 to 8.0 in men. Check the balloon cuff of the tube for leaks. Lubricate the tube with lidocaine jelly or similar lubricant.
3. Use the largest nares or use the right side if the nares are equal. Some operators recommend dilating the nares with a lubricated nasal airway. The patient may be sitting up or supine.
4. Have an assistant immobilize the patient's neck. Stand to the patient's side, with one hand on the tube and with the thumb and index finger of the other hand straddling the larynx (Fig. 1-1). Advance the tube slowly, using steady gentle pressure. Twist the tube to help to move past obstructions in the nose and nasopharynx. Advance the tube until you hear maximal airflow through the tube; you are now close to the larynx.
5. Listen carefully to the rhythm of inspiration and expiration. Then gently but swiftly advance the tube during the beginning of inspiration. Entrance into the larynx may initiate a cough, and most expired air should exit the tube even though the cuff is uninflated. Look for fogging of the tube; inflate the cuff.
6. If intubation is unsuccessful, carefully look for a bulge lateral to the larynx (usually the tip of the tube is in the pyriform fossa on the same side as the nares used). If found, retract the tube until you hear maximal breath sounds and reattempt intubation, manually displacing the larynx toward the bulge. If no bulge is seen, it is possible that the tube has gone posteriorly into the esophagus. In this case, withdraw the tube until you hear maximal breath sounds and again reattempt intubation after extending the patient's head and performing a Sellick's maneuver. Another option is using a

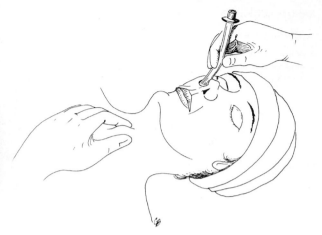

FIG. 1-1. Blind nasotracheal intubation while displacing the larynx to the patient's right.

directional control tip (Endotrol) or fiberoptic laryngoscope. Do not move the head if you suspect C-spine injury.

Complications other than local bleeding are rare. Occasionally, marked bleeding will prompt the need for orotracheal intubation or cricothyrotomy.

CRICOTHYROTOMY

Indications for immediate cricothyrotomy include severe, ongoing tracheobronchial hemorrhage, massive midface trauma, and inability to control the airway with the usual less-invasive maneuvers. Cricothyrotomy is relatively contraindicated in patients with acute laryngeal disease due to trauma or infection or recent prolonged intubation and should not be used in children below age 10.

Technique

1. Use sterile technique. Palpate the cricothyroid membrane, digitally stabilize the larynx. With a #11 scalpel, make a vertical 3 to 4 c incision, start at the superior border of the thyroid cartilage and incise caudally toward the suprasternal notch.
2. Repalpate the membrane and make a horizontal stab through its inferior aspect (Fig. 1-2). Keep the blade temporarily in place.
3. Stabilize the larynx by inserting the tracheal hook into the cricothyroid space and retracting the inferior edge of the thyroid cartilage

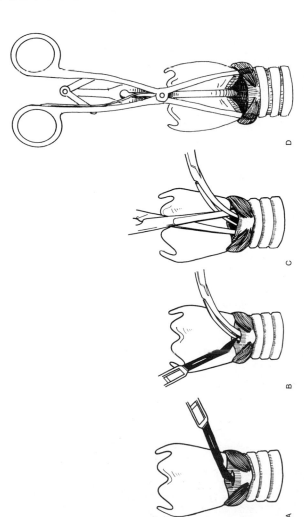

FIG. 1-2. Cricothyrotomy. **A.** Horizontal stab of the cricothyroid membrane following a vertical skin incision. **B** and **C.** Dilation with hemostat. **D.** Dilation with LaBorde dilator.

7

(assistant should hold after you place the hook). Leaving the blade tip in the space, insert a slightly open hemostat straddling the blade and spread open horizontally.

4. Remove the scalpel and insert and spread a dilator (LaBorde or Trousseau). Remove the tracheal hook.

5. Introduce a #4 Shiley tracheostomy tube (or the largest tube that will fit). Alternatively, a small cuffed ET tube may be used (#6, or the largest tube that will fit). Inflate the balloon. Secure the tube in place.

6. Check for bilateral breath sounds. Make sure you are not introducing subcutaneous air.

RAPID SEQUENCE INDUCTION

Complex airway emergencies in select nonfasted patients may require rapid sequence induction. This technique couples sedation to induce unconsciousness (induction) with muscular paralysis. Intubation follows laryngoscopy while maintaining cricoid pressure to prevent aspiration. The principal contraindication is any condition preventing mask ventilation or intubation.

1. Set up monitor, oximetry, and capnography, if available. Check equipment.

2. Preoxygenate with 100% oxygen.

3. **Lidocaine** (1.5 mg/kg IV) should be considered in head trauma patients to prevent increased ICP (intracranial pressure). Atropine (0.2 mg/kg IV) should be considered to prevent reflex bradycardia, but it is not essential.

4. Consider medication for sedation or analgesia, if not using such agents for induction.

5. A defasciculating dose of a nondepolarizing agent (i.e., vecuronium at 0.02 mg/kg) is used if succinylcholine is given for paralysis.

6. Induce with **thiopental** (3–5 mg/kg), **methohexital** (1 mg/kg), or **midazolam** (0.1 mg/kg with 5 mg max). Barbiturates should not be used in patients with hypotension or reactive airway disease (caution in head injury). Benzodiazepines may be inadequate for induction, however, midazolam is an excellent amnestic agent.

7. In patients needing analgesia in addition to sedation, consider opiates for induction. These agents are reversible with naloxone. **Fentanyl** 2 to 10 micrograms/kg is commonly used.

8. Cricoid pressure should be applied before paralysis and maintained until intubation is accomplished.

9. **Succinylcholine** (1.0 mg/kg) is chosen for paralysis in many cases because of its rapid onset and short duration of action; do not use in patients with pre-existing paralysis or hours after severe burns, as hyperkalemia will occur. A nondepolarizing agent such as **vecuronium** (0.2 mg/kg) may be chosen for patients with increased

intracranial pressure, those in status asthmaticus, or at operator discretion.
10. Intubate the trachea and release cricoid pressure.
11. Be prepared to bag the patient if intubation proves unsuccessful. Consider invasive airway techniques as indicated.

WHEN STANDARD TREATMENT FAILS

Alternative drugs for rapid sequence induction are listed in the textbook. Airway management alternatives to the above-described methods include retrograde tracheal intubation, translaryngeal ventilation, digital intubation, transillumination, fiberoptic assistance, and formal tracheostomy. Translaryngeal ventilation may be used to temporarily provide ventilation until a more definitive procedure is possible. When oral intubation is indicated but has been unsuccessful, and the patient can be temporarily ventilated with a bag–valve–mask unit, the following assist methods are warranted. Retrograde tracheal intubation, digital intubation, transillumination, or fiberoptic assistance may be helpful. Formal tracheostomy is reserved for those experienced in the technique when less invasive or more rapid methods (cricothyrotomy) are unsuccessful. These techniques are described in the textbook.

For further reading in *Emergency Medicine, A Comprehensive Study Guide,* see Chapter 11, Advanced Airway Support, by Daniel F. Danzl.

David M. Cline

SUPRAVENTRICULAR ARRHYTHMIAS

Sinus Arrhythmia

Clinical Significance

Some variation in the sinus node discharge rate is common, but if the variation exceeds 0.12 s between the longest and shortest intervals, sinus arrhythmia is present. The electrocardiogram (ECG) characteristics of sinus arrhythmia are: (1) normal sinus P waves and PR intervals; (2) 1:1 AV conduction; and (3) variation of at least 0.12 s between the shortest and longest P–P interval (Fig. 2-1). Sinus arrhythmias are primarily affected by respiration and are most commonly found in children and young adults, disappearing with advancing age.

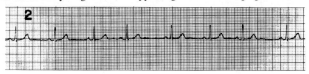

FIG. 2-1. Sinus arrhythmia.

Emergency Department Care

None is required.

Sinus Bradycardia

Clinical Significance

Sinus bradycardia occurs when the sinus node rate falls below 60. The ECG characteristics of sinus bradycardia are: (1) normal sinus P waves and PR intervals; (2) 1:1 AV conduction, and (3) atrial rate below 60 (Fig. 2-2). Sinus bradycardia represents a suppression of the sinus node discharge rate, usually in response to three categories of stimuli: (1) physiologic; (2) pharmacologic; and (3) pathologic (acute inferior myocardial infarction, increased intracranial pressure, carotid sinus hypersensitivity, hypothyroidism).

Emergency Department Care

1. Sinus bradycardia usually does not require specific treatment unless the heart rate is below 50 and there is evidence of hypoperfusion.
2. Initial therapy should begin with atropine 0.5 to 1 mg IV, may repeat up to 3 mg.

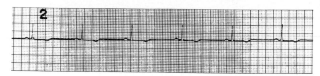

FIG. 2-2. Sinus bradycardia, rate 44.

3. External cardiac pacing can be used in the patient refractory to atropine or isoproterenol.

   a. The patient should be attached to the monitor leads of the external pacing device.
   b. Attach the pacing pads on the patient. The anterior pad should be placed over the precordium, which may require retracting a woman's breast superiorly. Place the posterior pad at the level of the heart, between the spine and the left scapula. Do not use the multifunction pacing defibrillation pads unless the patient is unconscious, as these pads cause more discomfort with pacing.
   c. Turn the pacing rate from 0 to between 60 and 80.
   d. Slowly turn the pacing output from 0 to the lowest point where continuous pacing is observed, usually in the range of 50 to 80 milliamps.
   e. Look for electrical capture on the monitor, recognized by a widened QRS following each pacing spike.
   f. The patient may require sedation with lorazepam (1–2 mg IV) or similar agent, or pain control with morphine (1–2 mg IV) or similar agent.

4. Epinephrine or dopamine drips may be used if external pacing is not available.
5. Internal pacing is required for the patient with symptomatic recurrent or persistent sinus bradycardia.

Sinus Tachycardia

Clinical Significance

The ECG characteristics of sinus tachycardia are: (1) normal sinus P waves and PR intervals; (2) an atrial rate usually between 100 and 160; and, (3) normally, 1:1 conduction between the atria and ventricles (although rapid rates can occur with AV blocks) (Fig. 2-3). Sinus tachycardia is in response to three categories of stimuli: (1) physiologic; (2) pharmacologic; or (3) pathological (fever, hypoxia, anemia, hypovolemia, pulmonary embolism). In many of these conditions, the increased heart rate is an effort to increase cardiac output to match increased circulatory needs.

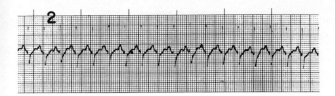

FIG. 2-3.   Sinus tachycardia, rate 176.

Premature Atrial Contractions (PACs)

Clinical Significance

The ECG characteristics of premature atrial contractions (PACs) are:
(1) ectopic P wave appears sooner (premature) than the next expected
sinus beat; (2) the ectopic P wave has a different shape and direction;
and (3) the ectopic P wave may or may not be conducted through
the AV node (Fig. 2-4). Most PACs are conducted with typical QRS
complexes, but some may be conducted aberrantly through the infranodal system. The sinus node is often depolarized and reset so that,
while the interval following the PAC is often slightly longer than the
previous cyclers length, the pause is less than fully compensatory. PACs
are common in all ages and are often seen in the absence of heart
disease.

Emergency Department Care

1. Any precipitating drugs (alcohol, tobacco, or coffee) or toxins should
   be discontinued.
2. Underlying disorders should be treated (stress, fatigue).
3. PACs that produce symptoms or initiate sustained tachycardias can
   be suppressed with quinidine, procainamide, or ß-adrenergic antagonists.

Multifocal Atrial Tachycardia (MFAT)

Clinical Significance

Multifocal atrial tachycardia (MFAT) is caused by at least two different
sites of atrial ectopy. The ECG characteristics of MFAT are: (1) three
or more differently shaped P waves; (2) varying PP, PR, and RR
intervals; and (3) atrial rhythm usually between 100 and 180 (Fig.
2-5). MFAT can be confused with atrial flutter or fibrillation. MFAT
is most often found in elderly patients with decompensated chronic

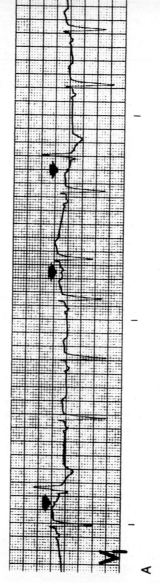

FIG. 2-4. Premature atrial contractions (PACs). Ectopic P' waves (arrows).

A

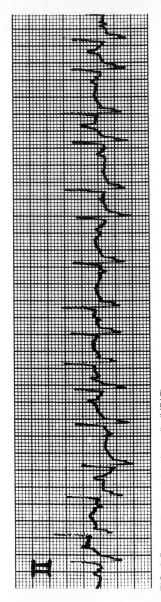

FIG. 2-5. Multifocal atrial tachycardia (MFAT).

14

lung disease, but it also may be found in patients with congestive heart failure or sepsis, or be caused by methylxanthine toxicity.

Emergency Department Care

1. Treatment is directed toward the underlying disorder.
2. Specific antiarrhythmic treatment is uncommonly indicated.
3. **Magnesium sulfate** 2 g IV over 60 s, followed by a constant infusion of 1 to 2 g/h.
4. Maintain the serum potassium levels above 4 mEq/L. Intravenous verapamil (5–10 mg) slows the ventricular response in most patients, decreases atrial ectopy in some patients, and is associated with conversion to sinus rhythm in many patients.
5. Cardioversion has no effect.

Atrial Flutter

Clinical Significance

Atrial flutter is a rhythm that originates from a small area within the atria. The exact mechanism—whether reentry, automatic focus, or triggered arrhythmia—is not yet known. ECG characteristics of atrial flutter are: (1) regular atrial rate between 250 and 350 (most commonly 280 and 320); (2) sawtooth flutter waves directed superiorly and most visible in leads II, III, aV_F; and (3) AV block, usually 2:1, but occasionally greater or irregular (Fig. 2-6). Carotid sinus massage is a useful technique to slow the ventricular response, increase the AV block, and unmask flutter waves. Atrial flutter is most commonly seen in patients with ischemic heart disease or acute myocardial infarction. Less common causes include congestive cardiomyopathy, pulmonary embolus, myocarditis, blunt chest trauma, and, rarely, digoxin toxicity. Atrial flutter may be a transitional arrhythmia between sinus rhythm and atrial fibrillation.

Emergency Department Care

1. Low-energy cardioversion (25–50 J) is very successful in converting more than 90% of cases of atrial flutter into sinus rhythm.
2. If cardioversion is contraindicated, ventricular rate control can be achieved with **diltiazem,** 0.25 mg/kg IV over 2 min; may repeat at 0.35 mg/kg.
3. Intravenous esmolol will convert up to 60% of patients with new onset atrial flutter to sinus rhythm.
4. Alternatives include **digoxin** (0.5 mg IV), **verapamil** (5–10 mg IV), or procainamide.

Atrial Fibrillation

Clinical Significance

Atrial fibrillation occurs when there are multiple small areas of atrial myocardium continuously discharging and contracting. The ECG char-

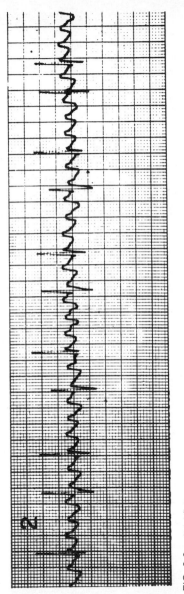

FIG. 2-6. Atrial flutter.

16

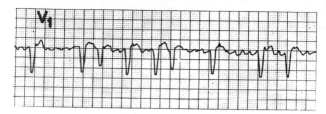

FIG. 2-7. Atrial fibrillation.

acteristics of atrial fibrillation are: (1) fibrillatory waves of atrial activity, best seen in leads V_1, V_2, V_3, and V_F; and (2) irregular ventricular response, usually around 170 to 180 in patients with a healthy AV node (Fig. 2-7). Disease or drugs (especially digoxin) may reduce AV node conduction and markedly slow ventricular response. Atrial fibrillation can occur in a paroxysmal or sustained manner. Predisposing factors for atrial fibrillation are increased atrial size and mass, increased vagal tone, and variation in refractory periods between different parts of atrial myocardium. Atrial fibrillation is usually found in association with four disorders: rheumatic heart disease, hypertension, ischemic heart disease, and thyrotoxicosis.

In patients with left ventricular failure, left atrial contraction makes an important contribution to cardiac output. The loss of effective atrial contraction, as in atrial fibrillation, may produce heart failure in these patients. Conversion from chronic atrial fibrillation to sinus rhythm also carries up to a 1% to 2% risk of arterial embolism.

Emergency Department Care

1. Atrial fibrillation with a rapid ventricular response and acute hemodynamic deterioration should be treated with synchronized cardioversion. Over 60% can be converted with 100 J, and over 80% with 200 J.
2. In more stable patients, the first priority is to achieve ventricular rate control. **Diltiazem** 20 mg (0.25 mg/kg) IV over 2 min is extremely effective. An infusion of 10 mg/h is usually started after the initial dose to maintain control and a second dose of 25 mg (0.35 mg/kg) can be given at 15 min if rate control is not achieved. Alternatives include **digoxin** (0.5 mg IV), and **verapamil** (5–10 mg IV).
3. Once ventricular rate control has been achieved, chemical conversion can be considered with procainamide, quinidine, or verapamil.

Supraventricular Tachycardia (SVT)

Clinical Significance

Supraventricular tachycardia is a regular, rapid rhythm that arises from either reentry or an ectopic pacemaker above the bifurcation of the

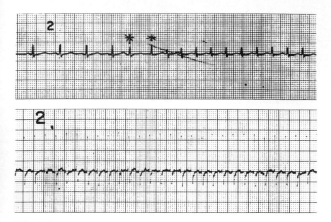

FIG. 2-8.   Reentrant supraventricular tachycarida (STV). Top: 2d PAD (*) initiates run of PAT. Bottom: SVT, rate 286.

bundle of His. The reentrant variety is clinically the most common (Fig. 2-8). These patients often present with acute, symptomatic episodes termed paroxysmal supraventricular tachycardia (PSVT). Ectopic SVT usually originates in the atria with an atrial rate of 100 to 250 (most commonly 140–200) (Fig. 2-9). In patients with bypass tracts, reentry can occur in either direction. It usually occurs in a direction that goes down the AV node and up the bypass tract, producing a narrow QRS complex.

Ectopic SVT may be seen in patients with acute myocardial infarction, chronic lung disease, pneumonia, alcoholic intoxication, and digoxin toxicity. Reentrant SVT can occur in a normal heart, or in association with rheumatic heart disease, acute pericarditis, myocardial infarction, mitral valve prolapse, or one of the pre-excitation syndromes.

Emergency Department Care

1. First attempt vagal maneuvers. These maneuvers can be done by themselves or after administration of drugs.

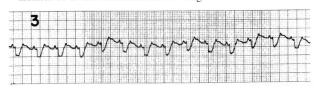

FIG. 2-9.   Ectopic supraventricular, tachycardia (STV) with 2:1 AV conduction.

    a. Carotid sinus massage attempts to massage the carotid sinus and its baroreceptors against the transverse process of C6. Massage should be done for 10 s at a time, first on the side of the nondominant cerebral hemisphere, and should never be done simultaneously on both sides.

    b. Facial immersion in cold water for 6 to 7 s with the nostrils held closed (diving reflex). This maneuver is particularly effective in infants.

    c. The Valsalva maneuver done in the supine position appears to be the most effective vagal maneuver for the conversion of reentrant SVT. For maximum effectiveness, the strain phase must be adequate (usually at least 10 s).

2. **Adenosine,** initially 6 mg rapid IV bolus. If there is no effect within 2 min, a second dose of 12 mg can be given.
3. **Verapamil,** 0.075 to 0.15 mg/kg (3–10 mg) IV over 15 to 60 s, with a repeat dose in 30 min, if necessary. Whenever verapamil is used intravenously, calcium should be readily available.
4. **Diltiazem,** 20 mg (0.25 mg/kg) IV over 2 min.
5. Further alternatives include **esmolol** (300 mcg/kg/min), **propranolol** (0.5–1 mg IV) or **digoxin** (0.5 mg IV).
6. Synchronized cardioversion should be done in any unstable patient with hypotension, pulmonary edema, or severe chest pain. The required dose is usually small, less than 50 J.

VENTRICULAR ARRHYTHMIAS

Aberrant Versus Ventricular Tachyarrhythmias

Differentiation between ectopic beats of ventricular origin and those of supraventricular origin, but conducted aberrantly, can be difficult, especially in sustained tachycardias with wide QRS complexes (WCT). In general, the majority of patients with WCT have ventricular tachycardia and should be approached as ventricular tachycardia, until proved otherwise. Several guidelines follow:

1. A preceding ectopic P wave is good evidence favoring aberrancy, although coincidental atrial and ventricular ectopic beats or retrograde conduction can occur. During a sustained run of tachycardia, AV dissociation favors a ventricular origin of the arrhythmia.
2. Postectopic pause: A fully compensatory pause is more likely after a ventricular beat, but exceptions occur.
3. Fusion beats are evidence for ventricular origin but, again, exceptions occur.
4. A varying bundle branch block pattern suggests aberrancy.
5. Coupling intervals are usually constant with ventricular ectopic beats, unless parasystole is present. Varying coupling intervals suggest aberrancy.

6. Response to carotid sinus massage or other vagal maneuvers wll slow conduction through the AV node and may abolish reentrant SVT and slow the ventricular response in other supraventricular tachyarrhythmias. These maneuvers have essentially no effect on ventricular arrhythmias.
7. A QRS duration of longer than 0.14 s is usually found only in ventricular ectopy or tachycardia.
8. Historical criteria also have been found to be useful: a patient over 35 years old, or history of myocardial infarction, congestive heart failure, or coronary artery bypass graft strongly suggest ventricular tachycardia in patients with WCT.

Emergency Department Care

1. As with ventricular tachycardia, start with **lidocaine** 1 to 1.5 mg/kg IV; may repeat up to 3 mg/kg.
2. **Adenosine** 6 mg IVP may be tried prior to procainamide (see Ventricular Tachycardia Management).

Junctional Rhythms

Clinical Significance

Under normal circumstances, the sinus node discharges at a faster rate than the AV junction, so the pacemaker function of the AV junction is overridden. If sinus node discharges slow or fail to reach the AV junction, junctional escape beats may occur, usually at a rate between 40 to 60, depending on the level of the pacemaker. Generally, junctional escape beats do not conduct retrograde into the atria, so a QRS complex without a P wave usually is seen (Fig. 2-10). Junctional escape beats may occur whenever there is a long enough pause in the impulses reaching the AV junction, such as in sinus bradycardia, slow phase of sinus arrhythmia, AV block, or following premature beats. Sustained junctional escape rhythms may be seen with congestive heart failure, myocarditis, hyperkalemia, or digoxin toxicity. If the ventricular rate is too slow, myocardial or cerebral ischemia may develop.

Emergency Department Care

1. Isolated, infrequent junctional escape beats usually do not require specific treatment.

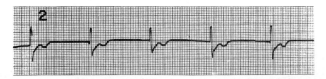

FIG. 2-10.   Junctional escape rhythm, rate 42.

2. If sustained junctional escape rhythms are producing symptoms, the underlying cause should be treated. Atropine can be used to accelerate temporarily the sinus node discharge rate and enhance AV nodal conduction.

Premature Ventricular Contractions (PVCs)

Clinical Significance

Premature ventricular contractions are due to impulses originating from single or multiple areas in the ventricles. The ECG characteristics of PVCs are: (1) a premature and wide QRS complex; (2) no preceding P wave; (3) the ST-segment and T wave of the PVC are directed opposite the major QRS deflection; (4) most PVCs do not affect the sinus node, so there is usually a fully compensatory postectopic pause, or the PVC may be interpolated between two sinus beats; (5) many PVCs have a fixed coupling interval (within 0.04 s) from the preceding sinus beat; and (6) many PVCs are conducted into the atria, producing a retrograde P wave (Fig. 2-11).

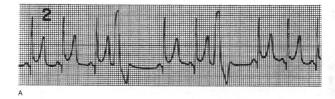

A

B

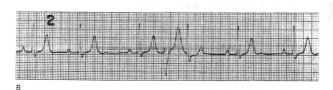

C

FIG. 2-11.   Premature ventricular contractions (PVCs). Top: unifocal PVC. Center: interpolated PVC. Bottom: multifocal PVCs.

PVCs are common, occur in most patients with ischemic heart disease, and are universally found in patients with acute myocardial infarction. Other common causes of PVCs include digoxin toxicity, congestive heart failure, hypokalemia, alkalosis, hypoxia, and sympathomimetic drugs.

Emergency Department Care

Most acute patients with PVCs will respond to intravenous **lidocaine** (1 mg/kg IV), although some patients may require procainamide. Although single studies have suggested benefits, pooled data and meta-analysis find no reduction in mortality from either suppressive or prophylactic treatment of PVCs.

Accelerated Idioventricular Rhythm (AIVR)

Clinical Significance

The ECG characteristics of accelerated idioventricular rhythm (AIVR) are: (1) wide and regular QRS complexes; (2) rate between 40 and 100, often close to the preceding sinus rate; (3) most runs of short duration (3–30 beats); and (4) an AIVR often beginning with a fusion beat (Fig. 2–12). This condition is found most commonly with an acute myocardial infarction.

Emergency Department Care

Treatment is not necessary. On occasion, AIVR may be the only functioning pacemaker, and suppression with lidocaine can lead to cardiac asystole.

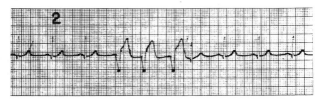

FIG. 2-12.   Accelerated idioventricular rhythms (AIVR).

Ventricular Tachycardia

Clinical Significance

Ventricular tachycardia is the occurrence of three or more beats from a ventricular ectopic pacemaker at a rate greater than 100. The ECG characteristics of ventricular tachycardia are: (1) wide QRS complexes; (2) rate greater than 100 (most commonly 150–200); (3) rhythm is

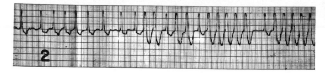

FIG. 2-13. Ventricular tachycardia.

usually regular, although there may be some beat-to-beat variation; and (4) QRS axis is usually constant (Fig. 2-13).

Ventricular tachycardia is rare in patients without underlying heart disease. The most common causes of ventricular tachycardia are ischemic heart disease and acute myocardial infarction. Ventricular tachycardia cannot be differentiated from SVT with aberrancy on the basis of clinical symptoms, blood pressure, or heart rate. Patients who are unstable should be cardioverted, which is effective for both arrhythmias. In general, it is best to treat all wide complex tachycardias as ventricular tachycardia with lidocaine or procainamide. Adenosine appears to cause little harm in patients with ventricular tachycardia and has potential merit for the treatment of wide QRS complex tachycardias.

Emergency Department Care

1. Unstable patients, or those in cardiac arrest, should be treated with synchronized cardioversion. Ventricular tachycardia can be converted with energies as low as 1 J, and over 90% can be converted with less than 10 J. ACLS guidelines recommend that pulseless ventricular tachycardia be *defibrillated* (unsynchronized cardioversion) with 200 J.
2. Clinically stable patients should be treated with intravenous antiarrhythmics.

   a. **Lidocaine** 75 mg (1.0–1.5 mg/kg) IV over 60 to 90 s, followed by a constant infusion at 1 to 4 mg/min (10–40 μg/kg/min). A repeat bolus dose of 50 mg lidocaine may be required during the first 20 min to avoid a subtherapeutic dip in serum level due to the early distribution phase.
   b. **Procainamide** IV at less than 30 mg/min until the arrhythmia converts, the total dose reaches 15 to 17 mg/kg in normals (12 mg/kg in patients with congestive heart failure), or early signs of toxicity develop, with hypotension or QRS prolongation. The loading dose should be followed by a maintenance infusion of 2.8 mg/kg/h in normal subjects.
   c. **Bretylium** 500 mg (5–10 mg/kg) IV over 10 min, followed by a constant infusion at 1 to 2 mg/min.

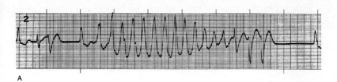

A

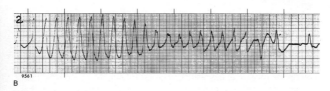

B

FIG. 2-14. Two examples of short runs of atypical ventricular tachycardia showing sinusoidal variation in amplitude and direction of the QRS complexes: "le torsades de pointes" (twisting of the points). Note that the top example is initiated by a late-occurring PVC (lead II).

Torsades de Pointes

Atypical ventricular tachycardia (torsades de pointes, or twisting of the points) is where the QRS axis swings from a positive to negative direction in a single lead (Fig. 2-14).

Drugs that further prolong repolarization—quinidine, disopyramide, procainamide, phenothiazines, tricyclic antidepressants—exacerbate this arrhythmia.

1. Recent reports have revealed that **magnesium sulfate** 1 to 2 g IV over 60 to 90 s, followed by an infusion of 1 to 2 g/h, is effective in abolishing these runs of torsade de pointes.
2. To date, treatment for torsades de pointes consists of accelerating the heart rate (thereby shortening ventricular repolarization) with **isoproterenol** (2–8 µg/min), while making arrangements for a ventricular pacemaker to overdrive the heart at rates of 90 to 120. Temporary pacing is the most effective and safest method to treat torsades de pointes and prevent its recurrence.

Ventricular Fibrillation

Clinical Significance

Ventricular fibrillation is the totally disorganized depolarization and contraction of small areas of ventricular myocardium—there is no effective ventricular pumping activity. The ECG of ventricular fibrillation shows a fine-to-coarse zigzag pattern without discernible P waves or QRS complexes (Fig. 2-15). Ventricular fibrillation is never accompanied by pulse or blood pressure.

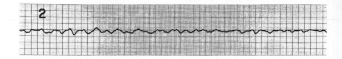

FIG. 2-15. Ventricular fibrillation.

Ventricular fibrillation is most commonly seen in patients with severe ischemic heart disease, with or without acute myocardial infarction. Primary ventricular fibrillation occurs suddenly, without preceding hemodynamic deterioration, whereas secondary ventricular fibrillation occurs after a prolonged period of left ventricular failure or circulatory shock.

Emergency Department Care

1. Current ACLS guidelines recommend immediate electrical defibrillation with 200 J. If ventricular fibrillation persists, defibrillation should be repeated immediately, with 200 to 300 J at the second attempt, increased to 360 J at the third attempt.
2. If the initial three attempts at defibrillation are unsuccessful, CPR and intubation should be initiated; further electrical defibrillations should be done after the administration of various intravenous drugs, according to ACLS guidelines.
3. **Epinephrine** in standard dose should be administered, 1 mg IV. If this is not successful, high-dose epinephrine may be given subsequently, 0.1 mg/kg. Repeat every 3 to 5 minutes.
4. Defibrillation should be attempted after each drug administration, at 360 J, unless lower energy levels have been previously successful.
5. Successive antiarrhythmics should then be administered with defibrillation attempted after each drug. The recommended sequence is **lidocaine,** 1.5 mg/kg, **bretylium,** 5 mg/kg, then consider **magnesium,** 2 g IV, and procainamide.

CONDUCTION DISTURBANCES

Atrioventricular (AV) Block

First-degree atrioventricular (AV) block is characterized by a delay in AV conduction, manifested by a prolonged PR interval. First-degree AV block needs no treatment and will not be discussed further. Second-degree AV block is characterized by intermittent AV conduction—some atrial impulses reach the ventricles and others are blocked. Third-degree AV block is characterized by complete interruption in AV conduction.

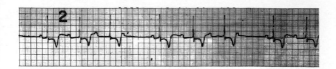

FIG. 2-16.   Second-degree Mobitz I (Wenckebach) AV block with 4.3 AV conduction.

Second-Degree Mobitz I (Wenckebach) AV Block

Clinical Significance

With this block there is progressive prolongation of AV conduction (and the PR interval) until atrial impulse is completely blocked. Usually, only a single atrial impulse is blocked. After the dropped beat, the AV conduction returns to normal and the cycle usually repeats itself, with either the same conduction ratio (fixed ratio) or a different conduction ratio (variable ratio).

The Wenckebach phenomenon has a seeming paradox. Even though the PR intervals progressively lengthen prior to the dropped beat, the increments by which they lengthen decrease with successive beats; this produces a progressive shortening of the R–R interval prior to the dropped beat (Fig. 2-16).

This block is often transient and is usually associated with an acute inferior myocardial infarction, digoxin toxicity, myocarditis, or is seen after cardiac surgery.

Emergency Department Care

1. Specific treatment is not necessary unless slow ventricular rates produce signs of hypoperfusion.
2. **Atropine,** 0.5 mg, repeated every 5 min, as necessary, titrated to the desired effect or until the total dose reaches 3.0 mg.
3. Although rarely needed, transcutaneous pacing may be used. (See sinus bradycardia section.)

Second-Degree Mobitz II AV Block

Clinical Significance

With this block, the PR interval remains constant before and after the nonconducted atrial beats (Fig. 2-17). One or more beats may be nonconducted at a single time.

The QRS complexes are usually wide. When second-degree AV block occurs with a fixed conduction ratio of 2:1, it is not possible to differentiate between a Mobitz type I (Wenckebach) or Mobitz type II block.

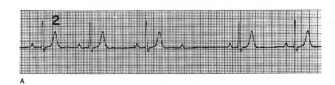

A

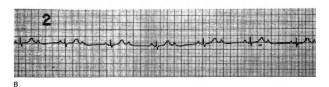

B

FIG. 2-17. Top: second-degree Mobitz II AV block. Bottom: second-degree AV block with 2:1 AV conduction.

Type II blocks imply structural damage to the infranodal conducting system, are usually permanent, and may progress suddenly to complete heart block, especially in the setting of an acute myocardial infarction.

Emergency Department Care

1. **Atropine** (0.5–1 mg IVP, may repeat up to 3.0 mg total dose) should be the first drug used.
2. Transcutaneous cardiac pacing is a useful modality in patients unresponsive to atropine. See sinus bradycardia section for technique.
3. Most cases, especially in the setting of acute myocardial infarction, will require permanent transvenous cardiac pacing.

Third-Degree (Complete) AV Block

Clinical Significance

In third-degree AV block, there is no atrioventricular conduction. The ventricles are paced by an escape pacemaker at a rate slower than the atrial rate (Fig. 2-18). When third-degree AV block occurs at the AV node, a junctional escape pacemaker takes over with a ventricular rate

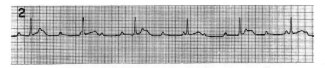

FIG. 2-18. Third-degree AV block.

of 40 to 60 and, since the rhythm originates above the bifurcation of the bundle of His, the QRS complexes are narrow.

When third-degree AV block occurs at the AV node, a junctional escape pacemaker takes over with a ventricular rate of 40 to 60 and, since the rhythm originates above the bifurcation of the bundle of His, the QRS complexes are narrow.

When third-degree AV block occurs at the infranodal level, the ventricles are driven by a ventricular escape rhythm at a rate of less than 40. Third-degree AV block located in the bundle branch or Purkinje system invariably have escape rhythms with wide QRS complexes.

Nodal third-degree AV block may develop in up to 8 percent of acute inferior myocardial infarctions where it is usually transient, although it may last for several days.

Infranodal third-degree AV blocks indicate structural damage to the infranodal conducting system, as seen with an extensive acute anterior myocardial infarction. The ventricular escape pacemaker is usually inadequate to maintain cardiac output and is unstable with periods of ventricular asystole.

Emergency Department Care

Third-degree AV blocks should be treated the same as second-degree Mobitz II AV blocks with atropine or ventricular demand pacemaker, as required. External cardiac pacing can be performed before transvenous pacemaker placement.

Pre-excitation Syndromes

Clinical Significance

Pre-excitation occurs when some portion of the ventricles are activated by an impulse from the atria sooner than would be expected if the impulse were transmitted down the normal conducting pathway. All forms of pre-excitation are felt to be due to accessory tracts that bypass all or part of the normal conducting system, the most common form being Wolff–Parkinson–White syndrome (WPW) (Fig. 2-19).

There is a high incidence of tachyarrhythmias in patients with WPW—atria flutter (about 5%), atrial fibrillation (10%–20%), and paroxysmal reentrant SVT (40%–80%).

Emergency Department Care

1. Re-entrant SVT (orthodromic, narrow QRS complex) in the WPW syndrome can be treated like other cases of reentrant SVT. **Adenosine,** 6 mg IV, or **verapamil,** 5 to 10 mg IV, are very successful at terminating this arrhythmia in patients with WPW, but ß-adrenergic blockers usually are ineffective.
2. Tachycardia with a wide QRS complex is usually associated with a short refractory period in the bypass tract; patients with this type

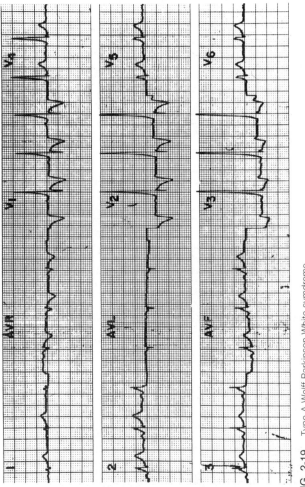

FIG. 2-19. Type A Wolff-Parkinson-White symdrome.

29

of tachycardia are at risk for rapid ventricular rates and degeneration into ventricular fibrillation. Stable patients should be treated with intravenous procainamide and unstable patients should be cardioverted. ß-adrenergic or calcium channel blockers should be avoided.
3. Atrial flutter or fibrillation with a rapid ventricular response is best treated with cardioversion.

PHARMACOLOGY OF ANTIARRHYTHMIC AND VASOACTIVE MEDICATIONS

This section of the chapter discusses the pharmacokinetics, indications, dosing, and adverse affect profile of antiarrhythmic and vasoactive agents that are pertinent to emergency medicine practice. (Vasodilating agents such as phentolamine, hydralazine, and clonidine, together with other drugs used in hypertension management, are discussed in Chapter 34.)

Class I Antiarrhythmic Agents

Procainamide

Procainamide is a second-line agent, generally used to treat and prevent recurrence of ventricular arrhythmias, specifically stable ventricular tachycardia (VT) and premature ventricular contractions (PVCs), that are not responding to lidocaine. Procainamide may also be used for slowing or converting supraventricular tachycardias (SVT), including atrial flutter and fibrillation (especially in Wolff–Parkinson–White [WPW] syndrome), paroxysmal supraventricular tachycardia (PSVT), paroxysmal atrial tachycardia, and paroxysmal AV junctional rhythm. Contraindications include complete AV heart block, second- or third-degree heart block, long QT intervals, and torsades de pointes.

Dosing and administration. Procainamide should be given by continuous infusion until the arrhythmia is controlled, hypotension develops, the QRS complex widens greater than 50%, QT interval prolongation develops, or a total of 17 mg/kg (1.2 g for a 70 kg patient) has been given. The recommended infusion rate is 20 mg/min, but, in urgent situations, 30 mg/min may be given cautiously. Blood pressure and QRS complex must be monitored during IV administration. If procainamide suppresses the VT, initiate a continuous infusion, at 1 to 4 mg/min, to maintain the suppression. Lower doses generally are necessary for patients with CHF, hypotensive states, and hepatic or renal failure.

Adverse effect profile. Adverse effects of procainamide include myocardial depression, prolongation of the QRS and QT interval, impairment of AV conduction, VF, torsades de pointes, and hypotension.

Lidocaine

Indications. Lidocaine is the drug of choice for suppression of ventricular arrhythmias and ventricular ectopy (frequent multifocal PVCs, couplets, salvos, and, especially, long runs of VT) in suspected acute myocardial ischemia or unstable angina. The drug also is indicated for control of VT and VF refractory to defibrillation and epinephrine. Prophylactic routine use of lidocaine is not recommended.

Dosing and administration. Lidocaine is given as an initial bolus of 1 mg/kg, followed by additional bolus doses of 0.5 mg/kg q5–10 min as needed, up to a cumulative dose of 3 mg/kg. When VF is present and defibrillation and epinephrine have failed, an initial bolus of 1.5 mg/kg is recommended for all patients. Conscious patients should receive lidocaine at a rate not exceeding 50 mg/min to minimize adverse CNS effects (25 mg/min if infused through a central line). In pulseless VT or VF, however, lidocaine can be given by rapid IV push. When IV lines are not available, the drug may be instilled endotracheally (ET), two to two and one-half times the IV dose, up to a total volume of 10 mL. Maintenance infusions should be started at 2 mg/min and titrated up to 4 mg/min as needed.

Patients older than 70, those with CHF, liver disease, or impaired hepatic blood flow, should have their loading dose and maintenance infusion rate lowered by 50%.

Adverse effect profile. Adverse effects from lidocaine usually occur when the drug is administered too rapidly in a conscious patient, when excessive doses are administered, or when a drug interaction potentiates toxicity. Symptoms of mild lidocaine toxicity that correlate with levels greater than 5 µg/mL include slurred speech, drowsiness, confusion, nausea, vertigo, ataxia, tinnitus, paresthesias, and muscle twitching. An abrupt change in mental status is a classic symptom of lidocaine toxicity. Serious symptoms occurring at plasma levels greater than 9 µg/mL may include psychosis, seizures, respiratory depression, and high degrees of sinoatrial (SA) or atrioventricular (AV) block.

Class II Antiarrhythmics: ß Blockers

Propranolol

Indications. Propranolol is indicated for a wide variety of supraventricular arrhythmias. These include paroxysmal atrial tachycardia (PAT), refractory sinus tachycardia, and tachyarrhythmias associated with thyrotoxicosis. Other indications for propranolol include the management of angina and acute myocardial ischemia, the treatment of idiopathic hypertrophic subaortic stenosis, and prophylaxis for common migraine headaches.

Dosing and administration. For life-threatening arrhythmias, the IV dose of propranolol is 0.5 to 1 mg, given as an IV bolus up to 5 mg at a rate not exceeding 1 mg/min.

Adverse effect profile. The drug is generally not given to patients with asthma or allergic rhinitis and is contraindicated in those with sinus bradycardia or advanced SA or AV block. Propranolol should also not be used in CHF or cardiogenic shock, unless these conditions are due to tachyarrhythmias.

Esmolol

Indications. Esmolol is currently indicated to control ventricular rate for the short term when the termination of SVT is desired. Esmolol also can be used to maintain normal sinus rhythm in post-AMI patients who cannot tolerate oral medications.

Dosing and administration. A loading dose of esmolol is given as an IV bolus of 500 μg/kg over 1 min, followed by IV infusion starting at 50 μg/kg per min infused over 4 min. Assess for therapeutic and adverse effects immediately following the infusion. If there is no response, give another loading dose over 1 min and increase the infusion rate to 100 μg/kg per min for 4 min. If there is still no response, repeat this procedure, using the same bolus dose each time and increasing the infusion rate by increments of 50 μg/kg per min until the rate of infusion reaches 200 μg/kg per min, the desired response is achieved, or adverse effects appear.

Adverse effect profile. The most common adverse effect associated with esmolol use is hypotension, which occurs in approximately 20% to 50% of patients being treated for SVT.

Labetalol

Indications. Labetalol is used in emergency medicine primarily for its antihypertensive actions, causing only minimal alterations in heart rate and cardiac output. It is a good alternative for treating the hypertensive patient with myocardial ischemia.

Dosing and administration. Labetalol can be administered IV through multiple IV boluses or a continuous IV infusion. When initiating IV bolus, the clinician should start with 20 mg (0.25 mg/kg in an 80 kg patient) and repeat with 40 mg to 160 mg every 10 min until the desired effect is reached, or until a total cumulative dose of 300 mg has been given. Alternatively, labetalol may be given via continuous infusion at a rate of 0.5 to 2 mg/min until the desired response or a total cumulative dose of 300 mg has been reached.

Adverse effect profile. The most common adverse effect associated with labetalol use is orthostatic hypotension. Adverse CNS effects that may occur include lightheadedness, drowsiness, dizziness, fatigue, and lethargy. Avoid the use of IV labetalol in patients with risks for intracranial bleeding as a hypotensive episode can induce CNS herniation.

Class III Antiarrhythmic Agents

Bretylium

Indications. The three indications for bretylium are treatment of VF refractory to repeated countershocks, epinephrine and lidocaine bolus doses; when lidocaine and procainamide have failed to control VT associated with a pulse; or when adenosine and lidocaine have failed to control wide-complex tachycardias.

Dosing and administration. The initial dose of bretylium for VF or pulseless VT is 5 mg/kg (500 mg = 1 ampule) administered by rapid IV push. If VT persists, the dose can be increased to 10 mg/kg and repeated at 15- to 30-min intervals, up to a maximum dose of 35 mg/kg. For recurrent or refractory ventricular tachyarrhythmias, 5 to 10 mg/kg should be infused over a period of 8 to 10 min. If these arrhythmias persist, repeated boluses of 5 to 10 mg/kg can given q1 to 2h as necessary. The standard dose for a bretylium infusion is 2 mg/min, with a dosing range of 1 to 2 mg/min.

Adverse effect profile. Postural hypotension is the most common adverse reaction and may occur within 15 to 30 min in as many as 60% of patients. If this occurs, the patient should be placed in a supine or Trendelenburg position and be resuscitated with crystalloid fluids. Bretylium should be avoided, if possible, in the setting of digoxin toxicity, since catecholamines are believed to exacerbate the toxic effects of digoxin.

Class IV Antiarrhythmic Agents: Calcium Channel Blockers

Verapamil

Indications. Verapamil is as effective as adenosine and diltiazem for terminating narrow-complex PSVT and for controlling the ventricular rate in atrial fibrillation/flutter, but not if it is associated with an accessory bypass tract, since ventricular tachyarrhythmias may be precipitated. The drug also may be used for patients presenting with narrow complex PSVT from WPW syndrome. Diagnosis of PSVT should be confirmed by 12-lead ECG and should be managed with vasovagal maneuvers (e.g., the Valsalva maneuver) prior to administering verapamil whenever possible.

Dosing and administration. When managing patients with PSVT, give 5 mg IV over 2 to 3 min. This may be repeated or doubled in 10 min. Lower initial doses of verapamil and slower administration techniques should be considered in older patients and those with hepatic dysfunction. Pretreatment with calcium chloride, gluconate, or gluceptate (500–1000 mg) can be given before or after verapamil infusion to prevent or reverse hypotension.

For the prevention of recurrent PSVT, oral administration of verapamil, 240 to 480 mg daily, should be given in three to four divided doses. Control of ventricular rate in digitalized adults with chronic atrial fibrillation or flutter is 240 to 320 mg daily in three or four divided doses. Maximum antiarrhythmic effects are generally seen within 48 h after initiating a verapamil dose.

Adverse effect profile. Incidence of hypotension is 5% to 10% with IV administration and may rarely require treatment with IV calcium salts or vasopressors. Conduction disturbances, such as bradycardia, AV block, and bundle branch block, occur in approximately 2% or fewer of patients and usually respond to a dosage reduction or discontinuation of the drug. Noncardiac side-effects with verapamil include constipation, dizziness, headache, and nausea.

Diltiazem

Indications. IV diltiazem is as effective as verapamil and adenosine for rapid conversion of PSVT to NSR and to slow ventricular rate in atrial fibrillation or atrial flutter. It should not be used in patients with a wide complex ventricular tachyarrhythmia, suggesting an accessory bypass tract (e.g., WPW syndrome).

Dosing and administration. The IV bolus dose for control of PSVT, atrial fibrillation, or atrial flutter is 0.25 mg/kg, using actual body weight (average adult dose, 20 mg), over 2 min. If further response is desired, a second IV bolus of 0.35 mg/kg actual body weight can be given at the same rate (average adult dose, 25 mg). Diltiazem maintenance IV infusion may be started immediately following the bolus dose(s). The recommended initial rate is 10 mg/h, yet some patients may respond to a 5 mg/h dose.

Nifedipine

Indications. The primary use of nifedipine in emergency medicine is to rapidly lower the blood pressure in hypertensive crisis. The drug can be given sublingually or orally and is therefore particularly convenient when IV lines cannot be started and the blood pressure needs to be lowered immediately.

Dosing and administration. The initial dose of nifedipine for hypertensive crisis is 10 mg. The patient should chew and then swallow the capsule. A repeat dose can be administered 10 min later.

Adverse effect profile. Side-effects occurring with nifedipine include lightheadedness, flushing, headache, and hypotension. Nifedipine may also cause dose-related peripheral edema in 10% to 30% of patients. Nifedipine should be used with caution in hypertensive crisis in patients who are already tachycardic.

Nimodipine

Indications. Nimodipine is indicated for the treatment of recent (within 96 h) subarachnoid hemorrhage SAH from ruptured congenital intracranial aneurysm in patients whose neurologic condition is good (e.g., Hunt and Hess grades I to III).

Dosing and administration. The dose is 60 mg q4h for 21 days for managing patients with SAH.

Adverse effect profile. The most common adverse effect is hypotension, which is often dose-related. In addition, edema and headache have been reported in patients with SAH.

Other Antiarrhythmic Agents

Adenosine

Indications. Adenosine, approved as an antiarrhythmic drug for the emergency management of PSVT involving the AV node, has been shown to be as efficacious as IV doses of verapamil or diltiazem. The drug has also been used as a diagnostic agent for distinguishing supraventricular from ventricular tachycardia, as well as diagnosing broad QRS complex tachycardias. Although it is extremely effective in *initial* conversion of reentrant PSVTs, recurrence of the arrhythmia (within minutes after initial conversion) may occur. It is contraindicated in second- or third-degree AV heart block or sick-sinus syndrome. Adenosine is not effective in converting atrial tachyarrhythmias (e.g., atrial fibrillation or flutter) or VT to NSR.

Dosing and administration. The initial dose for the treatment of acute PSVT is 6 mg/2 mL, given as a rapid IV bolus over 1 to 2 s directly into the vein or into the most proximal port of the IV tubing on the peripheral IV site.

Adverse effect profile. When adverse effects occur due to adenosine, they are minor and well tolerated because they last less than 1 min due to the drug's short half-life. The most common are dyspnea, cough, syncope, vertigo, paresthesias, numbness, nausea, and metallic taste. Cardiovascular adverse effects may include facial flushing, headache, diaphoresis, palpitations, retrosternal chest pain, sinus bradyarrhythmias (i.e., bradycardia, sinus arrest, AV block), atrial tachydysrhythmias (i.e., atrial fibrillation or flutter), PVCs, and hypotension.

Digoxin

Indications. Digoxin is indicated to improve cardiac output in CHF and to control heart rate in atrial fibrillation, atrial flutter, and paroxysmal atrial tachycardia. Use of digoxin in the treatment of CHF should be considered only when diuretics and vasodilators fail to improve cardiac output.

Dosing and administration. For control of supraventricular tachycardia, digoxin should be administered IV in a dose of 10 to 15 µg/kg (up to a total of 0.75–1.5 mg given over the first 24 h). This dose should be divided, with 0.25 to 0.5 mg given as the initial dose, and 0.125 to 0.25 mg q2 to 6h as subsequent doses until the entire dose is administered or the heart rate is sufficiently lowered.

Adverse effect profile. Symptoms of digoxin toxicity include mental depression, confusion, headache, drowsiness, anorexia, nausea, vomiting, weakness, visual disturbances (green or yellow vision or halo effects), delirium, EEG abnormalities, and seizures. Patients may also present with diarrhea and abdominal discomfort. Almost any type of arrhythmia may manifest in digoxin toxicity. The most common arrhythmias include an increased number of unifocal or PVCs, VT, junctional tachycardia, high-degree AV block, PSVT with block, and sinus arrest.

Magnesium

Indications. Magnesium is indicated for intractable VT/VF and torsades de pointes, regardless of prearrest serum magnesium levels. Also it has been studied and shown to be useful in managing refractory PVCs, MAT, PSVT, and for ventricular arrhythmias associated with cardiac arrest or digoxin toxicity that occur in patients who are, or are likely to be, hypomagnesemic. Magnesium also may be considered as a prophylactic/antiarrhythmic in the post-AMI patient.

Dosing and administration. An IV loading dose of magnesium sulfate is administered as 1 to 2 g mixed in 50 or 100 mL D_5W, using either 10% (100 mg/mL) or 50% (500 mg/mL) solutions. In cardiac-arrest scenarios, the IV dose can be injected over 1 to 2 min. If time permits, however, a safer method is to administer 2 to 4 g as an IV infusion over 20 to 60 min.

Adverse effect profile. Hypotension is the predominant adverse effect. Other signs of hypermagnesemia include flushing, sweating, CNS depression, depression of reflexes, flaccid paralysis, depression of cardiac function, circulatory collapse, hypothermia, and fatal respiratory paralysis.

Vasoactive Drugs—Vasoactive and Inotropic Agents

Epinephrine

Indications. Epinephrine is considered a first-line agent in the treatment of cardiac arrest and may be used in pulseless VT/VF (that has not responded to electrical countershock), asystole, and electromechanical dissociation (EMD). Epinephrine is also used as a vasopressor to increase blood pressure and as an antidote to reverse bronchospasm due to anaphylactic and hypersensitivity reactions.

Dosing and administration. Current American Heart Association (AHA) guidelines recommend that an epinephrine 1 mg IV bolus continues to be the initial dose in cardiac arrest. It is now recommended that the dosing frequency be increased to 3 to 5 min from a 5-min interval. The AHA recognizes that higher doses of epinephrine are acceptable, but it can neither recommend nor discourage their use. They do say, however, higher doses should only be used after the 1-mg dose has failed. The intermediate epinephrine dose suggestion is 2 to 5 mg IV push, also given every 3 to 5 min; the escalating regimen is 1 mg to 3 mg to 5 mg IV push, 3 min apart; the high dose reflects use of a bolus of 0.1 mg/kg every 3 to 5 min. Epinephrine may be given through a peripheral vein, through a central line, or endotracheally. Endotracheal administration is performed by placing no more than 10 mL at a time of a 1:10,000 solution (preload syringe) down the ET tube, then performing several rapid ventilations to disperse the drug throughout the airways for maximal absorption.

Adverse effect profile. Adverse effects are of minimal importance in the setting of cardiac arrest. Epinephrine does increase myocardial oxygen consumption significantly and thus can exacerbate ventricular irritability in the setting of myocardial ischemia.

Dopamine

Indications. Dopamine is indicated for reversing hemodynamically significant hypotension due to myocardial infarction, trauma, sepsis, overt heart failure, renal failure, and chronic CHF when fluid resuscitation is unsuccessful.

Dosing and administration. The range for low-dose dopamine is 1 to 2 μg/kg per min, whereas the moderate dose is 2 to 10 μg/kg per min. High dose begins at 10 μg/kg per min and should be titrated to adequate blood pressure response. As with all vasoactive infusions, dopamine should be discontinued by tapering the dosage. Most patients can be managed on 20 μg/kg per min or less. If higher doses are needed, an IV norepinephrine infusion should be added.

Adverse effect profile. Dopamine may produce dose-dependent adverse effects, including hypotension at low infusion rates, hypertension at high infusion rates, ectopic beats, headache, nausea, vomiting, angina pectoris, and tachycardia. Gangrene of the extremities has occurred in patients with occlusive vascular disease or diabetes, as well as in those who receive prolonged high-dose infusions.

Norepinephrine

Indications. Norepinephrine is used primarily as a vasopressor for the treatment of severe hypotension refractory to fluids and other pressor agents, specifically dopamine.

Dosing and administration. The initial adult dose is 0.5 to 1 μg/min, whereas the pediatric dose is 0–1 μg/kg/min.

Adverse effect profile. Large doses of norepinephrine may result in ventricular irritability, cardiac depression, decreased renal blood flow, and reflex bradycardia. If extravasation occurs, phentolamine, 5 to 10 mg in 10 to 15 mL of normal saline solution, should be infiltrated as soon as possible to prevent necrosis and sloughing.

Isoproterenol

Indications. Isoproterenol is now indicated only for refractory torsades de pointes and immediate temporary management of hemodynamically significant bradycardias in the denervated hearts of heart transplants.

Dosing and administration. Isoproterenol should be administered only by IV infusion. The infusion rate, 2 to 10 μg/min, should be titrated to the desired heart rate.

Adverse effect profile. It must be emphasized that the ß1-agonist action of isoproterenol will cause an increase in chronotropic effect. This effect raises myocardial oxygen requirements and could possibly precipitate or exacerbate myocardial ischemia, inducing serious arrhythmias (e.g., VT and VF).

Dobutamine

Indications. Dobutamine is used to increase inotropic activity in the short-term management of cardiac decompensation due to depressed contractility resulting either from organic heart disease or from cardiac surgical procedures. The drug should be used to increase cardiac output in the chronic CHF patient when standard therapy fails to improve symptoms or in the patient with pulmonary congestion and low cardiac output.

Dosing and administration. Dobutamine is administered only by IV infusion. The dosage range is 2 to 20 μg/kg/min; however, most patients can be maintained on 10 μg/kg/min or less.

Adverse effect profile. The primary adverse effects of dobutamine are increased heart rate, blood pressure, and ectopic arrhythmias. Heart rate increases greater than 10% may induce or exacerbate myocardial ischemia.

Atropine

Indications. Atropine is the treatment of choice for increasing heart rate in hemodynamically unstable bradycardias (e.g., decreased heart rate with hypotension, altered mental status, escape beats, and chest pain.

Dosing and administration. The dose of atropine for hemodynamically unstable bradycardias is 0.5 mg *rapid* IV push, repeated as necessary q3 to 5 min until a desired heart rate is achieved. Bolus doses of 1 mg can be given for asystole and repeated once if necessary. A total dose of 3 mg (0.04 mg/kg) results in full vagolytic blockade in humans. Atropine can be administered IV push, IM, and through the ET tube.

Adverse effect profile. Atropine is not indicated for bradycardia in hemodynamically stable patients. If administered, marked increases in heart rate can increase myocardial oxygen consumption, possibly inducing ischemia and precipitating ventricular tachyarrhythmias (including VT and VF).

Vasodilator Agents

Nitroglycerin

Indications. Nitroglycerin is approved for the prophylaxis, treatment, and management of angina pectoris. Intravenous nitroglycerin is used to control hypertension associated with surgery and is also used in CHF associated with acute myocardial infarction.

Dosing and administration. Nitroglycerin can be administered sublingually, lingually, intrabuccally, orally, topically, or by IV infusion. Sublingual tablets or sprays can be given every 5 min. Topical paste can be applied to the chest 1 to 2 inches, as needed, q4 to 8 hours. Start IV infusion at 5 to 10 µg/min and titrate in increments of 5 to 10 mg/min to desired response. Most doses range between 50 and 200 mg/min.

For further reading in *Emergency Medicine, A Comprehensive Study Guide*, see Chapter 22, Disturbances of Cardiac Rhythm and Conduction, by J. Stephan Stapczynski, and Chapter 23, Pharmacology of Antiarrhythmic and Vasoactive Medications, by David Levy and Elizabeth Lyons.

3 | Resuscitation of Children and Neonates

Charles J. Graham

Respiratory and cardiac arrest in children is most commonly due to primary respiratory conditions and shock. Because of age and size differences in children, drug dosages, compression and respiratory rates, and equipment sizes vary considerably (Table 3-1).

PEDIATRIC CARDIOPULMONARY RESUSCITATION

Securing the Airway

The airway is smaller, variable in size, and more anterior in the child than in the adult.

1. Mild extension of the head (sniffing position) opens the airway. Chin lift or jaw thrust maneuvers may relieve obstruction of the airway related to the tongue.
2. Oral airways are not commonly used in pediatrics but may be useful in patients whose airway cannot be maintained manually. Oral airways are inserted with a tongue blade as in adults.
3. A bag–valve–mask system is commonly used for ventilation. Minimum volume for ventilation bags for infants and children should be of 450 ml. The tidal volume necessary to ventilate children is 10 to 15 ml/kg. In emergency situations, however, observation of chest rise and auscultation of breath sounds will ensure adequate ventilation.
4. Endotracheal intubation is usually performed using a Miller (straight) blade with a properly sized tube. The internal diameter of the tube should be the same size as the end of the patient's little finger. The formula, 16 + age ÷ 4 gives approximate tube size. Uncuffed tubes are used in children up to 7 to 8 years.

Rapid Sequence Induction

Rapid sequence induction (RSI) is used to produce muscle paralysis and protect against effects of airway manipulation such as reflex bradycardia or increased intracranial pressure (ICP). Cardiac monitor and oximetry should be used.

1. RSI begins with preoxygenation with 100% oxygen.
2. **Lidocaine** (1.5 mg/kg IV) is used in head trauma patients to prevent increased ICP. **Atropine** (0.1 mg/kg IV) is given to prevent reflex bradycardia in children under 5 years old.
3. A defasciculating dose of a nondepolarizing agent (i.e., vecuronium at 0.02 mg/kg) is used in children over 5 years if succinylcholine is given for paralysis.

TABLE 3-1. Length-Based Equipment Chart

Length, cm

Item	54–70	70–85	85–95	95–107	107–124	124–138	138–155
ET tube size (mm)	3.5	4.0	4.5	5.0	5.5	6.0	6.5
Lip-tip length (mm)	10.5	12.0	13.5	15.0	16.5	18.0	19.5
Laryngoscope	1 Straight	1 Straight	2 Straight	2 Straight or curved	2 Straight or curved	2–3 Straight or curved	3 Straight or curved
Suction catheter	8F	8–10F	10F	10F	10F	10F	12F
Stylet	6F	6F	6F	6F	14F	14F	14F
Oral airway	Infant/small child	Small child	Child	Child	Child/small adult	Child/adult	Medium adult
Bag-valve-mask	Infant	Child	Child	Child	Child	Child/adult	Adult
Oxygen mask	Newborn	Pediatric	Pediatric	Pediatric	Pediatric	Adult	Adult
Vascular access catheter/butterfly	22–24/23–25, intraosseous	20–22/23–25, intraosseous	18–22/21–23, intraosseous	18–22/21–23, intraosseous	18–20/21–23	18–20/21–22	16–20/18–21
Nasogastric tube	5–8F	8–10F	10F	10–12F	12–14F	14–18F	18F
Urinary catheter	5–8F	8–10F	10F	10–12F	10–12F	12F	12F
Chest tube	12–12F	16–20F	20–24F	20–24F	24–32F	28–32F	32–40F
Blood pressure cuff	Newborn/infant	Infant/child	Child	Child	Child	Child/adult	Adult

Directions for use
1. Measure patient length with cm tape.
2. Using measured length in cm, access appropriate equipment column.

Adapted from Luten RD, Wears RL, Broselow J. et al: Length-based endotracheal tube sizing for pediatric resuscitation. *Ann Emerg Med* 21(8):900, 1992.

4. Cricoid pressure should be applied before paralysis and maintained until intubation is accomplished.
5. Either **thiopental** (3–5 mg/kg), **ketamine** (1–2 mg/kg), or **midazolam** (0.1–0.2 mg/kg, 5 mg max) should be chosen. Thiopental should not be used in patients with hypotension or reactive airway disease. Ketamine is contraindicated in increased intracranial pressure and can induce laryngospasm.
6. **Succinylcholine** (1.0 mg/kg in children >12 kg; 2.0 mg/kg in children <12 kg) is chosen in most cases for paralysis because of its rapid onset and short duration of action. A nondepolarizing agent such as vecuronium (0.2 mg/kg) may be chosen for patients with increased intracranial pressure or in those in status asthmaticus.
7. Intubate the trachea and release cricoid pressure.

Vascular Access

Vascular access can be challenging in a critically ill child. Airway management is paramount in pediatric arrest and should not be delayed while obtaining vascular access in the most rapid, least invasive manner possible. Peripheral venous access is attempted first (scalp, arm, hand, or antecubital sites). Intraosseous access is a quick, safe route for resuscitation medications and may be tried next. Percutaneous access of the femoral vein or access of the saphenous vein through cutdown can also be used, but they are more time consuming.

Technique for insertion of an intraosseous line is as follows. The bone most commonly used is the proximal tibia (Fig. 3-1). The anterior tibial tuberosity is palpated with the index finger, and the medial aspect of the tibia is grasped with the thumb. An imaginary line is drawn

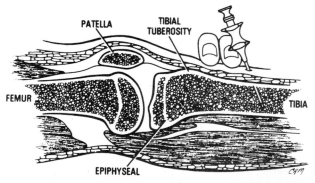

FIG. 3-1. The needle is inserted 2-cm distal to the tibial tuberosity on the medial aspect of the tibia. It is inserted in a caudal direction, away from the joint space.

between the two, and the needle is inserted 1 cm distal to the midpoint of this line. An 18-gauge spinal needle is used in infants up to 18 mo, whereas older children require a bone marrow needle. Using strict sterile technique, the needle is inserted in a slightly caudal direction until the needle punctures the cortex (see Fig. 3-1). The stylet is removed and blood or marrow contents are aspirated to confirm position. Fluids or drugs may then be administered (saline, glucose, epinephrine, dopamine, sodium bicarbonate, diazepam, or antibiotics).

Fluids

In shock, intravenous isotonic fluid (i.e., normal saline) boluses of 20 ml/kg should be given as rapidly as possible and should be repeated, depending on response. If hypovolemia has been corrected and shock or hypotension still persist, a pressor agent should be considered. (For Maintenance Fluids, see Chapter 17.)

Drugs

The indications for resuscitation drugs are the same for children as in adults. Drug dose calculations are a problem particular to pediatrics (Table 3-2). Using a drug dosage chart will reduce dosage errors. The Broselow tape is a length-based system for estimating the weight of children in emergency situations. The tape has drug dosages, equipment sizes, fluid volumes, and basic life-support techniques displayed. A drug-dose and equipment-size chart or Broselow tape should be readily accessible in emergency settings. Equipment should be stored so that appropriate sizes are readily accessible.

The *rule of six* may be used to quickly calculate continuous infusions. The rule of six calculation is: 6 mg $\times$ wt in kg, fill to 100 ml with D_5W. The infusion rate in ml/hr will equal the mcg/kg/min (i.e., an infusion running at 1 ml/h = 1 mcg/kg/min; at 5 ml/h = 5 mcg/kg/min).

Epinephrine is the only drug proven effective in cardiac arrest. It is indicated in pulseless arrest and in slow rates that are hypoxia induced and unresponsive to oxygenation and ventilation. If the initial dose of epinephrine (0.01 mg/kg of a 1:10,000 concentration) is not effective, 10 to 20 times the dose (0.1–0.2 mg/kg of a 1:1,000 concentration) may be given subsequently. Primary cardiac causes of bradycardia are rare and may be treated with **atropine** (0.02 mg/kg, min dose 0.1 mg).

TABLE 3-2. Essential Drugs

Drug	Concentration	Dose
Epinephrine: first dose	1:10,000 (0.1 mg/mL)	0.01–0.02 mg/kg
Epinephrine: high dose	1:1000 (1 mg/mL)	0.1–0.2 mg/kg
Atropine	1:10,000 (0.1 mg/mL)	0.02 mg/kg
Sodium bicarbonate	1 mEq/mL	1.0 mEq/kg

Sodium bicarbonate is no longer recommended as a first-line resuscitation drug. It is recommended only after epinephrine administration has been ineffective or as guided by arterial blood gases. Calcium is not recommended in routine resuscitation, but may be useful in hyperkalemia, hypocalcemia, and calcium channel blocker overdoses.

Arrhythmias

Arrhythmias in infants and children are most often the result of respiratory insufficiency or arrest, not primary cardiac events as in adults. Careful attention to oxygenation and ventilation are, therefore, cornerstones of arrhythmia management in pediatrics.

1. The most common rhythm seen in pediatric arrest situations is bradycardia leading to asystole. Oxygenation and ventilation are often sufficient in this situation; epinephrine may be useful if unresponsive to ventilation.
2. Outside of the arrest situation, the most common arrhythmia is supraventricular tachycardia (SVT). It presents with a narrow complex tachycardia with rates between 250 and 350 beats/min. **Adenosine** (0.1 mg/kg) is the current recommended drug for SVT in children.

It is sometimes difficult to distinguish between a secondary sinus tachycardia and SVT. Small infants may have sinus tachycardia with rates above 200/min. Patients with sinus tachycardia may have a history of dehydration or shock, examination evidence of dehydration or pallor, and have a normally sized heart on chest x-ray. Infants with SVT often have a nonspecific history, an exam with rales, enlarged heart or liver, and an enlarged heart on chest x-ray. Treatment of the unstable patient with SVT is with synchronized cardioversion at ¼ to ½ J/kg.

Defibrillation and Cardioversion

Ventricular fibrillation is rare in children but may be treated with defibrillation at 2 J/kg. If this attempt is unsuccessful, the energy is doubled to 4 J/kg. If two attempts at defibrillation at 4 J/kg are unsuccessful, epinephrine should be given and oxygenation and acid-base status should be reassessed. Cardioversion is used to treat unstable tachyarrythmias, at a dose of ¼ to ½ J/kg.

Use the largest paddles which still allow contact of the entire paddle with the chest wall. Electrode cream or paste is used to prevent burns of the chest wall. One paddle is placed on the right of the sternum at the second intercostal space and the other is placed at the left midclavicular line at the level of the xiphoid.

Neonatal Resuscitation

Most newborns do not require specific resuscitation after delivery, but about 6% of newborns require some form of life support in the delivery room. Emergency departments, therefore, must be prepared to provide neonatal resuscitation in the event of delivery in the emergency department.

1. The first step in neonatal resuscitation is to maintain body temperature. The infant should be dried and placed under a radiant warmer.
2. The airway should be cleared by suctioning the nose and mouth with a bulb syringe or a DeLee trap.
3. Next, a 5 to 10 second examination should assess heart rate, respiratory effort, color, and activity. If the infant is apneic or the heart rate is slow (<100/minute), administer positive pressure ventilation with bag–valve–mask and 100% oxygen. The rate should be 40 breaths/min. In mildly depressed infants, a prompt improvement in heart rate and respiratory effort usually occur.
4. If no improvement is noted after 30 sec and the condition deteriorates, endotracheal intubation should be performed. For infants under about 3000 grams, a #0 laryngoscope blade should be chosen; in infants over 2000 grams, #1 blade will work well.
5. If the heart rate is still below 50/min after intubation and assisted ventilation, cardiac massage should be initiated at 120 compressions/min. Cardiac compressions and ventilation should be synchronized in a 3:1 ratio.
6. If there is no response to these efforts, drug therapy may be used. Most neonates will respond to appropriate ventilation, therefore, drug therapy rarely is needed. Circulatory access may be obtained peripherally or through the umbilical vein or artery. The most expedient procedure to obtain access in the newborn is to insert a catheter into an umbilical vein and advance it 10 to 12 cm.
7. Medications that are useful in neonatal resuscitation include epinephrine, naloxone, isoproterenol, and bicarbonate. **Epinephrine** (0.01 mg/kg of 1:10,000 concentration) may be used if the heart rate is still below 120/min after all above measures have been taken.
8. **Naloxone** (0.1 mg/kg IV) may be useful to reverse narcotic respiratory depression.
9. **Isoproterenol** (0.05–0.1 mcg/min) may be infused if epinephrine fails to raise the heart rate.
10. **Sodium bicarbonate** therapy should be guided by blood gases and used in cases of significant metabolic acidosis after adequate ventilation is assured.

Meconium Staining

Aspiration of meconium stained amniotic fluid is associated with a high morbidity and mortality. With proper management, however, it is almost entirely preventable.

1. If meconium is noted at the time of delivery, the nose, mouth, and pharynx of the infant should be suctioned with a DeLee trap prior to delivery of the infant's shoulders.
2. Repeat suctioning of the airway should be performed after delivery with the infant under a radiant warmer.
3. The trachea should be visualized and meconium aspirated through an endotracheal tube, as many times as needed to clear the trachea. The infant may then be ventilated with positive pressure, if needed.

Neonatal Emergencies

Seizures

It is important to distinguish seizures from tremors or jitteriness associated with hypocalcemia, hypoglycemia, drug withdrawal, or no identifiable morbidity. Tremors are fine movements that respond to sensory stimuli, stop with manual stabilization, and are not accompanied by eye, oral, or lingual movements. A careful history and physical examination should be performed to see if drug withdrawal, birth asphyxia, or metabolic disorders are causing neonatal seizures. Laboratory studies should include blood sugar, electrolytes (including calcium, magnesium, and blood urea nitrogen [BUN]), and spinal fluid cell count, chemistries, culture and Gram stain. Additional studies such as EEG and imaging studies may be performed after in the infant is stabilized.

1. Treatment of neonatal seizures begins with assuring an intact airway. Intravenous access should be obtained and blood samples obtained.
2. Hypoglycemia is treated with 5 ml/kg IV of 10% glucose solution.
3. Drugs useful in neonatal seizures include phenobarbital and diphenylhydantoin. **Phenobarbital** is given in a loading dose of 20 mg/kg slow IV (over 10 min). If the initial 20 mg/kg dose is not effective, additional 5 mg/kg doses may be given every 5 min until seizures cease or until a total dose of 40 mg/kg has been reached.
4. In cases unresponsive to phenobarbital, **diphenylhydantoin** may be given at a dose of 15 to 20 mg/kg slow IV.
5. Lorazepam may be used in status epilepticus at a dose of 0.01mg/kg IV.
6. Infants with **pyridoxine** dependence respond immediately to 50 to 100 mg IV pyridoxine.

Diaphragmatic Hernia

Left-sided hernias are more common than right-sided hernias. Clinical signs include auscultating bowel sounds in the chest, respiratory distress, cyanosis, and vomiting. Chest radiographs demonstrate air-filled loops of bowel in the chest and an absent diaphragmatic margin. Emergency department management is directed toward stabilization prior to surgical repair. Surgical consultation should be obtained immediately. The infant should be intubated using as little bag–valve–mask ventilation as possible, as introducing more air into the gastrointestinal GI tract is deleterious. An NG tube should be placed, at low continuous suction. Intravenous fluids should be given to correct hypovolemia.

Gastroschisis and Omphalocele

An omphalocele is a defect in the umbilical ring, which allows the intestines to protrude in a sac outside the abdominal cavity. A gastroschisis is a defect in the abdominal wall that allows the antenatal evisceration of abdominal structures without an overlying sac. The emergency management of both conditions is the same: the eviscerated bowel should be wrapped in saline-soaked gauze and placed in a plastic bag to protect against hypothermia and evaporative losses. Immediate surgical consultation should be obtained. An NG tube should be placed to decompress the stomach. Intravenous fluid therapy may be needed to correct hypovolemia.

For further reading in *Emergency Medicine, A Comprehensive Study Guide,* see Chapter 16, Neonatal Resuscitation and Emergencies, by Seetha Shankaran and Eugene E. Cepela; Chapter 17, Pediatric Cardiopulmonary Resuscitation, by Robert Luten; and Chapter 18, Vascular Access in Infants and Children, by William H. Spivey and Dee Hodge, III.

Fluids, Electrolytes, and Acid-Base Disorders

Vincent Nacouzi

FLUIDS

The most commonly used fluid in the emergency department is 0.9% normal saline (NS). Because the osmolarity of the fluid matches that of serum, it is an excellent fluid for volume replacement. D_5W is mainly used as an IV drug route, however, certain drugs can be given only with normal saline, such as phenytoin. Hypotonic fluids such as D_5W should never be used to replace volume. Rapid administration of D_5W can cause cerebral edema. Lactated Ringer's solution is commonly used for surgical patients or trauma patients, however, only normal saline can be given in the same line with blood. $D_5 45$ normal saline, with or without potassium, is given as a maintenance fluid. The more concentrated dextrose solutions, $D_{10}W$ or $D_{20}W$ are used for patients with compromised ability to mobilize glucose stores, such as patients with hepatic failure, or as part of total parental nutrition (TPN) solutions. Table 4-1 lists the components of common IV solutions.

Maintenance Fluids

Adult: $D_5 45$ NS at 75 to 125 cc/h + 20 mEq/L of potassium chloride for an average adult (approximately 70 kg).

Pediatrics: 100 ml/k/d for first 10 kg of above solution
50 ml/kg/d for second 10 kg
20 ml/kg/d for every kg thereafter

(For more information about pediatric fluid management, see Chapter 17.)

ELECTROLYTE DISORDERS

It should be noted that with electrolyte and acid-base abnormalities, laboratory errors are not uncommon. Results should be double checked when the clinical picture and the laboratory analysis conflict. Following is a formula to calculate osmolarity:

Osmolarity

Use measured serum values in mEq/L.

$$\text{Osmolarity in mosm/L} = 2Na + \frac{\text{glucose}}{18} + \frac{\text{BUN}}{2.8} + \frac{\text{ETOH}}{4.6}$$

General Approach

Address the ABCs first, then in order correct fluid and perfusion deficits, pH, and electrolytes. Correct abnormalities at the same rate they were

TABLE 4-1. Components of Common IV Solutions

| | Cations | | | Anions | | | |
Solutions	Na$^+$ (mEq/L)	K$^+$ (mEq/L)	Ca^{++} (mEq/L)	Cl$^-$ (mEq/L)	HCO$_3^{3-}$ (mEq/L)	Dextrose (gm/L)	Osmolarity (mEq/L)
Extracellular Fluid	142	4	5	103	27		280–310
Lactated Ringer's	130	4	3	109	28*		273
0.9% NS	154	0	0	154	0	0	308
D$_5$.45% NS	77	0	0	77	0	0	407
D$_5$W	0	0	0	0	0	50	253
D$_{10}$W	0	0	0	0	0	100	506
3% NS	513	0	0	513	0	0	1026

*Lactate, converts to bicarbonate

produced, however, slower correction is usually safe unless the condition warrants rapid intervention (i.e., hypoglycemia, hyperkalemia).

Hyponatremia ($Na^+ < 135$ mEq/L)

Clinical Findings

The clinical presentation of hyponatremia is often dominated by the underlying disease process. Signs and symptoms of hyponatremia usually begin when the serum sodium level drops below 120 mEq/L and includes: abdominal pain, headache, agitation, hallucinations, focal neurologic signs, confusion, and seizures.

Diagnosis and Differential

The diagnosis of hyponatremia can be made from the electrolyte panel, and for some patients a urine sodium level is needed. The most common cause is dilutional, and may be brought on by trauma, sepsis, cardiac failure, cirrhosis, or renal failure. Hyponatremia may also be factitious (false elevation in the measured sodium) due to hyperglycemia, elevated protein, or hyperlipidemia. True hyponatremia (low osmolarity) can be classified by ECF (extracellular fluid) and urine sodium level. Syndrome of inappropriate antidiuretic hormone (SIADH) is a diagnosis by exclusion, when low plasma osmolarity and concentrated urine appear in a patient with normal volume when no diuretics have been given. Causes of hyponatremia are listed in Table 4-2.

Emergency Department Care

1. First correct the volume or perfusion deficit, if any. Use normal saline if there is a volume deficit. (See Chapter 30 for discussion on using vasopressors in CHF.)
2. In stable patients, restrict fluids (500–1500 ml of water daily).
3. In severe hyponatremia ($Na^+ < 120$ mEq/L, with CNS changes), give **hypertonic saline,** 3% NS (513 mEq/L) at 25 to 100 ml/h. Administer with **furosemide,** in small repeated doses of 20 to 40 mg. An alternate treatment method is giving normal saline with furosemide. The sodium deficit can be calculated by taking the patient's weight in kg times 30% (140—measured Na^+). The rate of correction should be less than 0.5 mEq/L/hr. Complications of rapid correction include CHF and central pontine myelinolysis, which can cause alterations in consciousness, dysphagia, dysarthria, and paresis.

Hypernatremia ($Na^+ > 145$ mEq/L)

Clinical Features

The clinical picture is usually dominated by the underlying disease process. Symptoms attributable to hypernatremia, however, usually be-

TABLE 4-2. Causes of Hyponatremia

Hyponatremia with decreased ECF
  Extrarenal losses; urinary Na < 20 mEq/L
    Sweating, vomiting, diarrhea
    Third-space sequestration (burns, peritonitis, pancreatitis)
  Renal losses: urinary Na > 20 mEq/L
    Loop or osmotic diuretics
    Aldosterone deficiency (Addison's disease)
    Ketonuria
    Salt-losing nephropathies; renal tubular acidosis
Hyponatremia with normal ECF: urinary Na > 20 mEq/L
  Inappropriate ADH secretion
  Sick-cell or reset osmostat syndromes
  Physical and emotional stress or pain
  Myxedema, Addison's disease, Sheehan's syndrome
Hyponatremia with increased ECF
  Urinary Na > 20 mEq/L
    Renal failure
  Urinary Na < 20 mEq/L
    Cirrhosis
    Cardiac failure
    Renal failure
Pseudohyponatremia (hyperproteinemia, hyperlipidemia, hyperglycemia)

---

gin when the serum sodium is greater than 158 mEq/L and include irritability (expect osmolality of 350–375) and brain hemorrhage (mostly seen with neonates after a large IV sodium load [i.e., with sodium bicarbonate]). An osmolality increase of 50 or more is associated with 50% death rate.

Diagnosis and Differential

The most frequent cause of hypernatremia is a decrease in total body water due to decreased intake or excessive loss. The more common causes are diarrhea, vomiting, hyperpyrexia, and excessive sweating. The causes of hypernatremia are listed in Table 4-3.

Emergency Department Care

Treat dehydration/fluid deficits with NS or LR. Switch to 0.5 NS after obtaining a urine output of greater than 0.5 ml/kg/h. Avoid lowering the Na^+ more than 10 mEq/L/day. Monitor central venous pressure and pulmonary capillary wedge pressure. Use the formula below to calculate the total body water deficit.

$$\text{Water deficit} = \text{TBW} \left(1 - \frac{\text{measured Na}^+}{\text{desired Na}^+} \right) = \text{water needed to correct the hypernatremia}$$

If no urine output is observed after NS/LR rehydration, rapidly switch

TABLE 4-3 Causes of Hypernatremia

Loss of water
  Reduced water intake
    Defective thirst
    Unconsciousness
    Inability to drink water
    Lack of access to water
  Increased water loss
    Vomiting, diarrhea
    Sweating, fever
    Hyperventilation
    Diabetes insipidus, osmotic diuresis
    Thyrotoxicosis
    Severe burns
Gain of sodium
  Increased intake
    Hypertonic saline ingestion or infusion
    Sodium bicarbonate administration
  Renal salt retention (usually because of poor perfusion)

to 0.5 NS: unload the body of the extra sodium by using a diuretic (i.e., furosemide, 20–40 mg IV).

If Standard Treatment Fails

In children with a serum sodium level greater than 180 mEq/L, consider peritoneal dialysis, which may be lifesaving.

Hypokalemia ($K^+ < 3.5$ mEq/L)

Clinical Features

Signs and symptoms include weakness, ileus, and its associated nausea and vomiting. Patients have an increased sensitivity to digitalis. ECG shows U waves (potassium level below 2.7 mEq/L), prolonged QT, and flat, depressed T waves.

Diagnosis and Differential

The most common cause is the use of loop diuretics. Table 4-4 lists the causes.

Emergency Department Care

Patients should be monitored continuously for dysrhythmias.

1. Administer 10 to 15 mEq of **potassium chloride** per hour in 50 to 100 mL of dextrose in water (D_5W), piggyback into saline over 3 to 4 hours. No more than 40 mEq of $K+/h$ replacement and no more than 40 mEq in a liter of IV fluids. It takes 40 to 50 mEq of $K+$ to raise the serum concentration by 1 mEq/L.

TABLE 4-4. Causes of Hypokalemia

Shift into the cell
   Raising the pH of blood
   Administration of insulin and glucose
Reduced intake
Increased loss
   Renal loss
      Primary hyperaldosteronism
      Secondary hypoaldosteronism associated with diuretics, malignant
      hypertension, Bartter syndrome, renal artery stenosis
      Miscellaneous
         Hypercalcemia
         Liddle syndrome
         Magnesium deficiency
         Renal tubular acidosis
         Acute myelocytic and monocytic leukemias
   Gastrointestinal loss (vomiting, diarrhea, fistulas)

2. Oral replacement (in the awake, asymptomatic patient) is as rapid as and safer than IV therapy. Use 20 to 40 mEq/L of KCL or similar agent.

Hyperkalemia ($K^+ > 5.0$ mEq/L)

Clinical Features

Signs and symptoms include weakness, increased deep tendon reflexes (DTR), and confusion. As the serum potassium level rises, the ECG progressively changes with peaked T waves (precordial) at 6 mEq/L, prolonged PR and QT at 6.5 mEq/L, diminished P waves, and depressed ST segments at 7 mEq/L, BBB-like pattern above 7 mEq/L, irregular rate and sine wave pattern at levels above 8 mEq/L.

Diagnosis and Differential

Renal failure with oliguria is the most common cause. Appropriate tests for management include an ECG, electrolytes, calcium, magnesium, ABG (check for acidosis), UA, and a digoxin level. Causes of hypernatremia are listed in Table 4-5.

Emergency Department Care

Patients must be monitored closely for ECG changes and adequate ventilation should be assured. Maintaining diuresis is very important.

1. For severe hyperkalemia (level over 7.0 mEq/L) give calcium gluconate or **calcium chloride,** 10 mL of a 10% solution over 10 min. Do not use in digoxin toxic patients. Hyperkalemia in the presence of digoxin toxicity is an indication for digoxin specific antibodies, and calcium should be withheld since it will exacerbate the dysrhythmias in these patients. For patients on digoxin without dysrhythmias

TABLE 4-5. Causes of Hyperkalemia

Factitious
Laboratory error
Pseudohyperkalemia: hemolysis, thrombocytosis, leukocytosis
Metabolic acidemia (acute)
Increased intake into the plasma
Exogenous: diet, salt substitutes, low-sodium diet, medications
Endogenous: hemolysis, GI bleeding, catabolic states, crush injury
Inadequate distal delivery of sodium and decreased distal tubular flow
Oliguric renal failure
Impaired renin–aldosterone axis
Addison's disease
Primary hypoaldosteronism
Other (heparin, β blockers, prostaglandin inhibitors, captopril)
Primary renal tubular potassium secretory defect
Sickle cell disease
Systemic lupus erythematosus
Postrenal transplantation
Obstructive uropathy
Inhibition of renal tubular secretion of potassium
Spironolactone
Digitalis
Abnormal potassium distribution
Insulin deficiency
Hypertonicity (hyperglycemia)
Beta-adrenergic blockers
Exercise
Succinylcholine
Digitalis

who are in need of calcium add 10 mL of a 10% solution to 100 mL of D5W and give over 20 to 30 min.

2. For patients with levels above 5.5 mEq/L (especially in acidotic patients), give 1 amp of **sodium bicarbonate,** 50 ml of an 8.4% (50 mEq/L) or 7.5% (44 mEq/L) solution over 10 min.

3. Give 1 amp of **D$_{50}$W,** 50 cc of a 50% solution with 10 u regular **insulin** IVP (5 units in dialysis patients). This can be followed with 1000 mL of D20W with 40 u insulin over the next 2 to 4 h.

4. **Kayexalate** (PO or PR) 1 gm binds 1 mEq of K+ over 10 min. Administer 15 to 25 gm of kayexalate PO with 50 ml of 20% sorbitol every 4 h (sorbitol used because kayexalate is constipating). Per rectum, give 20 gm in 200 ml 20% sorbitol over 30 min. Kayexalate can exacerbate CHF.

5. Maintain diuresis with **furosemide,** 20 to 40 mg IV push.

6. If above measures fail or the patient has complications, use dialysis.

Hypercalcemia (Ca$^+$ > 10.5)

The ionized fraction of calcium is the physiologically active one; that fraction is approximately 40 to 50% of the total calcium reported by most laboratories (normal total calcium is 8.5–10.5 mg/dL). Total calcium levels, especially in the presence of hypoalbuminemia, may be low and yet be associated with normal ionized calcium levels. Several factors affect the serum calcium level: parathyroid hormone (PTH) increases calcium and decreases phosphate; calcitonin and vitamin D metabolites decrease calcium.

Clinical Findings

A mnemonic to aid recall of common hypercalcemia symptoms is *stones* (renal calculi), *bones* (bone destruction secondary to malignancy), *psychic moans* (lethargy, weakness, fatigue, confusion) and *abdominal groans* (abdominal pain, constipation, polyuria, polydipsia). On the ECG you may see depressed ST segments, widened T waves, shortened QT intervals, and bradyarrhythmias. Levels above 20 mEq/L can cause cardiac arrest.

A mnemonic to aid recall of the common causes is *PAM P. SCHMIDT:* Parathyroid hormone, Addison's disease, Multiple myeloma, Paget's disease, Sarcoidosis, Cancer, Hyperthyroidism, Milk-alkali syndrome, Immobilization, excess Vitamin D, and Thiazides.

Emergency Department Care

Emergency treatment is important in the following conditions: a calcium level above 12 mg/dL, a symptomatic patient, a patient who cannot tolerate PO fluids, or a patient with abnormal renal function.

1. Correct dehydration with normal saline, 5 to 10 L, may be required.
2. Administer **furosemide,** 40 mg, but do not exacerbate dehydration if present. Correct the concurrent hypokalemia or hypomagnesemia. Do not use thiazide diuretics (worsens hypercalcemia).
3. If above treatments are not effective, administer **calcitonin** 0.5 to 4 MRC units/kg IV over 24 hours or IM divided every 6 hours.
4. **Hydrocortisone** 25 to 100 mg IV every 6 h.

Hypocalcemia ($Ca^+ < 8.5$)

Clinical Features

The signs and symptoms of hypocalcemia are paresthesias, increased DTR, spasms, cramps, weakness, confusion, and seizures. Patients may also demonstrate Chvostek's sign (twitch of the corner of mouth on tapping with finger over cranial nerve VII at zygoma) or Trousseau's sign (more reliable, carpal spasm when the blood pressure cuff is left inflated at a pressure above the systolic BP for greater than 3 min). If the patient is alkalotic, ionized calcium (physiologically active) may be very low, even with a normal total calcium.

Diagnosis and Differential

Most common causes: shock, sepsis, renal failure, pancreatitis, drugs. Physiologic effects seen when the level of total calcium falls below 6.5 mg/dL. Consider checking calcium levels in refractory CHF. Included in the differential is strychnine poisoning, hypomagnesemia, and tetanus toxin.

Emergency Department Care

1. If asymptomatic use oral **calcium gluconate** tablets, 1 to 4 g/day divided q6 h, with or without **Vitamin D,** (calcitrol, 0.2 mcg, bid).
2. In more urgent situations with symptomatic patients, **calcium gluconate,** or **calcium chloride,** 10 mL of a 10% solution can be given over 10 min, slow IV.
3. In massive blood transfusions when given more rapidly than 1 unit every 5 min, give 10 mL of 10% solution after 4 units of blood. Newer blood bank preparations, however, avoid citrate; check with your blood bank.

Hypomagnesemia

Clinical Findings

Signs and symptoms of hypomagnesemia include: CNS—depression, vertigo, ataxia, seizures, increased DTR, tetany; cardiac—arrhythmias, prolonged QT, worsening of digitalis effects, and hypothermia.

Diagnosis and Differential

Most common cause is alcoholism (in the U.S.), followed by poor nutrition, cirrhosis, pancreatitis, or excessive gastrointestinal fluid losses.

Emergency Department Care

1. Must correct volume deficit and other electrolyte abnormalities, such as decreased potassium, decreased calcium, and decreased phosphate, first.
2. If the patient is an alcoholic in delirium tremens (DTs) or pending DTs, administer 2 gm **magnesium sulfate** over the first hour, then 6 gm over the next 24 h. Check DTR every 15 min. DTR disappear when the serum magnesium level rises above 3.5 mEq/L, at which time the magnesium infusion should be stopped, at least momentarily.

Hypermagnesemia

Clinical Findings

Signs and symptoms manifest progressively; DTR disappear with a serum magnesium level above 3.5 mEq/L, muscle weakness at a level above 4 mEq/L, hypotension at a level above 5 mEq/L, and respiratory paralysis at a level above 8 mEq/L.

Diagnosis and Differential

Most common cause is renal failure and magnesium containing preparations, such as common antacids.

Emergency Department Care

1. Rehydrate with normal saline and **furosemide** 20 to 40 mg IV.
2. Correct acidosis with ventilation and sodium bicarbonate 50 to 100 mEq, if needed.
3. Five mL of a 10% solution of CaCl IV antagonizes the effects of magnesium.

Phosphate and Chloride Abnormalities

Hypophosphatemia rarely occurs, except in patients receiving TPN. Hyperphosphatemia occurs mainly with renal failure and can be treated with hydration, acetazolamide, or dialysis. Chloride abnormalities usually occur in association with other metabolic disorders, such as metabolic alkalosis (hypochloremia) or dehydration (hyperchloremia). Treatment for chloride disorders is the correction of the volume deficit with normal saline, the acid-base abnormality, or the potassium deficit.

ACID-BASE DISORDERS

Acid-base regulation involves the interplay of several body systems, but primarily the lungs and the kidneys. *Acidosis* is due to gain of acid or loss of alkali; causes may be metabolic (fall in serum HCO_3) or respiratory (rise in pCO_2). *Alkalosis* is due to loss of acid or addition of base and is either metabolic (rise in serum HCO_3) or respiratory (fall in pCO_2). The body attempts to limit the change in pH. Metabolic disorders prompt an immediate compensatory change in ventilation, either venting CO_2 or retaining it, however, the compensation will not correct the pH completely in the acute situation. In response to respiratory disorders, the kidney attempts to excrete hydrogen ion (with chloride) or retain it, but this takes 48 to 72 h.

Several conditions should alert the clinician to possible acid-base disorders: history of renal, endocrine, or psychiatric disorders (drug ingestion), or signs of acute disease: tachypnea, cyanosis, Kussmaul respirations, respiratory failure, shock, changes in mental status, vomiting, diarrhea, or other acute fluid losses.

General Approach

The type of acid-base disturbance the patient has can be determined by several steps, drawing blood, then determining the presumptive type of acid-base disorder from the pH, the pCO_2, the CO_2 content (serum bicarbonate), then confirming the presumptive type. We can confirm the presumptive type by comparing the patient's actual lab values to values calculated by formulas that predict the anticipated compensatory changes.

1. **Blood Draw.** After initial attention to the ABC's, a complete history (including ROS), and physical examination, send blood for arterial blood gas measurement, electrolytes, BUN, creatinine, serum osmolality, and dip urine for ketones and glucose. If a patient has a normal pH, normal pCO_2, and a normal CO_2 content, the patient does not have an acid-base problem.

   Use as normals: pH = 7.4, HCO_3 = 24 mm/L, pCO_2 = 40 mmHg

2. **Presumptive Type.** Determine the type of acid-base disorder from the following: Any listed increase or decrease uses the above normals as reference points.

Type	pH	pCO_2	HCO_3
Respiratory acidosis	Decreased	Increased	Increased
Respiratory alkalosis	Increased	Decreased	Decreased
Metabolic acidosis	Decreased	Decreased	Decreased
Metabolic alkalosis	Increased	Increased	Increased
Mixed disorder	Variable	Variable	Variable

Now move to the appropriate step below to confirm the presumptive type.

Respiratory Acidosis

Using historical information, respiratory acidosis can be further divided into acute respiratory acidosis, (e.g., hypoventilation from narcotic overdose) and chronic respiratory acidosis (e.g., COPD with CO_2 retention). Only in chronic conditions does the kidney have time to compensate for the respiratory changes (takes 48–72 hours). Formulae to calculate the expected changes in pH (from 7.4) and HCO_3 (from 24 mm/L) using the observed change in pCO_2 (from 40 mmHg) are:

Acute respiratory acidosis. Predicted decrease in pH = (0.007) × (observed change in pCO_2); predicted increase in HCO_3 = (0.1) × (observed change in pCO_2).

Chronic respiratory acidosis. Predicted decrease in pH = (0.003) × (observed change in pCO_2); predicted increase in HCO_3 = (0.35) × (observed change in pCO_2).

   If these conditions do not hold true, you do not have a primary respiratory disorder. (See Simple Metabolic Acidosis, below.)

Respiratory Alkalosis

Using historical information, respiratory alkalosis can be further divided into acute respiratory alkalosis (e.g., hyperventilation from anxiety) and chronic respiratory alkalosis (e.g., untreated hyperthyroidism). Only in chronic conditions does the kidney have time to compensate for the respiratory changes (takes 48 to 72 hours). Formula to calculate the expected changes in pH (from 7.4) and HCO_3 (from 24 mm/L) using the observed change in pCO_2 (from 40 mmHg) are:

Acute respiratory alkalosis. Predicted increase in pH = (0.007) × (observed change in pCO_2); predicted decrease in HCO_3 = (0.2) × (observed change in pCO_2). Usually the HCO_3 is not less than 18 in acute conditions.

Chronic respiratory alkalosis. Predicted increase in pH = (0.0017) × (observed change in pCO_2); predicted decrease in HCO_3 = (0.5) × (observed change in pCO_2). Usually the HCO_3 is not less than 14 in chronic conditions.

If these conditions do not hold to be true, you do not have a primary respiratory disorder. (See Simple Metabolic Alkalosis below.)

Simple metabolic acidosis. If the acid-base disorder is a simple metabolic acidosis, you should be able to predict the decrease in pCO_2 (from 40 mmHg) using the observed change in HCO_3 (from 24 mm/L) with the following formula:

Predicted decrease in pCO_2 = (1.0 to 1.5) observed decrease in HCO_3

If these conditions do not hold to be true, you have a mixed disorder.

Simple metabolic alkalosis. If the acid-base disorder is a simple metabolic acidosis, you should be able to predict the increase in pCO_2 (from 40 mmHg) using the observed change in HCO_3 (from 24 mm/L) with the following formula:

Predicted increase in pCO_2 = (0.25 to 1.0) observed increase in HCO_3

If these conditions do not hold to be true, you have a mixed disorder. If you have determined that you have a mixed disorder, you will need to consider treatments listed in both the respiratory and metabolic sections that follow.

Respiratory Acidosis

Clinical Presentation

Respiratory acidosis may be life-threatening and a precursor to respiratory arrest. The clinical picture is often dominated by the underlying disorder. Typically, respiratory acidosis depresses the mental function, which may progressively slow the respiratory rate. Patients may be confused, somnolent and, eventually, unconscious.

Diagnosis

Although frequently hypoxic, in some disorders the fall in oxygen saturation may lag behind the elevation in pCO_2. Pulse-oximetry may be misleading, therefore, making arterial blood gases essential for the diagnosis. The differential diagnosis includes: COPD, drug overdose, CNS disease, chest wall disease, pleural disease, and trauma.

Emergency Department Care

1. Increase ventilation. In many cases, this requires intubation. The hallmark indication for intubation in respiratory acidosis is depressed mental status. Only in opiate intoxication is it acceptable to await treatment of the underlying disorder (rapid administration of naloxone) before reversal of the hypoventilation.

2. Treat the underlying disorder. Remember that high-flow oxygen therapy may lead to exacerbation of CO_2 narcosis in patients with COPD and CO_2 retention. Monitor these patients closely when administering oxygen to them and intubate if necessary.

Respiratory Alkalosis

Clinical Presentation

Hyperventilation syndrome is a problematic diagnosis for the emergency physician, as a number of life-threatening disorders present with tachypnea and anxiety: asthma, pulmonary embolism, diabetic ketoacidosis and others. Symptoms of respiratory alkalosis often are dominated by the primary disorder promoting the hyperventilation. Hyperventilation by virtue of the reduction of pCO_2, however, lowers both cerebral and peripheral blood flow, causing distinct symptoms. Patients complain of dizziness, painful flexion of the wrists, fingers, ankles and toes (carpal–pedal spasm) and, frequently, a chest pain described as tightness.

Diagnosis and Differential

The diagnosis of hyperventilation due to anxiety is a diagnosis of exclusion. Arterial blood gases can be used to rule out acidosis and hypoxia. (See Chapter 33, Pulmonary Embolism, for discussion of calculating the alveolar–arterial oxygen gradient.) Causes of respiratory alkalosis to consider include: hypoxia, fever, hyperthyroidism, sympathomimetic therapy, progesterone therapy, liver disease, and anxiety.

Emergency Department Care

1. Treat the underlying cause. Only when more serious causes of hyperventilation are ruled out should you consider the treatment of anxiety. Anxiolytics may be helpful, such as lorazepam 1 to 2 mg, IV or po.

2. Rebreathing into a paper bag can cause hypoxia. If you choose this method, monitor with pulse oximetry.

Metabolic Acidosis

When considering metabolic acidosis, causes should be further divided into elevated and normal anion-gap acidosis. The term anion gap is misleading because in serum, there is no gap between total positive and negative ions, however, we commonly measure more positive ions than negative ions. The anion gap, therefore, is measured as follows:

Anion gap = $Na+ - (Cl^- + HCO_3^-)$ = approx 10 to 12 mEq/L

Clinical Presentation

No matter what the etiology, acidosis can cause nausea and vomiting, abdominal pain, change in sensorium, and tachypnea, sometimes a Kussmaul pattern. It also leads to decreased muscle strength and force of cardiac contraction, arterial vasodilation, venous vasoconstriction, and pulmonary hypertension. Patients may present with nonspecific complaints or shock.

Diagnosis and Differential

Causes of metabolic acidosis can be divided into two main groups: (1) those associated with increased production of organic acids (increased anion gap metabolic acidosis, Table 4-6); and (2) those associated with a loss of bicarbonate or addition of chloride (normal anion-gap metabolic acidosis, Table 4-7). A mnemonic to aid the recall of the causes of increased anion-gap metabolic acidosis is: *A MUD PILES*—alcohol, methanol, uremia, DKA, paraldehyde, iron and isoniazid, lactic acidosis, ethylene glycol, salicylates, and starvation. A mnemonic that can aid the recall of normal anion-gap metabolic acidosis is *USED CARP*—ureterostomy, small bowel fistulas, extra chloride, diarrhea, carbonic anhydrase inhibitors, adrenal insufficiency, renal tubular acidosis, and pancreatic fistula.

TABLE 4-6. Causes of High Anion-Gap Metabolic Acidosis

Lactic acidosis
   Type A—Decrease in tissue oxygenation
   Type B—No decrease in tissue oxygenation
Renal failure (acute or chronic)
Ketoacidosis
   Diabetes
   Alcoholism
   Prolonged starvation (mild acidosis)
   High-fat diet (mild acidosis)
Ingestion of toxic substances
   Elevated osmolar gap
     Methanol
     Ethylene glycol
   Normal osmolar gap
     Salicylate
     Paraldehyde
     Cyanide

TABLE 4-7. Causes of Normal Anion-Gap Metabolic Acidosis

With a tendency to hyperkalemia	With a tendency to hypokalemia
Subsiding DKA	Renal tubular acidosis, type I
Early uremic acidosis	Renal tubular acidosis, type II
Early obstructive uropathy	Acetazolamide therapy
Renal tubular acidosis, type IV	Acute diarrhea (losses of HCO_3
Hypoaldosteronism	and K)
Potassium sparing diuretics	Ureterosigmoidostomy

Emergency Department Care

After the ABCs have been assured, the following general treatment is recommended.

1. Give supportive care by improving perfusion, administering fluids as needed, improving oxygenation and ventilation.
2. Correct the underlying problem. If the patient has ingested a toxin, lavage, administer activated charcoal, give the appropriate antidote, and perform dialysis, as directed by the specific toxicology chapters in this handbook. If septic, perform cultures and administer antibiotics, as directed by the appropriate chapters in this handbook. If in shock, administer fluids and vasopressors as directed by Chapter 8 on Hemorrhagic Shock, or Chapter 9 on Septic Shock. If the patient is in DKA, treat as directed in Chapter 117, Diabetic Emergencies, with IV fluids and insulin.
3. When pH <7.1 or HCO_3 <8 to 10, consider treatment with sodium bicarbonate (controversial). Raise the pH to approximately 7.25, using 1 mEq/kg of HCO_3 over 20–30 minutes. Beware of sodium overload, particularly in neonates and patients in pulmonary edema. Reassess pH, pCO_2, HCO_3 and determine the need for further therapy.

Metabolic Alkalosis

The two most common causes of metabolic alkalosis are excessive diuresis (with loss of potassium, hydrogen ion, and chloride) and excessive loss of gastric secretions (with loss of hydrogen ion and chloride). Other causes of hypokalemia also should be considered.

Clinical Features

Symptoms of the underlying disorder (usually fluid loss) dominate the clinical presentation, but general symptoms of metabolic alkalosis include muscular irritability, tachydysrhythmias, and impaired oxygen delivery.

Diagnosis and Differential

The diagnosis of metabolic alkalosis is made from laboratory studies revealing a bicarbonate level above 26 mEq/L and a pH above 7.45. In most cases, there is also an associated hypokalemia and hypochloremia. The differential diagnosis includes dehydration, loss of gastric acid, excessive diuresis, administration of mineralocorticoids, increased intake of citrate or lactate, hypercapnia, hypokalemia, and severe hypoproteinemia.

Emergency Department Care

1. Administer fluids in the form of normal saline in cases of dehydration.
2. Administer potassium as KCl, not faster than 20 mEq/h, unless serum potassium is above 5.0 mEq/L.

For further reading in *Emergency Medicine: A Comprehensive Study Guide*, see Chapter 19, Acid-Base Problems; Chapter 20, Blood Gases; and Chapter 21, Fluid and Electrolyte Problems, by Robert F. Wilson and Christopher Barton.

Acute Pain Relief and Conscious Sedation

Frantz R. Melio

The underutilization of sedation and analgesia in the ED has been well documented. Reasons for this include misunderstanding of a patient's response to pain, lack of knowledge of the pharmacokinetics of the various agents used, the fear of serious side-effects, and issues related to convenience. Patients at risk for receiving suboptimal treatment include children, the elderly, and the cognitively impaired. It is crucial not to confuse sedation and analgesia. Achieving both states often requires using multiple agents.

Clinical Features

Physiologic responses to pain and anxiety include increased heart rate, blood pressure, and respiratory rate. Behavioral changes include facial expressions, posturing, crying, and vocalization. Pain is best assessed using objective scales. Subjective impressions are often incorrect. Pain relief is a dynamic process and reassessment is mandatory.

Emergency Department Care

When treating anxious patients, or patients in need of uncomfortable procedures, one should begin with nonpharmacologic interventions. Communication should be appropriate for the developmental age of the patient. A gentle and unhurried approach is best. Procedures should be explained in a clear and honest manner with time given for questions and answers. With children, anticipation of painful procedures should be minimized by discussing the procedure just before it is performed. Environmental adjustments, such as dimmed lights, a quiet room, and audiovisual input, may be helpful. Parents should be included in interventions as their help may be crucial in comforting their child. Certain children will require restraints. Parents should be relieved of the responsibility of restraining their child. Once the necessity for pharmacologic interventions has been determined, consideration should be given to the need for sedation or analgesia, the route of delivery, and the desired duration of effects. Multiple agents may be needed to achieve the optimal state.

Systemic Analgesia and Sedation

Whenever systemic analgesia or sedation is used, the patient should be continuously monitored (cardiac monitor and pulse oximetry) and under constant observation by a dedicated health care provider who is trained in airway management. Oxygen, suction, and appropriately sized airway equipment should be readily accessible. Precalculated doses of reversal agents (**naloxone,** 0.1 mg/kg/dose) for opiates and **flumazenil** (0.01

mg/kg, with additional 0.005 mg/kg doses, to a maximum 0.2 mg/dose and 1 mg total) for benzodiazepines should be available. A baseline clinical assessment should be obtained, including blood pressure, heart rate, respiratory rate, and level of consciousness. This assessment should be made and documented every 5 to 10 minutes during the procedure and until the patient returns to baseline. Particular care should be taken when providing systemic analgesia or sedation to patients with underlying disease. Generally, administering medications intravenously is the best method for obtaining rapid and safe analgesia or sedation. Other routes may be appropriate (especially in children), but provide less reliable and slower clinical effects, limit the ability to titrate, and result in frequent under- or over-medication.

Analgesia for Brief Procedures

Opiates are the drugs of choice for analgesia. Fentanyl is a synthetic narcotic, which is 100 times more potent than morphine. It has almost immediate onset of action and an approximately 30-min duration when administered intravenously. Fentanyl and other narcotics are relatively contraindicated in patients with hemodynamic or respiratory compromise, as well as those with altered mental status. Fentanyl is less likely to cause respiratory depression, histamine release, and cardiovascular compromise than other opiates. Respiratory depression can be minimized by administering fentanyl slowly over 3 to 5 min. The dose of **fentanyl** is 2 to 3 μg/kg with additional doses titrated by 0.5 μg/kg until the desired level of analgesia is reached.

Nitrous oxide is an effective analgesic that produces a state of conscious sedation with euphoria and dissociation. It can be used alone or in conjunction with local anesthetics. Nitrous oxide is delivered as a 30% to 50% mixture with oxygen. It should be self-administered through a system that is fail-safe against delivery of an hypoxic mixture. Peak effects are reached within 1 to 2 min, and the patient is fully aroused within minutes of cessation of therapy. Since nitrous oxide must be self-administered, it is not practical for use in young children. Nitrous oxide has minimal respiratory or cardiovascular effects. It is contraindicated in patients who have recently been sedated with another agent, and those with altered mental status, dyspnea, severe COPD, pneumothorax, eye injury, or obstructed viscous.

Ketamine is a dissociative analgesic that also has sedative properties. Ketamine is usually given IM or IV to adults. Oral, rectal, intramuscular, and intravenous administration has been described in children. The dose of **ketamine** is 4 mg/kg when given PO, PR, and IM. A supplemental 2 mg/kg dose may be given. The IV dose is 1 mg/kg with additional 0.25 mg/kg doses titrated to the desired effect. **Atropine** (0.01 mg/kg) is often used as an adjunct to control hypersalivation. Although airway reflexes are usually protected and bronchodilation occurs, ketamine can cause laryngospasm. Ketamine has catecholamine-releasing properties.

It should be avoided in the setting of head trauma, or in patients with poor sympathetic tone or prolonged stress. Adults and older children may have unpleasant hallucinations when awakening from ketamine-induced sedation. This emergence reaction may be minimized by placing recovering patients in a darkened, quiet room. Low-dose **midazolam** (0.01 mg/kg IM or IV or 0.1 mg/kg PO) attenuates this experience, but it may lead to respiratory depression.

Analgesia for Longer Procedures

Morphine is the gold standard for this use. *Meperidine* is a synthetic derivative of morphine that is one tenth as potent and has a shorter duration. Meperidine also causes less respiratory depression than morphine in infants younger than 3 months old. Otherwise, meperidine offers no advantages over morphine. The IV dose of **morphine** is 0.1 mg/kg with additional doses of 0.05 mg/kg titrated to the desired effect. The dose of **meperidine** is 1 mg/kg with additional 0.5 mg/kg doses given, if necessary. Most adults will require a total dose of 1.5 to 3.0 mg/kg of meperidine for a painful procedure. The DPT cocktail (meperidine, 2 mg/kg; promethazine, 1 mg/kg; and chlorpromazine, 1 mg/kg) is unreliable, can cause respiratory depression, and has a duration of action of more than 7 h. More appropriate regimens should be used in its place.

Hydroxyzine is synergistic with opiates and has intrinsic analgesic properties. **Hydroxyzine,** 0.5 mg/kg, can be given PO or IM in conjunction with narcotics. Hydroxyzine will reduce the incidence of nausea and vomiting associated with opiate administration.

Phenothiazines do not enhance analgesia and produces nonreversible sedation. Their use in this setting should be limited to the treatment of nausea.

Ketorolac is a nonsteroidal anti-inflammatory agent which can be given orally, intramuscularly, or intravenously. The IM and IV doses are 0.5 to 1 mg/kg (max 60 mg, 30 mg in the elderly). It has been reported to be a potent analgesic with a long duration of action. Ketorolac does not cause respiratory depression. It can be used in combination with opiate analgesics. The most common side-effects are related to gastrointestinal irritation.

Sedation for Brief Procedures

Benzodiazepines are sedative agents that provide skeletal muscle relaxation, anxiolysis, and amnesia. They have no direct analgesic properties. When used in combination with opioids, it is generally safer to administer the benzodiazepine first for sedation or relaxation, followed by carefully titrating the opioid for analgesia. The dose of opioid required is usually lowered in these cases, and patients are more prone to developing respiratory compromise. Hypotension, another side-effect of benzodiazepines, can be avoided by administering these agents slowly. *Midazolam* is a short-acting benzodiazepine that has been successfully used by oral, rectal, nasal, subcutaneous, intramuscular, and intravenous routes. It is a potent sedative with excellent amnestic properties. **Midazolam**'s duration of action is 30 to 40 mins. An effective adult dosage regimen is 1 to 2 mg every 5 min, until sedation or muscle relaxation occurs. Lower dosages may be more appropriate for the elderly. (In children, dosage should be 0.15 mg/kg IV and IM.) The IV dose is titrated in 0.02 mg/kg increments, and the supplemental aIM dose is 0.1 mg/kg. Rectal and intranasal dosage is 0.2 to 0.4 mg/kg. Oral dose is 0.5 mg/kg, with a maximum dose of 12 mg.

The actions and side-effects of barbiturates are similar to those of benzodiazepines. Two important differences must be noted: (1) Barbiturates can increase airway tone and, therefore, should not be given to patients with moderate to severe airway disease; and (2) these agents must be used cautiously, as patients may rapidly progress from light sedation to deep sedation to general anesthesia.

Methohexital and *thiopental* are ultra-short acting barbiturates, with methohexital having a shorter duration of action. **Methohexital,** 0.5 to 1 mg/kg, or **thiopental,** 1 to 5 mg/kg, will produce sedation within 1 to 2 min. They are administered slowly by titrated incremental IV doses. Methohexital may be given rectally to children in doses of 20 mg/kg. Thiopental frequently causes hypotension, particularly when given rapidly. This effect is accentuated in the presence of hypovolemia, or preexisting heart disease.

Sedation for Longer Procedures

Diazepam is a longer acting benzodiazepine with anxiolytic and amnestic properties. It has been largely superseded by midazolam.

Pentobarbital is a barbiturate that induces sleep and can be administered by various routes. Intravenous administration can lead to sleep within 1 min, which lasts for 15 to 60 min. Recommended dosage varies greatly. An initial 2.5 mg/kg (max, 100 mg) intravenous dose can be given followed, as needed, every 5 min by an additional 1.25 mg/kg (maximum total 300 mg). Intramuscular dosage is 2 to 5 mg/kg, with a maximum dose of 100 to 200 mg. Pentobarbital can cause respiratory and cardiovascular depression, particularly when administered rapidly or in conjunction with a narcotic.

Chloral hydrate has been used successfully, particularly in children under 4 years old. It is unlikely to cause respiratory depression. Chloral hydrate can be administered orally or rectally at a dosage of 75 mg/kg. Its main disadvantage is its 30 to 60 min onset of action and its prolonged duration (up to several h).

Disposition. Patients are eligible for discharge only when fully recovered. When discharged, the patient must be accompanied by an adult and should not drive for at least 6 to 12 h. Instructions for care must be given to responsible accompanying adults, since many of these systemic agents impair recall.

For further reading in *Emergency Medicine, A Comprehensive Study Guide*, see Chapter 34, Systemic Analgesia and Sedation for Procedures in Adults, by Donald M. Yealy; and Chapter 38, Pediatric Analgesia and Sedation, by Elaine S. Pomeranz and Roy M. Kulick.

2 | ACUTE SIGNS AND SYMPTOMS IN ADULTS

Chest Pain

Sarah A. Stahmer

Patients with acute nontraumatic chest pain are among the most challenging patients cared for by emergency physicians. They may appear seriously ill, or they may appear completely well and yet remain at significant risk for sudden death or an acute myocardial infarction.

Clinical Features

The typical pain of myocardial ischemia has been described as retrosternal or epigastric squeezing, tightening, crushing, or pressure-like discomfort. The pain may radiate to the left shoulder, jaw, arm, or hand. In many cases, particularly in the elderly, the predominant complaint is not of pain, but of a poorly described visceral sensation with associated dyspnea, diaphoresis, nausea, light-headedness, or profound weakness. The onset of symptoms may be sudden or gradual, and symptoms usually last minutes to hours. In general, symptoms that last less than 2 min, or are constant over days, are less likely to be ischemic in origin. Symptoms that are new, occur with increasing frequency or severity, or occur at rest are called unstable and warrant urgent evaluation even if they are absent at the time of presentation.

Physical Examination

Patients with acute myocardial ischemia may appear clinically well or be profoundly hemodynamically unstable. The degree of hemodynamic instability is dependent on the amount of myocardium at risk, associated dysrhythmias, valvular compromise, and the patient's response to acute ischemia. Worrisome signs may be clinically subtle, particularly the presence of sinus tachycardia, which may be due to pain and fear, or may be an early sign of physiologic compensation for left ventricular failure. Patients with acute ischemia often have a paucity of significant physical findings. Rales, a third or fourth heart sound, cardiac murmurs, or rub are all clinically relevant and important findings. The presence of chest wall tenderness has been demonstrated in patients with acute MI, and so its presence should not be used to exclude the possibility of acute myocardial ischemia.

Diagnosis and Differential

Electrocardiography. Of all the diagnostic tools clinically used in assessing chest pain, the ECG is the most reliable when used and interpreted correctly. Patients with acute infarctions may have ECG findings that range from acute ST-segment elevations to unchanged from old ECG to completely normal. This means that the ECG is useful only if it has a positive, or diagnostic, finding. New ST-segment elevations,

Q waves, bundle branch block, and T-wave inversions or normalizations are highly suggestive of ischemia and warrant aggressive management in the ED. The presence of a normal or unchanged ECG does not rule out the diagnosis of acute myocardial ischemia (AMI).

Serum markers. Serum markers, if positive, are highly specific for AMI and include myoglobin, creatinine phosphokinase (CK) and its MB isoenzyme, troponin T, cardiac myosin light chains, and others. The timing of their release into the bloodstream following AMI is unpredictable, so the documentation of normal serum markers in the bloodstream does not exclude the diagnosis of AMI.

Echocardiography. Emergency two-dimensional echocardiography may have value in the evaluation of chest pain when the ECG is nondiagnostic, for example, in patients who are paced, have a bundle branch block, or have a baseline abnormal ECG. The finding of regional wall motion abnormalities in the acutely symptomatic patient is highly suggestive of active ischemia. Two-dimensional echo may also aid in the diagnosis of other conditions that may mimic ischemic disease, such as pericarditis, aortic dissection, or hypertrophic cardiomyopathy.

Provocative tests. A number of tests are now being performed in some EDs that will unmask otherwise unrecognized, clinically significant ischemic disease. Patients with atypical chest pain and a normal stress thallium have a very low incidence of subsequent ischemic events. For those patients who cannot exercise, stress testing with intravenous dipyridamole, dobutamine, or adenosine with thallium imaging are equally sensitive in screening for significant coronary artery disease CAD.

Differential diagnosis. The priority must always be to exclude life-threatening conditions, and the ED physician should organize their test-ordering strategy to screen for those conditions first. For a complete list of all possible causes of nontraumatic chest pain, see Table 6-1.

Cardiovascular Causes of Chest Pain

Angina pectoris. The pain of chronic stable angina is episodic and lasts 5 to 15 min. It is precipitated by exertion and relieved with rest or sublingual nitroglycerin within 3 min. The pain is typically visceral in nature (aching, pressure, squeezing) with radiation to the neck, jaw, arm or hand. In individual patients the character of each attack varies little with recurrent episodes. Most patients can differentiate their usual angina from other causes of pain. The physician evaluating the patient with stable angina should carefully screen for changes in the pattern that would suggest a shift from stable to unstable angina or even suggest a different diagnosis.

TABLE 6-1. Etiology of Nontraumatic Chest Pain

Cardiac causes
  Coronary artery disease
  Stable angina
  Unstable angina
  Variant angina
  Acute myocardial infarction
Pericarditis
Valvular disease
  Aortic stenosis
  Subaortic stenosis
  Mitral valve prolapse
Vascular causes
  Aortic dissection
  Pulmonary embolus
  Pulmonary hypertension
Pulmonary causes
  Pleural irritation from infection, inflammation, infiltration
  Barotrauma from pneumothorax, pneumomediastinum
  Tracheobronchitis
Musculoskeletal causes
  Costochondritis
  Intercostal muscle strain
  Cervical thoracic spine problems
Gastrointestinal causes
  Esophageal reflux/spasm
  Mallory Weiss syndrome
  Biliary colic
  Dyspepsia
  Pancreatitis
Miscellaneous causes
  Herpes zoster
  Chest wall tumors

Unstable angina. Patients who complain of a change in the character of their typical angina pain must be identified early because they are at risk for myocardial infarction (MI) or sudden cardiac death. The ED physician should look for patients who note any of the following: (1) new or recent onset of angina; (2) changing character of their angina (i.e., more frequent, more severe, precipitated by less exertion, or less responsive to nitroglycerin); or (3) angina at rest.

Variant (prinzmetal) angina. This form of angina is thought to be due to spasm of the epicardial vessels in patients with either normal coronary arteries (⅓ of patients) or in patients with underlying athero-sclerotic disease (⅔ of patients). Pain typically occurs at rest and may be precipitated by the use of tobacco or cocaine. The ECG typically shows ST-segment elevations during an acute attack.

Acute myocardial infarction. Ischemic pain that lasts longer than 15 min, is not relieved by nitroglycerin, or is accompanied by diaphoresis, dyspnea, nausea, or vomiting, suggests the diagnosis of acute myocardial infarctin (AMI). The clinician must understand the limitations of the screening tools used in the ED and should have a high level of suspicion for AMI in patients with risk factors and prolonged or persistent symptoms for whom there is no other clear diagnosis (Fig. 6-1). (See Chapter 29 for a complete discussion of Myocardial Ischemia and Infarction.)

Aortic dissection. This diagnosis should be suspected in the patient who complains of sudden onset of severe, tearing pain in the retrosternal or midscapular area. High-risk patients are also those at risk for AMI, specifically the middle-aged hypertensive male. The patient may be hypertensive, or hypotensive in shock. There may be a diastolic murmur of aortic regurgitation indicating a proximal dissection, or distal pulse deficits, indicating a distal dissection. The dissection may occlude coronary ostia, resulting in myocardial infarction, or the carotids, resulting in cerebral ischemia and stroke. The CXR is abnormal in 90% of cases. An ECG may show myocardial ischemia or infarct. Angiography remains the most definitive diagnostic tool. Contrast CT and transesophageal echocardiography (TEE) also have been shown to be helpful. TEE can also demonstrate wall-motion abnormalities, pericardial effusion, and valvular insufficiency, which may be associated findings in such patients. (See Chapter 35 for a complete discussion of Aortic Dissection.)

Pericarditis. The patient with pericarditis will typically complain of pain that is constant, retrosternal, and radiating to the back, neck, or jaw. Pain is classically worsened by lying supine and is relieved by sitting forward. The presence of a pericardial friction rub supports

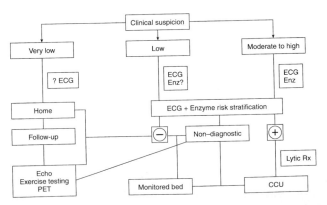

FIG. 6-1.   Disposition of patients with suspected acute myocardial ischemia.

the diagnosis. ECG may show PR depressions, diffuse ST-segment elevations or T-wave inversions that are typically diffuse. Echocardiography may reveal pericardial effusion. (See Chapter 32 for a complete discussion of pericarditis.)

Pulmonary embolus. Patients will complain of sudden onset of pleuritic chest pain associated with dyspnea, tachypnea, tachycardia, or hypoxemia. The absence of any of these findings does not preclude the diagnosis, and a high index of suspicion is essential. CXR and ECG are also essential in excluding other diagnoses. They may be normal or may have nonspecific findings in patients with PE. Arterial blood gas measurement will reveal an increased alveolar–arterial gradient in 95% of cases. Scintigraphic V/Q scanning is an extremely sensitive test for PE, and a normal study rules out the disorder. For patients with indeterminate scans, pulmonary angiography is the gold standard for PE. (See Chapter 33 for a complete discussion of Pulmonary Embolism.)

Musculoskeletal causes. Chest pain due to irritation or inflammation of structures in the chest wall is commonly seen in the ED. Possible causes include costochondritis, intercostal strain due to severe coughing, and pectoralis muscle strain in the setting of recent physical exertion. Patients will complain of sharp pain that is worsened with movement of the chest wall, coughing, and have pain that can be elicited by palpation of the chest wall. These findings in a patient without any other symptoms and no history of significant cardiac disease supports the diagnosis of musculoskeletal pain. This pain is generally responsive to nonsteroidal anti-inflammatory agents. It is important to emphasize that the presence of chest wall tenderness does not rule out the possibility of ischemia.

Gastrointestinal causes. Esophageal reflux, dyspepsia syndromes, and esophageal motility disorders can produce chest pain that is difficult to distinguish from ischemic pain. The patient may complain of burning, gnawing pain associated with an acid taste radiating into the throat. Pain may be exacerbated by meals, worse when supine and associated with belching. The clinician should determine whether the patient's symptoms are due to a gastrointestinal disorder based on the clinical presentation and the absence of findings suggesting an ischemic cause. Diagnostic decisions should not be made on the basis of a response to a therapeutic trial of antacids, GI cocktails, or nitroglycerin. When the history, physical examination, and diagnostic workup point to a gastrointestinal etiology of the pain, the patient may be treated with antacids and H_2 blockers and discharged home with followup with an internist or gastroenterologist ordered.

Emergency Department Care

It should be assumed that every patient complaining of chest pain may be having an AMI. Patients with suspicious histories should have a large-bore intravenous line established, a cardiac monitor, and an ECG obtained as soon as possible. Vital signs and pulse oximetry should be continuously monitored.

1. Ask the patient about cardiac risk factors, pre-existing CAD, quality of chest pain, time of onset and duration of symptoms, and whether the pattern has been stable, unstable, continuous, or intermittent. Ask specifically for clues to noncardiac causes of chest pain: ability to elicit pain by movement or cough; relationship to meals; pain that is of sudden onset, referred to the back, or pleuritic in nature.

2. Examine the patient, looking for evidence of heart failure or valvular insufficiency, pericardial rubs, or tenderness of the chest wall. Specifically, ask whether pain elicited on palpation of the chest wall exactly reproduces the patient's pain.

3. Obtain an ECG on all patients for whom there is a reasonable suspicion of ischemia. Remember that a normal ECG, although minimizing the likelihood of an AMI, does not definitively rule out the possibility of MI.

4. Patients for whom the etiology of chest pain remains unclear, consider obtaining arterial blood gases, CXR, and echocardiogram, as guided by clinical suspicion and findings.

5. Do not use the patient's clinical response to GI cocktails, nitroglycerin, or NSAIDs to exclude the possibility of myocardial ischemia.

6. In patients with nondiagnostic ECGs for whom there is a clinical suspicion for ischemia, consider provocative testing, echocardiography, or admission and observation. Do not rely on serum enzyme testing to rule out the possibility of clinically significant disease.

For further reading in *Emergency Medicine, A Comprehensive Study Guide*, see Chapter 24, Chest Pain, by Jay L. Falk and John F. O'Brien.

Michael E. Chansky

DYSPNEA

Dyspnea is a subjective feeling of difficult, labored, or uncomfortable breathing. Dyspnea does not result from a single pathophysiologic mechanism, yet two thirds of patients complaining of dyspnea have either a cardiac or pulmonary disorder.

Clinical Features

The patient presents with shortness of breath or breathlessness, and must be rapidly evaluated for tachypnea, tachycardia, use of accessory respiratory muscles, and stridor. Other signs and symptoms include agitation or lethargy due to hypoxia. In patients with any of the above signs or symptoms, airway control and mechanical ventilation must be anticipated. Lesser degrees of dyspnea allow for a detailed medical history, which often identifies the primary responsible process (Table 7-1).

Diagnosis and Differential

In addition to accurate interpretation of the history and examination, ancillary tests aid in determining the severity and specific cause of dyspnea. Pulse oximetry is a rapid but insensitive screen for disorders of gas exchange. Arterial blood gas analysis (ABG) is more sensitive but cannot evaluate the work of breathing. A chest x-ray may indicate the category of primary disease (infiltrate, effusion, pneumothorax) but may be normal. EKG, hemoglobin, and spirometry may help identify the specific process, though challenging cases may require cardiac stress testing, echocardiography, formal pulmonary function testing, neuromuscular tests (EMG), or pulmonary biopsy.

Emergency Department Care

There is no specific cause or treatment of dyspnea. Aggressive management of the underlying disorder is indicated after maintaining airway support and oxygenation. Provide supplemental oxygen with a goal of maintaining a PO_2 of over 60 mmHg. This can be lowered to 50 mmHg in patients with severe COPD and known hypoxia. All patients with unclear causes of dyspnea and hypoxia require admission to a monitored bed.

HYPOXIA

Hypoxia is defined as an insufficient delivery of oxygen to the tissue, and it results from any combination of five distinct mechanisms:

1. *Hypoventilation*—hypoxia and elevated pCO_2 (narcotic OD)
2. *Right-to-left shunt*—unoxygenated blood entering systemic arteries (atelectasis)
3. *Ventilation/perfusion mismatch*—regional alteration of ventilation or perfusion (PE, asthma)
4. *Diffusion impairment*—alveolar blood barrier abnormality (ARDS, sarcoid, CHF)
5. *Low inspired oxygen*—high altitude

Hypoxemia is defined as an abnormally low arterial oxygen tension, arbitrarily pO_2 <60 mmHg. Patients with hypoxemia may not be dyspneic and patients with dyspnea may not have hypoxemia.

Clinical Features

Signs and symptoms of hypoxemia are nonspecific. Tachypnea and tachycardia may be present, and CNS manifestations include agitation, headache, somnolence, seizures, and coma. At pO_2 <20 mmHg there is a central depression of respiratory drive. Dyspnea may be present, but cyanosis is not a sensitive or specific indicator of hypoxemia.

Diagnosis and Differential

The diagnosis of arterial hypoxemia requires clinical suspicion and objective measurement. Formal diagnosis requires ABG although pulse oximetry is useful for screening gross alterations in pO_2. Calculation of the arterial alveolar oxygen difference A-aO_2, where $A = FIO_2 (760-pH_2O) - 1.2 (pCO_2)$ and aO_2 = ABG value can further quantitate the degree of hypoxemia. The history and examination should help delineate the exact etiology of hypoxia (see examples above). Disorders causing dyspnea can lead to hypoxia (see Table 7-1).

TABLE 7-1. Most Common Disorders Causing Dyspnea

Airway	*Vascular*
Foreign body	Pulmonary embolism
Angioedema	Sickle cell
Cardiac	*Neuromuscular*
LV failure	CVA
Arrhythmia	Guillain–Barré
Tamponade	Myasthenia gravis
Ischemia	Neuropathy
Lung Parenchymal	Spinal cord trauma
Asthma	*Miscellaneous*
Pneumonia	Anemia
ARDS	Shock
Pleural and Chest Wall	CO poisoning
Pneumothorax	
Effusion	
Pregnancy	

Emergency Department Care

Regardless of the specific cause of hypoxemia, the initial approach remains the same: Aggressive management of the underlying disorder (if identified), while ensuring a patent airway and providing supplemental oxygenation, with a goal of maintaining an arterial O_2 >60 mmHg. All hypoxic patients require hospitalization and monitoring until control of the underlying process is achieved. An arterial line is indicated if multiple ABGs arc anticipated.

HYPERCAPNIA

Hypercapnia is arbitrarily defined as an arterial pCO_2 >45 mmHg, and is exclusively due to alveolar hypoventilation. It is almost never due to intrinsic lung disease and is never due to increased CO_2 production.

Clinical Features

The signs and symptoms of hypercapnia depend on the absolute value of pCO_2 and its rate of change. Acute elevations result in increased intracranial pressure, and patients may complain of headache, confusion, lethargy, seizures, and coma. Acute pCO_2 >100 mmHg can result in cardiovascular collapse, whereas chronic hypercapnia may be well tolerated.

Diagnosis and Differential

The diagnosis requires clinical suspicion and an ABG. Pulse oximetry can be normal. The ABG will reveal an acute respiratory acidosis with little metabolic compensation (low pH, high pCO_2, low pO_2, normal bicarbonate). The differential includes drug overdosages, hypoglycemia, severe asthma or COPD, neuromuscular disorders, severe obesity, and upper airway obstruction.

Emergency Department Care

Aggressive specific therapy, while maintaining airway/ventilatory support, is indicated. A heroin overdose will respond more rapidly than a patient with Guillain-Barré syndrome. Disposition depends primarily on the underlying etiology and severity. Many patients will require hospitalization.

For further reading in *Emergency Medicine, A Comprehensive Study Guide*, see Chapter 25, Dyspnea, Hypoxia, and Hypercapnea, by David Plummer.

| Hemorrhagic Shock

John E. Gough

Acute hemorrhage is defined as rapid blood loss and is seen with various medical and surgical conditions. Among the most common causes of significant hemorrhage are trauma, disorders of the GI and reproductive tracts, and vascular disease. Hemorrhagic shock occurs when the degree of blood loss overcomes the body's compensatory mechanisms and compromises tissue perfusion and oxygenation.

Clinical Features

Individual response to acute hemorrhage will be affected by many factors, including the patient's age, pre-existing state of health, medication use, as well as the etiology, duration, and severity of the hemorrhage. Clinical presentations often, but not always, correlate with the amount of acute blood loss. Blood loss of less than 20% of the circulating volume frequently presents with a narrow pulse pressure, cool clammy skin, and prolonged capillary refill. Tachycardia may be present, but the blood pressure is usually normal. Hemorrhages involving 20% to 40% of the circulating blood volume result in tachycardia, tachypnea, and orthostatic hypotension. If not treated, these symptoms worsen and oliguria and skin mottling develop. Acute hemorrhages exceeding 40% volume are associated with worsening of above symptoms, as well as decreased or absent peripheral pulses, profound hypotension, pallor, lethargy, or coma. Death often results from respiratory arrest due to fatigue of the respiratory muscles.

Diagnosis and Differential

Hemorrhage should be suspected in any patient presenting with the above clinical features. The possibility of occult hemorrhage should also be suspected in patients with abdominal pain, chest pain, back pain, dizziness, syncope, and GI disturbances. GI and vaginal bleeding are common causes of hemorrhage, and evidence of such bleeding should be carefully sought out in the history and physical exam. Any patient sustaining either penetrating or blunt trauma is at risk for significant hemorrhage and shock. In addition to obvious external hemorrhage, occult hemorrhage is seen with intrathoracic, intra-abdominal, pelvic, and skeletal injuries.

Diagnosis of acute hemorrhage will depend upon both the history and physical examination. Historical points, such as weakness, dizziness, syncope, change of color of stool or emesis, bruising, and, prolonged or abnormal menses are all important clues. A physical examination, with attention to the vital signs (including orthostatic changes), evidence of petechiae, and pelvic and rectal examination (including guaiac of stool), is indicated.

Laboratory tests, such as hemoglobin and hematocrit (H&H) should be obtained. Early in acute hemorrhage, the H&H may not accurately reflect the amount of hemorrhage. Re-evaluation with repeated measurements will more accurately reflect the amount of blood loss, as well as response to therapies rendered. The possibility of coagulopathies should be investigated if expected. All females of childbearing age should have a pregnancy test.

In the presence of trauma, modalities to determine the presence of hemorrhage (diagnostic peritoneal lavage, CT scanning, radiographs) should be obtained, as indicated.

Differential diagnoses include other medical and traumatic causes of shock. In the presence of trauma, acute hemorrhage should *always* be considered the cause of shock. Other potential traumatic causes include tension pneumothorax, cardiac tamponade, and severe head and spinal cord injuries. Nontraumatic causes include sepsis, cardiogenic, endocrine, and anaphylaxis.

Emergency Department Care

The ultimate goals of the ED management of hemorrhagic shock are to stabilize the patient, to control the bleeding, and to provide for adequate perfusion of oxygen. Often definitive hemorrhage control requires operative intervention, therefore, early appropriate referral is necessary. The approach to stabilization is best handled by addressing the ABCs of resuscitation:

1. Attain and maintain adequate patency of the airway. This may necessitate airway adjuncts, such as endotracheal intubation. Cervical spine precautions should be instituted.
2. All patients should receive high-flow oxygen.
3. Assess ventilations. Correct conditions that impair proper ventilations (e.g., decompression of tension pneumothorax).
4. Control hemorrhage. Most external hemorrhage can be controlled by direct compression. Rarely, clamping or tying off of vessels is needed. Use of tourniquets is discouraged.
5. Obtain venous access. At least two large-bore (14–16g) IV lines should be started. At this time, blood should be drawn for laboratory studies. Isotonic crystalloids (NS or LR) are the initial fluids of choice. Administer rapid boluses of 20 to 40 ml/kg in the unstable patient. (Ongoing research is examining the traditional role of attempting to restore blood pressure through the use of intravenous infusions.) If the patient fails to respond, blood administration is necessary. Fully crossmatched blood is desirable, however, type specific or type O blood may be used. Autologous blood may be given if the capabilities for autotransfusion exist. Fresh-frozen plasma or platelet use is best determined by clinical evidence and monitoring of coagulation parameters.

6. Continuous monitoring of patient status, including cardiac monitor, pulse oximetry, urine output, vital signs, capillary refill, and mental status.
7. Diagnostic tests, as noted above, should be obtained. Rapid referral will be dictated by the source of hemorrhage.
8. Medical anti-shock trousers (MAST) use has diminished, but they may be used to stabilize pelvic or femur fractures and to tamponade bleeding.

If Standard Treatment Fails

1. Synthetic high molecular weight colloids such as hydroxyethyl starch and dextran remain predominantly in the intravascular space and act as volume expanders.
2. A combination of 7.5% hypertonic saline and 6% dextran 70 has shown promise in animal studies.

For further reading in *Emergency Medicine, A Comprehensive Study Guide*, see Chapter 26, Hemorrhagic Shock, by Steven C. Dronen and Patricia L. Lanter.

9 | Septic Shock
John E. Gough

Sepsis and septic shock are common, potentially life-threatening complications of infectious diseases. Proliferation of the infecting organism or invasion of the bloodstream from the focus of infection results in the release of exogenous toxins. The host response to these toxins is a release of endogenous mediators (complement, kinins, etc.). This can lead to refractory hypotension, multiple organ system failure, and death. Gram-positive and gram-negative bacteria account for the majority of sepsis. Predisposing factors to bacterial sepsis include diabetes mellitus, lymphoproliferative disease, cirrhosis, burns, invasive procedures and devices, and chemotherapy. Other potential causes of sepsis include fungi, *rickettsiae*, viruses, and protozoans. Nonbacterial sepsis is more commonly seen in immunocompromised individuals.

Clinical Features

Hyperpyrexia is commonly seen with infectious diseases and may be seen with sepsis. Hypothermia is not uncommon, however, in sepsis and septic shock, particularly with very young, elderly, or immunocompromised patients. Other common abnormalities of the vital signs include tachycardia, tachypnea, and a wide pulse pressure.

Mental status changes are common and may range from mild disorientation to coma. Ophthalmologic manifestations include retinal hemorrhages, cotton wool spots, and conjunctival petechiae.

Early cardiovascular manifestations include peripheral vasodilatation, however, cardiac output is initially maintained through a compensatory tachycardia. Myocardial depression may be secondary to circulating myocardial depressant factors. As sepsis progresses, hypotension may occur. Patients in septic shock may demonstrate a diminished response to volume replacement.

Respiratory symptoms include tachypnea and hypoxemia. Sepsis is the most common condition associated with the development of acute respiratory distress syndrome (ARDS).

Renal manifestations include azotemia, oliguria, and active urinary sediment. Azotemia and oliguria often result from acute tubular necrosis (ATN). The development of ATN may be precipitated by hypotension, dehydration, aminoglycoside administration, and pigmenturia.

Liver dysfunction is common, and the most frequent presentation is cholestatic jaundice. Development of painless mucosal erosions may predispose the patient to upper GI bleeding. Cutaneous lesions may be the result of: (1) direct invasion (cellulitis, erysipelas, fasciitis); (2) a consequence of hypotension or disseminated intravascular coagulation (DIC) (acrocyanosis, necrosis); and (3) secondary to infective endocarditis (microemboli, vasculitis).

Laboratory abnormalities with sepsis include neutrophilic leukocytosis. A left shift, resulting from demargination and release of less mature granulocytes from the marrow, is common. Neutropenia occurs less frequently but is associated with higher mortality. Etiologies of neutropenia are increased peripheral utilization, damage by bacterial byproducts, and depression of production.

The hemoglobin and hematocrit may be decreased if there is associated GI bleeding. Red cell number usually is not affected but production and survival of RBCs is decreased. Isolated thrombocytopenia occurs in 30% of sepsis cases and may be an early clue to bacteremia. DIC occurs in <5% of cases of sepsis, with gram-negative infections precipitating DIC more readily.

Examination of liver enzymes often show increases in transaminase, alkaline phosphatase (up to 3 times normal), and bilirubin (usually not more than 10 mg/dL). Hyperglycemia may be the result of increased catecholamines, cortisol, and glucagon. Increased insulin resistance, decreased insulin production, and impaired utilization of insulin may further contribute to hyperglycemia. Rarely, depletion of glucagon and inhibition of gluconeogenesis leads to hypoglycemia.

Early in sepsis, blood gas determinations often reveal hypoxemia and a respiratory alkalosis. As perfusion worsens and glycolysis increases, a metabolic acidosis occurs. This acidosis is further exacerbated by lactic acid production.

Diagnosis and Differential

Septic shock should be suspected in any patient with a temperature >38° C or <36° C, systolic blood pressure <90 mmHg, and evidence of inadequate organ perfusion. Other symptoms include mental status changes, hyperventilation, warm or flushed skin, and a wide pulse pressure. Very young, elderly, and immunocompromised patients often have atypical presentations. History and physical examination, coupled with other diagnostic modalities, will often help identify the source of infection. Historical description of the above features, with particular attention to organ system dysfunction, is indicated.

Many diagnostic tests are available to help with the identification of the source of sepsis, but septic shock remains a clinical diagnosis. Laboratory tests such as a complete blood count, prothrombin time, partial thromboplastin time, electrolytes, liver function tests, renal function tests, urinalysis, and arterial blood gases (ABGs) are often utilized.

Cultures should be obtained from the blood and urine. Also cultures of the CSF, sputum, and other secretions should be obtained as indicated. The gram stain and counter immunoelectrophoresis (CIE) can help to quickly identify pathogens and guide initial therapy until definitive culture and sensitivities are available. Radiographs of suspected foci of infection (chest, abdomen, etc.) should be obtained. CT scanning may help identify areas of occult infection or abscesses in the cranium, thorax, abdomen, and pelvis.

Differential diagnosis should include other noninfectious types of shock, such as hypovolemic, cardiogenic, neurogenic, obstructive, endocrine, and anaphylaxis.

Emergency Department Care

1. Address ABCs of resuscitation. Aggressive airway management with endotracheal intubation may be needed.
2. Administer high-flow oxygen.
3. Correct hypotension. Initiate therapy with rapid infusions of crystalloid IV fluids (NS or LR). Often 4 to 6 L may be required. In addition to blood pressure, monitor mental status, pulse, capillary refill, CVP, and urine output (>30 cc/kg/h adult, >1 cc/kg/h pediatric).
4. **Dopamine** 5 to 20 μg/kg/min titrated to response.
5. If blood pressure remains <70 mmHg despite above measures, begin intravenous infusion of **norepinephrine** 8 to 12 μg/min loading dose, 2 to 4 μg/min constant infusion.
6. Ideally begin empiric antibiotic therapy after obtaining cultures, but do not unduly delay administration. Dosages should be the maximum allowed and given intravenously. When source is unknown, therapy should be directed against both gram-positive and gram-negative organisms, usually a third generation **cephalosporin** (e.g., ceftriaxone, 1 gm IV; cefotaxime, 2 gms IV; ceftazidime, 2 gms IV), or imipenum, 750 mg IV, and an aminoglycoside (gentamicin, 2 mg/kg IV, tobramycin, 2 mg/kg IV). Other choices should be directed by the suspected source of infection. (Initial or loading doses listed).
7. Remove source of infection (e.g., remove indwelling catheters or drainage of abscess).
8. Severe acidosis is treated with oxygen, ventilation, IV fluids, and sodium bicarbonate (1 mEq/kg, or as directed by ABGs).
9. Treat DIC with fresh-frozen plasma. Begin with 15 to 20 ml/kg.
10. If adrenal insufficiency is suspected, administer glucocorticoids (solucort, 100 mg IVP).

If Standard Treatment Fails

1. Monoclonal antibodies. E5 and HA–IA have shown promise in decreasing the time to organ recovery and improving survival in a subset of patients with gram-negative infections. Further trials are ongoing.
2. Anti-tumor necrosis factor (TNF) and IL-1ra (interleukin-1 receptor antagonist) use has shown decreased mortality in animal testing. No definitive conclusions for human use can be made at this time.

3. Nitric oxide synthetase inhibitors are being investigated to increase levels of nitric oxide. Nitric oxide functions as a neurotransmitter, regulator of vascular tone, and an inhibitor of platelet aggregation and leukocyte adhesion.

4. Pentoxifyline inhibits cytokine activation of neutrophils and production of TNF by endotoxin exposed monocytes.

5. Ibuprofen, a cyclo-oxygenase inhibitor, may attenuate flulike symptoms and decrease fever, tachycardia, and the metabolic rate in the septic patient.

For further reading in *Emergency Medicine, A Comprehensive Study Guide*, see Chapter 27, Septic Shock, by Jon Jui.

10

Anaphylaxis and Acute Allergic Reactions

Christian A. Tomaszewski

Allergic reactions can range from trivial appearing urticaria to full-blown shock (anaphylaxis), with cardiovascular collapse and respiratory compromise. The most common etiologies include hymenopteran stings and intravenous penicillin. Although most acute allergic reactions are Type I, when an antigen interacts with IgE on mast cells and basophils, other hypersensitivity reactions include: Type II—antigen interacts with IgG and IgM antibodies (e.g., blood transfusion reaction, ITP); Type III—deposition of antigen–antibody complexes (e.g., serum sickness, poststreptococcal glomerulonephritis); and Type IV—delayed hypersensitivity reaction from T lymphocytes (e.g., poison ivy, TB skin test).

Clinical Features

Anaphylaxis can occur within seconds, but can be delayed an hour, after a sensitized individual is exposed to such things as: (1) drugs (e.g., penicillin and trimethoprim–sulfamethoxazole); (2) foods (e.g., shellfish, nuts, eggs, and preservatives such as sulfites and tetrazine dyes); and (3) stings (especially hymenoptera). In addition, such things as aspirin, NSAIDs, codeine, and radiocontrast material can cause an anaphylactoid reaction, which has no immunologic basis but has the same final mediators as anaphylaxis.

Anaphylactic reactions range from local organ involvement to serious multisystem effects. Dermatologic features include pruritis, urticaria, erythema multiforme, and angioedema. The latter can be seen as an isolated response to ACE inhibitors. Respiratory features may include tracheal swelling, stridor, wheezing, and respiratory arrest. Gastrointestinal features include nausea, cramps, vomiting, and diarrhea. Untreated, anaphylaxis leads to shock with tachycardia and hypotension. Cardiac patients are susceptible to myocardial ischemia, as well as an exaggerated allergic response if on beta blockers.

Diagnosis and Differential

Diagnosis will be based on symptoms seen in any particular patient. Usually history will confirm exposure to a potential allergen, either a new drug, food, or insect sting. There is no specific test available in the ED to confirm the diagnosis. Working may, however, include CBC, glucose, electrolytes, urinalysis, and ABG, depending on presenting symptoms. The differential includes myocardial infarction, pulmonary embolism, asthma, hypovolemia, hereditary angioedema, and vasovagal reactions.

Emergency Department Care

The airway is the primary concern in the treatment of any allergic reaction. Patients with respiratory symptoms or abnormal vital signs should be placed on a cardiac monitor with intravenous access. The combination of oxygen and epinephrine can usually reverse any impending respiratory compromise.

1. Administer high flow oxygen, by face mask if necessary, to maintain adequate oxygenation. Endotracheal intubation, if required, can be difficult because of angioedema or laryngeal spasm, therefore, preparation should be made for transtracheal jet insufflation or cricothyroidotomy.

2. Any patient with unstable vital signs or airway symptoms should receive **epinephrine,** subcutaneously 0.3 to 0.5 mg (0.3–0.5 ml) in a solution of 1:1000. With shock, the same dose can be given intravenously, but diluted to 1:10,000.

3. There must be termination of further exposure. This may be as simple as stopping an intravenous line of drug or removing a stinger. If definitive medical care is delayed, a tourniquet may prevent allergen dissemination.

4. Most patients, especially if hypotensive, will require larger volumes of crystalloid fluids. If after 1 to 2 L, the patient is still hypotensive, intravenous **epinephrine** (0.1–1 mcg/kg/min) or **dopamine** (2–10 mcg/kg/min) can be used. If hypotension persists in spite of fluids and pressors, CVP or Swan–Ganz monitoring may be useful.

5. Every patient with allergic symptoms requires antihistamines. **Diphenhydramine** can be given, 50 mg IV in serious cases, or 25 mg orally or intramuscularly in mild cases. In addition, an H_2 blocker, such as **cimetidine,** 300 mg IV, can be helpful.

6. After treatment with epinephrine, any persistent bronchospasm can be treated with nebulized **beta agonists,** such as **albuterol** 0.5 ml in 3 ml saline.

7. **Steroids** may be useful in controlling persistent or delayed allergic reactions. They are also the mainstay of treatment in Type IV delayed hypersensitivity reactions. Severe cases can be treated with **methylprednisolone,** 125 mg IV. Most other reactions can be treated with oral **prednisone,** 60 mg to start.

In mild reactions, patients may be observed several hours prior to discharge. Severe cases, with any evidence of hypotension or respiratory compromise, deserve prolonged observation with repeated doses of antihistamines and steroids. Remember, all serious cases require **preventive therapy** upon discharge. This includes a self-administration epinephrine kit, as well as referral to an allergist for desensitization therapy.

If Standard Treatment Fails

If hypotension persists despite aggressive management with IV fluids and catecholamines, reconsider the diagnosis. If the patient is on beta blockers, glucagon (5 mg IV) may be useful. In recalcitrant cases of laryngeal or bronchial spasm, neuromuscular blockade or general anesthesia may be required for adequate ventilation.

For further reading in *Emergency Medicine, A Comprehensive Study Guide,* see Chapter 28, Anaphylaxis and Acute Allergic Reactions, by Joseph A. Salomone, III.

11 | Cyanosis

Gary D. Wright

Cyanosis is the physical finding of bluish discoloration of the skin and mucous membranes, resulting from elevated amounts of deoxygenated hemoglobin. Detection of cyanosis is subjective and cannot be considered a sensitive indicator of arterial oxygenation. A variety of factors other than the absolute amount of deoxygenated hemoglobin may influence this subjective detection. Unexplained cyanosis in the setting of normal arterial oxygenation should prompt further evaluation for abnormal hemoglobin, especially methemoglobin. The recreational use of nitrites has been well described, especially in the homosexual, juvenile, and deviant populations. These patients presenting with cyanosis should be highly suspicious for methemoglobinemia.

Clinical Features

Cyanosis can be divided into two categories, central and peripheral. The central type is seen when arterial blood is deoxygenated or abnormal hemoglobin exists. This central cyanosis is physically manifested by skin and mucous membrane involvement. Peripheral cyanosis is due to an abnormally high amount of oxygen extraction in the periphery due to slow peripheral blood flow. All physiologic states of decreased peripheral blood flow may lead to cyanosis (Table 11-1).

Diagnosis

When cyanosis is suspected, evaluation with pulse oximetry and arterial blood gas (ABG) sampling is indicated. Pulse oximetry may overestimate total oxygen saturation in the presence of met- or carboxyhemoglobin. In such circumstances, ABG analysis with cooximetry is indicated. In central cyanosis, the oxygen saturation of ABG is decreased due to underlying hypoxia. In peripheral cyanosis, the oxygen saturation should be normal. If met- or carboxyhemoglobin is present, the ABG can show a normal PaO_2, a normal calculated oxygen saturation, and a decrease in the measured oxygen saturation. In the presence of a measured or calculated oxygen saturation discrepancy, direct measurement of met- or carboxyhemoglobin is indicated.

Differential Diagnosis

Hypoxia, anemia, and polycythemia may masquerade as cyanosis, and can be diagnosed by hemoglobin, hematocrit, and ABG. Polycythemia leads to cyanosis by peripheral sludging. If ABG, hemoglobin, and hematocrit are normal, the cause of cyanosis may be abnormal skin pigment or abnormal hemoglobin. Cyanosis can also be mimicked by exposure to heavy metals. Carboxyhemoglobin does not cause cyanosis

TABLE 11-1. Causes of Cyanosis

Central Cyanosis
  Decreased arterial oxygen saturation
    Decreased atmospheric pressure—high altitude
    Impaired pulmonary function
      Alveolar hypoventilation
      Uneven relationships between pulmonary ventilation and
      perfusion
      Impaired oxygen diffusion
    Anatomic shunts
      Certain types of congenital heart disease
      Pulmonary arteriovenous fistulas
      Multiple small intrapulmonary shunts
    Hemoglobin with low affinity for oxygen
    Hemoglobin abnormalities
      Methemoglobinemia—hereditary, acquired
      Sulfhemoglobinemia—acquired
      Carboxyhemoglobinemia (not true cyanosis)
Peripheral Cyanosis
  Reduced cardiac output
  Cold exposure
  Redistribution of blood flow from extremities
  Arterial obstruction
  Venous obstruction

Braunwald E: Hypoxia, polycythemia, and cyanosis, in Wilson J, Braunwald E, Isselbacher JK, et al (eds.): *Harrison's Principles of Internal Medicine*, 12th, ed. New York, McGraw-Hill, 1991, pp. 224–228. Used by permission.

but occasionally does produce a cherry-red flushing of the skin, retina, and mucous membranes. Cyanosis may be caused by met- or sulfhemoglobin. Most are due to acquired states secondary to chemicals or medications. Benzocaine, nitrates and nitrites, acetanilid and aniline may cause met- or sulfhemoglobin. Patients on nitroglycerin and nitroprusside infusions for greater than 24 h should be monitored periodically for methemoglobin.

Emergency Department Care

The goal of treatment is restoration of normal oxygenation levels.

1. Hypoxia—The use of supplemental oxygen therapy should be used initially as a diagnostic and therapeutic tool. Titration of supplemental oxygen therapy is recommended in patients with chronic lung disease. If cyanosis in patients without cardiovascular or pulmonary disease is not corrected with supplemental oxygen, methemoglobin should be highly suspected. In cardiovascular or pulmonary disease patients who do not respond to oxygen therapy and methemoglobin is not present, rapid identification and treatment of the underlying disease is necessary.

2. Methemoglobinemia should only be treated in the symptomatic patient (angina, shortness of breath, dysrhythmia, hypotension, stupor, or coma). The antidote for methemoglobinemia is a 1% solution of **methylene blue** in a dose of 1 to 2 mg/kg IV over 5 min. Complications of methylene blue include hemolysis and precipitation of methemoglobinemia.

3. Sulfhemoglobin is irreversible and treatment is directed towards symptomatic and supportive therapy, in addition to identification and removal of the source agent.

If Standard Treatment Fails

Maintenance of the airway with supportive measures and admission for further diagnostic evaluation of the underlying physiologic abnormality is required in patients who do not respond to the above measures.

For further reading in *Emergency Medicine, A Comprehensive Study Guide*, see Chapter 29, Cyanosis, by Ann Harwood–Nuss and Tom Kunisaki.

12 | Syncope

Christian A. Tomaszewski

Syncope accounts for up to 3% of all ED visits. By definition, syncope is a transient loss of consciousness, accompanied by loss of postural tone. The most common cause of syncope is vasovagal, usually a benign paradoxic withdrawal of sympathetic tone during upright posture. Even with extensive history and diagnostic workup, however, up to one half of patients will never have a definite etiology established for their syncopal episode.

Clinical Features

Clinical features, which are extremely useful in workup and diagnosis, of the syncopal episode can be divided into three phases:

1. *Presyncopal phase*—A presyncopal episode marked by an aura or abrupt onset suggests a seizure. However, cardiac causes can occur abruptly as well. Associated events are helpful. A sudden change in posture after prolonged recumbency, especially in the presence of volume depletion or diseases of the capacitance vessels (e.g., diabetes, Shy–Drager syndrome) may suggest orthostatic syncope. The hallmark of vasovagal syncope is premonitory symptoms such as lightheadedness, feeling of warmth or nausea, and dimming of vision immediately prior to syncope. In addition, look for appropriate stimuli (i.e., blood drawing, injury, fear) in combination with standing before diagnosing vasovagal syncope. An elderly patient may say that they were wearing a tight collar, shaving, or turning their head immediately prior to fainting, thus suggesting carotid sinus hypersensitivity. If the patient relates that upper extremity exercise preceded the event, he may be suffering from obstruction of the brachiocephalic or subclavian artery (i.e., subclavian steal syndrome).
2. *Syncopal phase*—The common hallmarks of seizure, i.e. tongue biting and incontinence, can also be seen with convulsive syncope, which are brief clonic jerks due to cerebral anoxia.
3. *Post-syncopal phase*—A postictal phase with disorientation and slow return to normal is suggestive of seizure. In vasovagal syncope, recovery is usually within seconds. If primary cerebral ischemia (i.e., TIA) is the cause of syncope, the patient usually reports other neurologic deficits from brainstem ischemia associated with the drop attack.

Additional clues as to the etiology of a syncopal episode can be obtained from history and physical exam. Patients on cardiac medications, namely nitrates, diuretics, and antiarrhythmics, are susceptible to dysrhythmias and postural hypotension. Syncope from hypoglycemia is usually seen only in the presence of insulin or oral hypoglycemia use. The cardiac exam may reveal a ventricular flow obstruction problem as the source of syncope: a murmur from aortic or mitral stenosis, or an accentuated pulmonary gallop from pulmonary embolism or hypertension. Elderly patients are more susceptible to cardiac causes of syncope, partially due to atherosclerosis, but also because of numerous cardiovascular medications.

Diagnosis and Differential

Although an etiology for the syncopal episode may be difficult to establish, the most important tools in workup of syncope is a good history, physical examination, and EKG. The history should be directed to high-risk factors, including age, medications, and presyncopal events. Selected laboratory testing is the norm. The EKG may show signs of ischemia or dysrhythmias, although a short period of cardiac monitoring may be more useful for the latter. A glucose check may be useful if one suspects use of hypoglycemic agents. An elevated CPK or depressed bicarbonate may suggest a seizure episode. A hematocrit or rectal exam for occult GI bleeding may explain syncope associated with orthostatic hypotension. Because syncope is rarely associated with normal pregnancy, the differential should include ectopic pregnancy in any childbearing woman, especially with pelvic pain.

A variety of bedside tests may provide clues in selected cases, such as reproducing presyncopal symptoms with hyperventilation. A BP check in both arms, with more than a 20 mmHg difference, suggests subclavian steal syndrome. Carotid sinus massage in selected patients without bruits can be performed in the ED, with patient monitoring and atropine available, if one suspects carotid sinus hypersensitivity. Orthostatic hypotension can be used to rule out a 20% volume deficit or poor vascular tone (autonomic instability from drugs or disease) by a pulse increase of >30 beats/min, or systolic blood pressure drop of 25 mmHg after 2 min of standing from a supine posture.

The etiology of syncope includes one of three processes: lack of oxygen to the brain, lack of glucose to the brain, or seizure activity. If the latter two are ruled out, the differential is narrowed to the various causes of temporary oxygen deprivation to the brain (Table 12-1). Most worrisome among these are central cardiac problems, such as flow obstruction, dysrhythmias, or myocardial ischemia. Fortunately, peripheral vascular problems are more common, including vasovagal, orthostatic, or drug induced. Drugs may be responsible for a variety of syncopal etiologies: dysrhythmias may arise from tricyclic antidepressants, antiarrhythmics, beta or calcium channel blockers; orthostatic hypotension can result from volume depletion due to diuretics or vasodilation due to calcium channel blockers, nitrates, or antihypertensives.

TABLE 12-1. Cardiovascular Causes of Syncope

Cardiac

Dysrhythmias
  Bradycardia
  Tachycardia
Flow obstruction
  Left ventricle—valve stenosis or cardiomyopathy
  Right ventricle—valve stenosis or pulmonary embolism
Ischemia

Peripheral Vascular

Vasovagal
Orthostatic
Drug-induced
Situational—micturition or Valsalva
Carotid sinus sensitivity
Cerebrovascular—TIA or subclavian steal syndrome

Emergency Department Care

By definition, syncope results in spontaneous recovery of consciousness. The most difficult management problem in these patients, therefore, is disposition, especially without a definitive diagnosis. Patients can be divided into three classes for disposition:

1. *High-risk patients*, age >60 or with a history of cardiac disease, should be admitted for monitoring. With admission, the workup of these patients can be expedited to determine a possible structural or electrical cause of cardiac syncope.
2. *Young patients* with no obvious illness can be discharged after a single episode of syncope, with instructions to return if presyncopal symptoms recur.
3. *All other patients* require a weighing of relative age and medical condition, as well as number of syncopal episodes. Worrisome cases may benefit from outpatient Holter monitoring with early followup.

For further reading in *Emergency Medicine, A Comprehensive Study Guide*, see Chapter 30, Syncope, by Andrew G. Wilson.

13 | Abdominal Pain

Peggy E. Goodman

Abdominal pain is a challenging and common presenting complaint in the ED. Gastrointestinal, genitourinary, cardiovascular, pulmonary, and other sources need to be considered.

Intraabdominal sources of pain include: peritonitis due to disease or injury of the abdominal or pelvic viscera; obstruction of the intestine, ureter, or biliary tree producing visceral pain, often accompanied by nausea and vomiting; and vascular disorders, such as bowel infarction and aortic dissection, leakage, or rupture.

Other sources of pain perceived as abdominal can be extra-abdominal, metabolic, or neurogenic. Extra-abdominal sources of pain include abdominal wall, thoracic, and pelvic pain. Abdominal wall pain is usually traumatic in origin. Intrathoracic disease, including pneumonia, pulmonary embolism, pneumothorax, esophageal disease, and acute myocardial ischemia may be accompanied by vague abdominal distress, nausea, vomiting, and diaphoresis. Pelvic sources of pain, such as salpingitis, tubo-ovarian abscess, ovarian cyst torsion or rupture, abortion, and ectopic pregnancy also need to be considered in the differential diagnosis. Metabolic disorders, including diabetic ketoacidosis, sickle-cell crisis, porphyria, spider and scorpion bites, heavy metal intoxication, and autoimmune disease, as well as neurogenic disorders, such as pre-eruptive herpes zoster and spinal disk disease, may be interpreted as abdominal pain.

Diagnosis and Differential

When evaluating a patient with abdominal pain, it is important to consider immediate life threats that might require emergency intervention. Important aspects of the patient history include the time of onset, character and severity, location of pain and its referral, both initially and subsequently. Anorexia, nausea, vomiting, and changes in bowel habits are symptoms common to numerous abdominal disorders and are therefore of limited usefulness in diagnosis. Cardiorespiratory symptoms such as chest pain, dyspnea, and cough, genitourinary symptoms such as urgency, dysuria, and vaginal discharge, and history of trauma should be elicited. Past medical and surgical history should be elicited, and a list of medications, particularly steroids, antibiotics, or NSAIDs, should be noted. A thorough gynecologic history is indicated in female patients.

The physical examination should include the patient's general appearance. Patients with visceral pain tend to move about, whereas patients with peritonitis tend to lie still. The skin should be evaluated for pallor or jaundice. The vital signs should be inspected for signs of hypovolemia due to blood loss or dehydration, such as tachycardia or hypotension.

The abdomen should be inspected for contour, scars, peristalsis, masses, distension, or pulsation. Palpation is the most important aspect of the physical examination. The abdomen and genitals should be assessed for tenderness, guarding, masses, organomegaly, and hernias. A pelvic examination is recommended in all postpubertal females. During the rectal examination, the lower pelvis should be assessed for tenderness and masses.

Elderly patients often fail to manifest the same signs and symptoms as younger patients. Conditions more common in the elderly include: sigmoid volvulus, diverticulitis, acute mesenteric ischemia, and abdominal aortic aneurysm. Mortality is higher in the elderly because of difficulty in diagnosis, delays in seeking treatment, and pre-existing cardiovascular, respiratory, or other chronic disease.

Laboratory evaluation is supplementary to a careful history and physical examination. CBC values can be normal in the presence of disease, although serial hematocrit may be of value in patients with acute blood loss. Urinalysis may reveal hematuria in cases of renal colic or pyuria in urinary tract infection or other intra-abdominal inflammation near the urinary tract. Pregnancy test should be obtained in women of childbearing age and is useful in the assessment of ectopic pregnancy. Serum amylase elevation and electrolyte abnormalities are neither specific nor sensitive diagnostic tools. ECG should be considered in patients over 40, especially with upper abdominal or nonspecific symptomatology.

Imaging studies that may aid in diagnosis include: radiographic views of the abdomen and chest, which are most useful if one is specifically assessing for biliary or renal calculi, air in the biliary tree, abnormal vascular calcifications, abnormal gas patterns, air fluid levels, free intraperitoneal air, or intrathoracic pathology; and ultrasonography, which is a valuable diagnostic technique for the diagnosis of cholelithiasis, choledocholithiasis, cholecystitis, biliary duct dilatation, pancreatic masses, hydroureter, intrauterine and ectopic pregnancies, ovarian and tubal pathology, free intraperitoneal fluid, suspected appendicitis, and abdominal aortic aneurysm. Barium contrast and radioisotope studies are useful for several specific disorders, but may not be immediately available in the emergency situation. Adjuncts to diagnosis include laparoscopy and computer-aided decisionmaking.

Emergency Department Care

Resuscitative and stabilizing measures should be instituted, as appropriate. Unstable patients should be diagnosed clinically with immediate intervention and surgical consultation.

1. During the initial evaluation, the patient should have nothing by mouth until certain it will not worsen patient condition nor conflict

with diagnostic studies or surgical intervention. Consider intravenous hydration with normal saline or lactated Ringer's solution.

2. Upon completion of a thorough history and physical examination, the judicious use of analgesics is appropriate, although still controversial. IV narcotics can be reversed, if necessary, by naloxone. Recent studies support the use of NSAIDs in the treatment of renal colic.

3. Surgical or Ob/Gyn consultation should be obtained for patients with suspected acute abdominal or pelvic pathology requiring immediate intervention, including, but not limited to, abdominal aortic aneurysm, intra-abdominal hemorrhage, perforated viscus, intestinal obstruction or infarction, and ectopic pregnancy.

If Standard Treatment Fails

Despite a thorough history and physical examination with laboratory and imaging studies, approximately 40% of patients presenting to the ED with acute abdominal pain will receive no definite diagnosis. Misdiagnosis occurs in approximately 30% of patients; the emergency physician should avoid giving specific labels or diagnoses to patients with abdominal pain of uncertain etiology. Disposition options include discharge with followup in 24 h, admission for observation, or short-term observation with repeat assessment. Patients discharged from the ED should be told to have a low threshold for return if symptoms should worsen or not improve.

For further reading in *Emergency Medicine, A Comprehensive Study Guide,* see Chapter 31, Abdominal Pain, by William D. Fales and David T. Overton.

14 | Gastrointestinal Bleeding

Peggy E. Goodman

Gastrointestinal (GI) bleeding is potentially life-threatening. The most common causes of upper GI bleeding are peptic ulcer disease, erosive gastritis, esophagitis, and duodenitis. Less common but important causes of hemorrhage are esophageal and gastric varices, Mallory–Weiss syndrome, and aortoenteric fistula. The most common cause of apparent lower GI bleeding remains upper GI bleeding, but true lower GI bleeding is usually caused by diverticulosis or angiodysplasia.

Diagnosis and Differential

The bleeding source often can be identified by careful history. Coffee-ground or bloody emesis suggest a source proximal to the ligament of Treitz, whereas melena and hematochezia suggest a distal lesion. Weight loss or changes in bowel habits are classic symptoms of malignancy, and vomiting followed by hematemesis is suggestive of a Mallory–Weiss tear. Drug history, particularly ingestion of salicylates and glucocorticoids, nonsteroidal anti-inflammatory agents (NSAIDs), anticoagulants, and alcohol should be elicited.

The vital signs should be evaluated for hypotension, tachycardia, decreased pulse pressure, tachypnea, or orthostatic vital sign changes, although these may occur only after significant volume loss. The skin should be examined for signs of shock and decreased perfusion, as well as for signs of liver disease or coagulopathy. An ENT examination should be performed to look for occult nasopharyngeal bleeding, which could cause swallowed blood to mimic coffee-ground emesis or melena. The abdomen should be examined for tenderness, masses, ascites, and organomegaly. Rectal examination for masses and the presence of blood should be performed.

The most urgent tests are the type and crossmatching of blood products and the hemoglobin and hematocrit. Additional studies should include BUN, creatinine, coagulation studies, liver function studies, electrolytes, and serum glucose levels. The initial hematocrit level often will not reflect the actual amount of blood loss and therefore serial hematocrits should be evaluated. EKG should be considered in patients over 40, as silent ischemia can occur secondary to decreased oxygen delivery.

Routine abdominal radiographs and barium contrast studies are generally of limited value, and barium limits the use of endoscopy or angiography. Endoscopy can provide the most accurate diagnosis, as well as hemostatic intervention. If available, GI angiography and technetium-labeled red cell scans can localize the site of bleeding, and angiographic embolization or intravascular injection of vasopressors can be used to control hemorrhage.

Emergency Department Care

Primary. History, physical examination, and diagnosis often must occur simultaneously with resuscitation and stabilization of the patient.

1. High-flow oxygen should be administered to all patients. If there is a risk of aspiration, endotracheal intubation should be performed. Cardiac and urinary output monitoring to assess systemic perfusion should be initiated.
2. Volume replacement through large-bore intravenous lines should be instituted using normal saline or lactated Ringer's solution.
3. Indications for administration of blood products include continued active bleeding and failure to improve perfusion and vital signs after the infusion of crystalloid.
4. A nasogastric tube should be placed in all patients with significant GI bleeding. Gentle gastric lavage, using room temperature water or saline, should be performed if bright red blood or clots are aspirated. Over-vigorous suction can cause erosions and should be avoided. Iced solutions and levarterenol are of no proven benefit.

Secondary. Upper GI endoscopy is the most accurate technique for identification of bleeding sites. Endoscopic hemostasis by sclerotherapy, band ligation or electrocoagulation is the treatment of choice for acute GI hemorrhage. Proctoscopy, sigmoidoscopy, and colonoscopy are often diagnostic in patients with lower gastrointestinal hemorrhage, and may be used to provide hemostasis.

Emergency surgical consultation and intervention is indicated for patients who do not respond to medical therapy and in whom endoscopic hemostasis fails. Surgical consultation is advised for any patient admitted with GI hemorrhage.

If Standard Treatment Fails

Intravenous and intra-arterial infusions of vasopressin have been used as temporizing measures to control GI bleeding. Adverse reactions such as hypotension, cardiac arrhythmias, myocardial and splanchnic ischemia occur, although the addition of nitroglycerin may reduce their incidence.

Balloon tamponade, using the Sengstaken–Blakemore tube, can be used as a temporizing measure for variceal hemorrhages. The gastric balloon should be inflated first and, if bleeding continues, the esophageal balloon should be inflated. Radiologic confirmation of balloon placement should be performed, and the balloon should be kept in place for 24 h after bleeding has ceased. Complications of its use include mucosal ulceration, esophageal or gastric rupture, asphyxiation, tracheal compression, and aspiration pneumonia (see Chap. 43, Esophageal Emergencies). Histamine$_2$ antagonists remain of unproven benefit.

For further reading in *Emergency Medicine, A Comprehensive Study Guide,* see Chapter 32, Gastrointestinal Bleeding, by David T. Overton.

15 Coma and Altered States of Consciousness

John E. Gough

Coma is the most dramatic alteration of consciousness and represents the endpoint on a continuum of mental status changes. Mental status changes are the most sensitive indicators of advancing central nervous system (CNS) disease, and functional changes are greater than, and always precede, structural changes seen in the brain and spinal cord. A change in the level of consciousness is often the first sign of severe pathologic processes in the nervous system, however, changes may also be the result of a variety of medical and surgical conditions. To aid in the evaluation of a patient with mental status changes, the ED physician should develop differential diagnoses in two major groups: 1) metabolic and toxic—requiring primarily medical management; and 2) structural and focal—often necessitating surgical management. For the purposes of communication and documentation it is best if nonspecific terms such as *stuporous, lethargic* and *semi-comatose* are abandoned and less subjective terminology (e.g., the AVPU system) are utilized.

Clinical Features

Depending on the initial presentation, it may be necessary to perform certain lifesaving interventions to stabilize the patient before beginning the history and physical examination. The history, as always, is an important tool in the evaluation of the patient with an alteration in mental status. The evolution of the changes should be sought, as well as the presence of chronic diseases, medication (prescribed or illicit) use, toxin exposure, and history of recent or remote trauma. Unfortunately, the patient will often be unable to provide much of the history Additional history should be obtained from any available source, such as family, friends, and EMS personnel. Further information can be obtained from medic alert tags, medication bottles, and review of available medical records. Table 15-1 lists potential causes for coma and may be a useful mnemonic aid in the evaluation of the patient presenting with profound mental status changes and coma.

With the above causes in mind, a complete physical examination should be performed. Severe hypothermia and CNS-depressant drug use may significantly alter the patient's responses. Frequent re-evaluation is recommended. The possibility of trauma should always be suspected. The patient should be carefully evaluated for any signs of trauma, particularly head injuries (CSF oto- or rhinorrhea, hemotympanum, mastoid hematomas, raccoon eyes). The vital signs should be obtained and frequently re-evaluated. Hypo- or hyperthermia may be either the cause of the altered mental status or associated with the underlying

TABLE 15-1. Mnemonic Aid for Coma Causes

TIPS	Vowels
T— Trauma (all types), temperature	A—Alcohol (other ingested drugs or toxins)
I— Infection (neurologic and systemic)	E— Endocrine (all types), exocrine (liver, electrolytes)
P—Psychiatric, porphyria	I— Insulin (DM)
S— Space occupying lesions, SAH, stroke, shock, seizures	O—Oxygen, opiates
	U—Uremia, renal causes, including hypertension

etiologies (e.g., sepsis, structural lesions). Alterations of the pulse may represent a primary cardiac etiology (dysrhythmia) or be precipitated by other causes (increased intracranial pressure [ICP]). Alterations in normal respiratory function must be carefully monitored, as they may help identify the etiology of coma (increased ICP, hypoxia, drug use). In a patient with shock, hypo- and hypertension should be considered to have a non-neurologic cause until proven otherwise.

A careful examination of the skin may reveal needle tracks suggesting drug use. Other cutaneous abnormalities may help identify the cause of the alteration of mental status, such as cyanosis (hypoxia, polycythemia), pallor (blood loss), cherry-red mucous membranes (CO exposure), cellulitis, abscesses, and uremic frost.

Examination of odors on the breath may also help indicate possible etiologies. The presence of the odor of alcohol is common, however, one should never assume that simply because a patient has been drinking, the coma is secondary to alcohol use alone. Specific odors such as acetone (DKA), halitosis (infections), and almonds (cyanide) should be noted.

Dysrhythmias may either be the etiology of coma or secondary to other causes of coma. Continuous cardiac monitoring is essential, and dysrhythmias should be treated as indicated. The patient should be evaluated for evidence of endocarditis. The presence of bruits, pulsatile masses, organomegaly, and ascites also should be noted. The rate and pattern of respirations should be evaluated and documented. Cheyne-Stokes respirations, characterized by periodic, regularly increasing then decreasing depths of respirations followed by short periods of apnea, indicate diencephalic control of respiration. Hyperventilation may represent hypoxemia, a compensatory effort to correct metabolic acidosis, or a brain injury (e.g., upper brainstem damage). Apneustic breathing presents with long pauses at the end of inspiration and is seen with fifth cranial nerve lesions. Cluster breathing, breathing in short bursts, is associated with lesions in the pons. Ataxic breathing is irregular with no specific pattern, and often precedes agonal respirations and death.

Mental status changes may range from mild disorientation to coma. An objective description of the patient's highest level of function is helpful. The physician should evaluate and record the ability of the patient to follow commands, to respond to voice, and to respond to noxious stimuli. Further, the inability to respond to any of the above should be documented. Detailed testing of all the cranial nerves may be unrealistic depending on the patient's level of consciousness, however, attempts to evaluate cranial nerve function should be performed and documented.

Pupil size, shape, and reactivity should be evaluated. It is important to remember that other factors (e.g., drug use, trauma, previous surgery) can affect the results obtained. At this time, a fundoscopic examination looking for papilledema, hemorrhages, and venous pulsations should be performed.

Ocular movements may be difficult to test, but spontaneous movements should be noted in the comatose patient. Without cortical control, most comatose patients will have roving eye movements. If both eyes cross the midline there is no evidence of brainstem damage. Abnormal deviation of the eyes may be a diagnostic clue. Generally the eyes will deviate toward the side of physiologically inactive lesions and away from active irritable foci. Doll's eye movement, the involuntary movement of the eyes upward and downward upon passive flexion of the neck, is an indication that the cause of the coma is in the cortex and not the brainstem. This maneuver should not be performed if there is suspicion of a cervical spine injury. Oculovestibular testing is utilized to determine the integrity of the brainstem. To perform this test 50cc of ice water is instilled against the tympanic membrane. If prominent nystagmus of both eyes occurs, the brainstem is normal. If no response occurs, however, the brainstem is considered to be functionless.

Other important cranial nerve functions to test are corneal and gag reflexes. Other nerve function testing will be dictated by the ability of the patient to cooperate in the testing.

The initial portion of motor exam testing is through observation, and the presence or absence of spontaneous movements should be noted. If the patient can move a body part to command, a high-level motor system function exists. If no spontaneous movements occur, the patient's response to stimuli should be tested. Abduction of the limbs or movement toward noxious stimuli show motor system involvement at the level of diencephalon or higher. Decorticate posturing, hyperextension of the legs, flexion of the elbows, and hands directed toward the center of the body, is seen with lesions of the internal capsule and upper midbrain. Decerebrate rigidity, arms extended and teeth clenched, is caused by severe disease of the midbrain. Total paralysis is a grave finding that can be seen with deep comas, but is more commonly associated with structural lesions that affect the brainstem nuclei. While motor function is being evaluated, the sensory exam can be performed.

Hemisensory lesions and specific sensory level abnormalities should be documented. Reflexes should be tested and abnormalities, as well as differences between the sides and the upper and lower half of the body, should be noted.

Diagnosis

The need for x-ray and laboratory studies will be guided by the history and physical examination. Common laboratory examinations include CBC, BUN, electrolytes, glucose, calcium, arterial blood gases, and toxicologic screening. Other diagnostic tests include radiographs (C-spine, skull, CXR), CT scanning, and lumbar puncture. Further testing, including MRI, EEG, echocardiography, and carotid Doppler ultrasonography, may be indicated but are more commonly performed as part of an inpatient workup.

Emergency Department Care

1. Aggressive airway control, maintaining cervical spine precautions. Endotracheal intubation may be necessary to protect against aspiration and provide means of hyperventilation. To guard against iatrogenically increasing ICP, rapid sequence induction with administration of lidocaine 1 mg/kg may be indicated.
2. Oxygenation and hyperventilation. Administer high flow O_2. The pCO_2 should be lowered to approximately 25 mmHg if increased ICP is suspected.
3. Control hemorrhage.
4. Intravenous access should be obtained, and blood should be drawn for appropriate laboratory studies.
5. Obtain and record vital signs. Continuously monitor patient status, including cardiac monitor, pulse oximetry, blood pressure, temperature, and mental status.
6. Empirically administer **thiamine,** 100 mg IV, **naloxone,** 2 to 4 mg IV (larger doses of naloxone may be necessary with synthetic narcotic use). As the patient may become combative after naloxone administration, restraints should be readily available.
7. Perform fingerstick glucose analysis and, if hypoglycemic, administer 50g of a 50% **dextrose** solution IV (in adults).
8. If benzodiazepine overdose is suspected, give **flumazenil** 0.2 mg IV over 15 sec. This dose may be repeated every 60 sec, to a total dose of 1.0 mg.
9. Appropriate laboratory and diagnostic tests, as noted above, should be obtained as indicated by the patient assessment. CT scans and lumbar puncture are critical tests in the management of these patients.
10. Essential emergency treatments, as indicated by diagnostic tests, include antibiotics for suspected meningitis, **mannitol,** 1 gm/kg

IV, for recent transtentorial, central, or cerebellar herniation, and immediate surgery for operable lesions (e.g., subdural, epidural, or other hematomas with shift of the midline structures).
11. Referral to appropriate subspecialty (medical, neurologic, neurosurgical), as indicated by patient condition and results of above diagnostic modalities.

If Standard Treatment Fails

Free radical scavengers, such as polyethylene glycol superoxide dismutase, are under investigation. It is postulated that free radical scavengers may decrease sequelae seen after head injuries.

For further reading in *Emergency Medicine, A Comprehensive Study Guide*, see Chapter 33, Coma and Altered States of Consciousness, by Gregory L. Henry.

3 | LIFE-THREATENING SIGNS AND SYMPTOMS IN CHILDREN

16 | Fever

Juan A. March

Fever is the single most common complaint of children presenting to the ED and accounts for about 30% of all pediatric outpatient visits. The physician evaluating the febrile child must differentiate the mildly ill from the seriously ill child. Many factors, such as clinical assessment, physical findings, age of the patient, and height of the fever, can influence evaluation and management decisions.

Clinical Features

It is important to recognize that fever represents a symptom of some underlying disease, and one must determine the actual disease process. Body temperature normally varies from morning to evening with the body's circadian rhythm. In general, higher temperatures are associated with a higher incidence of bacteremia. A retrospective study of hyperpyrexia reported that the incidence of meningitis was twice as high in children with fever above 41.1°C (105.9°F), compared to children with fever between 40.5° and 41.0°C (104.9° and 105.8°F).

Diagnosis and Differential

Infants up to 3 months. The age of the patient influences the extent of the workup. Early studies suggested that infants under the age of 3 mo are at high risk for serious life-threatening infection. Clinical assessment of the severity of illness in a young, febrile infant is problematic. Young infants lack social skills, such as the social smile, and lack the ability to interact with the examiner.

The history and physical examination may provide clues to the diagnosis. A history of lethargy, irritability, or poor feeding suggests a serious infection. The physical examination may reveal a focus of infection such as an inflamed eardrum. Inconsolable crying, or increased irritability when handled is frequently seen in infants with meningitis. Cough or tachypnea with a respiratory rate over 40 might suggest a lower respiratory infection and the need for a chest x-ray.

The absence of any diagnostic abnormalities on history or physical examination suggests the need for extensive laboratory tests to detect occult infection. These tests would include a complete blood count and differential, erythrocyte sedimentation rate (ESR), blood culture, lumbar puncture, chest x-ray, urinalysis and culture, and a stool culture if there is a history of diarrhea. Urinary tract infections may not produce symptoms other than fever, so a urinalysis and culture should be included routinely in the evaluation. Antibiotic therapy and hospitalization should be instituted as suggested by the results of these studies.

The recognition of occult serious infection in the well appearing young, febrile infant is problematic. No single variable can correctly identify these infants. Combinations of variables are more helpful in the differentiation process, ESR greater than 30 mm/hr, white blood cell count (WBC) over 15,000/mm^3, band cell count at or over 500/mm^3, evidence of soft-tissue infection, pyuria (WBC >10/hpf), or leukocytes in the stool. The absence of these variables is usually (but not always) associated with the absence of serious illness.

The appropriate management of the young febrile infant presents another area of disagreement. Some physicians hospitalize all febrile infants under 3 mo old, whereas others hospitalize only those under 1 mo of age. Because the differentiation between a sick and well infant is so difficult, all such febrile infants need extensive septic workups. The decision not to hospitalize must be made after careful assessment and after ensuring the reliability of followup.

Infants 3 to 24 months. Clinical judgment appears to be more reliable in the assessment of the older infant. Characteristics to note are willingness to make eye contact, playfulness, response to noxious stimuli, alertness, and consolability. The history and physical examination will frequently reveal the source of the infection. Otitis media is generally caused by *Streptococcus pneumoniae* or *Haemophilus influenza* and antibiotic therapy should be directed at these organisms. Pneumonia is commonly of viral etiology, however, it is appropriate to institute antibiotic therapy to ensure coverage of *H. influenzae*. Nuchal rigidity or Kernig or Brudzinski signs may not be apparent in the child under 2 years old. A bulging fontanelle, vomiting, irritability that increases when the infant is held, inconsolability, or a febrile seizure may be the only signs suggestive of meningitis. About 20% of children with petechiae will have bacteremia or meningitis most frequently with *Neisseria meningitidis* or *H. influenzae*. The incidence of bacteremia in children 3 to 24 mo with a temperature of 39.5°C (103.1°F) or more is about 5 to 6%. The organism most commonly causing bacteremia in this age group is *S. pneumoniae*. It is apparent that bacteremia patients do better if they receive antibiotics early. The blood culture appears to be useful for following a patient who may not be returning for periodic evaluations. Controlled trials investigating efficacy have demonstrated a reduction in the incidence of meningitis in bacteremic children treated with ceftriaxone compared to those treated with oral or no antibiotics. Parenteral ceftriaxone, however, should never be initiated without appropriate antecedent diagnostic studies.

Older febrile children (>24 months). Children over 2 are easier to evaluate because they can specify their complaints. The risk of bacteremia appears lower in this age group, but the incidence of streptococcal pharyngitis is higher. Pneumonia in this age group may be caused by *Mycoplasma pneumoniae*, but these children present with cough and fever.

Emergency Department Care

Aside from febrile seizures, fever is not known to produce any harmful effects in children. One can facilitate heat loss in a child using any combination of measures.

1. *Increasing heat loss.* Unwrapping a bundled child increases heat loss through radiation. Sponging also helps to reduce fever by evaporation, however, this should be done slowly using tepid water only. Studies have shown that sponging and antipyretics used together are more effective than either modality used alone.
2. Drug dosage for **ibuprofen** is 5 to 10 mg/kg per dose at 6 h intervals (max dose, 600 mg) and dosage for **acetaminophen** is 10 to 15 mg/kg per dose at 4 h intervals. Alternating these two drugs in an effort to avoid the recrudescence of fever is common practice.

All patients with positive blood cultures should be recalled for repeat evaluation. If clinically well and afebrile, they should be instructed to complete the course of therapy. Any patient who remains febrile, however, or does poorly even on antibiotics should receive a complete septic evaluation (CBC, blood culture, lumbar puncture, chest film, urine culture), be hospitalized, and receive parenteral antibiotics.

For further reading in *Emergency Medicine, A Comprehensive Study Guide*, see Chapter 35, Fever, by Carol D. Berkowitz.

Fluid and Electrolyte Therapy

Juan A. March

Important differences exist between young children and adults in fluid and electrolyte metabolism and homeostasis. The physiologic consequences of fluid and electrolyte disturbances are more pronounced in children due to their higher metabolic rate. The turnover of fluid and solute per kg of body weight is three times that of adults. Also a higher percentage of their body weight is from water.

Clinical Features

Deficits or Dehydration

The most common mechanism for fluid deficits or dehydration in children is excessive fluid loss. It is imperative to recognize the child with a fluid deficit and treat accordingly in order to prevent cardiovascular collapse. The most accurate way of assessing the degree of dehydration is by weight.

Often an accurate pre-illness weight is not available, and the degree of dehydration must be estimated clinically. The history should include intake (quantity and type of fluid), output (site, type, and amount), and other medical problems (pre-existing and acute). Vital signs, including weight, temperature, heart rate, respiratory rate, blood pressure, and capillary refill time, should be taken. Physical examination should be performed, with emphasis on the general appearance of the child, anterior fontanelle, skin elasticity, and mucous membranes.

Dehydration is divided into three groups, according to the degree of the fluid deficit: mild (<5% dehydration), moderate (5%–10% dehydration), and severe (>10% dehydration). Mild dehydration is usually made from the history, as physical signs are minimal or absent. Pulse rate may be slightly increased, but blood pressure is normal.

The clinical signs of moderate dehydration are much more obvious. The skin may be dry, with tenting and loss of turgor. Mucous membranes are tacky or dry. The anterior fontanelle and eyeballs will be sunken. The child will usually have an altered sensorium with lethargy, restlessness, or irritability, and prolonged capillary refill time (>2 s). Patients are in the early stage of compensatory shock (evidence of marked intravascular volume depletion with normal blood pressure).

In severe dehydration there is uncompensated shock and evidence of circulatory collapse. The skin is cold, clammy, and mottled. Capillary refill time is significantly delayed (>3 to 5 s). Peripheral pulses may be absent, and evidence of poor CNS perfusion, with varying degrees of altered sensorium, may be present.

Differential Diagnosis

Types of dehydration. The types of dehydration refers to the osmolar load of the plasma relative to the degree of fluid loss. Since the main solute in plasma is sodium, serum osmolality is mainly a reflection of sodium concentration. The types of dehydration are isonatremic (isotonic), hyponatremic (hypotonic), and hypernatremic (hypertonic). Each type of dehydration is associated with special problems. Defining the type of dehydration will direct management.

The majority of pediatric patients will present with isonatremic dehydration with a proportionate loss of water and electrolytes, with serum sodium of 130 to 150 mEq/L.

In hyponatremic dehydration, serum sodium is less than 130 mEq/L, and the sodium deficit is greater than the water deficit. This typically occurs when sodium-poor fluids (e.g., tap water) are given to replace GI losses. In hypernatremic dehydration, serum sodium is greater than 150 mEq/L. Hypernatremia occurs when free water replacement is inadequate (incorrectly diluted formulas) or if sodium intake is abnormally high (boiled skim milk or use of baking soda).

Emergency Department Care

Replacement of the fluid deficit occurs in three phases: (1) correction of shock; (2) restoration of ECF volume; and (3) replacement of ICF stores or maintenance fluid.

Correction of Shock

The treatment of shock is directed towards preventing circulatory failure. Children may be in a compensated shock state and still maintain normal blood pressure. Hypotension is a very late and ominous sign. Accurate weight should be obtained for all pediatric patients.

1. Vascular access should be started and blood obtained for immediate analysis of electrolytes, glucose, BUN or creatinine, and pH. A bedside glucose measurement should be done. If peripheral access cannot be obtained, percutaneous cannulation of the femoral or external jugular vein is an alternative. For children less than 6 years old, an intraosseous infusion needle may be placed for initial volume expansion.
2. All patients in shock should receive supplemental oxygen.
3. For correction of shock from all types of dehydration, the initial fluid bolus is the same—20 mL/kg of isotonic crystalloid (0.9% NS or lactated Ringer's solution) over 5 to 20 minutes. Glucose-containing solutions should be avoided as they are poor volume expanders and, in addition, bolus amounts can lead to hyperglycemia and resulting osmotic diuresis.
4. If hypoglycemia is present, administer 0.5 to 1.0 gm/kg of glucose using $D_{25}W$.

Although crystalloids provide good volume expansion, if the child has underlying cardiac, pulmonary, or renal disease, 10 mL/kg boluses of colloids should be used. Rapid delivery of bolus fluids can be achieved by attaching a three-way stopcock to the extension tubing of the intravenous line. A 20 to 50 mL syringe can then be used to push fluid aliquots. This allows for rapid bolus infusion without disrupting fragile veins. After the fluid bolus is completed, reassess the patient. If perfusion remains compromised, the fluid bolus should be repeated. In general, few patients require more than 40 to 60 mL/kg of isotonic crystalloid during the first hour of therapy.

The next phase of therapy is restoration of ECF volume. The aim of this phase is correction of the fluid deficit with restoration of the fluid compartments over 24 to 48 h. Fluid therapy for this phase depends on the degree and type of dehydration present.

Isonatremic dehydration. For the patient with isotonic dehydration, the initial fluid boluses given are subtracted from the calculated fluid deficit. The remaining deficit is replaced over 24 h: one half is given over the first 8 h, and the other half over the subsequent 16 h. For example, a 7-kg patient with 10% dehydration has a fluid deficit of 100 mL/kg, or 700 mL. If an initial fluid bolus of 20 mL/kg of normal saline were given, the remaining fluid deficit is 700 mL − 140 mL = 560 mL. One half of the 560 mL, or 280 mL, is given over the first 8 h (35 mL/h). This is added to the child's maintenance fluid rate, which is 30 mL/hr. Thus, the total rate of fluid for the first 8 h is 35 mL/h + 30 mL/h = 65 mL/h. The rate for the following 16 h is 45 mL/h (15 mL/h + 30 mL/h = 45 mL/h. The IV solution used is $D_5 0.2NS$ or $D_5 0.45NS$. Forty mEq/L of potassium chloride should be added after adequate urine output is established.

Hyponatremic dehydration. In hypotonic dehydration, the water deficit is calculated and replaced as above. The sodium deficit, however, is different. Initial fluid boluses are given as normal saline or lactated Ringer's solution, which are relatively hypertonic solutions. The remainder of the fluid deficit, as well as the maintenance fluid, is given as D_5 0.45 NS. Forty mEq/L of potassium chloride is added after adequate urine output is established. If initial serum sodium is less than 120 mEq/L, 3% saline can be administered to correct the sodium deficit acutely since central pontine myelinolysis has not been reported in children.

Hypernatremic dehydration. In hypertonic dehydration, serum sodium must be lowered slowly. Rapid rehydration leads to rapid expansion of intracellular volume, especially in the CNS, and this may cause abrupt cellular swelling and cerebral edema. The goal is to decrease the serum sodium by approximately 10 to 15 mEq/L/day. Replacement of the fluid deficit is accomplished evenly over 48 h, or 72 h if the initial sodium is greater than 175 mEq/L. For initial serum sodium greater than 210 mEq/L, dialysis may be required. Patients may not appear dehydrated and may appear not to require initial fluid boluses. If in doubt, however, a bolus of normal saline should be administered. The remaining fluid deficit is added to the maintenance fluid requirement for the next 48 h.

Maintenance. The goal of maintenance fluid and electrolyte therapy is to provide the body with water, sodium, potassium, chloride, and bicarbonate, in order to maintain a state of normal homeostasis. Normal maintenance requirements provide water and electrolytes to replace those that are lost through urine, stool, and insensible routes. There is a 1:1 relationship between calories expended and body water required. In other words, the body needs 1 mL of water for every kilocalorie (kcal) expended (Table 17-1).

TABLE 17-1. Bodily Water Requirements

Weight, kg	Water Requirement/24 Hour
≤10	100 mL/kg
11–20	1000 mL + 50 mL/kg for each kg <10
≥20	1500 mL + 20 mL/kg for each kg <20

Daily maintenance requirements of sodium and potassium are 2 to 3 mEq/kg/24 h. Five grams of glucose per 100 kcal expended provides approximately 20% of the total daily caloric expenditure and will prevent ketosis. Newborn infants may require 10 grm of glucose per 100 kcal expended. Standard intravenous solutions that meet these requirements are 5% dextrose in 0.2 or 0.25 normal saline (D_5 0.2NS or D_5 0.25NS), with 20 mEq/L of potassium chloride added. Many conditions can alter a child's metabolic rate. Maintenance fluid and electrolyte requirements may need to be adjusted accordingly.

For further reading in *Emergency Medicine, A Comprehensive Study Guide*, see Chapter 36, Fluid and Electrolyte Therapy, by Bonnie Sowa.

Upper Respiratory Emergencies

Juan A. March

Diseases that cause upper respiratory tract (URT) obstruction account for a significant percentage of pediatric emergency visits. Some are common and quite benign, whereas others are much less common and are true pediatric emergencies.

Clinical Features

Physical Examination

Cyanosis, although dramatic, has inherent limitations as a diagnostic tool. Also, cyanosis depends to a great extent on the amount of hemoglobin in the blood and the status of peripheral circulation. Conversely, a very young infant whose hemoglobin is normally high and whose peripheral circulation is normally somewhat sluggish may show varying degrees of peripheral cyanosis despite a normal pO_2. For these reasons, cyanosis has limited diagnostic value. When present, however, cyanosis can be an ominous sign.

Labored respirations consist of a triad of signs: tachypnea, chest retractions, and nasal flaring. Each has specific limitations in the infant less than 6 mo old. They appear early in the course and worsen, thus serving as prognostic as well as diagnostic signs.

Tachypnea, an increased respiratory rate, is not specific for respiratory tract disease and is seen in cardiac disorders as well as diseases that cause metabolic acidosis. Chest retractions and nasal flaring are more specific for respiratory tract disorders than is tachypnea, and both appear early in the course of the disease. Coughing is uncommon in young infants and, if there is a persistent cough, pertussis, Chlamydia pneumonia, or cystic fibrosis should be considered. Sneezing is more common and is much less significant. Sneezing occurs quite often, usually in the absence of any respiratory disease.

Grunting is an extremely valuable diagnostic sign. Grunting localizes the respiratory disease to the lower respiratory tract and correlates with disease severity. Stridor is similar to grunting as a sign of respiratory distress. It appears early and correlates with severity. Stridor on inspiration is indicative of obstruction at or above the larynx. Biphasic stridor places the obstruction in the trachea, whereas expiratory stridor usually means obstruction below the carina. Only isolated expiratory stridor is referred to as *wheezing,* however; isolated inspiratory stridor is simply called *stridor.*

Differential Diagnosis

When confronted with a stridorous child, the physician should ascertain the age of the patient and the duration of symptoms. A child under 6 mo old with a long duration of symptoms characteristically has a congenital cause of stridor. The patient over 6 mo old with a relatively short duration characteristically has an acquired cause of stridor, such as viral croup, epiglottitis, or foreign-body aspiration. The most common causes of acquired stridor are epiglottitis, viral croup, foreign body aspiration, and retropharyngeal abscess.

EPIGLOTTITIS

Clinical Features

Epiglottitis is a life-threatening disease; age range in which it occurs is 2 to 7, and the etiology is almost always Haemophilus influenzae. Classically, there is an abrupt onset of high fever, sore throat, stridor, dysphagia, and drooling. Physical examination reveals a toxic-appearing child, ashen gray in color, apprehensive, anxious, but with minimal movements, in the characteristic sniffing position. Absence of a spontaneous cough differentiates epiglottitis from viral croup.

Epiglottitis also occurs in teenagers and young adults. Epiglottitis should be considered whenever symptoms of sore throat, dysphagia, and drooling are out of proportion to the visible pharyngeal pathology.

Diagnosis

An acceptable approach is to obtain portable lateral neck x-ray. The physician *must* stay with the child at all times and *not* send the patient to the x-ray department unattended. If total airway obstruction or apnea occurs, children with epiglottitis can be effectively bagged.

Lateral neck x-rays must be taken with the neck extended and should be taken during inspiration. The epiglottis is normally tall and thin but, in epiglottitis, it is very swollen and appears squat and flat, like a thumbprint.

Emergency Department Care

1. Until recently, attempted visualization of the epiglottis in the ED was considered a totally unacceptable approach to diagnosis. Current literature, however, argues that direct visualization is safe and accurate. Although still controversial, it is prudent to ensure the availability of a person skilled in intubation before attempting direct visualization. It is *unacceptable* to carefully observe the patient with epiglottitis for signs of deterioration. What will surely be observed is sudden and total obstruction. The objective of airway management is to prevent this from occurring.
2. Supportive therapy should include IV hydration, humidification of the air to the ETT, administration of oxygen, as necessary,

3. Choices for IV antibiotics include cefuroxime, 50 mg/kg q 8h IV, cefotaxime, 50 mg/kg q 8h, or ceftriaxone, 50 mg /kg/ q 24h. Steroids are not necessary.

VIRAL CROUP

Clinical Features and Diagnosis

Viral croup is usually a benign, self-limited disease. Age range is 6 mo to 3 years; the etiology is usually parainfluenza virus. The typical history is 2 to 3 days of URI with a gradually worsening cough, especially at night. By day four, barking cough, stridor, and dyspnea, as well as varying degrees of anxiety, are present. Physical examination reveals marked stridor, retractions, tachypnea, hoarseness, and mild cyanosis on room air. A typical case of croup can be differentiated from epiglottitis on clinical grounds, so x-rays are not necessary in every patient.

Emergency Department Care

Treatment is basically symptomatic: cool mist, oxygen when needed, and hydration either, IV or PO. Antibiotics are not needed.

1. Steroids have been shown to be beneficial in croup, **prednisone,** 1 to 2 mg/kg day, or dexamethasone 0.25 to 0.5 mg/kg/dose q6h.
2. Although **racemic epinephrine** can be used to treat severe cases, due to rebound stridor it is recommended these patients be admitted or watched at least 6 to 12 h prior to discharge.
3. Spasmodic croup, usually without a preceding URI or fever, almost always occurring at night, is thought to be due to allergy and is very sensitive to mist.

Bacterial tracheitis, a more severe form of croup, has been increasing in the past few years. Also referred to as membranous laryngotracheobronchitis, it is usually caused by *Staphylococcus aureus*. The patient has more respiratory distress than with epiglottis and may present similar to it, however, x-ray shows the typical findings of croup. The patient may need intubation as well as antibiotics.

FOREIGN BODY ASPIRATIONS

Clinical Features

Foreign body aspirations cause over 3000 deaths each year, over half of which are children under 4 years old. The most common foreign bodies (FB) are peanuts and sunflower seeds, but almost any object may be aspirated.

The patient may present with a variety of signs, depending on the location of the FB and the degree of obstruction—wheezing, persistent pneumonia, stridor, coughing, or apnea. As many as one third of the aspirations may *not* be witnessed or remembered by the parent. The physician must highly suspect an FB. If it is opaque, the FB can be easily seen on x-ray, but most airway FBs are radiolucent. FBs will cause air trapping, which leads to hyperinflation of the obstructed lung and a shift of the mediastinum during expiration away from the obstructed side. Mediastinal shift also may be seen on bilateral decubitus x-rays of the chest. A single negative x-ray does not rule out the presence of an FB.

Emergency Department Care

Treatment of airway FBs is laryngoscopy or bronchoscopy in the operating room under anesthesia. The patient with an airway FB will require respiratory care for 24 to 72 h after FB removal. Antibiotics, steroids, oxygen, mist, and chest physiotherapy all may be necessary.

RETROPHARYNGEAL ABSCESS

Clinical Features and Diagnosis

Retropharyngeal abscess formation usually occurs in children aged 6 mo to 3 years. It begins with a URI, which localizes to the retropharyngeal lymph nodes over several days. Dysphagia and refusal to feed occur before significant respiratory distress. Patients usually appear toxic, also presenting febrile, drooling, and with inspiratory stridor and dysphagia. They assume an almost opisthotonic posture.

The diagnostic test is a lateral neck x-ray performed during inspiration, which shows a widened retropharyngeal space. Physical examination may show a retropharyngeal mass often seen with a tongue blade and a flashlight. Palpation of the mass is dangerous as it may lead to rupture of the abscess.

Emergency Department Care

Treatment includes high-dose IV antibiotics, usually **penicillin** G, 250,000 units/kg/day divided q4h.

For further reading in *Emergency Medicine, A Comprehensive Study Guide*, see Chapter 37, Upper Respiratory Emergencies, by Nick Relich.

Hypoglycemia in Children

Juan A. March

Hypoglycemia is a relatively common condition in pediatrics, particularly in acutely sick infants and children. The diagnosis and treatment of hypoglycemia in the ED should be prompt because persistent or recurrent hypoglycemia may have permanent catastrophic effects on the brain, particularly in infants. Hypoglycemia is defined as a serum or plasma glucose concentration less than 45 mg/dL. The values of serum or plasma glucose concentration are 10% to 15% higher than those for whole blood.

Clinical Features

Hypoglycemia occurs as a primary or secondary feature of a large number of clinical conditions. In addition, ingested substances such as insulin, salicylates, beta blockers, oral hypoglycemics, ethanol, and quinidine, can cause hypoglycemia. The symptomatology is variable and may be overshadowed by the dramatic appearance of the primary disease, such as meningococcemia. It is prudent, therefore, to assess for and treat hypoglycemia immediately.

Patients become symptomatic from hypoglycemia because of compensatory heightened adrenergic activity and the cerebral metabolic perturbances directly attributable to glucose deprivation. Older children usually have the same signs as adults. Manifestations tend to be subtler and nonspecific in infants and include poor feeding, lethargy, apnea, hypotonia, and hypothermia. Infants and children with unexplained respiratory or cardiac arrest should be tested immediately for hypoglycemia. Clinical signs of hypoglycemia include adrenergic excess, such as anxiety, tachycardia, perspiration, nausea, tremors, pallor, chest pains, weakness, abdominal pain, hunger, and irritability. Neuroglycopenic effects, such as confusion, ataxia, headache, depressed consciousness, blurred vision, lightheadedness, focal neurologic deficits, seizures, strabismus, staring, and paresthesia may also be apparent.

Diagnosis

In those suspected, or at risk, to be hypoglycemic, bedside glucose measurement can be diagnostic within 2 min. Take care to ensure the testing strip is completely covered with blood and that isopropyl alcohol does not contaminate the specimen. When bedside glucose is unavailable, it is better to treat unnecessarily than to delay appropriate treatment.

Emergency Department Care

There are three important aspects of emergency patient care: (1) rapid diagnosis of hypoglycemia; (2) acquisition of germaine blood and urine specimens; and (3) prompt restoration and maintenance of euglycemia. Clearly it is imperative to replete the serum with glucose, but it is short-sighted to neglect the first two objectives.

1. After specimen collection, a bolus of 10% **dextrose** in water ($D_{10}W$) is given intravenously or intraosseously.
2. Follow the bolus with a continuous infusion of $D_{10}W$ in an age- and weight-appropriate fashion. When dosing dextrose, it is helpful to recall that $D_{50}W$ can easily injure a peripheral vein, causing extravasation, therefore, it should be diluted. Furthermore, neonates are less tolerant of a rapid osmotic load and should be given only $D_{10}W$ when possible. When standard therapy fails, however, hydrocortisone is useful for those who cannot achieve euglycemia despite adequate dextrose administration. This is especially true of patients with hypopituitarism and adrenal insufficiency.

For further reading in *Emergency Medicine, A Comprehensive Study Guide*, see Chapter 39, Hypoglycemia in Children, by Mark Goetting and Bassam Gebara.

Altered mental status in children is the failure to respond to the external environment after appropriate stimulation, in a manner consistent with the child's developmental level. These patients require simultaneous stabilization, diagnosis, and treatment often with aggressive resuscitation.

Clinical Features

The spectrum of altered mental status ranges from confusion to lethargy, stupor, and coma. The lethargic patient has decreased awareness of his surroundings, the stuporous patient can be aroused with noxious stimuli, whereas the comatose patient is unresponsive to any stimuli. Conditions that affect level of alertness can be divided into three pathologic categories: supratentorial lesion, subtentorial lesion, and metabolic. Presentation of supratentorial lesions include focal motor abnormalities, rostral to caudal progression of dysfunction, and slow nystagmus towards the lesion with cold calorics. Subtentorial lesions produce rapid loss of consciousness, cranial nerve abnormalities, abnormal respiratory patterns, and asymmetric or fixed pupils. Metabolic etiologies produce depressed consciousness before exhibiting motor signs. When motor signs are present, they are typically symmetric. Pupillary reflexes are intact except with profound anoxia, opiates, barbiturates, and anticholinergics.

Diagnosis and Differential

A thorough history and physical examination is paramount in determining diagnosis. The history should include inquiries regarding fever, headache, weakness, head tilt, abdominal pain, vomiting, diarrhea, hematuria, weight loss, rash, gait disturbances, and palpitations. The examination should look for signs of occult infection, trauma, toxicity, or metabolic disease. A useful tool for organizing diagnostic possibilities is the mnemonic AEIOU TIPS (Table 20-1).

Diagnostic adjuncts include electrolytes, glucose, and renal and liver function studies, which may provide important clues. A blood culture is indicated whenever sepsis is suspected. Toxicology screens are warranted if ingestion is a possibility. Lumbar puncture should not be delayed if meningitis is suspected. A twelve-lead EKG may be helpful if there are auscultatory findings or rhythm disturbances on the monitor. Chest x-ray can confirm pneumonia or a foreign body, whereas abdominal films are helpful in patients with signs of acute abdomen, intussusception, or ingestion of radiopaque material. CT scans should be ob-

TABLE 20-1. AEIOU TIPS:

A **Alcohol**—Changes in mental status can occur with serum levels less than 100 mg/dL. Concurrent hypoglycemia is common.
Acid-base and metabolic—Hypotonic or hypertonic dehydration, diabetic ketoacidosis, hepatic failure, inborn errors of metabolism
Arrhythmia/cardiogenic—Stokes–Adams, aortic stenosis, SVT

E **Encephalopathy**—Reyes syndrome. Hypertensive encephalopathy may occur in childen with diastolic pressures of 100–110 mmHg.
Endocrinopathy—In general, altered mental status is a rare presentation of this category. Thyrotoxic children may present with ventricular dysrhythmias. Pheochromocytoma may present with hypertensive encephalopathy.
Electrolytes—Hyponatremic children become symptomatic with levels around 120 mEq/L. Hypernatremia and disorders of calcium, magnesium, and phosphorus can produce changes in mental status.

I **Insulin**—Hypoglycemia, ketotic hypoglycemia. Irritability, confusion, seizures, and coma can occur with blood glucose levels 40 mg/dL or less.
Intussusception

O **Opiates**—Common household exposures are Lomotil, Imodium, and dextromethorphan.

U **Uremia**—Renal failure, hemolytic uremic syndrome.

T **Trauma**—Remember to look for signs of child abuse, particularly shaken baby syndrome with retinal hemorrhages.
Tumor—Primary, metastatic, or meningeal leukemic infiltration.
Thermal—Hypo- or hyperthermia.

I **Infection**—One of the more common causes of altered mental status in children and meningitis, which should be high on the differential list.
Intracerebral vascular disorders—Subarachnoid, intracerebral or intraventricular hemorrhages can be seen with trauma, ruptured aneurysm, or AV malformation. Venous thrombosis can follow severe dehydration or pyogenic infection of the mastoid, orbit, middle ear, or sinuses.

P **Psychogenic**—Rare in the pediatric age group.
Poisoning

S **Seizure**

tained before lumbar puncture and can aid in the diagnosis of increased intracranial pressure, bleeding, and vascular or mass lesions. Miscellaneous laboratory tests that can be helpful include blood ammonia level, serum osmolality, blood alcohol level, thyroid function tests, and blood lead level.

Emergency Department Care

The first priority is patient stabilization. Airway, breathing, and circulation should be immediately addressed. Supplemental oxygen, continuous pulse oximetry, and cardiac monitor should be employed in all cases.

1. Administer sufficient oxygen to maintain a pulse oximetry reading of at least 95%. Assisted ventilations and endotracheal intubation may be necessary. Care must be taken to protect the cervical spine, if trauma is suspected.
2. Crystalloid IV fluids should be given for hypotension with an initial bolus of 20 ml/kg. Repeat boluses up to a total of 60 ml/kg may be given.
3. Bedside blood sugar determinations should be made and glucose, 0.25 g/kg IV of 10% or 25% dextrose, should be given if the patient is hypoglycemic.
4. Seizures should be aborted with benzodiazepines (i.e., **lorazepam,** 0.05 mg/kg), followed by phenytoin or phenobarbital, if seizures persist.
5. Control core body temperature, maintaining euthermia with radiant heat sources if necessary. Acid-base status should be normalized. Sodium bicarbonate should be used sparingly and only in circumstances where the pH is less than 7.0. Empiric IV antibiotics should be given quickly in septic-appearing patients, especially those with possible intracranial infections.

Once the patient is hemodynamically stabilized, further workup to determine the causative process may proceed using clues gathered from the initial assessment, and definitive treatment may proceed using the appropriate chapters in this handbook to guide further management. In general, patients who present with altered mental status should be admitted to an intensive care unit (ICU) or transferred to a tertiary care center for pediatric intensive care. Only those patients with transient, reversible causes may be treated and discharged home with disease-specific instructions. All patients discharged should have a repeat evaluation within 24 h.

If Standard Treatment Fails

Persistent hypotension unresponsive to fluid boluses should be treated with pressor agents. Naloxone may be given if opiate or clonidine overdose is suspected. The standard naloxone dose is 0.1 mg/kg for those less than 5 years old or 20 kg, and 2 mg/kg in children over 5 years old. Remember to ask about ingestions and look for clues of common toxicological syndromes.

For further reading in *Emergency Medicine, A Comprehensive Study Guide*, see Chapter 40, Altered Mental Status in Children, by Nancy Pook, Natalie Cullen, and Jonathan Singer.

Syncope and Breath Holding

Debra G. Perina

Syncope is common in children and is a sudden brief loss of consciousness that may be accompanied by seizure-like activity. At least 15% of children will experience a syncopal episode before they complete adolescence. In fact, vasovagal syncope is estimated to occur in 15% to 25% of adolescents. By definition, this condition is transient and usually self-limited.

Clinical Features

Most cases of childhood syncope are benign, but the child must be evaluated carefully to rule out serious underlying conditions. Etiologies causing syncope may be divided into cardiac, neurologic, metabolic, autonomic, respiratory, and unknown. (Reviewing the Altered Mental Status in Children, Chapter 20, may also be helpful when evaluating a child who presents with syncope.)

Diagnosis and Differential

A thorough history and physical examination will most often lead to the correct diagnosis. Each major etiology of syncope, along with its salient diagnostic points, are provided below.

Cardiac syncope. Syncope due to cardiac problems is usually caused by arrhythmias or ventricular outflow obstruction. This is the most serious form of syncope in children. A suggestive history includes a family history of unexplained sudden death, prior history of Kawasaki disease, prior cardiac surgery, recent unexplained change in exercise tolerance, or known congenital pulmonary outflow obstruction. Physical findings suggestive of aortic stenosis may include a systolic ejection click, a harsh systolic ejection murmur over the base of the heart radiating to the carotids, and a palpable thrill in the suprasternal notch. Syncope associated with exercise is worrisome and one should consider the possibility of idiopathic hypertrophic subaortic stenosis (IHSS). A systolic murmur enhanced by standing or a Valsalva maneuver may be due to IHSS. Chest pain in an adolescent is often not serious but, in a young child, palpitations often are reported as chest pain. An arrhythmia should be strongly considered if this report is accompanied by complaints of dizziness, lightheadedness, or syncope.

Neurologic syncope. Seizures are the most common cause of neurologic syncope. Distinguishing a true seizure disorder from the activity that results from a breath-holding spell can be problematic. In general, activity resulting from breath holding will be transient with a rapid return to the patient's normal status, whereas a true seizure results in a prolonged loss of consciousness with a delay in return to a normal state. A family history of seizures is not helpful in distinguishing the two. Any child with a focal physical finding after a syncopal episode should be evaluated for a true seizure disorder, neurotrauma, or unsuspected CNS lesion or infection.

Respiratory syncope.   Causes of respiratory syncope include hyperventilation, prolonged hypoxia, such as that seen with severe pneumonia or asthma, and post-tussive syncope. Hyperventilation is by far the most common cause inducing hypocapnia that results in cerebral vasoconstriction, reduced delivery of oxygen and glucose to the brain, and syncope. Post-tussive syncope is seen with prolonged, severe, frequent coughing episodes, as with pertussis.

Autonomic syncope.   Vasovagal, or vasodepressor, syncope is the most common cause of syncope in children and is responsible for at least 50% of cases. Vasovagal syncope occurs from a decrease in peripheral vascular resistance that leads to a drop in arterial pressure and cerebral perfusion. Vasovagal syncope usually occurs in response to emotional stress and is more likely if one is tired, hungry, or recovering from a recent illness. Environmental conditions, such as crowding, warmth, or enclosed space, can also promote an episode. Prodromal symptoms of palpitations, nausea, and diaphoresis may be reported. Brief seizure-like activity may also occur. Orthostatic hypotension is another form of autonomic syncope, which results from a gravity mediated loss of blood from the brain and thorax on standing. Orthostatic hypotension is uncommon in the healthy child, and underlying causes such as hypovolemia and anemia should be considered.

Breath holding.   Breath-holding spells are a form of autonomic syncope resulting from transient cerebral anoxia. These spells are most common in infancy and early childhood. A careful history is paramount to making the diagnosis. Breath-holding spells are associated with an outburst of crying, anger, or pain, followed by a brief loss of consciousness and sometimes even a short burst of seizure-like activity. There are two types of breath-holding spells—pallid and cyanotic. The cyanotic type is more commonly associated with vagally mediated hypotension occurring after vigorous crying. The pallid type is more likely to occur after a fright or injury and is caused by a vagally mediated severe bradycardia or a brief period of asystole. Reassurance is generally all that is necessary, however, in any uncertain situation it is wise to obtain an ECG to eliminate conduction defects as an underlying cause.

Metabolic syncope.   This is a relatively uncommon cause of syncope in children. The prodrome is gradual in onset, unlike many of the other types of syncope. Associated symptoms include weakness, diaphoresis, confusion, and hunger. These symptoms are unrelated to position and are not associated with changes in pulse or blood pressure. Hypoglycemia is a rare cause of syncope in children except in insulin-dependent diabetics. Drug ingestion, unfortunately, is a much more common cause. Alcoholism is a major problem in adolescents and should be considered in any adolescent with a history of unexplained blackout spells.

Hysteria. Perhaps a *swoon* would be better terminology for hysterical syncope, as it involves no changes in vital signs or derangement of cerebral perfusion. It generally occurs in front of an audience. The patient remains calm, falls gracefully to the floor, and may variably respond to the surroundings. Hysterical syncope is most common in adolescents and is usually for attention-getting or secondary gain. Hysteria is a diagnosis of exclusion, however, and other causes of syncope should be considered and eliminated before arriving at this diagnosis.

Emergency Department Care

Most causes of syncope can be diagnosed with a thorough history and physical examination. When there is an obvious cause, such as breath holding or vasovagal syncope, laboratory testing is not necessary and only reassurance is needed.

1. Laboratory studies such as glucose, electrolytes, drug screens, and complete blood count need only be done if the history and physical examination produce findings suggestive of metabolic syncope or orthostatic hypotension. CT scans are seldom helpful, but they may be indicated in cases when tonic–clonic activity is observed or return to consciousness is prolonged and neurologic syncope is suspected. If cardiac syncope is suspected, an ECG and chest x-ray should be done and an outpatient echocardiogram and Holter monitor may be of value. If IHSS is suspected, an echocardiogram should be done, if possible, in the ED.
2. If an arrhythmia is thought to be the cause of the syncopal episode, the patient should be admitted, otherwise most patients presenting with syncope and breath holding may be discharged after arranging appropriate referral.
3. When tonic–clonic activity is observed or return to consciousness is prolonged after an apparent syncopal event, EEGs may be indicated along with referral to a pediatric neurologist.

For further reading in *Emergency Medicine, A Comprehensive Study Guide*, see Chapter 41, Syncope and Breath Holding, by David A. Poleski.

4 | EMERGENCY WOUND MANAGEMENT

22 | Evaluation of Wounds

Michael J. Utecht

Traumatic wounds are common problems encountered in the ED. When caring for wounds, the ultimate goal is to restore the physical integrity and function of the injured tissue without infection.

When treating a wound the emergency physician should consider the time and mechanism of injury, as well as its location, as all play roles in the wound's potential for infection. In most soft-tissue injuries, a shearing force applied by a piece of glass, a metal edge, or a knife result in a linear laceration producing a wound that exhibits considerable resistance to infection. Wounds caused by compression or tension forces, such as the collision of two bodies, absorb greater energy resulting in stellate lacerations, which are one hundred times more susceptible to infection than those caused by shear forces.

An infective dose of bacteria may be derived from either an exogenous source or the endogenous microflora of the patient. Over most of the body surface, the density of bacteria is quite low (trunk, upper arms, and legs). Moist areas harbor millions of bacteria, as do exposed anatomic areas (head, face, hands, and feet). As these organisms reside in the most superficial layers of the skin, topically applied antiseptic agents provide sterility or near sterility in most skin areas of the body. Lacerations contacting the oral cavity usually are heavily contaminated with facultative and anaerobic organisms. The largest number of organisms is encountered in the gingival crevices, plaque on the teeth accounting for the reported high infection rate of wounds resulting from human and animal bites. Wounds contacted by human or animal fecal contaminants also run a high risk for infection, despite therapeutic intervention.

Wound Examination

Examination of the injured site must begin by detecting any sensory, motor, and vascular complications or injuries to specialized ducts. When the injury occurs to an extremity and bleeding complicates thorough inspection of the wound, a sphygmomanometer placed proximal to the injury and inflated to a pressure greater than the patient's systolic blood pressure will provide excellent hemostasis. Palpation of the bone adjacent to the wound may detect tenderness or instability consistent with an underlying bone injury, which can be confirmed by roentgenograms. Injuries requiring open reduction of fractures, neurorrhaphy, vascular anastomosis, tendon juncture, or repair of specialized ducts are best treated in the operating room by the appropriate specialist. In the absence of these underlying injuries, wound treatment can be undertaken in the ED.

Clinical observation of the wound in the ED is a reliable method of predicting the ultimate appearance of the healing scar after closure.

Wounds with retraction of their edges ≥5 mm generally result in fine scars. In uneven, jagged-edged wounds, the perimeter of the wound is considerably longer than that of a linear incision, resulting in less static tension per unit length of the wound. By electing to convert the jagged wound edges into a straight wound, the potential benefits of the long wound perimeter are lost. Reapproximation of the edges of the debrided wound requires greater closing forces than would have been needed prior to debridement, resulting in a wide scar. The physician must take this into consideration, especially when wounds involve cosmetic areas (e.g., face) and should debride as little of the wound as possible.

For further reading in *Emergency Medicine, A Comprehensive Study Guide*, see Chapter 42, The Evaluation of Wounds in the Emergency Department, by Richard F. Edlich, George T. Rodeheaver, and John G. Thacker.

23 | Wound Preparation, Local and Regional Anesthesia

Michael J. Utecht

LOCAL ANESTHESIA

Cleansing bacteria and other debris from a laceration followed by debridement and wound closure cannot be accomplished without local or regional anesthesia often complemented by sedation. (The technique of conscious sedation for adults and children is covered in Chapter 5, therefore, attention in this chapter will focus on local anesthesia.)

Selection of Anesthetic Agent

The selection of the anesthetic for infiltration anesthesia is based on pharmacologic and toxicologic considerations. The pharmacologic properties of these agents include severity of pain elicited by injection, onset and duration of activity, and frequency of adequate anesthesia. Toxicologic manifestations of local anesthetic agents are almost exclusively local (e.g., damage to tissue defenses).

Lidocaine

Lidocaine injection is less painful when the drug is buffered and warmed first; it must be buffered immediately prior to use. A simple way to buffer a 30-mL vial containing 1% lidocaine is to add 3 mL of 4.2% sterile solution of sodium bicarbonate (1 mEq/mL), using single-dose vials, at a 10:1 dilution. A simple way to warm the vial or bottle is to place it in the IV solution warmer heated to 40°C.

Antimicrobial preservatives have been added to local anesthetic contained in multidose vials. These preservatives are potent allergens and have been implicated in allergic reactions to local anesthetic agents.

The addition of epinephrine, with its vasoconstrictive properties, enhances the duration of anesthetic activity by slowing the clearance of the agent from tissue and providing improved hemostasis. This benefit must be weighed against its effects on tissue defenses. The local vasoconstrictive action of epinephrine may result in hypoxic conditions that limit white blood cell function potentially impairing the killing of bacterial contaminants. Some authors, therefore, argue against the use of epinephrine in heavily contaminated wounds.

Bupivicaine, with duration of anesthesia nearly four times longer than that of lidocaine, recommended for prolonged anesthesia.

TOPICAL ANESTHESIA

One painless way to anesthetize lacerations is to use a topical solution or gel containing 0.5% tetracaine, 0.5% epinephrine (adrenalin), and

11.8% cocaine (TAC). Another advantage is vasoconstriction, resulting in improved hemostasis. It is most effective when applied 20 min before suturing to wounds involving the scalp, forehead, and eyebrow. Anesthesia is usually evidenced by complete blanching of the skin within 1 cm of the wound edges. TAC cannot be used in lacerations involving the ear, penis, and digits, nor can it be used on, or applied to, mucous membranes as a toxic reaction to cocaine might develop. In an effort to avoid the toxic effects of cocaine, recent investigators have studied several additional topical anesthetics, including LET (lidocaine 4%, epinephrine .1%, and tetracaine .5%). The two agents were similar in adequacy and duration of anesthesia except in children over the age of 6 years, who had a greater proportion of incomplete anesthesia. Other topical agents are currently under investigation.

Side Effects of Anesthetic Agents

Side-effects of local anesthetic agents are divided into allergic reaction and systemic toxicity. True allergic reactions are rare. Because the aminoamide compounds are believed to be incapable of stimulating antibody formation, true anaphylaxis should not be encountered. Some patients presumed to be allergic to the amide-type compound have had responses to the preservative (e.g., methylparaben) or stabilizers added to the local anesthetic agents but not to the agent itself. When treating a patient with a known history of allergy to an amide-type agent, the physician should try a subcutaneous challenge with a local anesthetic agent different from the one causing the previous reaction. An alternative approach is to inject an antihistamine such as 1% diphenhydramine hydrochloride into the wound, which should achieve anesthesia for approximately 30 min.

Usually systemic toxicity is due to either a rapid inadvertent intravenous injection or an excessive amount of the local anesthetic. Adverse signs include CNS manifestations, such as dizziness, tinnitus, periorbital tingling, nystagmus, and fine skeletal muscle twitching. Treatment is to discontinue the administration of the agent and to provide supportive care and hyperventilation. Overt convulsions, usually self-limited, may follow. If convulsions persist, diazepam or lorazepam may be administered in small incremental doses. Signs and symptoms of cardiovascular collapse indicate the final stage and require aggressive treatment with intravenous fluids and a vasopressor or positive inotropic agent.

INFILTRATION ANESTHESIA

The simplest and most practical technique of anesthetizing most lacerations is infiltration anesthesia by injecting into intact skin at the periphery of the wound. A reliable method of minimizing the discomfort of infiltration anesthesia is to use a warmed (40°C) and buffered anesthetic

(10:1 solution of 10 mL 1% lidocaine: 1 mEq/mL of sodium bicarbonate) in a syringe fitted with a 30-gauge needle and to inject the smallest amount of agent slowly (>10 S) into the deep dermal-subcutaneous tissue, as the needle is slowly withdrawn.

REGIONAL NERVE BLOCKS

In certain situations, a regional nerve block offers several advantages over infiltration anesthesia. First, it does not distort the wound, facilitating reapproximation of the wound edges. Secondly, when there is a need to anesthetize sensitive areas, such as the palm of the hand or sole of the foot, a regional block may be accomplished by passing the needle through more proximal skin, which has a considerably higher pain threshold. This section will cover only the techniques for finger and toe blocks. (The reader is referred to the textbook for a more comprehensive review of other techniques.)

Finger Blocks

Metacarpal blocks are used to anesthetize either the index, ring, long, or small finger (Fig. 23-1). The block is performed on each side of the affected finger by inserting a 27-gauge needle at a 90° angle to the dorsum of the hand, approximately 1 cm proximal to the metacarpophalangeal joint, midway between each metacarpal bone. The needle is then advanced at a 90° angle to the skin until its tip is at the level of the lateral volar surface of the metacarpal head, or until resistance of the palmar aponeurosis is detected. Three mL of anesthetic is injected slowly.

A digital nerve block is more efficacious than a metacarpal block and requires less time to anesthetize the injured finger. Insert a 27-gauge needle into one side of the extensor tendon of the affected finger, just proximal to the web (Fig. 23-2). Approximately 1 mL of anesthetic is injected superficially into the subcutaneous tissue lying on the dorsal surface of the extensor tendon to block the dorsal digital nerve. The needle is then advanced toward the palm, just distal to the web, and another 1 mL is injected to block the volar digital nerve. Before removing the needle, redirect it across the extensor tendon to the opposite side of the finger, and inject approximately 1 mL of solution to block the other dorsal digital nerve. Then reintroduce the needle on the opposite side and repeat the same technique. The total volume of anesthetic agent should not exceed 4 mL. Epinephrine must not be used.

Toe Blocks

A 27-gauge needle should be introduced on the dorsal aspect of the base of the midpoint of the involved toe (Fig. 23-3). Angle the needle

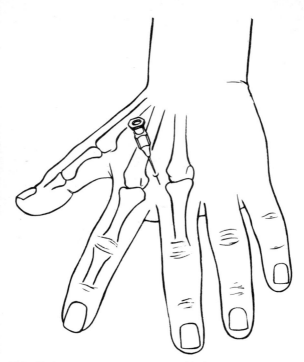

FIG. 23-1.   Regional metacarpal nerve block.

around the bone until the skin blanches on the plantar surface. While withdrawing the needle, inject 1.5 mL of anesthetic. Before withdrawing the needle, it should be redirected to the opposite side of the toe for injection. The total volume should not exceed 3 mL, and epinephrine should not be used.

For the hallux, a modified collar (ring) block is employed (see Fig. 23-3). The 27-gauge needle is inserted on the dorsolateral aspect of the base of the toe. When the plantar skin blanches, inject 1.5 mL of anesthetic. Before withdrawing the needle, pass it under the skin on the dorsal aspect of the toe and inject another 1.5 mL of anesthetic as the needle is withdrawn. Then introduce the needle on the dorsomedial aspect of the toe and apply as on the opposite side. The total volume is usually 4.5 mL. Again, epinephrine should not be used.

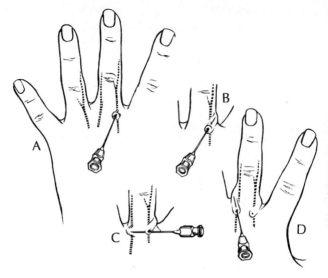

FIG. 23-2.   Digital nerve block.

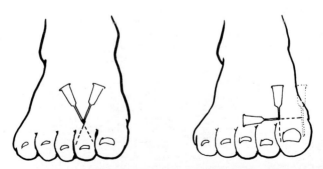

FIG. 23-3.   (*Left*) Regional block of toe. (*Right*) Regional block of hallux (great toe).

WOUND PREPARATION

Careful wound preparation involves appropriate removal of hair that may interfere with wound closure, skin antisepsis, hemostasis, selected debridement of devitalized tissue, mechanical cleansing, and antibiotics when indicated.

Hair is a source of wound contamination, and removal prevents hair from becoming entangled in suture and the wound during closure. Minimize hair removal by clipping with scissors around the wound edges or by applying lubricant or ointments such as bacitracin to keep hair out of the wound edges. A surgical clipper with a disposable clipper blade can be used for large amounts of hair. Eyebrows should never be removed.

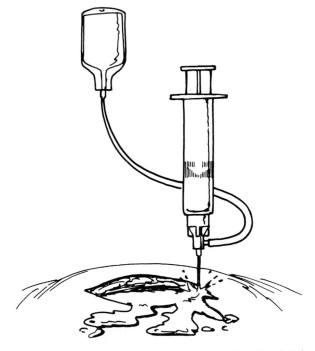

FIG. 23-4.   High-pressure syringe irrigation assembly. Note that the needle is held as close as possible and perpendicular to the surface of the wound during wound irrigation.

Disinfection the skin around the wound without contacting the wound itself. Superiority of one antiseptic agent over another has not been shown. Since inadvertent spillage of these agents into the wound can damage wound defenses and invite infection, spillage should be avoided.

Good hemostasis is important to ensure visualization of the wound and prevent unwanted hematomas, which can interfere with wound healing. Fortunately, most bleeding is controlled by applying direct pressure. Persistent bleeding, however, may require the use of electro-surgical coagulation or careful ligation of some larger vessels (>2 mm).

Heavily contaminated wounds or those that contain devitalized tissue will need to undergo careful debridement. Although the extent of such debridement is wound specific, as little tissue as possible should be debrided. Following debridement, heavily contaminated wounds and those with extensive amounts of devitalized tissue are best left to heal by using delayed primary or secondary closure. Open wound management should be employed for high-energy-depositor missile injuries.

Two techniques are employed for cleansing: irrigation and scrubbing. Low-pressure irrigation (.5 psi) can be used for clean wounds by using a bulb syringe. High-pressure irrigation (7 psi) should be reserved for dirty or heavily contaminated wounds; it is achieved by delivering fluid from a 19-gauge needle or angiocath attached to a 30 mL syringe. Continuous high pressure can be obtained through an irrigation assembly as depicted in Figure 23-4.

Although scrubbing is an effective means of removing bacteria from wounds, tissue trauma inflicted by scrubbing impairs the wound's infec-

---

TABLE 23-1. Indications for Antibiotic Prophylaxis in Wounds

High-risk anatomic site—i.e., forefoot, hand
Contaminated wounds
    Bodily fluids
    Organic matter or dirt
Wounds with devitalized tissue
Extensive soft-tissue injury
Stellate lacerations
Lacerations >5 cm
Indwelling prosthetic devices
Endocarditis prophylaxis needed for
    Prosthetic heart valves
    Arteriovenous fistula
    Patent ductus arteriosus
    Tetralogy of Fallot
    Ventricular septal defect
    Coarctation of the aorta
    Valvular heart disease
Lymphedema
Immunocompromised patients
Peripheral vascular disease

tion resistance. To minimize tissue damage, while maintaining bacterial removal efficiency, use a fine pore sponge and a nontoxic surfactant such as poloxamer 188.

Antibiotic use also needs consideration. Table 23-1 lists indications for antibiotic prophylaxis in wounds. (Suggestions for prophylaxis of infective endocarditis can be found in Chapter 31.)

For further reading in *Emergency Medicine, A Comprehensive Study Guide,* see Chapter 43, Local and Regional Anesthesia for Wound Repair, by Richard F. Edlich, George T. Rodeheaver, and John G. Thacker; and Chapter 44, Wound Preparation, by Richard F. Edlich, George T. Rodeheaver, and John G. Thacker.

Methods for Wound Closure,
Difficult Wounds

Michael Utecht

SUTURES

Suture material is broadly categorized as absorbable and nonabsorbable. The most common nonabsorbable suture materials include monofilament nylon, polymer polypropylene, and the newer polybutester. Nylon is still the most frequently used and has good application for surface percutaneous closures. Four to five knots are required for good knot security. Polymer polypropylene is stronger than nylon but may be more difficult to work with. Polybutester can stretch, which allows some swelling, and reportedly has better knot security. The most commonly used absorbable suture in emergency medicine is polyglycolic acid (PGA). This material has excellent knot security and maintains 50% of its tensile strength for 25 days. PGA has a high friction coefficient, however, which requires more force to pull in through tissue. PGA is also available in a coated form that snags less but requires more knots to be secure. Chromic gut has less tensile strength than PGA, but has application for intra-oral laceration repair.

There are two techniques for sutural closure of skin: percutaneous and dermal (subcuticular). Percutaneous sutures are passed through the epidermal and dermal layers of the skin. Dermal sutures reapproximate the divided edges of the dermis without penetrating the epidermis. Some wound closures require both techniques. Either type can be used as a continuous or an interrupted suture. Sutural closure of the adipose tissue beneath the skin should be avoided, as sutures beneath the skin increase the incidence of infection. To prevent needle puncture scars, skin sutures must be removed before the eighth day after wound closure, and skin tape should be applied to reinforce the edges as needed. Most facial sutures are removed by the fifth day

NEEDLES

Needles are available in a variety of dimensions, geometries, and needle points. A 135 needle (3/8 circle) is used to reapproximate thin planar structures such as skin. The 180 needle (1/2 circle) is used in deeper tissue because a limited arc of wrist rotation will pass the entire needle through the tissue. The compound curved needle is ideally suited for dermal skin closure.

Generally, needles have cutting edges, are taperpoint, or are a combination of the two. Cutting needles have at least two opposing edges designed to penetrate tough tissue. A third cutting edge categorizes a needle as a conventional, or reverse, cutting edge needle. The conventional cutting edge needle has an apical cutting edge located on the inner surface that cuts tissue beneath the surface and directs the needle

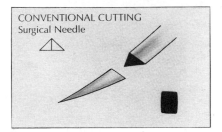

FIG. 24-1.   Conventional cutting edge surgical needle. **Top left.** Front view of point. The point of the needle has three cutting edges, with its apical cutting edge on the inside, concave surface of the needle. **Side view.** Its apical cutting edge is positioned on the inside, concave surface of the needle. **Bottom right.** The body of the needle has a side-flattened cross-sectional configuration.

point toward the skin (surface seeking) (Fig. 24-1). It produces a triangular defect, the apex of which is directed toward the laceration. This can cause skin cut-through when positioning the suture ligature. In contrast, the reverse cutting edge needles have a third cutting edge on the outer curvature of the needle. The advantage of this needle is a flat surface closest to the wound edge, which limits tissue cutout and directs the point of the needle toward the depth of the wound (depth seeking).

The taperpoint needle tapers to a sharp tip (Fig. 24-2). It spreads tissue without cutting and is used in soft tissue that does not resist needle penetration, such as fascia and muscle. It is preferred when the smallest possible hole in tissue is desirable and to avoid cutting small

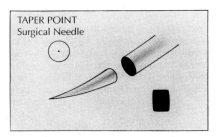

FIG. 24-2.   Taperpoint surgical needle. **Top left.** Front view of point. The geometry of this needle tapers to a point and has no cutting edges. **Side view.** The point of his needle has a narrow taperpoint geometry. **Bottom right.** The body of the needle has a side-flattened, cross-sectional configuration.

incisions extending from the hole periphery. Tapercut needles combine features of taperpoint and cutting edge needles. They are ideal for oral mucous membranes.

Tape

For certain wounds, tape offers the advantage over sutures of superior resistance to infection. Unfortunately, for wounds under tension injudicious use of tape can lead to wound edge inversion unless dermal sutures are used prior to taping. Tape is especially valuable for closing transverse lacerations over the brow, under the chin, or across the malar prominence. Benzoin tincture can be applied to the wound edges to improve adherence but should not be spilled into the wound as it may increase infection.

Staples

Metal staples also offer superior infection resistance but they do not provide the same meticulous coaptation as sutures. Skin staples, therefore, should be used in areas where the healing scar is not too apparent, such as the scalp.

SUTURING TECHNIQUES

The wound should be prepared as described in Chapter 23. Bleeding should be controlled by gentle compression with gauze sponges applied to the wound surface using aseptic technique. If this fails, use electrocoagulation. Larger vessels should be clamped with a curved hemostat and tied off using a 5-0 synthetic absorbable suture. The wound should be irrigated as outlined in Chapter 23.

Simple Interrupted Sutures

Before passing the needle through tissue, lay the free end of the suture away from you. Starting with the hand prone, introduce the needle through the tissue toward you. Because the ratchet mechanism of most needle holders is designed for right-handed people, most physicians prefer to hold the needle holder with the right hand, allowing them to hold the tissue forceps with the left. Be careful not to crush the tissue with the forceps. Rather than pinching, use one arm of the forceps to elevate the tissue as with a skin hook. (Figs. 24-3–24-10).

Dermal sutures

Dermal sutures are recommended for wounds subjected to strong skin tensions. They maintain the wounds' strength and prevent the development of wound dehiscence after suture removal. Dermal repair is accomplished with the least possible number of interrupted sutures using absorbable suture material with a compound-curved needle. Be sure to bury the knot (Fig. 24-11).

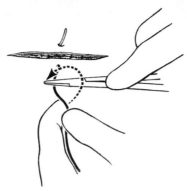

FIG. 24-3. Formation of first throw; position the needle holder. The instrument tie is performed with a needle holder held in the right hand. The left hand holds the fixed suture end between the tips of the thumb and index finger. The needle holder is positioned perpendicular to and above the fixed suture end. By keeping the length of the free suture end relatively short (<2 cm), it is easy to form suture loops **(arrow),** as well as to save suture material. Because the needle holder passes the free suture end through the suture loop, knot construction can be safely accomplished without detaching the needle from the fixed suture end.

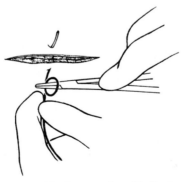

FIG. 24-4. Formation of the first suture loop. The fixed suture end held by the left hand is wrapped over and around the needle holder jaws to form the first suture loop. (If the suture is wrapped twice around the needle holder jaws, the first, double-wrap throw of the surgeon's knot square will be formed. A double-wrap, first throw displays a greater resistance to slippage than a single-wrap throw, accounting for its frequent use in instrument ties in wounds subjected to strong, static skin tensions.)

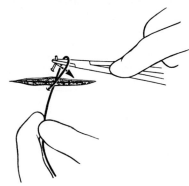

FIG. 24-5.   The free suture end is clamped and withdrawn through the suture loop to form the first, single-wrap throw. The tips of the needle holder jaws grasp the suture end and withdraw it through the first suture loop **(arrow).** The resulting first throw will have a figure-eight shape.

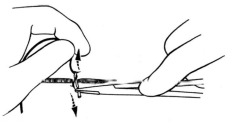

FIG. 24-6.   The first single-wrap throw is advanced to the wound surface. The figure-eight-shaped throw will be converted into a rectangular-shaped throw by reversing the direction of the hand movement. The left hand moves away from the physician, while the needle holder held in the right hand advances towards the physician. This single-wrap throw is advanced to the wound surface by applying tension in a direction that is perpendicular to that of the wound **(arrows).** Once the first throw of the square knot contacts the skin, the edges of the midportion of the wound are approximated.

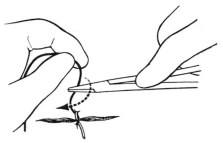

FIG. 24-7.   Formation of the second throw; position the needle holder. The needle holder releases the free suture end. The right hand holding the needle holder moves away from the physician to be positioned perpendicular to and above the fixed suture ends. The second throw will be formed by the left hand as it wraps the fixed suture end over and around the needle holder jaws **(arrow).** If the needle holder is placed beneath the fixed suture end, the ultimate knot construction would be a granny knot (1 × 1).

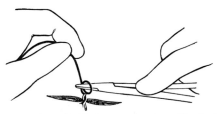

FIG. 24-8.   Formation of the second suture loop. The fixed suture end held by the left hand is wrapped over and around the needle holder to form the second suture loop. With the suture wrapped around the needle-holder jaws, the needle holder is moved to grasp the free suture end, after which it is withdrawn through the suture loop.

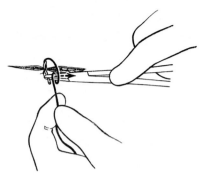

FIG. 24-9.   The suture end is clamped and withdrawn through the suture loop to form the second, single-wrap throw. The tips of the needle-holder jaws grasp the free suture end and withdraw it through the second suture loop **(arrow).** By withdrawing the free suture end through the loop, a rectangular-shaped second throw is formed. The physician applies tension to the suture ends in a direction perpendicular to that of the wound.

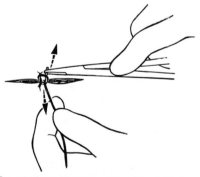

FIG. 24-10.   The square knot (1 = 1) is advanced to the wound surface. The second throw is advanced and set against the first throw by applying tension to the suture ends in a direction perpendicular to that of the wound. Advancement of the second throw is complete when it contacts the first throw and forms a square knot. Ideally, the physician should be able to advance the two-throw square knot to allow meticulous approximation of the edges is accomplished, the physician will construct a knot using this instrument technique, with a sufficient number of throws and 3-mm cut ears so that knot security is determined by breakage rather than by slippage.

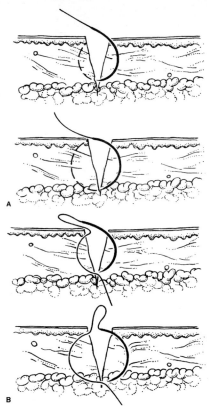

FIG. 24-11.   Dermal suture closure. **A. Top.** Dotted line is pathway of compound curved needle through left dermal wound margin. **Bottom.** Dotted line is pathway of standard needle with one radius of curvature through the left dermal wound margin. Note that the diameter of the pathway of the compound curved needle through tissue is smaller than that of the standard needle. **B. Top.** Pathway of compound curved needle through the right dermal wound margin. **Bottom.** Pathway of the standard needle, with one radius of curvature through the right dermal wound margin.

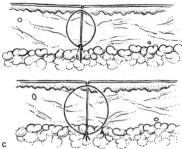

FIG. 24-11 continued. **C. Top.** Tied suture loop following tissue passage of compound curved needle. **Bottom.** Tied suture loop following
tissue passage of standard needle. Note that the diameter of the tied
suture loop constructed by a compound curved needle is smaller than
that of one constructed by a standard needle with a single radius of
curvature.

Continuous Percutaneous Sutures

These sutures can accomplish closure more rapidly than interrupted
sutures and accommodate better to the developing edema of the wound
edges during healing. Interrupted suture closure, however, permits a
more meticulous approximation of the wound edges. Two different
techniques are generally employed. In the first technique, the needle
pathway is at a 90° angle to the wound edges, resulting in a visible
suture that crosses the wound edges at a 45° angle (Fig. 24-12). In the

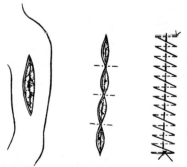

FIG. 24-12. Linear laceration of the arm subjected to strong skin tensions, with marked retraction of wound edges. **Center.** Three interrupted
dermal sutures markedly reduce the retraction of the skin edges. **Right.**
Continuous percutaneous suture.

second technique, the process is reversed—the needle pathway is at a 45° angle to the wound edges so that the visible suture is at a 90° angle to the wound edges.

Continuous Subcuticular Sutures

These sutures are attractive alternatives for wounds subjected to strong skin tensions, in patients prone to keloid formation, in children frightened by suture removal, and by people who are unable to contact a health professional for suture removal. Each suture is passed just beneath the dermal–epidermal junction. The suture is started as an interrupted dermal suture with its knot buried (Fig. 24-13). The next stitch is passed horizontally through the superficial dermis and, on exiting, is pulled across the wound at a right angle to the wound. Slight backtracking of

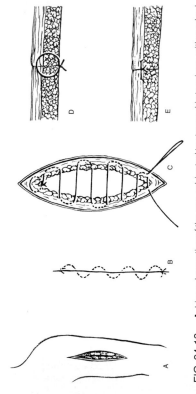

FIG. 24-13. **A**. Linear laceration of the arm subjected to strong skin tensions, with marked retraction of wound edges. **B**. Continuous subcuticular suture. **C**. Construction of continuous subcuticular suture. **D**. The subcuticular suture starts as an interrupted dermal suture with its knot buried in the subcutaneous tissue. **E**. The subcuticular suture ends by constructing a knot located within the dermis.

each bite will position accurately. One bite from the end of the wound, a small horizontal bite is passed toward the end of the wound, leaving a small loop. The suture passes horizontally through a small bite in the opposite wound edge, and a 5-throw knot is constructed using the loop.

Closure of U-shaped and V-shaped flaps requires special techniques, as shown in Figures 24-14 and 24-15.

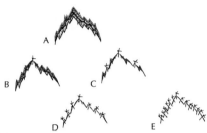

FIG. 24-14. **A.** V-shaped laceration with irregular wound edges. **B.** An interrupted percutaneous suture approximates the midportion of the wound. **C.** Two additional percutaneous sutures are used to approximate the lateral sids of the wound. **D.** Additional percutaneous sutures are positioned between the percutaneous sutures. **E.** The interrupted percutaneous sutures allow the wound to be reconstructed like a jigsaw puzzle.

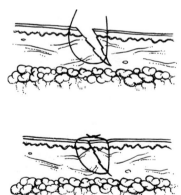

FIG. 24-15. **Top.** The edges of the V- or U-shaped laceration often have a beveled edge. Wound closure is accomplished by first passing the suture through one side of the wound, then through the other. This maneuver allows the suture to be passed through the same depth on either side of the wound. **Bottom.** After the knot is constructed, meticulously approximate the wound edges.

RING TOURNIQUET SYNDROME

Acute or chronic digital swelling can leave a finger ring tightly trapped at the base of the proximal phalanx, resulting in nerve damage, ischemia, and digital gangrene if not promptly removed. Several techniques are available for removing a ring. The finger involved first must be assessed for major lacerations or neurovascular compromise. Reduced sensory perception or diminished pulses call for immediate ring cutting. In the absence of neurovascular compromise, use ring-sparing techniques.

The string technique is especially useful in removing rings from a swollen finger. Wrap the finger in a spiral ligature from the distal interphalangeal joint over the proximal interphalangeal joint and to the ring (Fig. 24-16). Then pass the needle beneath the ring and advance the proximal free end beyond the ring, followed by slow unwinding of the suture until the ring passes over the PIP joint and can be pulled off the finger.

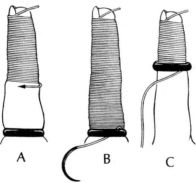

A   B   C

FIG. 24-16.   String technique.

An alternative to the string technique is the rubber glove technique. Remove a finger from the appropriately sized surgical glove and pull onto the involved digit. Position a curved forcep proximal to the ring; pass it distally to grasp the latex and draw it between the ring and the finger. The latex compresses the finger uniformly until the ring can be passed over the finger glove.

Embedded Fishhook

Several techniques are available to remove an embedded fishhook. Hook wounds do not require suture closure and are considered tetanus-prone. Antibiotic therapy is not warranted. The simple pull is utilized when the hook is superficially embedded in the epidermis or has a small barb.

Enlarge the entry wound 1 to 2 mm to help to pull the barb out (Fig. 24-17).

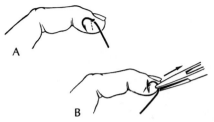

FIG. 24-17. Simple pull technique.

The string pull is well suited for hooks embedded beneath the dermis (Fig. 24-18). Pass the suture around the bend of the hook. Then direct the eye of the hook toward the skin and apply a sharp pull to the suture in the direction parallel to the shank.

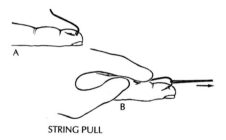

STRING PULL

FIG. 24-18. String-pull technique.

Push-and-clip is used when the hook is embedded deeply within a joint, cartilage, tendon, or deep subcutaneous tissue, or when the other techniques have failed. First anesthetize the overlying skin. Then advance the hook through the skin and cut the bend with wire cutters; withdraw the shank in a retrograde fashion (Fig. 24-19).

If Standard Treatment Fails

When standard wound closure methods fail to achieve hemostasis or the desired appearance, consultation should be obtained from a plastic surgeon or appropriate surgical specialist. Pressure dressings can be used on a temporary basis to stop bleeding while awaiting consultation.

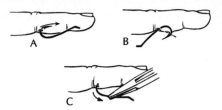

FIG. 24-19.   Push-and-clip technique.

For further reading in *Emergency Medicine, A Comprehensive Study Guide,* see Chapter 45, Methods for Wound Closure, by Richard F. Edlich, George T. Rodeheaver, and John G. Thacker; and Chapter 46, Technical Considerations in Wound Repair, by Richard F. Edlich and John M. Eggleston.

Soft Tissue Injuries to the Face

David M. Cline

SCALP

Emergency Department Care

The scalp and forehead are parts of the same anatomic structure (Fig. 25-1). Eyebrows should never be clipped or shaved because their delicate contour and form are valuable landmarks for the meticulous reapproximation of the wound edges. After the wound has been cleansed and hemostasis achieved, the base of the wound should always be palpated. Physical examination is often a more accurate technique for diagnosing injuries to the underlying bone than is x-ray examination.

When the edges of a laceration of either the eyebrow or the scalp are devitalized, debridement is mandatory. When debriding these sites, the scalpel should cut an angle parallel to that of the hair follicles. Wound closure should be initiated first with approximation of the galea aponeurotica with buried, interrupted absorbable 4-0 sutures. The divided edges of muscle and fascia must also be closed with buried, interrupted, braided absorbable 4-0 synthetic sutures to prevent further development of depressed scars. Some authors recommend single-layer closure with 3-0 nylon sutures.

The skin edges of anatomic landmarks should be approximated first with key stitches, using interrupted, nonabsorbable monofilament 5-0 synthetic sutures (Fig. 25-2). Accurate alignment of the eyebrow,

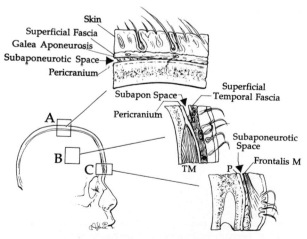

FIG. 25-1. Diagram of five layers of the scalp.

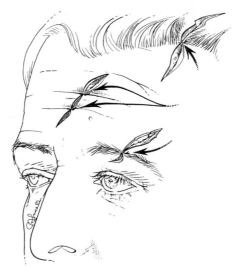

FIG. 25-2.   Key stitches in the eyebrow.

transverse wrinkles of the forehead, and the hairline of the scalp is essential. It may necessary to have younger patients raise their eyebrows to create wrinkles for accurate placement of the key stitches. A firm pressure dressing placed around the head can close any potential dead space, encourage hemostasis, and prevent hematoma formation. This pressure dressing should be left in place for 48 h.

EYELIDS

Injuries and Treatment

A superficial laceration of the skin parallel to the lid margin may require no closure, especially if aligned with the lid fold. If the laceration is not aligned with the skin fold, approximation of the skin edges with a running, subcuticular nonabsorbable, monofilament 5-0 synthetic suture is recommended. The suture should be removed 72 h after injury to avoid the development of epithelial cysts at the entrance and exits of the suture. Because the direction of this laceration is perpendicular to that of the dynamic skin tensions, wound repair will usually result in a narrow, aesthetically pleasing scar. In contrast, lacerations to skin the direction of which is perpendicular to the lid margin will heal with a conspicuous scar, often developing a linear contracture that causes an upward pull on the lid. A Z-plasty revision of the healing scar 6 to 12 mo later will lengthen the contracture and prevent this deformity.

Closure of a laceration that extends through the entire eyelid requires a three-layer closure, with meticulous approximation of each layer (Fig. 25-3). This technique should only be performed or guided by experienced operators; all others should consult an ophthalmologist or a plastic surgeon. After a protective lens is positioned in the conjunctival sac, closure should begin with a marginal, nonabsorbable, monofilament 5-0 synthetic suture, aligning and approximating the gray line, which is the end of a sheet of fascia between the orbicularis oculi muscle and the tarsal plate (Fig. 25-3). If the gray line is not approximated accurately, notching of the eyelid often results, with possible inversion of the eyelashes. Traction of the long untied ends of the marginal suture approximates the wound edges and aligns the anterior and posterior lid margins.

The conjunctiva and tarsal plate are then closed with interrupted, braided, absorbable 6-0 synthetic sutures; the knots are buried so they do not abrade the cornea. The orbicularis oculi muscle is approximated by interrupted, braided absorbable, 6-0 synthetic sutures. The eyelid skin is closed with interrupted, nonabsorbable, monofilament 6-0 synthetic sutures, the knots of which lie on the surface. A skin suture 2 mm from the lashes is tied over the long ends of the marginal suture, which prevents it from irritating the conjunctiva. The skin and marginal sutures are removed on the fourth postoperative day. In the following 6 mo, linear contraction of the vertical scar may be encountered, resulting in a pull on the lid margin. In such cases, lengthening of the skin scar with a Z-plasty corrects the deformity.

Injuries of the lacrimal system occur most frequently in naso-orbital fractures and soft-tissue lacerations. They may be difficult to diagnose because of severe ecchymosis of the eyelids. The location of the laceration and physical findings, however, can alert the emergency physician to a possible injury to this system, which may be caused by a laceration medial to the punctum from a knife, razor, or even a coat hanger (Fig. 25-4). Severance of the lower lacrimal canaliculus results in widening of the palpebral fissure. The orbicularis oculi muscle tends to enlarge the laceration and produce ectropion. Laceration of either canaliculus displaces the injured lid laterally. Proper management of injuries to this system is necessary to prevent subsequent complications, such as annoying epiphora and dacryocystitis. These injuries should be immediately referred to an ophthalmologist.

NOSE

Injuries and Treatment

Lacerations of the nose may be limited to skin or may involve the deeper structures (sparse nasal musculature, cartilaginous framework,

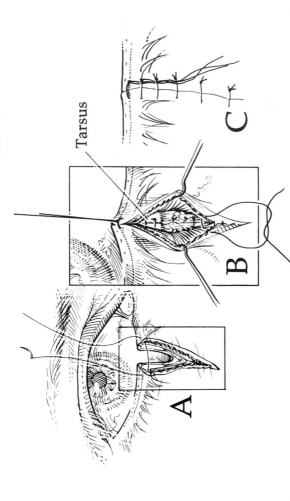

FIG. 25-3. Repair of lacerations through the lid. A scleral lens has been placed in the conjunctival sac. **A.** The first suture is passed through the gray line of the eyelid. **B.** The conjunctiva and tarsal plate are then closed. **C.** A skin suture is tied over the long ends of the marginal suture.

Tarsus

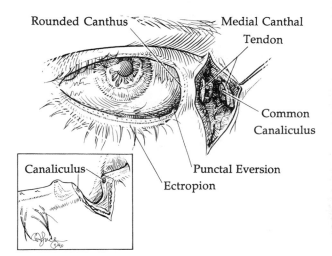

FIG. 25-4. The orbicularis oculi muscle exerts traction in a lateral direction on the medial canthus when the medial canthal tendon is severed. This results in a characteristic deformity with a rounded medial canthus and a decreased distance between the medial and lateral canthi. Insert: Laceration of the lower lid through the lacrimal canaliculus.

and nasal mucous membrane). They are repaired by accurate reapproximation of each tissue layer (Fig. 25-5). Inexperienced operators should refer such cases to an otolaryngologist or a plastic surgeon.

When the laceration extends through all tissue layers, closure should begin with a marginal, nonabsorbable, monofilament 5-0 synthetic suture that aligns the skin surrounding the entrances of the nasal canals, to prevent malapposition and notching of the alar rim (see Fig. 25-5). Traction on the long, untied ends of the marginal suture approximates the wounds and aligns the anterior and posterior margins of the divided tissue layers. The mucous membrane should then be repaired with interrupted, braided, absorbable 5-0 synthetic sutures, with their knots buried in the tissue. The divided edges of the cartilage should then be approximated with interrupted, braided, absorbable 5-0 synthetic sutures. The cut edges of the skin, with its adherent musculature, are closed with interrupted, nonabsorbable, monofilament 5-0 synthetic sutures. After wound closure, linear lacerations of the alar rim may shorten and result in notching of the rim 3 to 6 mo later. A Z-plasty at the alar rim will correct this deformity.

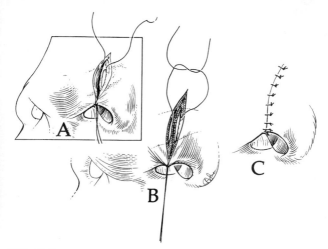

FIG. 25-5. Repair of a linear laceration extending through all tissue layers of the nose. **A.** A marginal suture should be placed through the alar rim to align the nasal canal. Traction should be applied to the marginal suture to align the individual tissue layers. **B.** The divided nasal mucosa and cartilage should be approximated separately. **C.** The skin edges are approximated by interrupted, nonabsorbable, monofilament 5-0 synthetic sutures.

A hematoma often develops between the septal mucoperichondrium and the cartilage after either fracture or dislocation of the septum or excessive bending of the septal cartilage. If not detected, fibrosis may develop in the hematoma, resulting in permanent thickening of the nasal septum, with partial obstruction of the nasal airway. Consequently, following any nasal injury the septum should be inspected for hematoma formation using a nasal speculum.

The presence of bluish swelling in the septum confirms the diagnosis of septal hematoma. Treatment of the hematoma is evacuation of the blood clot. Drainage of a small hematoma can be accomplished by aspiration of the blood clot through a #18 needle. A larger hematoma is drained through a horizontal incision in the mucoperichondrial layer along the floor of the nose. In bilateral hematomas, resection of a portion of the septal cartilage in the operating room is recommended to allow communication between both hematomas. Reaccumulation of blood can be prevented by nasal packing. Antibiotic treatment is recommended to prevent infection that may cause necrosis of cartilage.

LIPS

Injuries and Treatment

The technique of closure will depend largely on the type of lip wound. Superficial lacerations involve the skin and subcutaneous tissue. Deep lacerations may extend through the muscle and underlying mucosa. Each tissue layer of the laceration must be reapproximated meticulously (Fig. 25-6). The vermilion–cutaneous and the vermilion–mucosal margins are important anatomic landmarks that must be apposed by key stitches to prevent the development of a step-off deformity difficult to correct at a later date.

Repair of a laceration through the lip requires a three-layered closure (Fig. 25-6). Using skin hooks, apply traction to align the anterior and posterior borders of the laceration. Closure of the wound should start at the vermilion–skin junction with a nonabsorbable, monofilament 6-0 synthetic suture (see Fig. 25-6). The orbicularis oris muscle is then repaired with interrupted, braided, absorbable 4-0 synthetic sutures. The vermilion–mucous membrane junction is approximated with a braided, absorbable 5-0 synthetic suture. The suture ligature's knot is buried in the subcutaneous tissue. The divided edges of the mucous membrane and vermilion are then closed using interrupted, braided, absorbable 5-0 synthetic sutures with a buried-knot construction. Skin edges of the laceration are usually jagged and irregular, but they can be fitted together as the pieces of a jigsaw puzzle using interrupted, nonabsorbable, monofilament 6 0 synthetic sutures with their knots formed on the surface of the skin. During healing, a linear wound of the lip may undergo contraction, resulting in notching of the lip. The deformity can be corrected by a Z-plasty revision of the linear scar.

CHEEKS

Injuries and Treatment

Lacerations of the cheek are of great concern because they may be associated with injury to the facial nerve or parotid duct (Fig. 25-7). The site of injury to the facial nerve can be assessed accurately by assessing the functionality of the nerve's various branches. During its passage through the facial canal, the facial nerve divides into several important branches: the greater superficial petrosal nerve, the chorda tympani, and the nerve to the stapedius muscle. The greater superficial petrosal nerve, which innervates tear production, can be evaluated by a modification of Schirmer's test. A strip of filter paper is hooked over the lower lid and acts as a wick. The patient is given a whiff of ammonia, and the rate of flow along the wick is compared to that of a similar strip applied to the opposite conjunctival sac. Loss of stapedius muscle function may be detected by an acoustic impedance bridge. The chorda tympani, which supplies the anterior two thirds of the tongue and

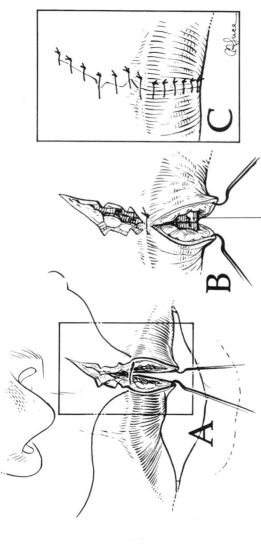

Orbicularis Oris Muscle

FIG. 25-6. Irregular-edged vertical laceration of the upper lip. **A.** Traction is applied to the lips and closure of the wound is begun first at the vermilion–skin junction. **B.** The orbicularis oris muscle is then repaired with interrupted, braided, absorbable 4-0 synthetic sutures. **C.** The irregular edges of the skin are then approximated.

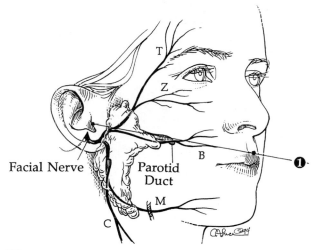

FIG. 25-7. The course of the parotid duct is deep to a line drawn from the tragus of the ear to the midportion of the upper lip.

innervates the submandibular gland, can be assessed by evaluating taste and salivary production. In cases of facial paralysis following blunt trauma without soft-tissue disruption, the prognosis for recovery is good and exploration is generally not needed.

Division of the submandibular glands and ducts does not require repair. The glands will drain through a fistula that usually develops after injury to the floor of the mouth. Lacerations of the cheek should be reapproximated with interrupted, nonabsorbable, monofilament 5-0 synthetic sutures in a manner similar to that of putting together a jigsaw puzzle.

EAR

Injuries and Treatment

A laceration of the skin on the lateral aspect of the auricle should get minimal debridement because skin deficits in this site are not easily closed without distortion of the cartilage. In through-and-through lacerations, approximating the skin with minimal cartilaginous suturing will restore contour without numerous buried sutures (Fig. 25-8). Notching the helical rim can be prevented by Z-plasty, which is best performed 6 to 12 mo after wound closure. Circular lacerations through the external

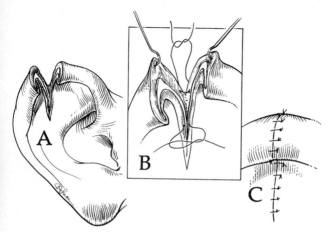

FIG. 25-8.   **A.** Laceration through auricle **B.** One or two interrupted, braided 6-0 synthetic sutures will approximate divided edges of cartilage. **C.** Interrupted, nonabsorbable, monofilament 6-0 synthetic sutures approximate the skin edges.

auditory canal should be closed carefully with interrupted, nonabsorbable, monofilament 6-0 synthetic sutures. After wound closure, the canal should be packed tightly with an impregnated gauze. A prosthetic appliance should be worn for 4 mo to prevent the development of stenosis of the canal. Specialist (ear, nose, and throat [ENT]) consultation may be required.

EAR LOBE CLEFTS

As with any laceration to the skin of the lateral surface of the lobule, debridement of the margins of a cleft wound should be minimal because deficits in this area are difficult to close without distortion of the cartilage. Any epithelial growth over the cleft borders, however, should be removed (Fig. 25-9). Using a sterile marking pen, a 1-mm margin is outlined around the wound, indicating the ultimate margins of the primary repair of the cleft. The margins are then anesthetized with 1% lidocaine, using a 30-gauge needle. After marking the skin, a #11 knife blade is used to excise the cleft tissue completely to a point just above the superior aspect of the cleft. The edges are approximated by interrupted 6-0 polypropylene sutures. ENT consultation may be appropriate.

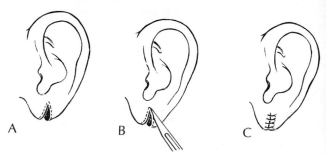

FIG. 25-9.   **A.** A 1-mm margin is outlined around the wound edges. **B.** A #11 knife blade completely excises the cleft margins. **C.** The wound edges are approximated by interrupted percutaneous sutures.

For further reading in *Emergency Medicine, A Comprehensive Study Guide,* see Chapter 47, Soft Tissue Injuries to the Face, by Richard F. Edlich.

| Fingertip Injuries

Stephanie B. Abbuhl

Fingtertip injuries can be divided into four categories: (1) digital tip amputation with skin or pulp loss only; (2) digital tip amputation with exposed bone; (3) injury to the perionychium; and (4) fracture of the distal phalanx. Successful repair of fingertip injuries require a knowledge of anatomy (Fig. 26-1) and an understanding of techniques of reconstruction.

DIGITAL TIP AMPUTATION WITH SKIN OR PULP LOSS ONLY

There are many techniques for management of digital tip amputations with skin or pulp loss only. Healing by secondary intention is the simplest. In children under 12, conservative management is preferred because spontaneous regeneration of the fingertip occurs, usually with excellent results. Alternative treatments use a nonadhering dressing, which is changed periodically until healing is complete. In adults, recent studies also suggest that conservative management may yield results similar to those in children, despite the decreased regenerative potential of soft tissues in adults.

Skin graft repair of a fingertip is frequently associated with induration and fissuring of the skin, reduced sensitivity in the area, and problems involving the donor site. In patients who have had split-thickness skin grafts, tenderness and cold sensitivity at the graft site are common complaints. Regardless of what technique is used, patients will experience some cold intolerance and aberration in sensitivity approximately 30% to 50% of the time.

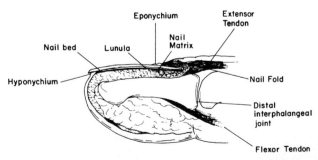

FIG. 26-1. The anatomy of the tingertip is shown in sagittal section.

DIGITAL TIP AMPUTATION WITH EXPOSED BONE

There are two additional treatment considerations when bone is exposed in a digital tip amputation. Rongeuring of a small protruding portion of the phalanx may be performed to shorten the fingertip and allow healing by secondary intention. Another choice is microsurgical reimplantation, when the amputated part is at the level of the distal interphalangeal joint or proximal to it. In a child, reimplantation of a sharply amputated single digit at this level should always be considered. Due to the thumb's critical importance to hand function, even amputations distal to the interphalangeal joint should be treated by reimplantation if suitable vessels are found distally.

INJURY TO THE PERIONYCHIUM

The perionychium includes the entire complex of the nail plate, nail bed, nail matrix, and surrounding paronychium. A force than can break the durable nail plate can disrupt the nail matrix and bed and will heal by scar formation (Figure 26-2). Scar formation in the matrix results in a split or absent nail, and scars in the nail bed produce a split or nonadherent nail. Meticulous repair of the nail matrix and bed will reduce the scar formation and should be done as soon as possible after the injury. The decision as to whether a nail bed or matrix laceration is severe enough to warrant suturing is often further complicated by an overlying hematoma, which makes assessing the nail bed difficult. In general, hematomas that have separated over 25% of the nail plate from the nail bed or matrix require removal of the nail plate for complete inspection of the nail bed.

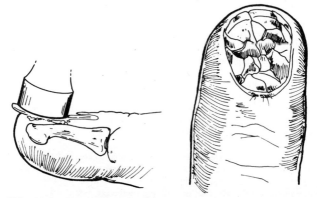

FIG. 26-2.   A hammer applies force over a large area, resulting in multiple stellate lacerations of the nail bed and matrix.

Small Hematomas

Hematomas involving less than 25% of the visible nail plate often cause throbbing pain, requiring evacuation of the hematoma. Regardless of the method of evacuation, the hole made in the nail plate must be large enough to allow prolonged drainage. Common techniques used include a microcautery unit or a paper clip heated until red hot by either a Bunsen burner or an alcohol lamp.

Large Hematomas

With large hematomas, the nail plate must be removed to allow visualization of the bed and matrix. Using appropriate anesthesia, a cleavage plane is developed between the nail plate and bed by opening and closing the blades of iris scissors. Using the same technique, a similar plane is also developed between the eponychium and the nail plate (Fig. 26-3). Gentle distal traction on the nail plate will then separate the plate from the proximal nail sulcus. The nail bed and matrix should be washed with a fine-pore cell-sized sponge soaked in poloxamer 188 or normal saline. Linear and stellate lacerations are repaired with 7-0 chromic gut interrupted sutures.

Occasionally lacerations of the nail bed are associated with partial avulsions of the nail matrix from the sulcus (Fig. 26-4). A suture placed from the proximal portion of the sulcus into the free margin of the nail matrix will bring the matrix back into position beneath the nail fold. Two incisions can be made perpendicular to the lateral curved margin of the eponychial fold to better visualize the injured matrix (Fig. 26-5).

After the nail bed and matrix are reapproximated, the nail plate should be thoroughly cleansed and replaced back into the proximal sulcus to serve as a stent and protective covering for the bed and matrix. A hole is burned through the nail plate at a point not directly over the repair site to allow drainage of any blood. The nail plate is held in place with an interrupted, monofilament 5-0 nylon suture passed through the distal end of the nail plate to fingertip skin. The fingertip is dressed with nonadherent gauze, and a volar splint is placed to protect the injured part and restrict movement. The dressing can be removed 5 days later to check for hematoma formation, which should be evacuated if present. The suture is removed in 3 weeks, although the nail plate will frequently adhere to the nail bed and matrix for 1 to 3 mo, until dislodged by the new nail.

If the nail plate is destroyed or too damaged to be used as a splint, several synthetic materials can be used. A nail-shaped silicone sheet can be sutured in place, although there is potential for mechanical interference with nail-plate growth and increased risk of infection; or simply cover the nail bed and matrix with a nail-shaped, nonadherent dressing extending beneath the proximal nail fold. After dressing

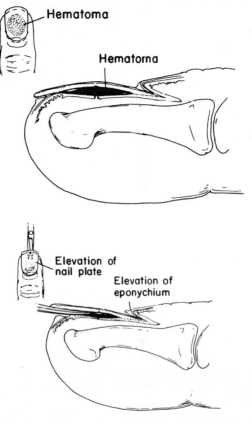

FIG. 26-3. A large hematoma involves more than 25% of the visible nail plate B. The nail plate must be removed to permit appropriate examination and repair of the nail bed and matrix.

the wound, a volar splint should be applied and left in place for 7 to 10 days. The gauze dressing can be removed 5 to 10 days after repair.

It is important to explain to the patient that nail-plate growth takes 6 to 12 mo. Patients should also understand that when there has been a severe nail-bed and matrix injury, nail deformity may be unavoidable and surgical revision may be considered in the future.

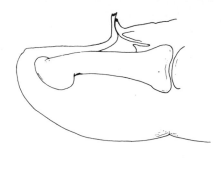

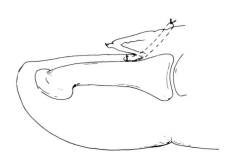

FIG. 26-4. **Top.** Partial avulsion of the nail matrix from the sulcus.
Bottom. A horizontal mattress suture through the proximal nail fold to the
avulsed segment of the nail matrix returns the matrix into the fold.

LACERATIONS ASSOCIATED
WITH A FRACTURE OF THE DISTAL PHALANX

Approximately 50% of nail bed injuries have an associated fracture of
the distal phalanx. If a fracture of the tuft or distal phalanx is present,
it must be reduced and the nail bed and matrix should be repaired, as
already described. If stable anatomic reduction cannot be maintained,
fixation with a .028-in. Kirschner wire is recommended.

Avulsion of the Nail Bed and Matrix

When a nail plate is avulsed, fragments of the nail bed can remain
attached to the nail plate. These fragments, along with other retrievable

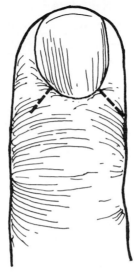

FIG. 26-5.   Incisions in the eponychium enhance visualization and repair of injury of the nail matrix.

fragments unattached to the nail plate, should be replaced as free grafts (Fig. 26-6). Even when the bare cortex of the distal phalanx is exposed, a graft will often survive. The graft should be carefully approximated to the nail bed segments using 7-0 chromic sutures attached to a microsurgical spatula needle. Pressure dressing is applied to prevent accumulation of blood and serum beneath the graft.

FRACTURE OF THE DISTAL PHALANX

When a fracture of the distal phalanx has occurred, any associated injury to the nail bed and matrix must be repaired. There is usually soft-tissue support of a distal phalanx fracture due to the dorsal nail plate and the volar pulp and fibrous septa. When the soft tissue support is lost, fixation of the fracture with a Kirschner wire is required. Splinting of the fracture is necessary for 10 to 14 days.

When a child is struck on the fingertip, the injury that often results is an open fracture of the base of the distal phalanx with the nail plate lying superficially to the eponychium. Because the epiphyseal plate is weaker than the insertion of the extensor tendon, an epiphyseal separation occurs, rather than a mallet finger. Management includes closed

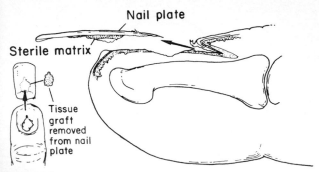

FIG. 26-6. Avulsion of a segment of nail bed and matrix is be treated by retrieving the avulsed tissue and replacing it as a graft. If the avulsed nail bed is not avilable, grafts of nail bed can be used to repair the nail bed and matrix.

reduction by hyperextension and replacing the nail plate back under the proximal nail fold after thorough cleansing.

Hospital Care

Reimplantation of a sharply amputated part proximal to the nail should be considered if suitable vessels are identified distally. In patients with nail-bed avulsions and no retrievable fragments, nail-bed grafting is indicated and is best done in the operating room. A full-thickness or split-thickness nail-bed graft from an adjacent amputated finger is a good choice for cover coverage of the avulsion. Split-thickness nail-bed grafts from an adjacent finger or from a toe nail bed also provide excellent donor sites.

For further reading in *Emergency Medicine, A Comprehensive Study Guide*, see Chapter 48, Fingertip Injuries, by Richard F. Edlich and Raymond F. Morgan.

| Puncture Wounds and Animal Bites

Stephanie B. Abbuhl

PUNCTURE WOUNDS

In evaluating puncture wounds, the major concerns are the potential injury to underlying structures, foreign body retention, and infection. Infection occurs in up to 15% of puncture wounds, with *Staphylococcus* and *Streptococcus* species predominating. Other organisms include *Aerobacter aerogenes* and *Mycobacterium fortuitum*. *Pseudomonas aeruginosa* is the most frequent etiologic agent in post-puncture wound osteomyelitis, particularly when foreign body penetration occurs through the sole of footwear.

Clinical Features

The history should document risk factors associated with an increased incidence of infection: larger wounds with deeper penetration; obvious contamination with foreign matter and debris; wounds occurring outdoors; wounds distal to the metatarsal necks in the forefoot; wounds penetrating through footwear; time interval greater than 6 to 12 h from injury; and wounds in patients with underlying diseases, including immunocompromised states, diabetes mellitus, and peripheral vascular disease. The potential for retained foreign body can be partially assessed by asking patients who removed the object and whether it appeared to remain intact.

Puncture wounds involving the forefoot carry the highest risk of infectious complications, as it has little overlying soft tissue compared with the heel and the arch of the foot.

On physical examination, the likelihood of injury to structures beneath the skin must be determined. The neurovascular status of the extremity distal to the site of injury, the function of all flexor and extensor tendons, sensation to light touch, and two point discrimination must be documented. The presence of infection is suggested when there is evidence of pain, swelling, erythema, warmth, fluctuance, decreased range of motion, or evidence of drainage from a puncture wound site.

A high index of suspicion should be maintained for the possibility of a retained foreign body. Materials such as wood, glass, and plastic and thin objects, such as pins and needles, can easily break and are common foreign bodies in puncture wounds. Development of an infection should prompt the search for a potential foreign body.

Diagnosis

Two-view plain-film radiographics should be obtained in all infected puncture wounds and in any wound suspicious for a retained foreign body. Many organic substances, such as wood splinters, cactus spines, thorns, and vegetable matter may not be seen on plain films. If suspicion for a foreign body remains high, other imaging modalities may be employed. Ultrasound has identified objects as small as 1 by 2 mm, with sensitivity as high as 95% to 98%, and specificity from 89% to 98%. CT scan and MRI are both good at contrasting between soft tissues and differentiating densities. MRI, however, cannot be used with metallic objects or with substances such as gravel, which produce significant artifacts.

Emergency Department Care

1. All puncture wounds require good local wound care. Irrigation is recommended, whenever possible, to decrease the risk of infection and to remove foreign matter.
2. Uncomplicated, clean puncture wounds in reliable, healthy patients do not appear to require prophylactic antibiotics. Although there have been no definitive studies to clearly outline which patients would benefit from prophylactic antibiotics, they should be considered for puncture wounds that are at high risk for infection, including: contaminated wounds; wounds occurring outdoors; wounds to the forefoot, particularly distal to the metatarsal neck; wounds penetrating through footwear; delay in treatment greater than 6 to 12 h from injury; larger wounds with deeper penetration; and wounds in patients with underlying diseases, such as peripheral vascular disease, diabetes mellitus, and immunocompromised states.
3. Wounds that are infected at presentation need to be cultured and have antibiotics initiated as soon as possible. Coverage should be directed at gram-positive organisms, especially *Staphylococcus aureus*, so that dicloxacillin, first-generation cephalosporins (e.g., cefalexin), or erythromycin are good choices.
4. Any patient who relapses or fails to improve after initial therapy for a puncture wound should be suspected of having osteomyelitis. Radiographs are indicated and any wound drainage should be cultured. A bone scan will be abnormal 48 to 72 h after the onset of symptoms. Broad coverage that includes activity against *Staphylococcus* and *Pseudomonas* is recommended. A reasonable regimen would be parenteral nafcillin, 1 to 2 gm IV q4h, and ceftazidime, 1 to 2 gm IV q8h.
5. Conditions for admission include wound infection in patients with diabetes mellitus, peripheral vascular disease, or other immunocompromised states; wounds with progressive cellulitis and lymphangitic spread; osteomyelitis; septic arthritis; and deep foreign bodies necessitating operative removal.
6. Outpatient management includes instructions for elevation and close followup. Patients with plantar puncture wounds should initially be nonweight bearing.

7. Tetanus prophylaxis should be provided according to standard guidelines.

HUMAN BITES

Human bites cause injury from direct tissue destruction, injury to underlying structures, and infection. Infection is due to the inoculation of tissues with normal human oral flora, which consists of gram positive and gram negative aerobic and anaerobic organisms.

Clinical Features

The evaluation of human bites should include the time interval since the injury, mechanism, location, depth of penetration, tetanus immunization status, medication allergies, and underlying medical conditions predisposing to poor wound healing. Of particular concern is the clenched fist injury (CFI), which occurs at the metacarpophalangeal (MCP) region as the fist strikes the mouth and teeth of another individual. These hand injuries are at increased risk for serious infection and any questionable injury in the vicinity of the MCP joint should be considered a CFI until proven otherwise.

The physical examination should include assessment of the direct injury and a careful evaluation of the underlying structures, including tendons, vessels, nerves, deep spaces, joints, and bone. Local anesthesia is usually required to perform a careful wound exploration. In a CFI, the wound must be examined through a full range of motion at the MCP joint to detect extensor tendon involvement, which may have retracted proximally in the unclenched hand. The examination must also assess a potential joint-space violation. Radiographs are recommended, particularly of the hand, to delineate foreign bodies and fractures.

Human bites to locations other than the hand appear to have similar rates of infection as nonbite lacerations. Human bites in children and bites to the face have exhibited low rates of infection, often less than 5%. Human bites to the hand, however, are frequently complicated by infection including cellulitis, lymphangitis, abscess formation, tenosynovitis, septic arthritis, and osteomyelitis. Frequent organisms in human bite infections are *Streptococcus viridans, Staphylococcus aureus, Haemophilus* species, *Bacteroides* species, *Fusobacterium* species and *Peptostreptococcus* species. *Eikenella corrodens* has been associated in up to 25% of wounds due to CFI and is a common cause of osteomyelitis.

Diagnosis and Differential

A good history and physical exam usually will reveal a straightforward diagnosis. There are times, however, when a patient may try to conceal or deny the true etiology of a human bite and a high degree of suspicion is warranted, particularly when the wound is on the hand. It is important to keep in mind that viral diseases can also be transmitted by human bites (i.e., herpes simplex, herpetic whitlow, and hepatitis B). The potential risk of acquiring HIV through a human bite appears to be negligible.

Emergency Department Care

1. Copious wound irrigation with a normal saline solution and debridement of devitalized tissue are critical to initial management.
2. Human bite wounds to the hand should initially be left open. Other sites can undergo primary closure unless there is a high degree of suspicion for infection.
3. Prophylactic antibiotics should be administered in hand wounds as soon as possible. In bites to other locations, antibiotics are recommended only when there is a risk factor, such as asplenia, diabetes mellitus, immune deficiency, and the like. Dicloxacillin, 500 mg po qid, plus penicillin, 500 mg po qid, is the best low-cost choice for coverage of both aerobic and anaerobic pathogens. Cefuroxime, 500 mg po bid, amoxicillin/clavulanic acid, 500 mg po tid, or erythromycin 500 mg po qid are reasonable alternatives. A 3- to 5-day course of antibiotics is recommended.
4. Wounds that are infected at presentation require systemic antibiotics after cultures are obtained. Unless the infection is quite mild, these patients also require admission for parenteral antibiotics and possible surgical intervention. Penicillin (or ampicillin), plus a penicillinase-resistant penicillin (nafcillin, 1–2 gm IV q6h), or a second-generation cephalosporin (i.e., **cefoxitin,** 1–2 gm IV q6h) provides reasonable coverage. Diabetics should receive a parenteral aminoglycoside (i.e., **gentamicin** 2 mg/kg IV loading dose).
5. Other patients who require admission are those with wounds involving joint or bone.
6. Outpatient management of human bite wounds to the hand can be reliable patients who present without delay (<18–24 h). They must be instructed to return in 24 h for re-examination of the wound.
7. All wounds should be bandaged with a bulky dressing and be elevated and immobilized.
8. All patients with human bite wounds should receive tetanus immunization according to standard guidelines.

ANIMAL BITES

As with human bites, dog and cat bites can cause injury from direct tissue destruction, injury to underlying structures, and infection.

Dog Bites

Clinical Features and Diagnosis

A thorough history and physical exam as outlined in the section on human bites are required to assess the extent of the wound and the likelihood of infection. Radiographs are recommended if there is evidence of infection, suspicion of foreign body, bony involvement, or large dog intracranial penetration bites to the heads of small children.

Infections from dog bite wounds are often polymicrobial and include both aerobic and anaerobic bacteria. *Staphylococcus aureus, Pasteurella multocida,* alpha-hemolytic streptococci, *Actinomyces,* and *Bacteroides* species are among the most frequent isolates. *Capnocytophaga canimorsus* is a fastidious, gram-negative bacillus that has been associated with severe infection, causing sepsis, DIC, and cardiopulmonary failure.

Emergency Department Care

1. All dog bite wounds require appropriate local wound care with copious irrigation and debridement of devitalized tissue.
2. Primary closure has been successful in wounds to the head and neck, torso, and extremities other than the hands. Hand wounds should be left open initially, followed by delayed primary wound closure in 3 to 5 days.
3. Prophylactic antibiotics should be considered for wounds that are at high risk for infection, including: puncture wounds; hand or lower extremity wounds; delay in treatment greater than 24 h; wounds requiring debridement; wounds involving joints, ligaments, tendons or fractures; wounds in patients who are high risk hosts or over the age of 50. A first-generation cephalosporin (e.g., **cephalexin,** 25–50 mg/kg/day divided qid; 500 mg in adults) or an antistaphylococcal penicillin (e.g., **dicloxacillin** 12–25 mg/kg/day divided qid; 500 mg in adults) is a good first choice. Erythromycin or trimethoprim/sulfamethoxazole are alternatives in the penicillin-allergic patient. **Penicillin** (500 mg qid) is the drug of choice for *C. canimorsus* and should be used prophylactically in high-risk patients, such as those with asplenia, alcoholism, chronic lung disease, or other debilitating diseases. Cephalosporins, tetracyclines, erythromycin, and clindamycin are reasonable alternatives.
4. Wounds that are infected at presentation need to be cultured and have antibiotics initiated as soon as possible. Reliable, low-risk patients with only a local cellulitis and no involvement of underlying structures can be managed as outpatients with close followup. Infection developing within 24 h of injury suggests *Pasteurella multocida* and treatment with penicillin VK is recommended. Tetracycline in adults and erythromycin in children or pregnant females are alternatives. A wound infection that develops after 24 h often implicates staph and strep, and these patients should receive dicloxacillin or cephalexin (dosed as above).
5. Significant wound infections require admission and parenteral antibiotics. Examples include infected wounds with evidence of lymphangitis, lymphadenitis, tenosynovitis, septic arthritis, osteomyelitis, systemic signs, and injury to underlying structures, such as tendons,

joints or bone. Intravenous penicillin G (250,000 units/kg/day) and nafcillin (1–2 gm IV q4h) are good initial antibiotics while waiting for wound culture results. If gram-negative organisms are suspected, an aminoglycoside should be added. If an aminoglycoside is contraindicated, a second- or third-generation cephalosporin can be added. When sepsis is a consideration, broad coverage with imipenum/cilastin or ampicillin/sulbactam is appropriate.

6. Bandaging and tetanus immunization are the same as for human bites.

Cat Bites

Clinical Features

Cat bites are often puncture wounds because of the animal's long, slender fangs. The major pathogen is *Pasteurella multocida*, which causes a rapidly developing infection with prominent symptoms of pain and swelling. Many patients with septic arthritis due to *P. multocida* have altered host defenses due to glucocorticoids or alcoholism.

Emergency Department Care

1. All cat bite wounds require appropriate local wound care with copious irrigation and debridement of devitalized tissue.
2. Primary wound closure is usually indicated, except in puncture wounds and lacerations smaller than 1 to 2 cm, as they cannot be adequately cleaned. Delayed primary closure can be employed in cosmetically important areas.
3. Prophylactic antibiotics should be administered to high-risk patients, which includes patients with: puncture wounds, particularly to the hand; those with deeper wounds or a; delay in treatment; immunocompromised patients, and patients with arthritis or prosthetic joints. **Dicloxacillin** (12–25 mg/kg/day divided qid, 500 mg in adults) or **cephalexin** (25–50 mg/kg/day divided qid up to 500 mg) is a good regimen and covers *Pasteurella*. Penicillin-allergic patients can be treated with erythromycin, or tetracycline in nonpregnant females.
4. Wounds that are infected at presentation need to be cultured and have antibiotics initiated as soon as possible. When the etiology of the infection is unknown, dicloxacillin or cephalexin are good outpatient regimens. Penicillin is the drug of choice for known *P. multocida* infections.
5. Indications for admission and the choice of parenteral antibiotics (penicillin G and nafcillin) are similar to those outlined for dog bites.
6. Bandaging and tetanus immunization are the same as for human bites.

Cat-Scratch Disease

Clinical Features

Cat-scratch disease occurs most often in young patients and presents with persistent regional lymphadenopathy in the area of the body draining the site of a recent cat scratch or bite. Often this is preceded by an erythematous papule or pustule at the inoculation site. Although most patients with cat-scratch disease are not seriously ill and spontaneous resolution is common, up to 2% can suffer from involvement in the CNS, liver, spleen, bone, and skin. The precise etiologic agent has been difficult to determine.

Diagnosis and Differential

Diagnosis usually requires three of the following four criteria: (1) a history of a scratch or primary lesion from cat contact; (2) a positive cat-scratch skin-test antigen response; (3) negative laboratory results for other causes of lymphadenopathy; (4) characteristic pathologic findings of lymph nodes, which may include organism detection by Warthin–Starry staining. Serologic testing may soon be routinely available to aid in diagnosis.

Emergency Department Care

Several antibiotics have been suggested, including erythromycin 250 to 500 mg po qid, clarithromycin 250 to 500 mg po bid, or ciprofloxacin, 250 to 500 mg po bid. A 28-day course of therapy has been described with successful resolution of symptoms.

For further reading in *Emergency Medicine, A Comprehensive Study Guide*, see Chapter 49, Puncture Wounds and Animal Bites, by Robert P. Wahl, John Eggleston, and Richard Edlich (particularly the section on Exotic Animal Bites in this chapter).

This chapter outlines general principles of wound dressings and prophy-lactic antibiotic administration.

WOUND DRESSING

The type of dressing applied depends on its intended purpose. Debride-ment of open wounds may be accomplished through the use of dry, or wet-to-dry, absorbent dressings. The larger the size of the interstices of the cotton gauze dressing, the more absorbent the dressing will be. Absorbent dressings will remove fibrinous exudate, the bacteria it contains, and prevent tissue maceration. If fluid strike-through occurs, the dressing no longer provides a barrier to bacterial contamination and should be replaced.

Sutured wounds (except face and scalp) require dressings during the first 48 h post repair, when they are most vulnerable to contamination. A topical antibacterial ointment may be helpful. Facial suture lines should be cleansed with half strength peroxide every 6 h until the wound edges are free from blood. Wounds closed with tape do not require additional gauze dressings.

Occlusive dressings prevent drying of the dermis, promoting epithe-lial migration, but excessive accumulation of exudate under occlusive dressings provide a culture medium for bacteria.

Pressure dressings minimize accumulation of intercellular fluid and provide immobilization. Elevation of the wound above the patient's heart will further reduce edema. Distal circulation should be assessed after pressure dressings are applied.

Abraded skin should be protected from the sun for 6 months to avoid permanent hyperpigmentation.

ANTIBIOTICS

The effectiveness of antibiotic therapy depends upon the time of admin-istration, wound contamination, and mechanism of injury. Preoperative antibiotic treatment is most effective but, when this is impossible as in traumatic injuries, early intravenous antibiotic administration should be instituted, followed by parenteral therapy.

Wounds should not be left open while awaiting repair, as further contamination may occur. Open wounds develop a fibrinous coagulum, which limits antibiotic penetration, although this coagulum may have a protective effect by plugging lymphatic flow and spread of bacteria. Cover open wounds with moist gauze dressings to avoid dessication and contamination.

Some wounds are at high risk of infection, despite antibiotic use. These include those contaminated with pus, feces, saliva, or vaginal

secretions. Wounds contaminated by soil fractions that contain negatively charged particles must be treated with acidic antibiotics, such as
the cephalosporins and penicillin.

Antibiotic Prophylaxis

Patients with prosthetic valves, arteriovenous fistula, patent ductus arteriosus, tetralogy of Fallot, ventricular septal defect, coarctation of the
aorta, or valvular disease, require antibiotic prophylaxis for bacterial
endocarditis. A broad-spectrum bacteriocidal agent should be used. A
preoperative or intraoperative intravenous dose is followed by an oral
course. *S. aureus* and *S. epidermidis* are the most frequent pathogens
causing endocarditis. *S. aureus* prevention is accomplished with a penicillinase-resistant penicillin or a cephalosporin. Vancomycin is used
for penicillin-allergic patients. *S. epidermidis* has developed many methicillin-resistant strains and is difficult to treat. An aminoglycoside combined with a cephalosporin or vancomycin may be helpful. (See Chap.
31 for dosages of antibiotics.)

Lymphedematous patients are especially prone to soft-tissue infections and should be given intravenous antibiotics prior to wound closure.
Immunocompromised patients, including those with diabetes, are also
at risk for wound infection and may require antibiotic prophylaxis.

The nature and anatomic site of the wound is important in determining
the need for antibiotics. Forefoot wounds, deep palmar lacerations, and
any extremity wound involving exposed bone merit antibiotic prophylaxis. Missile injuries, crush injuries, wounds >6 h old, lacerations
greater than 5 cm in length, and stellate lacerations are all at increased
risk of infection. Wounds contaminated with saliva, feces, or vaginal
secretions will need antibiotic treatment, however, a large amount of
bacteria will remain in the wound, so open wound management should
be considered.

Generally, a broad spectrum antibiotic is indicated for prevention of
wound infection, with consideration of the normal bacterial flora of the
anatomic site and the pathogens usually encountered in various disease
states and conditions (see Chaps. 26 & 27).

Tetanus Prophylaxis

Wounds at high risk for bacterial infection also may be tetanus-prone.
(See Chap. 85 for recommendations on tetanus prophylaxis.) (see table
28-1)

Drains

Drains potentiate the risk of wound infection by serving as a conduit
for bacteria into the deep layers of the wound. Due to the high risk of
infection, their use is generally discouraged.

For further reading in *Emergency Medicine, A Comprehensive Study
Guide*, see Chapter 50, Post Repair Wound Care, by Richard F. Edlich,
George T. Rodeheaver, and John G. Thacker.

TABLE 28-1. Identifying Tetanus Prone Wounds

Clinical Features	Tetanus-Prone Wounds	Non-Tetanus-Prone Wounds
Age of wound	>6 h	≤6 h
Configuration	Stellate	Linear wound
Depth	>1 cm	≤1 cm
Mechanism of injury	Missile, crush, burn, frostbite	Sharp surface (e.g., knife)
Signs of infection	Present	Absent
Devitalized tissue	Present	Absent
Contaminants (dirt, feces, soil, saliva)	Present	Absent
Denervated and/or ischemic tissue	Present	Absent

5 | CARDIOVASCULAR DISEASES

Myocardial Ischemia, Myocardial Infarction, and their Management

Frantz Melio

MYOCARDIAL ISCHEMIA

Ischemic heart disease and its complications is the leading cause of death in the United States. Approximately 1.3 million nonfatal acute myocardial infarcts (MI) and 500,000 to 700,000 deaths occur yearly. Fifty to sixty percent of these patients will die prior to hospital arrival. The majority of additional deaths will occur early during initial hospitalization. Risk factor modification and improved medical care has decreased mortality by 40% over the last 30 years. Currently, the greatest potential for decreasing mortality and morbidity is by minimizing the time between injury and treatment.

Clinical Features

Myocardial ischemia results from the imbalance between myocardial oxygen supply and demand. The most common cause is narrowing of the epicardial coronary arteries by atherosclerotic plaques (coronary artery disease, CAD). The etiology of CAD is multifactorial. Seven major risk factors have been identified: age, male sex, family history, cigarette smoking, hypertension (HTN), hypercholesterolemia, and diabetes (DM). Cocaine is directly myotoxic, accelerates atherosclerosis and CAD, and causes MI in patients with no coronary artery disease. The progression from ischemia to infarction is a continuum. The process usually starts when an existing atheromatous plaque is disrupted (fissured). This results in platelet aggregation, thrombus formation, fibrin accumulation, and hemorrhage into the plaque, further compromising blood flow. Progression of this process to the point of total occlusion leads to cell death (infarction). Other causes of complete occlusion are nonruptured plaques, coronary arterial vasospasm, or coronary arterial embolism occurring at sites of narrowing. After acute coronary occlusion, ischemia and infarction progresses from the subendocardium to the epicardium over a 6-h period. Reperfusion within these 6 h has the potential to salvage myocardium and decrease morbidity and mortality.

Angina pectoris represents cardiac ischemia. Anginal pain is retrosternal and may radiate to the neck, jaw, shoulders, or the inside of the left or both arms. Associated symptoms include dizziness, palpitations, diaphoresis, dyspnea, nausea, and vomiting. Stable angina is characterized by episodic chest pain, usually lasting 5 to 15 min. The pain is provoked by exertion or stress and relieved by rest or nitroglycerin (NTG). Stable angina is usually due to a fixed coronary lesion. Unstable angina represents a clinical state between stable angina and MI. Physiologically, unstable angina is due to plaque rupture and thrombosis. There are three forms of unstable angina: (1) new onset angina (4–8 wk);

(2) worsening angina (decreased response to NTG, increased severity, or duration); (3) angina at rest. The natural history of unstable angina is 40% incidence of MI and 17% incidence of death within 3 months.

Variant (Prinzmetal) angina occurs primarily at rest (without provocation), but can be provoked by cocaine or tobacco use. Coronary artery spasm is thought to cause variant angina. MI patients present with severe anginal pain of 15 to 30 min duration. Elderly patients and diabetics may present with silent ischemia (painless) or atypical presentations (nonretrosternal chest pain, atypical radiation, weakness, dizziness, or dyspnea). Patients with inferior MIs may present with abdominal pain, nausea, or vomiting.

Ischemia alters normal cellular contractility and electrical activity. This leads to the major complications of cardiac ischemia or infarction, arrhythmias, and impaired ventricular function. The major determinant of prognosis in MI is the amount of infarcted myocardium. Heart failure usually develops when 25% of left ventricular (LV) muscle is impaired. When 40% of the LV myocardium is injured, cardiogenic shock occurs. Right ventricular (RV) MI occurs with 20 to 40% of inferior MIs. RV MI may cause hypotension, which is worsened by NTG, and signs of rightsided heart failure. MI leads to ventricular remodeling. Unaffected areas hypertrophy, infarcted area enlarge and may become hypo-, a-, or dys-kinetic. This may result in stasis of blood flow with resultant mural thrombosis and systemic arterial embolism (strokes, etc.). Cardiac output may drop, resulting in congestive heart failure. Infarcted areas may also undergo autolysis leading to rupture of the ventricular wall (cardiac rupture), ventricular septum, or papillary muscle (inferior MI). These complications can lead to pulmonary edema, cardiogenic shock, and death.

Arrhythmic complications are frequent and can be fatal. The incidence of lethal arrhythmias is greatest in the early phases of MI. The type of arrhythmia, but not the incidence, appears to be influenced by the site of infarction. PVCs are seen in virtually all MIs. Tachyarrhythmias are noted more frequently in anterior MI. Sinus bradycardia, first-degree atrioventricular blocks (AVB), and Mobitz I AVB are usually due to increased vagal tone seen in inferior MI. Mobitz II and complete AVB are usually due to structural damage to the conduction system seen in large anterior MI.

Pericarditis can occur during the first week post-MI. Dressler's syndrome occurs in the post-MI period and is characterized by chest pain, fever, pericarditis, and pleural effusions.

Diagnosis and Differential

The diagnosis of angina is based on history. Physical examination of patients with ischemia or infarction is often unremarkable. The clinician must determine if complications are present (arrhythmias, heart failure,

TABLE 29-1. Localization of MI Based on ECG Findings

II, III, AVF - inferior
V_1–V_3 - anteroseptal
I, aVL, V_4–V_6 - lateral
V_1–V_6 - anterolateral
V_{4R}-V_{6R} - right ventricular
Posterior MI have large R waves and ST depression in V_1 and V_2

and shock). New systolic murmurs may represent papillary muscle rupture. Friction rubs may be heard in the presence of pericarditis.

The most important diagnostic test is the ECG. Only half of MI patients, however, will have diagnostic changes on initial ECG. A normal or nonspecific ECG does not rule out ischemia or negate the need for hospitalization. The diagnostic yield of ECGs can be improved by recording additional leads (rightsided, 22 lead) and by obtaining serial recordings. Acute ischemia can be subendothelial (ST-segment depression) or transmural (ST-segment elevation). Ischemic T waves are deep, symmetrical, and invert. Infarcted, electrically dead tissue eventually produces Q waves. In the setting of MI, ST-segment changes are seen early, T-wave changes are variable, and Q waves take hours to develop. Infarcts can be localized by determining the ECG leads affected (Table 29-1). Prehospital ECGs can easily be obtained and transmitted, which can lead to earlier diagnosis and treatment of the MI patient.

Injured cardiac muscle cells release cardiac enzymes. Serial measurement of these enzymes is used to diagnose MI, but the role of these markers is limited in the ED. Many of the enzymes are not specific to myocardial injury (CK, LDH, myoglobin). Patients presenting early in the course of MI may not have elevated creatine kinase-myocardial band or LDH. The sensitivity of CK–MB immunoassays is 50% on presentation to the ED and rises to 90% if the duration of pain is greater than 9 h. Myoglobin, troponin, and CK–MB isoforms are released earlier than CK–MB. Monoclonal antibody measurements of these enzymes may lead to more rapid diagnosis. Patients with unstable angina will generally not show serial elevations of enzymes.

Echocardiography (ECHO) is useful in diagnosing impaired wall motion and anatomic complications of MI (ruptured papillary muscle or ventricular wall, pericardial effusion). Nuclear scans may also be used to diagnose MI. These modalities have been shown to be sensitive, but not specific, in the ED diagnosis of MI.

Differential diagnosis of cardiac ischemia or infarction includes pericarditis, cardiomyopathies, cardiac valvular disease, pulmonary embolism, pneumonia, pneumothorax, asthma or COPD, gastrointestinal disorders (especially esophageal disease), chest trauma, chest wall disorders, hyperventilation, aortic aneurysm and dissection, and mediastinal disorders.

Admission

Patients with acute MI or unstable angina who have either ongoing chest pain, ECG changes, arrhythmias, or hemodynamic compromise often require cardiac intensive care. Patients with unstable angina with resolved chest pain, normal or nonspecific ECG changes, and no complications should be admitted to a monitored bed. Chest-pain-free patients with normal or nonspecific ECGs can be admitted to a step-down unit. Chest-pain patients with low likelihood of MI can undergo serial ECG and cardiac enzyme testing in chest-pain observation unit and MI can be ruled out within 24 h.

Emergency Department Care

Most fatalities due to cardiac ischemia or infarction occur early. Optimum treatment depends on minimizing time delay to treatment. Strict attention should be paid to the ABCs. All patients suspected of having cardiac pain should be placed on a cardiac monitor, have an intravenous line established, be administered supplemental oxygen, and have vital signs obtained. A rapid screening, including risk factors and indications or contraindications for thrombolytics, should be performed. ECGs should be obtained within 5 min of the patient's presentation to the ED. Many of these steps can be accomplished in the prehospital arena.

Treatment of angina starts with a correction of modifiable risk behavior (smoking, diet, controlling underlying diseases). Nitroglycerin, aspirin, ß-blockers, and calcium channel agonists are all useful in the treatment of cardiac ischemia. There are three facets to the treatment of MI patients: (1) establish early coronary patency; (2) maintain patency; and (3) protect myocardium from further damage. Patency is established by thrombolytic therapy, angioplasty, or coronary artery bypass surgery. Maintenance of patency is achieved by anticoagulation. Protection of the myocardium is accomplished by reducing the heart's oxygen demand and increasing the oxygen delivery. Arrhythmias should be treated if the effect on heart rate exacerbates oxygen supply or demand imbalance, or if the arrythmia seems capable of deteriorating into cardiac arrest. Again, treatment should begin prior to ED arrival.

1. Aspirin is an essential drug in the treatment of cardiac ischemia or infarction. It has been shown to reduce cardiac deaths by 20%, a reduction similar to that of streptokinase (when used in combination, the effects are additive). The dose of **aspirin** is 160 to 325 mg given as soon as possible, chewed for more rapid onset. Aspirin and Indocin are used to treat Dressler's syndrome.
2. Nitroglycerin (NTG) reduces cardiac mortality by 20 to 30%. Oral and transdermal NTG are useful in preventing angina. Sublingual NTG (spray or tablet) is usually effective for the treatment of acute anginal pain. Relief is usually felt within 3 min. A sublingual dose

TABLE 29-2. Indications and Contraindications to β Blockade

Indications

Transmural MI (ST elevation and /or Q waves)
Reflex tachycardia or tachyarrhythmias with rapid ventricular response
Hypertension
Continued or recurrent pain
In conjunction with thrombolytics
Possible benefit: non-Q-wave MI and pain of >6 h duration

Contraindications

Absolute
Heart rate <60
Systolic BP <100 mmHg
Moderate to severe LV dysfunction
Signs of peripheral hypoperfusion
Severe COPD
Second- or third-degree AVB

Relative
Asthma
Severe peripheral vascular disease
Concurrent use of Ca channel blockers
Difficult-to-control diabetes
First-degree AVB

---

should be repeated 3 times at 2 to 5 min intervals. If there is no improvement with sublingual NTG, intravenous NTG should be started. Initial dosage of NTG infusions should be 5 to 10 μg/min. The dose should be titrated to pain and hypotension by 5 to 10 μg/min increments every 3 to 5 min. Doses above 100 μg/min have been associated with paradoxically increased ischemia. Nitrates decrease mean arterial pressure. They should be used carefully in the setting of hypotension, as they may further worsen perfusion to ischemic myocardium. NTG is not indicated in the setting of RV infarcts. A common side-effect of NTG is headache.

3. ß-blockers can reduce both the short- and long-term mortality in patients with MI. ß₁ blocking (cardioselective) agents are preferred (metoprolol). ß-blockers are useful to prevent attacks of stable angina. Indications and contraindications to the use of ß-blockers are shown in Table 29-2. Used in a setting of MI, the greatest benefit is seen when treated within 8 h. The targeted optimal heart rate is 60 to 90 beats per min in the setting of MI. Dosage of **metoprolol** is 5 mg given IV over 1 min (smaller doses may be used in patients with relative contraindications). This bolus is repeated twice every 5 to 15 min, for a total of 15 mg. **Esmolol,**

a short-acting ß-blocker, also can be used. An initial 500 µg/kg bolus is infused over 1 min, and a 50 µg/kg/min infusion is then titrated to a maximum dose of 200 µg/kg/min.

4. Calcium channel blockers have little benefit in the treatment of unstable angina and MI. Nifedipine increases mortality when used in the setting of MI or unstable angina. Verapamil has no significant effect in the acute setting, but it may be useful in the postinfarction period in the absence of heart failure. Diltiazem started 24 to 72 hrs after the onset of pain decreases mortality in patients with non-Q wave MI and no heart failure. Intravenous diltiazem and verapamil may be used to control ventricular rate in patients with supraventricular tachycardia.

5. Meta-analysis of trials has demonstrated a 30% to 40% decrease in mortality (thought to be related to decreased incidence of arrhythmia) when intravenous magnesium is given in acute stage of MI. ISIS-4 showed no clear benefit of magnesium over placebo. Magnesium therapy, however, was started 12 h later in ISIS-4. The recommended dose of **magnesium** is 1 to 2 gm over 10 to 20 min, followed by a continuous infusion of 1 to 2 gm/h.

6. Prophylactic lidocaine is not recommended and has been shown to have a trend towards increased mortality. Ventricular fibrillation (V fib) is reduced by 33%, but fatal asystole is increased by 50%. Patients presenting early (<6 hrs) and who are <60 yrs old are at higher risk for V fib and may be more likely to benefit from lidocaine.

7. ACE inhibitors have been shown to decrease mortality when used in the setting of CHF and in the postinfarction period. Their use in the acute treatment of MI is more controversial. When used within 24 h of MI, enalapril increases mortality (in patients >70), whereas captopril decreases mortality.

8. Heparin is used for its anticoagulative properties, which prevent the progression of coronary artery and mural thrombosis. Heparin may be used as a third-line agent (after aspirin and NTG) in unstable angina. Heparin bolus given early in the course of MI is an effective alternative to thrombolytics. In addition, **heparin** is a mandatory adjunct to thrombolytic therapy. The recommended IV dose is 5,000 to 10,000 unit bolus followed by a 1,000 to 1,500 unit/h infusion. Weight-based nomograms may prove to be a more appropriate dosing schedule. Subcutaneous dosing can be used with streptokinase. The dose is 12,500 units twice a day. Heparin use is associated with an increased risk of bleeding.

9. Thrombolytic agents open occluded arteries, salvage ischemic myocardium, and reduce the morbidity and mortality of MI. The choice of thrombolytics used is less important than minimizing the time between onset of pain and drug administration. Maximum benefit occurs when thrombolytics are given within 1 to 2 h of symptom

TABLE 29-3. Indications for Thrombolysis

1. Symptoms consistent with MI with onset <12 h
2. ECG criteria:
   >1mm ST elevation in 2 or more contiguous limb leads
   >2mm ST elevation in 2 or more contiguous chest leads
   New left-bundle branch block
3. No contraindications (see Table 29-4)
4. Absence of cardiogenic shock, unless mechanical reperfusion will
   be delayed >60 min, then use tPA

onset, and they should be administered within 30 min of a patients'
ED arrival. Some studies have shown time benefit and reduced
mortality with prehospital administration of thrombolytics. As
thrombolytics have potentially fatal side effects, the appropriate
selection of candidates for use is very important. Indications for
thrombolytic administration are noted in Table 29-3, and contraindications are listed in Table 29-4. Because of this need for selection,
only 20% to 25% of all MI patients receive thrombolytics. Thrombolytics are not indicated in the treatment of unstable angina. In
general, those who gain the most from thrombolytic treatment are

TABLE 29-4. Contraindications for Thrombolysis

Absolute
   Active or recent (<10 days) internal bleeding
   Active bleeding
   History of CVA <2–6 mo or any hemorrhagic CVA
   Intracranial or intraspinous surgery or trauma <2 mo
   Intracranial or intraspinous neoplasm, aneurysm, AV malformation
   Known bleeding diathesis
   Severe uncontrolled HTN (SBP >200 mmHg and/or DBP >120
   mmHg)
   Trauma or surgery at a noncompressible site <10 days
   Suspected aortic dissection or pericarditis
   Pregnancy

Relative
   Active peptic ulcer disease
   Cardiopulmonary resuscitation >10 min
   Use of oral anticoagulants (prothrombin time >15 sec)
   Hemorrhagic ophthalmic conditions
   Ischemic or embolic CVA >6 mo
   Uncontrolled HTN (SBP >180 mmHg and/or DBP >110 mmHg)
   Puncture of noncompressible blood vessel <10 days
   Significant trauma or major surgery >2 wks but <2 mo
   Advanced liver/kidney disease
   LV thrombosis
   Infectious endocarditis
   Advanced age (>75 yrs)

patients who present early, with large infarcts (anterior), and without evidence of heart failure.

The decision to administer thrombolytics should be individualized. For example, elderly patients (>75 y) have more complications but benefit the most from thrombolytics. There is evidence that treatment 6 to 12 h after onset of symptoms may decrease mortality. The risk for CVA, CHF, and cardiac rupture, however, is also increased. Cardiology consultation before initiating thrombolytics in cases of delayed presentation is appropriate. Before administering thrombolytics, informed consent should be obtained (with particular attention paid to an understanding of the risks). Indications and contraindications should be sought and noted (this includes examination for equal pulses, stool guaiac, and pericardial rubs) and checklists may be very useful. Blood tests (cardiac enzymes, coagulation studies, type and screen, etc.) should be drawn when IV lines are started. Arterial puncture should be avoided, as should venipuncture or central line placement in areas which are not readily compressible. There are four thrombolytics currently being used in the United States. Streptokinase (SK) and tissue plasminogen activator (tPA) are the most commonly used. The other two agents (urokinase and anisoylated plasminogen streptokinase activator - APSAC) have distinct disadvantages limiting their use.

Streptokinase activates circulating plasminogen and is not fibrin specific. It is derived from ß-hemolytic streptococcus and is capable of generating an allergic reaction (minor 5%–5.7%, anaphylaxis 0.2%–0.7%). Hypotension, usually responsive to fluids and slowing drug infusion, occurs in 13.3% to 15% of patients. Antibodies may develop 5 days after treatment and persist for 6 mo. Repeated doses of SK or APSAC are not recommended within this time period. Other contraindications to the use of SK include the presence of hypotension, and streptococcal infections within 12 mo. The dose of SK is 1.5 million units given over 60 min. The half-life of SK is 23 min, and systemic fibrinolysis persists for 24 h. Heparin should be given within 4 h of starting SK. The GUSTO trial demonstrated no benefit of IV over subcutaneous heparin when used with SK. tPA is a naturally occurring human protein and is not antigenic. tPA is fibrin specific and has a half-life of 5 min. The dose of tPA is listed in Table 29-5. When compared with traditional dosing, front-loaded tPA has been shown to have superior 90-min patency rates and reocclusion rates without increased bleeding risk. IV heparin must be given simultaneously with tPA. Compared with SK, tPA is more expensive ($2000 vs $300), has a greater 90-min (but not 24 hr) patency rate, causes a higher incidence of intracranial bleeding (0.94% vs 0.52%), and *may* (there were flaws in the GUSTO study) be associated with a decrease in mortality (6.3% vs 7.3%).

TABLE 29-5. tPA Dosages

Front-loaded

15 mg IV over 2 min, followed by 0.75 mg/kg (50 mg max) IV over 30 min, followed by 0.5 mg/kg (35 mg max) IV over 60 min

Traditional

Total dose 1.25 mg/kg (max 100 mg) over 3 hrs—60% given over 1 hr [6–10% of the total dose] over 1–2 min, the rest over the h), then the remaining 40% given over the next 2 h

The most significant *complication* of thrombolytics is hemorrhage, especially intracranial bleeding. External bleeding can usually be controlled by prolonged external pressure. Significant bleeding, especially internal, requires cessation of thrombolytics, heparin, and aspirin. Crystalloid and red blood cell infusion may be necessary. Anticoagulation due to heparin can be reversed with protamine. Dosage is 1 mg of protamine/100 units of heparin (heparin given as a bolus or infused in the previous 4 h). Cryoprecipitate (cryo) and fresh frozen plasma (FFP) will reverse fibrinolysis due to thrombolytics. Ten units of cryo are initially given, and fibrinogen levels are obtained. If the fibrinogen level is <1 g/L, repeat the dose of cryo. If bleeding continues despite a fibrinogen >1 g/L, or if fibrinogen is <1 g/L after 20 units of cryo, then administer 2 units of FFP. If this does not control hemorrhage, then platelets or antifibrinolytic agents (aminocaproic acid or tranexamic acid) are indicated. Intracranial hemorrhage requires all of the above to be initiated.

10. Primary angioplasty refers to the practice of emergent coronary angiography followed by angioplasty (PTCA) in lieu of thrombolysis. This procedure is successful in reducing stenosis to <40% in 94% of patients. In-hospital mortality is 7.2% (1.8% in patients eligible for thrombolytics). Compared with tPA, PTCA has a lower incidence of reinfarction and recurrent ischemia, bleeding complications (including CVA), and death. PTCA is also associated with greater improvements in LV function. There are three subsets of patients for which primary angiography or PTCA is especially attractive: (1) patients with MI in cardiogenic shock; (2) patients with nondiagnostic ECG; and (3) patients with contraindications to thrombolysis. Angiography also has the advantage of identifying patients who require bypass surgery. Although hospitals must be equipped/staffed with a 24-hr catheterization laboratory, cost analysis has shown that primary PTCA shortens hospital stays and lowers overall costs.

11. **Morphine** sulfate (2–10 mg IV, give in 2-mg increments) can be used to reduce anginal pain. Morphine has not been consistently shown to affect preload. Morphine may decrease cardiac output.

Morphine should be used with caution in the presence of hypotension and in patients with inferior MI.
12. Dysrhythmias should be treated as per ACLS protocols (see dysrhythmia chapter).
13. Right ventricular infarcts are treated somewhat differently than LV infarcts. Patients with RV infarcts are dependent on elevated RV filling pressures to maintain cardiac output. Diuretics and NTG should be avoided. Volume infusion should be used to increase cardiac output. Dobutamine is indicated if an inotropic agent is needed.

Management of Cardiogenic Shock

Cardiogenic shock (pump failure) in the setting of MI must be treated cautiously. Ideally, patients should have invasive monitoring (Swan–Ganz catheter) and be taken emergently for angiography and PTCA.

1. Patients in cardiogenic shock may have significant hypoxemia and may require intubation and ventilation. High-flow oxygen by face mask should be used at a minimum. Continuous positive airway pressure by sealed face mask may be an alternative, however, the effects on blood pressure and cardiac output should be monitored.
2. Hypotension in the absence of hypovolemia should be treated with vasopressors. Dopamine, although it will increase afterload and myocardial work, is a good agent to treat hypotension in this setting. Start **dopamine** at 2 mcg/kg/min and tritrate to desired response (not to exceed 20 mcg/kg/min). **Dobutamine** (2.5–20 mcg/kg/min) is both a vasodilator and an inotrope and is effective in improving oxygen supply versus demand. Due to its inotropic actions, dobutamine is usually effective in treating mild hypotension. Dobutamine is not a vasoconstrictor, however, and will not treat severe hypotension and shock.
3. The addition of vasodialators may improve cardiac output. Intravenous **nitroglycerin** (5–100 mcg/min) is used to reduce both preload and afterload (primarily preload). Intravenous **nitroprusside** (0.5–10 mcg/kg/min) is a balanced venous and arterial dilator, but may cause deterioration in myocardial oxygen supply and demand.
4. **Furosemide** (20–40 mg IV) and other loop diuretics are used to decrease pulmonary wedge pressure through diuresis.

Nitroprusside, NTG, and diuretics must be used with extreme caution in the setting of hypotension.

If Standard Treatment Fails

MI patients with continued hemodynamic instability, pain, or those who have not reperfused after administration of thrombolytics are candidates for rescue angioplasty. Emergent coronary artery bypass surgery may also be indicated for these patients. Patients in refractory cardiogenic shock should undergo emergent angioplasty. Intra-aortic balloon pump or other LV assisting devices may also be indicated for these patients.

For further reading in *Emergency Medicine, A Comprehensive Study Guide*, see Chapter 51, Myocardial Ischemia and Infarction, by Gary P. Young and J. Stephan Stapczynski; Chapter 52, Prehospital and Emergency Department Thrombolytic Therapy, by Terry J. Mengert and Mickey S. Eisenberg; also Chapter 53, Acute Interventions in Myocardial Infarction, by Marcus L. Williams and David A. Tate.

| Congestive Heart Failure
and Pulmonary Edema

David M. Cline

Acute pulmonary edema is one of the most dramatic presentations of the many clinical effects of heart failure. The most common precipitating factors of heart failure are: (1) cardiac tachyarrhythmias, such as atrial fibrillation; (2) acute myocardial infarction or ischemia; (3) discontinuation of medications, such as diuretics; (4) increased sodium load; (5) drugs that impair myocardial function; and (6) physical overexertion.

Clinical Features

Patients with acute pulmonary edema usually present with symptoms of left heart failure, severe respiratory distress, frothy pink or white sputum, moist pulmonary rales, and an S_3 or S_4. Patients frequently are tachycardic, have cardiac dysrhythmias such as atrial fibrillation or PVCs, and are hypertensive. There may be a history of exertional dyspnea, paroxysmal nocturnal dyspnea, and orthopnea. Patients with right heart failure have dependent edema of the extremities and may have jugular venous distention, hepatic enlargement and, less commonly, ascites.

Diagnosis and Differential

The diagnosis of acute pulmonary edema is made with clinical findings and the chest x-ray; the severity of illness may demand that a portable anterior–posterior film be taken. Additional tests that should be ordered to help management include an electrocardiogram, electrolytes, BUN, creatinine, complete blood count, arterial blood gas, and possibly cardiac enzymes. The diagnosis of right sidedheart failure is made clinically, but, if the cause is left heart failure, the heart will be enlarged on chest x-ray. In the differential diagnosis, consider the common causes of acute respiratory distress: asthma, COPD, pneumonia, allergenic reactions, and other causes of respiratory failure. The second consideration is cause of interstitial edema: pulmonary edema associated with the precipitating factors listed above in the introduction and causes of noncardiac pulmonary edema, such as drug-related alveolar capillary damage, or that seen with ARDS.

Emergency Department Care

The treatment of patients in acute pulmonary edema includes oxygen, preload reducers, diuretics, afterload reducers, and inotropic agents.

1. Administer 100% oxygen by face mask to achieve an oxygen saturation of 95% by pulse-oximetry. Consider immediate intubation for unconscious or visibly tiring patients.

2. Administer **nitroglycerin** sublingually 0.4 mg (may be repeated every 5 min), or as a topical paste, 1–2 inches. If the patient does not respond, or the ECG shows ischemia, give nitroglycerin as an IV drip, 5 mcg/min and titrate.
3. Administer a potent intravenous diuretic such as **furosemide**, 40 to 80 mg IV, or bumetanide (bumex), 1 to 2 mg IV. Electrolytes should be monitored, especially serum potassium.
4. For patients with resistant hypertension, or those who are not responding well to nitroglycerin, **nitroprusside** may be used, starting at 2.5 mcg/kg/min and titrated.
5. For hypotensive patients or patients in need of additional inotropic support, begin **dopamine** at 5 to 10 mcg/kg/min and titrate to a systolic BP of 90 to 100. Dobutamine can be given in combination with dopamine or as a single agent, providing the patient is not in severe circulatory shock. Start **dobutamine** at 2.5 mcg/kg/min and titrate to the desired response.
6. Administer continuous positive airway pressure (CPAP) by face mask if the patient has not responded to the above therapy.

Coexisting dysrhythmias (see Chap. 2) or electrolyte disturbances (see Chap. 4) should be treated, avoiding therapies that impair the inotropic state of the heart. **Morphine** can be given (1 to 2 mg IV) and repeated as needed. Its use is controversial, however, and may cause respiratory depression and add little to oxygen, diuretics, and nitrates. Digoxin acts too slowly to be of benefit in acute situations. Rotating tourniquets do not reduce preload and should not be used. For anuric (dialysis) patients, sorbitol, and phlebotomy may have some benefit, but, dialysis is the treatment of choice in patients who prove resistant to nitrates.

Long-term treatment of congestive heart failure includes dietary salt reduction, chronic use of diuretics such as furosemide, 20 to 80 mg PO daily, afterload reducers such as captopril, 6.25 to 25 mg PO bid/tid, and digoxin, 0.125 to 0.25 mg PO daily.

Disposition

Patients with acute pulmonary edema should be admitted to the ICU and may require invasive hemodynamic monitoring. In the presence of new arrhythmias, uncontrolled hypertension, or suspected MI, the patient should be admitted for evaluation and optimization of drug therapy, usually to a telemetry bed. Patients with an exacerbation of chronic CHF without chest pain or complicating factors who respond to diuretics may be discharged home if followup is arranged.

If Standard Treatment Fails

Consider acute mitral valve or aortic valve regurgitation as a cause of the pulmonary edema, especially if the heart is a normal size. The patient may need emergency surgery. The initial ECG may fail to demonstrate AMI; for patients who deteriorate or fail to improve, consider repeating 12–lead ECG and giving thrombolytic therapy if indicated. The patient may have *cor pulmonale* and may not tolerate high-flow oxygen if hypercapnic.

For further reading in *Emergency Medicine, A Comprehensive Study Guide,* see Chapter 54, Congestive Heart Failure and Pulmonary Edema, by Charles B. Cairns.

31 | Valvular Emergencies and Endocarditis

David M. Cline

VALVULAR HEART DISEASE

The majority of valvular heart disease is chronic in nature. Acute life-threatening valvular incompetence, however, may occur in association with myocardial infarction (mitral incompetence), endocarditis (mitral and aortic incompetence), or aortic dissection (aortic incompetence). Acute right-sided valvular heart disease is most frequently found in association with endocarditis in IV drug users. Chronic valvular disease may present with acute symptoms due to increased demands on cardiac output, such as exertion, tachycardia, anemia, pregnancy, or infection. When considering treatment options to medically suppress tachycardia, remember that tachycardia can significantly reduce regurgitant flow and improve cardiac output in aortic regurgitation, whereas it compromises ventricular filling and cardiac output in aortic stenosis.

Clinical Features

Acute mitral incompetence presents with dyspnea, tachycardia, and pulmonary edema, with or without ischemic chest pain. Acute aortic incompetence may present with acute pulmonary edema, however, patients may also complain of fever and chills if endocarditis is the cause, or (tearing) chest pain radiating between the shoulder blades if aortic dissection is the cause. Aortic regurgitation may also present with systemic emboli, or persistent tachycardia.

The most common presenting symptom in chronic valvular heart disease is dyspnea, usually on exertion. Mitral stenosis may also present, with atrial fibrillation, systemic emboli, or hemoptysis. Aortic stenosis may present with syncope on exertion, angina, or myocardial infarction. Mitral valve prolapse is most commonly asymptomatic, but may present with atypical chest pain, palpitations, fatigue, and dyspnea unrelated to exertion. A comparison table of murmurs and signs is listed in Table 31-1.

Acute rightsided valvular heart disease presents with symptoms in association with endocarditis, including fever, chills, dyspnea, and sepsis.

Diagnosis

In the emergency department, diagnosis is often suspected by auscultatory findings. ECG is not confirmatory. Chest x-ray may show straightening of the left-heart border in mitral stenosis, pulmonary edema with less cardiac enlargement than expected in acute left-sided valvular incompetence or possibly, aortic dilation in cases of aortic dissection.

199

TABLE 31-1. Comparison of Heart Murmurs, Sounds, and Signs

Valve Disorder	Murmur	Heart Sounds and Signs
Mitral stenosis	Mid-diastolic rumble, crescendos into S_2	Loud snapping S_1. Apical impulse is small and tapping due to under-filled left ventricle
Mitral regurgitation	Acute: harsh, apical systolic murmur that starts with S_1 and may end before S_2 Chronic: High-pitched, apical holosystolic murmur that radiates to the axilla	S_3 and S_4 may be heard
Mitral valve prolapse	Click may be followed by a late systolic murmur, which crescendos into S_2	Midsystolic click. S_2 may be diminished by the late systolic murmur
Aortic stenosis	Harsh systolic ejection murmur	Paradoxic splitting of S_2, S_3, and S_4 may be present. Pulse of small amplitude. Pulse has a slow rise and sustained peak
Aortic regurgitation	High-pitched, blowing diastolic murmur immediately after S_2	S_3 may be present. Wide-pulse pressure.
IHSS	Harsh systolic crescendo–decrescendo, best heard at the apex or left sternal border	No opening snap. Apical impulse may be double. Pulse has a brisk rise and double peak

A clinically suspected diagnosis should be confirmed by echocardiography or consultation with a cardiologist. The urgency for an accurate diagnosis and appropriate referral depends on the severity of symptoms and the suspected diagnosis.

Acute mitral or aortic incompetence should always be suspected in a patient presenting with acute pulmonary edema, especially when the heart is smaller than expected on chest radiography, or the patient does not respond to conventional therapy. When aortic dissection is suspected as the cause of acute aortic incompetence and the patient is sufficiently stable, computerized tomography scanning of the chest is useful. Angiography may still be required after CT scanning.

Emergency Department Care

1. Pulmonary edema should be treated with oxygen and intubation for failing respiratory effort. Use diuretics (i.e., **furosemide**, 40 mg IV), and nitrates (**nitroglycerin** IV, start at 5 mcg/min and titrate up) if

tolerated. Patients with aortic stenosis will usually have normal-to-low BP and will not tolerate afterload reducers. In contrast, patients with mitral incompetence or aortic incompetence can benefit from IV nitroprusside or nitroglycerin even with normal blood pressures. In these patients, reducing afterload helps to reduce regurgitation and helps to relieve pulmonary edema.

2. The hypertension associated with aortic dissection should be controlled with beta adrenergic blockade (e.g., **labetalol**, 20 mg IV) or intravenous **nitroprusside** (start at 0.5 mcg/kg/min and titrate up).

3. Patients with valvular heart disease and acute pulmonary edema should be considered for Swan–Ganz catheter insertion. Valvular disease, especially stenosis, may complicate the procedure.

4. Rapid atrial fibrillation, which may precipitate symptoms in patients with silent valvular disease, should have rate control with intravenous **diltiazem** (20 mg IV). Emergency cardioversion may be needed in severely compromised patients, but recurrence is common. The most common cause of arrhythmia in valvular heart disease, a dilated atrium, remains unchanged by cardioversion. The danger of embolization is greater in patients with atrial fibrillation.

5. In the event of embolization, anticoagulation should be undertaken with IV heparin (5000 units IV, followed by 1000 units/h), provided there is no history of bleeding. This is especially needed in the setting of atrial fibrillation.

6. Prophylaxis for infective endocarditis is recommended during procedures that are prone to bacteremia in patients at risk for developing endocarditis. Patients considered at risk, include patients with a prosthetic heart valve, a history of endocarditis, rheumatic heart disease, acquired and congenital valvular disease, idiopathic hypertrophic subaortic stenosis, or mitral valve prolapse with a murmur. Common procedures requiring prophylaxis are listed in Table 31-2.

Patients with acute onset of valvular incompetence will be acutely ill and will require admission. Patients with aortic stenosis presenting with syncope on exertion should be considered for admission. Consultation with a cardiologist may be required to determine the need for hospital admission.

If Standard Treatment Fails

In patients that do not respond to medical management consider intra-aortic balloon counter pulsation, however, this is contraindicated in wide-open aortic regurgitation.

Emergency surgery should be considered in all cases of acute symptomatic valvular disease, especially mitral and aortic regurgitation. Because stenotic lesions are slowly progressive, emergency surgery is rarely needed for stenotic defects, but a patient with new onset of

TABLE 31-2. Antibiotic Prophylaxis for Infective Endocraditis

Procedure	Standard Regimen*	Alternative Regimen
Dental procedure known to cause bleeding Bronchoscopy with rigid bronchoscope	Amoxicillin 3.0 g orally 1 h prior to the procedure, then 1.5 g 6 h after first dose	Clindamycin 300 mg orally 1 h before procedure and 150 mg 6 h after 1st dose or Erythromycin ethylsuccinate 800 mg or Erythromycin stearate 1.0 g orally 2 h prior to procedure and one half the dose 6 h after the first dose
Urethral catheterization if infection is present Urethral dilation	Ampicillin 2.0 g IV/IM plus gentamicin 1.5 mg/kg IV/Im (not to exceed 80 mg) 30 min before procedure, fillowed by amoxicillin 1.5 g orally 6 h after first dose	Vancomycin 1.0 g IV over 1 h plus gentamicin 1.5 mg/kg IV/IM (not to exceed 80 mg) 1 h prior to procedure and repeat 8 h later For low-risk patient, amoxicillin 3.0 g 1 h before procedure and 1.5 g 6 h after first dose
Incision and drainage of infected tissue	Cefazolin 1.0 g IM/IM 30 min before procedure and cephalexin 500 mg orally 6 h after first dose	Vancomycin 1.0 g IV over 1 h plus gentamicin 1.5 mg/kg IV/IM (not to exceed 80 mg) 1 h prior to procedure and repeat 8 h later

*Includes patients with prosthetic heart valves and others at high risk. Initial pediatric doses are as follows: amoxicillin, 50 mg/kg; ampicillin 50 mg/kg; erythromycins 20 mg/kg; clindamycin 10 mg/kg; gentamicin 2 mg/kg; and vancomycin 20 mg/kg. Pediatric dose should not exceed listed adult dose.

syncope in association with aortic stenosis should be considered for urgent repair.

PROSTHETIC VALVE DISEASE

Patients who receive prosthetic valves are instructed to carry a card in their wallet that describes their valve. Prosthetic valves tend to be slightly stenotic and a very small amount of regurgitation is common because of incomplete closure. Systemic embolism, originating from a thrombus on the prosthetic valve, is the most important complication of mechanical models. Endocarditis occurs frequently during the first 2 mo postsurgery and *Staphylococcus epidermidis* **and** *Staphylococcus aureus* dominate. Late cases of endocarditis are similar to the those affecting native valves.

Clinical Findings

Many patients have persistent dyspnea and reduced effort tolerance after successful valve replacement. Mechanical valves have loud metallic-sounding closing sounds. Patients with bioprostheses usually have normal S_1 and S_2, with no abnormal opening sounds.

Diagnosis

New or progressive symptoms referable to the heart suggest a prosthetic valve disorder. Therefore, new or progressive dyspnea of any form, new onset or worsening of congestive heart failure, decreased exercise tolerance, or a change in chest pain compatible with ischemia all suggest valvular dysfunction.

Emergency Department Management

Patients with a prosthetic valve suspected of having acute valvular dysfunction or endocarditis require admission to the hospital and evaluation of the valve for possible replacement.

INFECTIVE ENDOCARDITIS

Infective endocarditis can be divided into acute and subacute forms, depending on the virulence of the infecting organism. Endocarditis can be further divided into left and right heart disease. Leftsided disease (aortic and mitral involvement) is the most common. The most common organisms include *Streptococcus viridans* (declining in frequency), *Staphylococcus aureus* (increasing in frequency), *Enterococcus*, and fungal organisms. *Pseudomonas* and *Serratia* are important etiologic agents in IV drug users in certain areas of the country, especially Detroit and San Francisco, respectively.

Rightsided disease is usually seen in IV drug abusers (60%) and is caused by *Staphylococcus aureus* (75%), *Streptococcus pneumonia* (20%), and gram-negative organisms (4%).

Clinical Features

Acute leftsided disease presents with sepsis, with or without cardiac failure. Typically patients appear ill with fever, chills, and tachycardia, and they may have significant congestive failure symptoms, such as dyspnea, frothy sputum, and chest pain. Patients may quickly deteriorate, with acute rupture of mitral or aortic valves. Murmurs are typically that of aortic or mitral regurgitation, however, the murmur is often absent or unable to be heard over lung sounds in acute cases. Neurologic symptoms secondary to aseptic meningoencephalitis and embolization of vegetations account for 29% of ED presentations. These complications most commonly are mental status changes, hemiplegia, aphasia, ataxia, or severe headache. Patients may have ophthalmic presentation complaining of monocular blindness.

Patients with subacute leftsided disease present with recurrent intermittent fever and constitutional symptoms, such as malaise, anorexia, or weight loss. The majority of patients with leftsided subacute disease have a murmur of aortic or mitral regurgitation or a change in their previous murmur at the time of their admission to the hospital. Many admitted patients, however, have murmurs not previously detected. Patients may have Roth spots, which are retinal hemorrhages with central clearing. Peripheral evidence of endocarditis includes Osler's nodes, tender nodules on the tips of the toes and fingers, and Janeway's lesions, nontender plaques on the soles of the feet and palms of the hands.

Rightsided disease is usually acute and presents with fever and respiratory symptoms: cough, chest pain, hemoptysis, and dyspnea. Chest radiography often reveals pulmonary effusions and multiple pulmonary infiltrates of variable size and shape.

Diagnosis

The diagnosis of endocarditis is based on positive blood cultures and evidence of valvular injury or vegetations. Three separate cultures from different veins should be obtained. Aerobic, anaerobic, and fungal cultures should be obtained before antibiotics are started. Echocardiography is helpful but should not delay appropriate stabilizing treatments. Nonspecific laboratory findings that support this diagnosis include leukocytosis, elevated C-reactive proteins, normocytic anemia, hematuria (25%–50%) and pyuria.

Emergency Department Care

The first priority in the care of patients with acute infective endocarditis is stabilization of respiratory and cardiac symptoms.

1. For patients with mental status changes and hypoxia or a compromised airway, control of the airway with oral intubation may be required. Cardiac decompensation is usually due to leftsided valvular incompetence or rupture.
2. Acute rupture of the mitral or aortic valve should be stabilized with afterload reducers, such as sodium nitroprusside, with insertion of a Swan–Ganz catheter for monitoring therapy as soon as possible. Preparation for emergency surgery should be made for patients sus-

pected of acute valvular rupture. Aortic balloon counterpulsation may be helpful for mitral valve rupture, but it is contraindicated for wide-open aortic valve rupture.

3. The second priority is drawing three blood cultures from different sites and then starting empiric antibiotic therapy.

4. For acute infective endocarditis, a penicillinase-resistant penicillin, such as **nafcillin** 1.5 g every 4 h, should be given with an aminoglycoside chosen on the basis of local patterns of susceptibility. In geographic areas where there is a high incidence of methicillin-resistant *Staphylococcus*, or in the case of a patient already taking oral antibiotics use **vancomycin** 1 g IV in addition to an aminoglycoside.

5. Patients with prosthetic valve endocarditis also should be treated with antibiotics that cover *Staphylococcus epidermidis*, usually vancomycin, 1 g IV, in addition to an aminoglycoside.

6. Although subacute cases are frequently caused by *Streptococcus viridans*, which is covered by penicillin G, patients with subacute presentations that require admission should be started on a newer cephalosporin, such as **ceftriaxone**, 1 gram IV, in addition to an aminoglycoside, until cultures and sensitivities are known.

In general, patients with suspected endocarditis should be admitted to the hospital.

For further reading in *Emergency Medicine, A Comprehensive Study Guide,* see Chapter 55, Valvular Emergencies and Endocarditis, by David M. Cline.

Cardiomyopathies, Myocarditis,
and Pericardial Disease

David Dubow

THE CARDIOMYOPATHIES

As a group, cardiomyopathies are the third most common form of heart disease in the United States. By definition, cardiomyopathy is a disease process that directly affects cardiac structure and impairs myocardial function. Primary cardiomyopathies originate in the myocardium. Secondary cardiomyopathies are the result of a systemic disease process or a toxin that affects the heart muscle. The cardiomyopathies can be further subdivided into three groups: (1) dilated; (2) hypertrophied; (3) restrictive.

Dilated Cardiomyopathy

Dilation and hypertrophy of the myocardium result in depressed systolic function and low cardiac output. Although no specific cause is found in 85% of patients, systemic processes that produce or are associated with dilated cardiomyopathy include: infections (viral, protozoal), metabolic (thyrotoxicosis, myxedema, acromegaly, hemochromatosis, glycogen storage diseases, thiamine deficiency), myocardial toxins (ethanol, heavy metals, emetine, adriamycin, cobalt), peripartum, amyloidosis, neuromuscular disorders, collagen vascular diseases, sarcoidosis.

Clinical Features

Depressed cardiac output results in signs and symptoms of congestive heart failure (CHF), including dyspnea on exertion, orthopnea, paroxysmal nocturnal dyspnea, and bibasilar rales. Because the left ventricular contractile force is diminished, mural thrombi can form. The patient may present with evidence of peripheral emboli, such as acute neurologic deficit, flank pain, and hematuria or extremity cyanosis. Murmurs may or may not be the result of valvular disruption secondary to ventricular dilation.

Diagnosis and Differential

Chest x-ray usually shows an enlarged cardiac silhouette and evidence of venous congestion. The electrocardiogram commonly demonstrates ventricular hypertrophy, left atrial enlargement, Q or QS waves, and poor R wave progression across the precordium. In addition, atrial fibrillation and ventricular ectopy are frequently seen. Echocardiography will verify the diagnosis. Other possible diagnoses include: acute myocardial infarction, restrictive pericarditis, acute valvular disruption, sepsis, or any other condition that could result in a low-output cardiac state.

Emergency Department Care

Patients with symptomatic dilated cardiomyopathy require admission to a monitored or ICU setting. ED management is symptom directed:

Supportive Measures

1. Establish intravenous access.
2. Place the patient on a continuous cardiac monitor.
3. Provide supplemental oxygen as indicated.

Specific Treatment

4. Intravenous diuretics (i.e., **Lasix**, 40 mg IV) and **digoxin** (max dose 0.5 mg IV), unless contraindicated.
5. Consider anticoagulation to reduce mural thrombus formation.

Hypertrophic Cardiomyopathy

This illness, including idiopathic hypertrohic subaortic stenosis, is characterized by increased left ventricular muscle mass without dilation. The result is reduced compliance of the left ventricle and impaired diastolic relaxation and filling of the left ventricle.

Clinical Features

The most common symptoms include dyspnea on exertion, palpitations, syncope, and chest pain. Chest pain is a result of inadequate oxygen supply to the hypertrophied left ventricular muscle. Patients may also be aware of forceful ventricular contractions and may call these palpitations. Because hypertrophic cardiomyopathy can be hereditary, there may be a family history of death due to cardiac disease. Physical exam will usually reveal an S_4 and a systolic ejection murmur heard best at the lower left sternal border. Maneuvers that will increase the murmur include: Valsalva, standing, amyl nitrate inhalation, and beta-agonist infusion. Interventions that decrease the intensity of the murmur are: passive leg elevation in a supine patient, forceful hand gripping, squatting, alpha agonist infusion.

Diagnosis and Differential

ECG will show left ventricular hypertrophy in 30% of patients. Left atrial enlargement will be evident on ECG in 25% to 50% of patients, and large septal Q waves will be present in 25%. Another ECG finding is upright T waves in those leads with QS or QR complexes (T-wave inversion in such leads is suggestive of ischemia). Chest x-ray is frequently normal. Echocardiography is the diagnostic study of choice.

Emergency Department Care

General supportive care as discussed above should be instituted. The mainstay of treatment is beta blockers. In patients who do not respond to beta blockers, calcium channel blockers may be beneficial. Patients who are going to have dental procedures or potentially unsterile surgery should receive antibiotic prophylaxis (see Chap. 31). It is appropriate to counsel the patient about limiting or stopping participation in competitive athletics, since sudden death with vigorous exercise has been reported with hypertrophic cardiomyopathy.

Restrictive Cardiomyopathy

This is the least common cardiomyopathy. Although no specific cause can be found in the majority of cases, some causes have been identified: idiopathic, including endomyocardial fibrosis and eosinophilic myocardial disease; and secondary, including hemochromatosis, amyloidosis, sarcoidosis, and scleroderma.

Clinical Features

Symptoms of CHF predominate, including decreased exercise tolerance, dyspnea on exertion, orthopnea, and paroxysmal nocturnal dyspnea. Complaints of chest pain, either typical of or atypical for angina, are common. Physical exam reveals cardiac gallop rhythms, systolic murmurs, pulmonary rales, and pedal edema.

Diagnosis and Differential

The chest x-ray is frequently normal. The ECG is commonly abnormal, but it lacks unique abnormalities. ECG changes may include ventricular or atrial enlargement, low-voltage QRS complexes and nonspecific ST–T wave changes.

Emergency Department Care

Treatment for restrictive cardiomyopathy, such as dilated cardiomyopathy, is directed at ameliorating the symptoms. Diuretics, digoxin, vasodilators, and antiarrhythmic agents, as needed, are the mainstays of therapy. Patients with amyloid-induced cardiomyopathy are especially sensitive to digoxin, so this medication should be used with caution in such patients.

MYOCARDITIS

Inflammation of the myocardium is the definition of myocarditis. Myocardial inflammation may be the result of an infectious agent or part of a systemic disease process. Common infectious causes of myocarditis include: viruses (Coxsackie B, echovirus, influenza, parainfluenza, Epstein–Barr, hepatitis B) and bacteria (*Corynebacterium diphtheriae, Neisseria meningitides, Mycoplasma pneumoniae*, ß-hemolytic streptococci). Pericarditis frequently accompanies myocarditis.

Clinical Features

Symptoms of a systemic illness such as fever, myalgias, headache, and rigors are common. Retrosternal or substernal chest pain is a common complaint and is usually due to associated pericarditis. Physical findings include fever and sinus tachycardia out of proportion to the degree of fever. In more severe cases, signs of CHF (cardiac gallop rhythms, pulmonary rales, pedal edema) may be present. In patients with accompanying pericarditis, a friction rub can be heard.

Diagnosis and Differential

ECG changes include: nonspecific ST–T-wave changes, ST-segment elevation (secondary to pericarditis), atrioventricular block, and prolonged QRS duration. Chest x-ray is usually normal. Echocardiography may demonstrate diminished systolic function.

Emergency Department Care

These patients require hospitalization in a monitored or intensive-care setting. Treatment for idiopathic myocarditis is purely supportive, as above. In patients with myocarditis due to bacterial infection, antibiotics directed at the cause is indicated.

ACUTE PERICARDITIS

Inflammation of the pericardium may be the result of several disease processes, including: viral infection (Coxsackie virus or echovirus), bacterial infection (staphylococcus, *Streptococcus pneumoniae*, β-hemolytic streptococci, *Mycobacterium tuberculosis*), fungal infection (*Histoplasma capsulatum*), malignancy (leukemia, lymphoma, metastatic breast cancer, melanoma), drug-induced (procainamide, hydralazine), connective-tissue disease, radiation-induced, uremia, myxedema, postmyocardial infarction (Dressler's syndrome), or idiopathic.

Clinical Features

Sudden or gradual onset of precordial or retrosternal chest pain described as sharp and stabbing is the most common complaint. Pain may radiate to the back, neck, left shoulder or arm, or be referred to the left trapezial ridge. Patients frequently state the pain is eased with sitting up and leaning forward and exacerbated by laying supine. Low-grade fever (especially if etiology is infectious), dyspnea, and dysphagia are other symptoms. Physical exam may demonstrate fever and a resting tachycardia. Paradoxical pulse, venous distention, and Kussmaul's sign (inspiratory neck-vein distention) are indicators of increased pericardial pressure secondary to pericardial effusion. A transient friction rub is the most common and important physical finding. The rub is best heard with the patient sitting up and leaning forward.

Diagnosis and Differential

ECG changes include: ST-segment elevation most prominent in leads V_5 and V_6 and limb lead I. PR-segment depression may be seen in leads II, aVF, and V_4 through V_6. In the later stages of pericarditis the ST segment will normalize, the T-wave amplitude decreases, and the T wave will invert in leads previously demonstrating ST-segment elevation. It is hard to distinguish between the ST- and T-wave abnormalities seen with early repolarization and those of pericarditis. Pericarditis without other associated cardiac disease (e.g., myocarditis) does not cause significant dysrhythmias. Chest x-ray should be done to check for other causes of pain. Echocardiography is the diagnostic test of choice to check for pericardial effusion. Other tests include: CBC with differential, BUN and creatinine (to assess for uremic etiology), streptococcal serology, blood cultures (if bacterial infection is suspected), appropriate viral serology, other serological studies (antinuclear antibodies, anti-DNA, rheumatoid arthritis latex fixation), thyroid function studies, erythrocyte sedimentation rate, and creatinine kinase with MB fraction (to assess for associated myocarditis).

Emergency Department Care

Patients with idiopathic or presumed viral pericarditis are treated with nonsteroidal anti-inflammatory agents (NSAID) (**ibuprofen,** 400–600 mg qid, or **indomethacin,** 25–50 mg q6h) for 1 to 3 wk. When a specific cause can be identified, treatment is directed at the underlying disease. Any patient with evidence of myocarditis or hemodynamic compromise should be admitted to a monitored bed or ICU.

CONSTRICTIVE PERICARDITIS

Following acute pericardial injury, fibrous thickening and loss of elasticity of the pericardium may occur. Constriction occurs when fibrosis interferes with passive diastolic filling of the ventricle. Cardiac trauma, pericardiotomy (open heart surgery), intrapericardial hemorrhage, fungal or bacterial pericarditis, and uremic pericarditis are the most common causes. Constrictive pericarditis is commonly a chronic process, but acute symptoms may develop if a pericardial effusion develops within a fibrotic pericardial sac.

Clinical Features

Gradual onset of the symptoms of CHF (exertional dyspnea and decreased exercise tolerance) are common. Orthopnea, paroxysmal nocturnal dyspnea, however, are uncommon. Physical exam will reveal jugular venous distention, Kussmaul's sign (inspiratory neck vein distention), hepatomegaly, ascites, and pedal edema. Although an early diastolic pericardial knock may be heard at the apex following the second heart sound, a friction rub is not usually auscultated.

Diagnosis and Differential

ECG findings are not diagnostic, but may include low-voltage QRS complexes and inverted T waves. Chest x-ray demonstrates pericardial calcification in up to 50% of patients. There is usually little or no evidence of pulmonary venous congestion on x-ray. Echocardiography might demonstrate pericardial thickening or an effusion, but it is not as useful as in acute pericarditis. Other causes of the patient's condition should be considered, including: acute myocardial infarction, acute pericarditis or myocarditis, exacerbation of chronic ventricular dysfunction, or a systemic process resulting in decreased cardiac performance.

Emergency Department Care

In symptomatic cases, pericardiectomy is the treatment of choice. General supportive care should be delivered pending surgical treatment.

For further reading in *Emergency Medicine, A Comprehensive Study Guide*, see Chapter 56, The Cardiomyopathies, Myocarditis, and Pericardial Disease, by James T. Niemann.

Pulmonary Embolism

David M. Cline

Pulmonary embolism (PE) is a common deadly disorder difficult to diagnose. Risk factors include CHF, acute MI, COPD, pregnancy, prolonged immobilization, previous history of PE, history of deep-vein thrombosis (DVT), marked obesity, malignancy, estrogen use, surgery in the last 3 mo, or lower extremity trauma.

Clinical Features

The diagnosis of PE should be considered in any patient at risk who experiences acute dyspnea, chest pain, syncope, or shock. Common symptoms in decreasing order of frequency include dyspnea, pleuritic chest pain, anxiety, cough, hemoptysis, sweats, nonpleuritic chest pain, and syncope. Common signs in decreasing order of frequency include respiration >16, rales, pulse >100, temperature >37.8 C (100.4 F), phlebitis or DVT, cardiac gallop, and diaphoresis. The presence or absence of any symptom or sign does not confirm or exclude the diagnosis of pulmonary embolism.

Diagnosis and Differential

First the clinician must suspect the diagnosis of PE in patients at risk. Second, supplementary tests, including an ABG, 12-lead ECG, and chest x-ray will help to direct further testing and treatment. The diagnosis can be excluded or confirmed only with more sophisticated tests, such as a ventilation–perfusion lung scan (V–Q scan) or pulmonary angiography. The ABG will demonstrate a PaO_2 less than 81 mmHg in 80% of patients with PE. As many as 5% of patients with PE will have a PaO_2 greater than 90 mmHg. The presence of an increased alveolar–arterial (A–a) gradient is more sensitive (95%) for PE and is calculated with the following formula:

$$A\text{–a gradient} = (150 - 1.2[PCO_2]) - PaO_2.$$

Compare the above value to the expected normal A–a gradient calculated with the following formula : ([patient age/4] − 4). Patients with an increased A–a gradient should have further testing. The classic $S_1Q_3T_3$ pattern on the ECG is highly suggestive of PE but is present in only 12% of patients. The most common ECG finding is nonspecific ST–T wave changes. A completely normal ECG is seen in less than 10% of cases. The chest x-ray may be normal, but an elevated dome of one diaphragm is seen in 50% of patients. The chest x-ray also should be used to correlate the abnormalities seen with radionuclide studies. Other supplemental tests include CBC to aid in the differential diagnosis, PT, and PTT in anticipation of possible anticoagulation.

Venography can be helpful, as radiographic evidence of DVT will be seen in 90% of patients with PE (clinical signs are seen in only 33%). Some centers achieve a 95% sensitivity for DVT with impedance plethysmography.

The V–Q scan is a very sensitive test for PE, and a completely normal study rules out the disorder. Pulmonary angiography is the gold standard for diagnosing PE and is a much more specific test than the V–Q scan. Angiography exposes the patient to more potential complications, especially in elderly patients. Angiography may be needed to confirm the diagnosis if the V–Q scan demonstrates equivocal results, such as medium or low probability for PE, in a patient at risk.

Disorders in the differential diagnosis include respiratory disorders, such as asthma, COPD, pneumonia, spontaneous pneumothorax, and pleurisy. Cardiac disorders that may mimic PE include MI and pericarditis. Musculoskeletal disorders that may mimic PE include muscle strain, rib fracture, costochondritis, and herpes zoster. Intra-abdominal disorders that irritate the diaphragm or stimulate breathing may also present similar to PE. Finally, hyperventilation syndrome may mimic PE, however, this is a diagnosis of exclusion.

Emergency Department Care

The treatment of PE consists of initial stabilization, anticoagulation with heparin, and thrombolytic therapy in extreme cases. Patients should be hooked up to a cardiac monitor, noninvasive blood pressure device, pulse oximetry monitor, and an intravenous line.

1. Administer sufficient oxygen to maintain a pulse–oximetry reading of 95% O_2 saturation. Lower O_2 saturation levels may be acceptable in patients with chronic hypoxia. If an ABG is desired off O_2, ensure that the patient is stable enough to endure the period of potential hypoxia.
2. Crystalloid IV fluids should be given initially for hypotension, and a CVP or Swan–Ganz catheter should be considered if the patient does not respond to the fluid bolus of 500 to 1000 cc of normal saline. If thrombolytic therapy is being considered, however, central lines should be avoided.
3. For hypotension in the absence of hypovolemia, **dopamine** can be started at 2 to 5 mcg/kg/min and titrated to maintain a systolic blood pressure of 90 mmHg.
4. Start **heparin** with an IV bolus of 10,000 to 20,000 units, followed by a continuous drip of 1000 units/h to be adjusted using the partial thromboplastin time, aiming for 1.5 to 2 times control. Contraindications to anticoagulation include active internal bleeding, uncontrolled severe hypertension, recent trauma, recent surgery, recent stroke, intracranial or intraspinal neoplasm. Heparin can be used safely in

the nonbleeding pregnant patient but must be discontinued prior to delivery.

Patients who demonstrate any degree of clinical instability should be admitted to the ICU. Stable patients may be admitted to a telemetry bed. Heparin does not prevent the embolization of existing clots. Further embolization and shock most commonly occur within 4 h of initial symptoms. Patients should be stable and beyond this initial high risk period if admission to a nonmonitored bed is considered.

If Standard Treatment Fails

For persistent hypotension despite medical management with above measures, consider thrombolytic therapy. Urokinase, 4400/kg as an IV bolus, or tPA, 50 to 100 mg IV over 2 to 6 h, have been recommended. Streptokinase can be given in a dose of 250,000 units IV over 30 min followed by a continuous IV infusion of 100,000 units/h for the next 12 to 24 h. Ideally, consultation with an intensivist and documentation of PE with angiography should be done prior to starting thrombolytic therapy. For patients with contraindications to anticoagulation or thrombolytic therapy, a Greenfield filter can be inserted percutaneously.

For further reading in *Emergency Medicine, A Comprehensive Study Guide,* see Chapter 57, Pulmonary Embolism, by Robert S. Hockberger.

David Dubow

Hypertension in the ED can be broken down into five categories: (1) *Hypertensive emergency:* Defined as increased blood pressure (BP) with evidence of end-organ (brain, heart, kidney) damage or dysfunction. There is no absolute BP at which an emergency is defined. The goal of treatment is to lower the pressure to the patient's normal within 30 to 60 min in a gradual, controlled fashion. (2) *Hypertensive urgency:* Elevation of blood pressure that may be potentially harmful without signs or symptoms of end-organ dysfunction. This usually occurs at a sustained diastolic pressure of 115 mmHg or higher. Treatment is directed at gradually lowering the patient's BP to an appropriate level over 24 to 48 h. (3) *Mild, uncomplicated hypertension:* A diastolic BP between 90 and 115 mmHg without symptoms of end-organ dysfunction. ED BP readings should not be the basis for the diagnosis or treatment of mild hypertension. (4) *Transient hypertension:* Anxiety, pain, stroke, dehydration, alcohol withdrawal, overdoses, and other conditions can cause a brief elevation of BP without evidence of ongoing hypertension. Treatment of the underlying condition is the solution to this cause of hypertension. (5) *Pregnancy-induced hypertension:* During the third trimester the upper limit of normal BP is 125/75 mmHg. BP greater than 140/90 mmHg is of concern. Eclampsia is an elevated BP accompanied by signs and symptoms of hyperreflexia, confusion, headache, epigastric pain, seizures, or coma. Primagravidas and multigravidas over age 35 (especially with a prior history of hypertension or renal disease) are at greater risk. This condition is usually seen in the third trimester unless there is a prior history of hypertension or renal disease or it is a molar pregnancy.

Clinical Features

A history of CNS symptoms (blurred vision, diplopia, hemiparesis, seizures), cardiac symptoms (anginal chest pain, CHF), renal dysfunction, or pregnancy are indicative of a hypertensive emergency. Complaints of headache or blurred vision are nonspecific. Sudden elevations of catecholamines can also trigger acute hypertensive states. Pheochromocytoma is an uncommon problem that presents with episodic hypertension, headache, flushing, and diarrhea. Concomitant use of MAO inhibitors and sympathomimetics (e.g., over-the-counter cold medications and diet pills) or tyramine-containing foods (Chianti wine, aged cheese, beer, pickled herring) can lead to acute elevations of BP. It is important to elicit a prior history of hypertension and medication use from the patient. Especially inquire about the patient's compliance with prescribed medications. Withdrawal from Clonidine, especially when done concurrently with a beta blocker, can lead to severe hypertension.

The physical exam should focus on neurologic, cardiac, and pulmonary assessment. Examine the fundi for evidence of grade 3 (hemorrhages, exudates, vascular changes) or grade 4 (papilledema) retinopathy. Also recheck the BP at least once and measure it in both arms. Palpate the peripheral pulses in all extremities. In stable patients consider performing orthostatic measurements to assess for dehydration.

Diagnosis and Differential

The diagnosis of hypertension is based on a complete history and physical. In all patients with hypertensive emergencies and in some with urgencies perform the following laboratory tests: CBC (microangiopathic hemolytic anemia may lead to shistocytes and red cell fragments); electrolytes (hypokalemia or hyperkalemia may be present); BUN and creatinine (elevated, it is evidence of renal dysfunction); urinalysis (may show proteinuria, red cells, or red cell casts); ECG (may show evidence of cardiac ischemia or left ventricular hypertrophy); and chest x-ray (may demonstrate pulmonary edema). In patients with CNS symptoms, cerebral ischemia or hemorrhage might be seen on CT scan of the head.

Emergency Department Care

Generally the treatment of hypertensive emergencies and urgencies is lowering the BP in a controlled manner appropriate to the patient's condition. All patients demonstrating signs and symptoms of end-organ dysfunction require hospital admission, sometimes to a critical care unit, depending on condition and response to treatment. Medications used to lower the BP depends on the organ system affected, but, all patients with emergent and urgent conditions require the following:

1. Establish intravenous access.
2. Continuous cardiac monitoring.
3. Supplemental oxygen as needed.

Central nervous system. The goal of treatment is to gradually lower the BP over 30 to 60 min and then to lower the BP below a mean arterial pressure of 120 mmHg. In preferred order, the drugs of choice are:

1. **Sodium nitroprusside**—50 mg of Nipride is mixed in 500 mL of 5% D$_5$W (10 mcg/mL). Start infusion at 0.5 mcg/kg/min and titrate to the desired BP. The average effective dose is 3 mcg/kg/min, with a range of 0.5 to 10 mcg/kg/min. An arterial line is not necessary to initiate the Nipride drip, but one should be inserted for long-term use.
2. Intravenous **labetalol**—Repeat incremental boluses starting at 20 to 40 mg IV. BP usually falls within 5 min, with a maximum response

in 10 min, and a duration of up to 6 h. If the initial response is inadequate, double the IV dose every 30 to 60 min up to a total dose of 300 mg until the desired effect is achieved. A continuous IV infusion can be given by mixing 200 mg of labetalol in 200 mL of D_5W and run at 2 mg/min (2 mL/min). A loading dose of 20 mg may be given before beginning the drip. After the desired BP is obtained, stop the infusion.

3. **Nimodipine**—In the case of acute subarachnoid hemorrhage, 60 mg of nimodipine orally is given every 4 h to reduce vasospasm associated with subarachnoid bleeding. Avoid the use of clonidine and pure beta blocking agents.

Cardiovascular system—left ventricular failure and coronary insufficiency. The goal of treatment is to reduce both preload and afterload, thereby decreasing myocardial workload and oxygen demand.

1. **Nitroglycerin**—Begin a continuous infusion at 20 to 30 mcg/min and increase by 10 mcg/min every 3 to 5 min, as needed to control BP.
2. **Sodium nitroprusside**—(See above.) Coronary steal syndrome has been reported with Nipride.
3. Oral **nifedipine**—Although not FDA approved for this use, 10 to 20 mg may be given orally. To achieve the most rapid onset, instruct the patient to bite, chew, and then swallow a punctured capsule. Onset of action begins within 5 min, and maximal effect occurs in 20 to 30 min. Duration of action is 4 to 5 h.
4. **Furosemide**—If there is evidence of volume overload, give a bolus of 40 mg IV. Double the dose in 30 to 60 min if needed.
5. **Bumetanide**—Another loop diuretic, bumetanide may be given in an initial dose of 1 to 2 mg IV in the patient with evidence of volume overload.

Avoid the use of diazoxide, hydralazine and minoxidil, as they will increase myocardial oxygen demand. Use beta-blocking agents and labetalol with caution in patients with a history of, or evidence of, severe congestive heart failure.

Cardiovascular system—thoracic aortic dissection. Pharmacologic therapy is directed at reducing the BP and the aortic pressure wave by controlling the pulse rate.

1. Intravenous labetalol—see the discussion above.
2. A combination of intravenous propranolol and nitroprusside may be used. Begin by first giving propranolol 1 mg IV every 5 min until the heart rate is lowered to a rate of 60 to 80. Begin nitroprusside infusion, as discussed above, after the first dose of propranolol.

Pregnancy-induced hypertension. Pre-eclampsia and eclampsia are true hypertensive emergencies. Such patients require aggressive management and hospital admission. Prompt consultation with an OB–GYN physician is indicated.

1. Intravenous **magnesium**—In addition to controlling BP, magnesium sulfate has antiseizure properties. A 4 to 6 gm bolus is given initially, followed by a 1 to 2 gm/h infusion. Monitor the deep tendon reflexes and stop the infusion if they disappear.
2. **Hydralazine**—Should be used in combination with magnesium. Give 10 to 20 mg IV push (the IM routine can also be used if necessary). Repeat the dose in 30 min if needed.

Sodium nitroprusside and labetalol have been used with efficacy. It is important to monitor thiocynate levels if the nitroprusside infusion is going to be prolonged. Avoid the use of angiotensin-converting enzyme inhibitors and diuretics.

Catecholamine-induced hypertension. Combined alpha and beta blockade with **labetalol** is the treatment of choice. (See the discussion above for administration of labetalol.)

If Standard Treatment Fails

Other agents that have been used successfully to control hypertension include:

1. **Clonidine**—Load with an oral dose of 0.2 mg and give an additional 0.1 mg/h until the diastolic pressure is below 115 mmHg, up to a maximum dose of 0.7 mg. Usually 0.3 to 0.4 mg is adequate. Patients do not necessarily need to continue clonidine on discharge from the ED if they have close followup.
2. **Captopril**—In patients with known renovascular hypertension, 25 mg can be given 3 times per day to control BP.
3. **Minoxidil**—10 to 20 mg can be given orally and repeated in 4 h if necessary. It is important to co-administer a beta blocker to control symptomatic tachycardia, but excessive hypotension may result. Diuretics must also be administered to control sodium and water retention.

For further reading in *Emergency Medicine, A Comprehensive Study Guide*, see Chapter 58, Hypertensive Emergencies, by Raymond E. Jackson.

Aneurysms of the thoracic and abdominal aorta may be discovered as an incidental finding or may be the cause of the patient's presenting complaint. No matter how they are discovered, aortic aneurysms always have significance, depending on the size of the aneurysm and its stability.

ABDOMINAL ANEURYSMS

Clinical Features

The most common presentation of abdominal aortic aneurysm (AAA) is as a painless, pulsatile abdominal mass found unexpectedly during a routine examination or during CT scan or ultrasound of the abdomen for an unrelated problem.

The second most common presentation is an acute rupture. Patients with an acute AAA rupture may present with sudden syncope followed by spontaneous recovery in association with abdominal or back pain. Flank or costovertebral angle pain, lower quadrant abdominal pain, or hip pain may also be presentations of AAA rupture. AAA rupture is frequently misdiagnosed as renal colic. Age over 60 years is a risk factor for AAA.

Physical exam may reveal a tender, pulsatile abdominal mass, although absence of such a finding does not rule out AAA. It is prudent to check for symmetry of peripheral pulses in the lower extremities and to listen for abdominal bruits, which are further indications of AAA. Vital signs may be completely normal on initial presentation or demonstrate hypotension and tachycardia.

The chronic contained AAA rupture is the least common and most subtle. This is the result of erosion of the posterior AAA wall and containment of the leak by the peritoneum. There is no significant blood loss. Presenting signs and symptoms include chronic, severe upper lumbar back pain with a nontender, palpable AAA and stable vital signs.

Diagnosis and Differential

The diagnosis of AAA hinges on maintaining a high index of suspicion. The differential for syncope or abdominal pain is long and includes: cardiac dysrhythmia, cerebrovascular occlusive disease, exaggerated vagal response, appendicitis, diverticulitis, GI tumors, cholecystitis, and ischemic bowel disease. In obese patients it is frequently difficult to adequately palpate the abdomen, much less distinguish between AAA and a mass overlying a normal abdominal aorta. These patients need a quick and noninvasive radiologic study to determine if they have an AAA. It is important to remember that patients with a ruptured or

219

leaking AAA may appear stable initially, however, they may develop sudden and refractory hypotension without warning. Such patients rarely survive, even with prompt surgical intervention. *These patients should never be left unattended while undergoing diagnostic studies.* Plain abdominal x-rays may demonstrate a curvilinear calcification to the left of the lumbar spine or a soft-tissue bulge anterior to the lumbar spine. Plain x-rays are not, however, adequately sensitive to rule out AAA. Abdominal ultrasound is another modality to identify AAA. In some institutions it can be performed at the bedside while the patient remains in the ED. Computed tomography (CT) is very sensitive and specific for identifying AAA and ruptured AAA. Its use in the emergency diagnosis of ruptured AAA is controversial because of the time it takes to perform and the need for the patient to leave the ED. Indications for CT are: (1) patients suspected of having chronic, contained rupture; (2) stable patients who have aneurysms but are suspected of having acute abdominal conditions other than AAA rupture; and (3) patients whom a surgeon has examined and requested CT to assist in diagnosis or preoperative planning. In patients with a clinical presentation consistent with AAA rupture (age >60 years, syncope, abdominal or back pain, and a pulsatile abdominal mass), presume acute rupture and get immediate surgical consultation before obtaining any imaging studies.

THORACIC ANEURYSMS

Clinical Features

Thoracic aortic aneurysms are most commonly discovered as an incidental finding on chest x-ray. Ruptured thoracic aortic aneurysm is catastrophic and patients usually die before reaching the hospital. *Dissecting thoracic aortic aneurysm* presents with the sudden onset of tearing chest pain. Dissections originating in the ascending aorta lead to pain in the precordium whereas those beginning at the ligamentum arteriosum cause pain in the intrascapular region. If the dissection progresses into the abdominal aorta it may cause pain in the abdomen, flank, or even leg (indications of iliac artery involvement). Proximal dissection may occlude the origin of the carotid arteries, leading to stroke or transient ischemic attack, or it may disrupt the aortic valve and produce sudden heart failure or cardiac tamponade. Rarely patients will present with paraplegia due to interference with blood supply to the spinal cord.

Physical examination should include an evaluation of peripheral pulses and bilateral upper extremity blood pressures. It is also important to listen for cardiac murmurs that may indicate aortic valve disruption.

Diagnosis and Differential

Thoracic aortic dissections are frequently misdiagnosed as myocardial infarctions (MI). Key differentiated features of acute dissection include:

(1) the pain of dissection is cataclysmic in onset and is classically described as tearing; (2) intrascapular pain strongly suggests dissection over MI; (3) MI pain usually builds up and is described as heavy, crushing, or squeezing. Spontaneous perforation of the esophagus may also produce pain similar to dissection. A history of violent vomiting preceding pain onset and the presence of mediastinal air on chest x-ray should help distinguish it from dissection. The diagnosis of thoracic aortic dissection is best made with CT scan with contrast, however, angiography may be required. One should also obtain an electrocardiogram and chest x-ray to help identify other causes of acute chest pain.

Emergency Department Care

Patients with incidentally discovered aneurysms may be discharged with prompt surgical and medical referral. Patients with symptomatic aneurysms or dissection should be presumed to be in the process of rupture and require immediate surgical consultation. The role of the emergency physician is to provide supportive care until the patient can be taken into the operating room for repair of the vascular defect.

1. Obtain IV access and administer crystalloid fluids to support BP. Prepare to administer blood products if necessary.
2. Hypertensive patients with dissection require control of BP and pulse rate with specific agents for aneurisms (see Chap. 34).
3. Continuous cardiac monitoring.
4. Supplemental oxygen and emergent intubation is necessary.

If Standard Treatment Fails

The only curative treatment for ruptured, leaking, or dissecting aneurysms is surgery. Once the diagnosis is established, anything that delays the patient's delivery to the operating room is contraindicated. Some authors have suggested that the Military Antishock Garment (MAST) can be used to help stabilize a leaking AAA. Although its use will not directly harm the patient, there is no clear evidence that it will help.

For further reading in *Emergency Medicine, A Comprehensive Study Guide,* see Chapter 59, Thoracic and Abdominal Aneurysms by John L. Glover.

Mesenteric Ischemia

David Dubow

Mesenteric ischemia is a rare condition seen primarily in the elderly and critically ill. Presentation is usually vague, and the diagnosis is frequently not considered until the patient is critically ill, so morbidity and mortality are high. The key to improving patient outcome is a high level of suspicion and early diagnosis. Risks include age over 50, atrial fibrillation, recent myocardial infarction, recent discontinuance of anticoagulant therapy, previous episode of venous thrombosis, birth control pills, history of malignancy, polycythemia, portal hypertension, and pregnancy.

Clinical Features

Initial presentation of mesenteric ischemia always involves abdominal pain. It is frequently described as "pain out of proportion to physical findings." Intestinal angina (abdominal pain after a large meal relieved by vomiting) is rarely seen. A history of chronic weight loss or a fear of food in order to avoid abdominal pain may be reported. Nonocclusive mesenteric ischemia can be seen in the critically ill patient with low-flow cardiac output states. Patients being treated for cardiac failure with aggressive diuresis and have concurrent hypokalemia and digitalis toxicity or near toxicity may develop nonocclusive ischemia.

Vital signs are usually normal until the patient becomes severely ill. Abdominal findings are highly variable, depending on the stage of the disease. Initially the exam may be unremarkable, but as the ischemia progresses to frank necrosis, abdominal distention, diffuse tenderness and, ultimately, rigidity and peritoneal signs will develop.

Diagnosis and Differential

The key to early diagnosis is to suspect mesenteric ischemia in at-risk patients. Most patients will have a WBC count greater than 15,000, and 50% will exhibit a metabolic acidosis. Hemoconcentration and, occasionally, an elevated serum amylase and phosphate may be seen.

Abdominal x-rays should be obtained primarily to look for other conditions. Thickening of the bowel wall (thumb-printing) and air in the bowel wall are frequently described but rarely seen. Arteriography is the test of choice in hemodynamically stable patients.

Emergency Department Care

Initial stabilization of patients with mesenteric ischemia consists of continuous cardiac monitoring, a non-invasive BP device, IV access, and pulse oximetry.

1. Administer crystalloid IV fluids for replacement of plasma volume. Close monitoring of hemodynamic parameters with an arterial line, CVP or Swan–Ganz catheter, and Foley catheter should be considered, especially in elderly or frail patients.
2. Supplemental oxygen should be administered as indicated by pulse oximetry.
3. Bowel decompression is accomplished with a nasogastric tube.
4. Broad spectrum antibiotics should be given (early, use **cefoxitan** 1–2 grams IV; late, add **ticarcillin/clavulanate** 3.1 gm IV) and have been shown to prolong the period between ischemia and necrosis in mesenteric ischemia.
5. Anticoagulation with heparin should be started as soon as possible after arteriography.
6. Surgical consultation should be requested at the time of arteriography in the event that the study demonstrates the need for an emergency operation. All patients with mesenteric ischemia require ICU admission and many require emergent surgery.

If Standard Treatment Fails

Because the presentation of mesenteric ischemia is often obscure, other intra-abdominal problems must be considered, including myocardial infarction, ruptured or leaking abdominal aortic aneurysm, perforated viscous, intestinal obstruction, acute pancreatitis, acute cholecystitis, appendicitis, diverticulitis, pyelonephritis, acute hepatitis.

The administration of vasodilating drugs through the arteriography catheter increases the amount of salvageable bowel in mesenteric ischemia. Consider using these drugs after consultation with the surgeons.

For further reading in *Emergency Medicine, A Comprehensive Study Guide,* see Chapter 60, Mesenteric Ischemia, by John L. Glover.

37 | Acute Extremity Ischemia and Thrombophlebitis

David Dubow

Acute extremity ischemia may be caused by embolism, thrombosis, trauma, or low-flow states and may involve arteries or veins. Peripheral arterial occlusion is most frequently embolic. Venous obstruction is usually due to thrombosis and is caused by a triad of stasis, mechanical injury, and hypercoagulability. Careful history and physical exam will help to distinguish the various causes of extremity ischemia and are critical to its management.

ARTERIAL OCCLUSION

Clinical Features

Patients with acute arterial occlusion present with extremity pain. Other common symptoms include paresthesia, hypesthesia, anesthesia, paresis, or paralysis of the involved limb. A history of cardiac disease (arrhythmia, myocardial infarction, or valvular heart disease) suggests embolic occlusion. Complaints of claudication, rest pain, ulceration, or a history of peripheral vascular disease indicates thrombosis in situ.

Physical examination usually demonstrates a pale, mottled, or cyanotic limb, depending on the duration of occlusion. Distal pulses are absent, the skin is cool or cold to touch, and muscle palpation may elicit tenderness or rigor. If microemboli are the cause, petechiae, cyanosis, gangrene, or ulcerations in the distal extremity may be seen. In that case, distal pulses may be palpable.

Diagnosis and Differential

In addition to a careful history and physical exam, a hand-held continuous wave Doppler is useful. In the upper extremity the axillary, brachial, ulnar, and radial arteries may be evaluated. The femoral, popliteal, dorsalis pedis, and posterior tibialis arteries can be checked in the lower extremity. Listen for the absence or presence of arterial flow and note the characteristics of the signal (triphasic, biphasic, or monophasic). If there is no flow over a proximal site but a signal can be detected distally, this denotes collateral circulation. In addition, obtain a CBC and PT, PTT in anticipation of surgical intervention and/or anticoagulation.

Emergency Department Care

Surgical therapy is the treatment of choice for arterial occlusion. Anticoagulation should be considered as an alternative (although there is no clearly proven benefit) in consultation with the surgeon. Arteriography or ultrasonography may be performed to identify the source of the emboli.

If Standard Treatment Fails

Thrombolytic agents (streptokinase and urokinase) infused through an arterial catheter have been successful in some cases. Contraindications to thrombolysis include the presence of neurologic deficits, internal bleeding, intracranial lesions, or severe ischemia.

VENOUS OCCLUSION—SUPERFICIAL THROMBOPHLEBITIS

Clinical Features

Superficial thrombophlebitis is seen primarily in the lower extremities and involves the greater or lesser saphenous veins or varicosities. It is characterized by redness, tenderness, and induration along the course of the vein.

Diagnosis and Differential

It is frequently difficult to distinguish superficial thrombophlebitis of the greater saphenous vein from lymphangitis because lymphatic drainage from the leg runs along that vein. The diagnosis can be established by evaluating venous flow with either continuous-wave Doppler or venography.

Emergency Department Care

Patients with superficial thrombophlebitis can be treated as outpatients with bed rest, elevation, local heat, and analgesics for pain. Patients should expect slow improvement over 3 to 6 wks. Thrombosis at the saphenofemoral junction should be treated more aggressively with full anticoagulation (see discussion of Deep Venous Thrombosis below).

VENOUS OCCLUSION—DEEP VENOUS THROMBOSIS

Clinical Features

Deep venous thrombosis (DVT) most commonly affects the lower extremities. Classical findings of DVT include edema, warmth, erythema, pain, tenderness, and Homan's sign (pain in the calf with passive dorsiflexion of the foot). Such signs and symptoms are present in only 23% to 50% of cases, and significant thrombosis may be present with minimal findings. Risk factors for DVT include: previous history of thrombotic disease; recent lower extremity surgery; treatment with estrogens; use of birth control pills; recent urologic, orthopedic, or gynecologic surgery; advanced age; recent myocardial infarction; congestive heart failure; carcinoma; and obesity.

Diagnosis and Differential

Although venography remains the best way to diagnose DVT, other noninvasive modalities are available. Duplex scanning with continuous wave color-flow Doppler and impedance plethysmography (IPG) have accuracies of 90% to 100%. IPG is insensitive to infrapopliteal or partially occluding thrombi. A hand-held continuous-wave Doppler may also prove useful in examining venous flow in the groin, popliteal fossa, and posterior tibial veins. Absent Doppler flow augmentation with Valsalva maneuver or compression of the distal musculature are indicative of venous thrombosis. Other supplemental tests include a CBC and PT, PTT for probable anticoagulation.

Emergency Department Care

Patients with DVT need hospitalization and anticoagulation.

1. Heparinize with an initial IV bolus of 5000 units, followed by a continuous drip adjusted to a partial thromboplastin time 1.5 to 2.5 times normal.
2. Administer local heat and analgesia, as needed.
3. Strict bed rest and elevation of the extremity for the first 3 to 4 days.

VENOUS OCCLUSION—MASSIVE DEEP VENOUS THROMBOSIS

Clinical Features

Extensive iliofemoral thrombosis will lead to extensive swelling of the entire lower extremity up to the groin. The leg frequently has a doughy consistency. If venous collateral circulation is compromised the leg will be tensely swollen and cyanotic, and skin bullae may be present. Arterial circulation may be compromised due to swelling within muscular compartments.

Diagnosis and Differential

Venography, duplex Doppler, or IPG are all appropriate.

Emergency Department Care

Initial treatment of massive DVT is similar to that for acute DVT. Treatment with streptokinase or urokinase should be considered if there are no contraindications. If muscle compartment swelling endangers arterial circulation, fasciotomy may be necessary.

VENOUS OCCLUSION—UPPER EXTREMITY THROMBOSIS

Clinical Features

Axillary and subclavian veins are most commonly involved in upper extremity thrombosis; it is usually the aftermath of catheterization. Young people who have a narrowing of the thoracic outlet may develop *effort thrombosis* following strenuous physical activity. The presentation is often mild swelling of the forearm (occasionally the entire arm), nonpitting edema, normal skin color, with good distal pulses.

Diagnosis and Differential

Venography and duplex Doppler are appropriate studies.

Emergency Department Care

DVT of the upper extremity is treated the same as lower extremity DVT with elevation, rest, anticoagulation and analgesia. Effort-induced thrombosis of the upper extremity is treated with catheter infusion of thrombolytics. Surgical correction of extrinsic vein compression (e.g., first or cervical rib) is necessary. Balloon angioplasty also has been used to treat venous stenosis.

For further reading in *Emergency Medicine, A Comprehensive Study Guide*, see Chapter 61, Acute Extremity Ischemia and Thrombophlebitis, by Joel Feldman.

6 | PULMONARY EMERGENCIES

David F. M. Brown

Pneumonia is the sixth leading cause of death in the United States. Bacterial etiologies are the most common, followed by respiratory viruses and mycoplasma. Pneumococcus is responsible for up to 90% of all bacterial pneumonia, with *E. coli, P. aeruginosa, K. pneumoniae, S. aureus, H. influenzae*, and group A streptococci accounting for most of the rest. Legionella species and anaerobes are less frequent causes of bacterial pneumonia, with the latter primarily the result of aspiration. Respiratory viruses, mycoplasma, and chlamydia account for the bulk of atypical pneumonia, which account for a third or more of all cases of pneumonia. Patients with chronic diseases, such as congestive heart failure, cancer, bronchiectasis, COPD, diabetes, sickle-cell anemia, AIDS, and other immunodeficiencies, are at greater risk for pneumonia, as are smokers and postsplenectomy patients. Aspiration pneumonia occurs more frequently in alcoholics and in patients with seizures, stroke, or other neuromuscular diseases. Pneumocystis pneumonia is a common complication of HIV infection and is discussed in Chapter 84.

Clinical Features

Patients with bacterial pneumonia generally present with some combination of fever, dyspnea, cough, pleuritic chest pain, and sputum production (Table 38-1). *Pneumococcus* classically causes a single rigor and rusty brown sputum; *H. influenzae* is more common in smokers, and *S. aureus* frequently follows a viral respiratory illness, especially influenza and measles. Pneumonia due to legionella is spread via airborne aerosolized water droplets rather than by person-to-person contact. This form of pneumonia presents like mycoplasma and viral pneumonia, with fever, chills, malaise, dyspnea, and a non-productive cough; gastrointestinal symptoms of anorexia, nausea, vomiting, and diarrhea are also very common. Legionella may also cause mental status changes.

Physical findings of pneumonia vary with the offending organism and the type of pneumonia each causes, although most are associated with some degree of tachypnea and tachycardia. Lobar pneumonias, such as those caused by *pneumococcus* and *Klebsiella*, exhibit signs of consolidation, including bronchial breath sounds, egophony, increased tactile and vocal fremitus, and dullness to percussion. A pleural friction rub and cyanosis may be present. Bronchopneumonias, such as those caused by *H. influenzae*, reveal rales and rhonchi on exam without signs of consolidation. A parapneumonic pleural effusion may occur in either setting; empyemas are most common with *S. aureus, Klebsiella*, and anaerobic infections. Legionella, which starts with findings of

TABLE 38-1. Characteristics of Bacterial Pneumonia

Organism	Symptoms	Sputum	Chest X-ray	Therapy
Streptococcus pneumoniae	Single rigor, pleuritic chest pain, productive cough, dyspnea	Rusty; gram positive encapsulated diplococci	Lobar, occasional patchy, occasional small pleural effusion	Phenoxymethyl penicillin 500 mg po qid x 10d OR Erythromycin 500 mg po qid x 10d OR aqueous penicillin G 10–20 million units per day IV q4–6h OR ceftriaxone 1 g IV qd
Group A Streptococci	Abrupt onset of fever, chills, productive cough and pleuritic chest pain	Purulent, bloody; gram-positive cocci in chains and pairs	Patchy, multilobar large pleural effusion	See above
Hemophilus Influenza	Fever, dyspnea, occasional pleuritic chest pain	Short, tiny, gram-negative encapsulated cocci-bacilli	Patchy, frequently basilar, occasional pleural effusion	Ceftriaxone 1 g IV qd or cefuroxime 0.75–1.5 g IV q8h or amoxacillin clavulante 500 mg po q8h x 10d
Klebsiella pneumonia	Sudden cough, rigors, dyspnea, pleuritic chest pain, cyanosis. Most common in patients with diabetes, alcoholism, or COPD	Brown jelly, thick; short, plump, gram-negative encapsulated paired cocci-bacilli	Upper lobes, bulging fissure sign, abscess formation	Cefazolin 0.5–1.0 g q8h IV OR Gentamicin 3–5 mg/kg/day IV q8h
Staphylococcus Aureus	Abrupt onset of productive cough, pleuritic chest pain, chills, fever, occurring just after a viral illness	Purulent; gram-positive cocci in clusters	Patchy, multicenter with early abscess formation, empyema, pneumothorax	Oxacillin 8–12 g/d IV OR Vancomycin 500 mg IV q6h

(continued on p. 233)

Organism	Clinical Features	Gram Stain	Radiographic	Treatment
Legionella Pneumophila	Fever, chills, headache, malaise, dry cough, dyspnea, anorexia, diarrhea, nausea, vomiting. Occasional pleuritic chest pain	Few polymorpho-nuclear leukocytes, and no predominant bacterial species	Multiple patchy nonsegmented infiltrates, progresses to consolidation, occ. cavitation and pleuritic effusion	Erythromycin 1g IV q6h +/- Rifampin 600 mg po qd
Escherichia Coli	Recently hospitalized, debilitated or immunocompromised patients with fever, dyspnea, cough	Gram-negative cocci-bacilli	Patchy bilateral lower lobes	Ampicillin 6–8 g/day IV q6h plus Gentamicin 3–5 mg/kg/day IV divided q8h
Pseudomonas Aeruginosa	As above (E. coli)	Gram-negative cocci-bacilli	Patchy with frequent abscess formation	Tobramycin 3–5 mg/kg/day div ded q8h IV AND Carbenicillin 5–6 g q4h IV
Mycoplasma Pneumoniae	Upper and lower respiratory tract symptoms, non-productive cough, bullous myringitis, headache, malaise, fever	Few polymorpho-nuclear leukocytes and no predominant bacterial species	Interstitial infiltrates, (reticulonodular pattern), patchy densities, occasional consolidation	Erythromycin 500 mg po qid for 10–14d

233

patchy bronchopneumonia and progresses to signs of frank consolidation, has other common signs, including a relative bradycardia and confusion. Interstitial pneumonias, such as those caused by viruses and mycoplasma, may exhibit fine rales or normal breath sounds. Bullous myringitis when present in this setting, is pathognomonic for mycoplasma infection.

Clinical features of aspiration pneumonitis depend on the volume and pH of the aspirate, the presence of particulate matter in the aspirate, and bacterial contamination. Although acid aspiration results in the rapid onset of symptoms of tachypnea, tachycardia, and cyanosis, and often progresses to frank pulmonary failure, most other cases of aspiration pneumonia progress more insidiously. Physical signs develop over hours and include rales, rhonchi, wheezing, and copious frothy or bloody sputum. The right lower lobe is most commonly involved due to the anatomy of the tracheobronchial tree and to gravity.

Diagnosis and Differential

The differential includes acute tracheobronchitis, pulmonary embolus or infarction, exacerbation of COPD, pulmonary vasculitides, including Goodpasture's disease and Wegener's granulomatosis, bronchiolitis obliterans, and endocarditis. The diagnosis of pneumonia is made on the presenting signs and symptoms, examination of the sputum, and a chest radiograph (see Table 38-1). Other tests include a WBC with differential, pulse oximetry, blood cultures, and pleural fluid examination. Arterial blood gases should be obtained in ill-appearing patients. If legionella is being considered, serum chemistries and liver-function tests should be taken, as hyponatremia, hypophosphatemia, and elevated liver enzymes are commonly found. Also when appropriate, urine should be tested for legionella antigen, and serologic testing for mycoplasma can be performed, although these tests will have no impact on the emergency management of the patient. Bedside cold agglutinins may be positive in cases of mycoplasma, but are nonspecific.

Emergency Department Care

The treatment of pneumonia in the ED depends on the severity of the clinical presentation and the gram-stain results.

1. Oxygen should be administered as needed, and antibiotic treatment should be initiated.
2. Therapies directed against specific organisms are listed in Table 38–1, although empirical antibiotic coverage is generally recommended unless the clinical features and sputum gram-stain strongly suggest a specific etiology. For outpatient management, **erythromycin**, 500 mg qid for 10 to 14 days, is an excellent choice for empiric therapy. **Clarithromycin**, 500 mg bid for 10 days, or **azithromycin**,

500 mg on day 1 followed by 250 mg qd for 4 additional days, are more expensive alternatives with fewer side-effects and better compliance.

3. Close followup is necessary, as gram-negative infections are not well covered by this approach and should be considered in patients who do not respond to therapy.

4. Hospital admission should be reserved for patients at the extremes of life, pregnant women, and those with clinical signs of toxicity (i.e., tachycardia, tachypnea, hypoxemia, hypotension, volume depletion) or serious comorbid conditions (i.e., renal failure, diabetes, cardiac disease).

5. Patients requiring admission generally also receive empiric antibiotic therapy. For those with community-acquired pneumonia at low risk for gram-negative infection, recommended treatments include **erythromycin**, 500 mg IV q6h, **ceftriaxone**, 1 to 2 g IV qd, or trimethoprim–sulfamethoxazole.

6. Patients at high risk for gram-negative pneumonia or Legionella (alcoholics, diabetics, institutionalized or intubated patients) should be treated with a combination of erythromycin, 1 g IV q6h, and either a third-generation cephalosporin, trimethoprim–sulfamethoxazole, ampicillin/sulbactam, or ticarcillin/clavulonic acid.

7. If Pseudomonas is suspected, double coverage with an antipseudomonal penicillin (i.e., ticarcillin) or cephalosporin (i.e., ceftazidime) AND either an antipseudomonal aminoglycoside (tobramycin) or a fluoroquinolone (ciprofloxacin) is recommended.

8. Local antibiotic sensitivities and resistance patterns, as well as local standards of care, should help determine final antibiotic selection.

9. Aspiration pneumonitides require a different therapeutic approach. Witnessed aspirations should be treated with immediate tracheal suctioning, and the pH of the aspirate should be ascertained. Bronchoscopy is indicated for the removal of large particles and for further clearing of the large airways. Irrigation of the tracheobronchial tree with neutral or alkaline solutions is contraindicated, as it is of no proven benefit and may promote spread of the aspirate deeper into the terminal airways. Oxygen should be administered, but steroids and prophylactic antibiotics are of no value and should be withheld.

If Standard Treatment Fails

Failure of outpatient therapy generally requires hospital admission and broader spectrum intravenous antibiotics. Patients with hypoxemia, despite oxygen therapy or impending respiratory failure, should be treated with endotracheal intubation and mechanical ventilation. This will improve oxygen delivery to the alveoli and facilitate pulmonary toilet. Patients with aspirations who require intubation should also be treated with positive end-expiratory pressure (PEEP), which has been shown to decrease mortality if initiated within 6 h after aspiration.

For further reading in *Emergency Medicine, A Comprehensive Study Guide*, see Chapter 64, Bacterial Pneumonias, by Georges C. Benjamin; Chapter 65, Viral and Mycoplasma Pneumonias, by K.P. Ravikrishnan; and Chapter 67, Aspiration Pneumonia, Empyema and Lung Abscess, by Georges C. Benjamin.

Amy J. Behrman

Since 1985 the incidence of tuberculosis (TB) and multidrug-resistant TB (MDR-TB) has risen significantly in the United States. Risk factors for active TB include history of infection with human immunodeficiency virus (HIV), homelessness, recent incarceration, nursing home residence, and immigration from areas with endemic TB. Patients with these histories often seek care in EDs and may present with unrecognized primary or reactivation TB.

Clinical Features

Primary TB. Primary TB is usually asymptomatic and noncontagious, presenting with only a new positive reaction to TB skin testing. Some people may present with pneumonitis or extrapulmonary disease. Immunocompromised patients are more likely to develop rapidly progressive primary infections.

Reactivation TB. The lifetime reactivation rate after primary infection is about 10% in the general population but is higher in the very young, the elderly, those with major systemic illness and, especially, those with compromised immune systems. Most patients with reactivation TB present subacutely with symptoms of fever, cough, weight loss, night sweats, and malaise. Over 80% have pulmonary involvement.

Pulmonary TB. Pulmonary TB usually presents with persistent cough; constitutional symptoms, sputum, and hemoptysis may be present. Physical examination usually shows normal lung until illness is severe.

Extrapulmonary TB. Pleural involvement with exudative effusion usually occurs when a peripheral parenchymal focus ruptures. *Pericarditis* may occur by extension of infection from the pleura or lymph nodes. Symptoms, physical findings, and complications are typical for pericarditis. *Peritonitis* usually presents insidiously after seeding from infected lymph nodes. Stains and cultures from pleural, pericardial, and peritoneal fluid are frequently nondiagnostic, and biopsy may be necessary. *Meningitis* usually occurs after hematogenous spread of primary infection. The course is generally more acute in children. Patients typically present with fever and meningeal signs; 30% have cranial-nerve deficits. CSF typically shows low glucose with a predominance of monocytes. Bone involvement usually presents with pain in a vertebral body or joint.

Miliary TB. Miliary TB is a multisystem disease that can occur after hematogenous spread of primary or reactivation TB. Common symptoms and findings include fever, cough, weight loss, adenopathy, hepato-

237

splenomegaly, anemia, and other cytopenias. Extrapulmonary TB is much more common in patients with HIV than in others.

Diagnosis and Differential

Consider the diagnosis of TB in any patient with respiratory complaints or constitutional symptoms in order to facilitate early diagnosis, protect hospital staff, and make appropriate dispositions.

Chest radiographs are extremely useful. Classic findings in primary TB infection are infiltrates with or without adenopathy. Lesions may calcify. Reactivation TB typically presents with lesions in the upper lobes or superior segments of lower lobes. Cavitation, calcification, scarring, atelectasis, and effusions may be seen. Unfortunately, TB can present with a wide range of additional radiographic abnormalities. HIV and TB coinfected patients are particularly likely to present with atypical or normal radiographs.

Microbiologic testing can be useful in the ED. Acid-fast staining of sputum is positive in 50% to 80% of patients presenting with pulmonary TB. New DNA probe techniques, when available, can yield definitive diagnoses in hours. New culture techniques (BACTEC system) can confirm diagnoses in days rather than the weeks necessary for traditional cultures.

Skin testing with purified protein derivative (PPD) identifies most, but not all persons with prior TB infection. Results are read 48 to 72 hours after placement; guidelines for interpretation are summarized in Table 39-1. All reactors should be evaluated for active disease and

---

TABLE 39-1. Interpretation of PPD Skin Test

>5 mm is positive* in:
  Patients with HIV infection
  Patients who have close contact with a TB-infected person
  Patients with abnormal chest radiograph suggestive of healed tuberculosis
>10 mm is positive in patients not meeting the above criteria but who have other risks:
  Intravenous drug users
  High-prevalence groups (immigrants, long-term care facility residents, persons in local high risk areas)
  Patients with conditions that increase the risk of progression to active disease
>15 mm is positive in all others
Detection of newly infected persons in a screening program:
  >10 mm increase within any 2-y period is positive if <35 years of age
  >15 mm increase within any 2-y period is positive if >35 years of age
If the patient is anergic, other epidemiologic factors must be considered.

*A positive reaction does not necessarily indicate disease.

possible preventive therapy. Patients with HIV or other immunosuppressed states and patients with disseminated TB may be anergic.

Emergency Department Care

ED infection control. Patients with history or symptoms indicating a risk of active TB should be identified as early as possible in their prehospital and ED course. Patients with suspected TB should be isolated. Specially-designed masks must be available for patient and healthcare-worker use, as specified by OSHA. Patients with known diagnoses of TB or MDR-TB should be treated as contagious even if currently on medication until their sputum is proved to be clear.

Treatment. Patients with new diagnoses of TB who are discharged from the ED must have immediate referral for long-term outpatient care with a physician or the Public Health Department. They must be educated about home isolation and screening of household contacts. Intermittent, directly observed therapy is often advisable. Patients suspected of having MDR-TB because of their histories or community prevalence data should receive four drugs INH, rifampin, pyrazinamide, and either streptomycin or ethambutol to which their infections are likely to be sensitive. Table 39-2 summarizes the initial daily drug doses and side effects.

TABLE 39-2. Dosages and Common Side Effects of Some Drugs Used in Tuberculosis

Drug	Daily Use	Some Potential Side Effects
INH	Adult: 5 mg/kg (max. 300 mg) Children: 10–20 mg/kg (max. 300 mg)	Hepatitis, neuritis, lupus syndrome, abdominal discomfort, hypersensitivity reaction, metabolic acidosis, CNS effects
Rifampin	Adult: 10 mg/kg (max. 600 mg) Children: 10–20 mg/kg (max. 600 mg)	Hepatitis, thrombocytopenia, drug interactions, GI disturbances
Pyrazinamide	Adult: 15–30 mg/kg (max. 2 g) Children: Same	Hepatitis, arthralgia, rash, hyperuricemia, GI disturbances
Ethambutol	Adult: 5–25 mg/kg (max. 2.5 g) Children: 15–25 mg/kg (max. 2.5 g)	Optic neuritis, GI disturbances
Streptomycin	Adult: 15 mg/kg (max. 1 g) Children: 20–30 mg/kg (max. 1 g)	8th cranial nerve damage, renal failure, proteinuria, eosinophilia, electrolyte disorders, neuromuscular blockade

Admission is indicated for clinical instability, unreliable outpatient followup and compliance, diagnostic uncertainty (such as a febrile AIDS patient with pulmonary infiltrates), and active, known MDR-TB. Admission to respiratory isolation is mandatory.

If Standard Treatment Fails

Patients who present with worsening disease on outpatient therapy may have missed diagnoses, including other pulmonary infections, malignancies, and inflammatory disorders. They may also be failing TB therapy because of noncompliance or unrecognized drug resistance. Consider admission.

For further reading in *Emergency Medicine, A Comprehensive Study Guide,* see Chapter 68, Tuberculosis, by Robert D. Welch.

40 | Pneumothorax

David C. Kolb

Pneumothorax is an abnormal collection of air in the pleural space. It may occur spontaneously or secondary to trauma and can cause malfunction of the thoracic pump, resulting in pulmonary and hemodynamic complications. Tension pneumothorax is a true emergency needing immediate intervention.

Spontaneous pneumothorax occurs without any recognizable local trauma. Primary spontaneous pneumothorax occurs in a person without underlying lung disease, whereas a secondary spontaneous pneumothorax occurs in patients with COPD or other underlying pulmonary disease.

Traumatic pneumothorax occurs secondary to both blunt and penetrating mechanisms, including iatrogenic causes.

IATROGENIC PNEUMOTHORAX

Iatrogenic pneumothorax can occur secondary to barotrauma or to the performance of invasive procedures. It is the most commonly described complication of subclavian vein catheterization. A chest film should be ordered routinely immediately after any invasive procedure to the neck or chest.

Lung inflation at high pressures can cause barotrauma, which introduces air into the pleural space resulting in pneumothorax. Pneumothorax should always be considered in the patient who deteriorates while on mechanical ventilation or postsubclavian vein catheterization.

Clinical Features

The most common symptoms of pneumothorax are chest pain on the side of the pneumothorax and dyspnea. Chest pain is sharp and pleuritic. Dyspnea, tachycardia, and tachypnea may be present if the degree of pneumothorax compromises pulmonary function. Physical exam shows decreased breath sounds, and hyper-resonance of the affected side may be present. Other physical findings include subcutaneous emphysema of the neck and chest wall and, if tension develops, tracheal deviation, cyanosis, and jugular venous distention.

Diagnosis

If tension pneumothorax is suspected, immediate treatment with needle thoracostomy is indicated before any diagnostic studies. In the stable patient a chest x-ray confirms the diagnosis. The expiratory chest film is most sensitive. This technique should be ordered.

Emergency Department Care

1. If the patient is relatively asymptomatic with a small (<15%–20%), spontaneous pneumothorax, inpatient or outpatient observation without intervention may be appropriate. Pleural space air is gradually absorbed; supplemental oxygen increases the rate of absorption.
2. Tube thoracostomy (a chest tube) is indicated in patients with complete lung collapse, severe underlying lung disease, significant dyspnea, or unsuccessful simple aspiration. Tube thoracostomy is described elsewhere.
3. If pneumothorax is increasing in size, if the patient is on mechanical ventilation, or if general anesthesia is contemplated, tube thoracostomy should be performed. If signs of tension pneumothorax are evident, needle thoracostomy by insertion of a large-bore needle into the second intercostal space is indicated, followed by tube thoracostomy.
4. Simple catheter aspiration may be performed as an alternative to tube thoracostomy in primary spontaneous pneumothorax. In the nonsequential catheter aspiration technique, a 14 to 16-gauge catheter is introduced into the pleural space at the level of the second or third intercostal space at the midclavicular line and air is aspirated with a syringe using a three-way stopcock. A chest x-ray is performed immediately after aspiration and again at 6 h. Patients with full expansion at 6 h may be discharged. Utilizing the sequential method, patients with persistent pneumothorax after simple aspiration should have a Heimlich flutter valve attached to the catheter for 1 h. If after 1 h re-expansion has been unsuccessful, the catheter should be connected to wall suction for 1 h. If pneumothorax persists, tube thoracostomy should be performed.

On occasion, rapid expansion of a pneumothorax with excessive negative pressure may result in the development of unilateral or even bilateral pulmonary edema.

Spontaneous Pneumothorax and AIDS

Spontaneous pneumothorax as a complication of pneumonia in the AIDS patient is rare, but when it occurs it is usually due to organisms such as *Pneumocystis carinii, Mycobacterium tuberculosis, Klebsiella pneumoniae,* and *Staphylococcus aureus*. Apparently these infections result in bronchopleural fistulae and fibrosis, which predisposes to pneumothorax. Recurrence is characteristic of pneumothoraces associated with PCP, and contralateral pneumothoraces develop in approximately 50% of patients. These patients are difficult to treat, and treatment decisions must be individualized.

For further reading in *Emergency Medicine, A Comprehensive Study Guide,* see Chapter 69, Spontaneous and Iatrogenic Pneumothorax, by Kimberlydawn Wisdom.

Hemoptysis

David F. M. Brown

Hemoptysis is the expectoration of blood from the bronchopulmonary tree. Massive hemoptysis is defined as greater than 200 mL/24h or greater than 100 ml /day for 3 to 7 days and requires prompt intervention to prevent asphyxiation from impaired gas exchange. Minor hemoptysis is the production of smaller quantities of blood, often mixed with mucus.

Clinical Features

Hemoptysis may be the presenting symptom for a variety of conditions. A careful history and physical exam will guide the clinician to the correct diagnosis and subsequent treatment. A history of underlying lung disease should be sought, as well as any history of tobacco use. The acute onset of fever, cough, and bloody sputum suggests pneumonia or bronchitis, whereas a more indolent productive cough indicates bronchitis or bronchiectasis. Dyspnea and pleuritic chest pain are hallmarks of pulmonary embolism. Fever, night sweats, and weight loss may reflect tuberculosis or bronchogenic carcinoma. Chronic dyspnea and minor hemoptysis may represent mitral stenosis or alveolar hemorrhage syndromes, with or without renal disease. The physical examination is aimed at assessing the severity of hemoptysis and the underlying disease process. Common signs include fever and tachypnea. Hypotension is uncommon except in extremely massive hemoptysis. The cardiac examination may reveal a diastolic rumble of mitral stenosis or a pronounced P2 suggesting pulmonary embolus. Pulmonary examination may reveal rales, wheezes, or focal consolidation. More commonly, however, the heart and lung exams are normal. The oral and nasal cavities should be carefully inspected to rule out an extrapulmonary source of bleeding.

Diagnosis and Differential

The diagnosis of hemoptysis, massive or minor, is made quickly from the history. The underlying etiology can be more difficult to ascertain. A careful history and physical, as described above, will generally be suggestive. A chest x-ray is the most important diagnostic test. PA and lateral projections should be performed except in the unstable patient. Other supplemental tests should include oxygen saturation, hemoglobin/hematocrit, platelet count, coagulation studies, ABG, urinalysis, and ECG. Less urgently, a PPD can be placed and sputum can be sent for gram stain, AFB smear, and appropriate cultures. The differential diagnosis includes infection (tuberculosis, bronchitis, bronchiectasis, bacterial pneumonia, fungal pneumonia, and lung abscess), neoplasms (bronchogenic carcinoma, bronchial adenoma), cardiogenic (mitral stenosis, LV failure), trauma and foreign body aspiration, pulmonary embolism, primary pulmonary hypertension, pulmonary vasculitis, and bleeding diathesis. The cause is unknown in 2% to 19% of cases.

Emergency Department Care

The treatment of hemoptysis in the ED depends on its severity and persistence. Initial management should focus on controlling the ABCs. Cardiac and pulse oximetry monitors, as well as noninvasive BP machines should be utilized and large-bore intravenous lines should be placed.

1. Supplemental oxygen should be administered to keep O_2 saturation above 90%.
2. IV crystalloid should be administered initially for hypotension.
3. Blood should be typed and cross-matched; packed red blood cells should be transfused as needed.
4. Fresh frozen plasma (2 units) should be given to patients with coagulopathies. Patients with ongoing massive hemoptysis should be placed in the decubitus position with the bleeding lung down to minimize spilling of blood into the contralateral lung.
5. Cough suppression with codeine (15–30 mg) or other opioids is indicated.
6. Indications for admission include massive or minor hemoptysis whose underlying cause carries a high risk of proximate massive bleeding. Some underlying conditions may warrant admission regardless. All admissions should include consultations with a pulmonologist or a thoracic surgeon and frequently will need ICU monitoring. If the appropriate specialists are unavailable, the patient should be transferred after stabilization.
7. Patients who are discharged should be treated with cough suppressants (i.e., **codeine** 15–30 mg q4–6h) for several days and, if an infectious etiology is suspected, antibiotics (**trimethoprim/sulfamethoxazole** 160 mg/800 mg bid, **amoxicillin** 250 mg qid, or **doxycycline** 100 mg bid).

If Standard Treatment Fails

For persistent hemoptysis and worsening respiratory status, endotracheal intubation should be performed with a large (8.0 mm) tube. This will allow for better suctioning and permits the passage of a flexible bronchoscope. Rarely, a double-lumen endotracheal tube can be placed to seal off the hemorrhaging lung and ventilate the functioning lung. These are difficult to place; the small lumens limit suctioning and airway clearance. If the bleeding is coming from the left lung, it is better to selectively intubate the right mainstem bronchus by simply advancing the endotracheal tube. Selective intubation of the left mainstem bronchus is more difficult due to anatomic differences and usually must be performed over a bronchoscope. Thoracic surgery should be consulted to help with further assessment and management, which may include bronchoscopy, CT scanning, or bronchial artery angiography, followed by embolization or surgery.

For further reading in *Emergency Medicine, A Comprehensive Study Guide*, see Chapter 70, Hemoptysis, by James R. Yankaskas.

42 | Asthma and Chronic Obstructive Pulmonary Disease (COPD)

Frantz R. Melio

Asthma is a common chronic affliction with wide clinical variability. Though most patients have mild disease, asthma can be rapidly fatal. Patients with COPD often present in distress, expending tremendous effort to combat hypoxia. Uncomplicated medical or surgical disease will become more serious or life-threatening as the impact of COPD is unmasked.

Clinical Features

Asthma is defined as reversible airway obstruction, associated with hyper-responsiveness of the tracheobronchial tree. An early component of an asthmatic attack is bronchial smooth-muscle contraction. Bronchial inflammation, edema, and mucus hypersecretion become more prominent as the attack progresses. Increased airway resistance leads to air trapping, increased airway pressures, ventilation–perfusion imbalance, increased work of breathing, hypoxemia and, in severe cases, hypercapnea. Although bronchospasm can be reversed within minutes, mucus plugging and inflammatory changes do not resolve for days to wks. Patients with attacks lasting more than several days, steroid-dependent patients, and those with prior attacks requiring intubation are at higher risk for respiratory failure.

The most common etiology of COPD is cigarette smoking. Other causes include environmental toxins, genetic aberrations, and sustained bronchospastic airflow obstruction. There are two dominant clinical forms of COPD: (1) pulmonary emphysema, characterized by abnormal, permanent enlargement and destruction of the air spaces distal to the terminal bronchioles; and (2) chronic bronchitis, a condition of excess mucus secretion in the bronchial tree, occurring on most days for at least 3 mos in the year for at least 2 consecutive years. Elements of both forms are often present, though one predominates. Airway resistance, especially to expiration, is a fundamental feature of either condition. Hypoxemia and hypercapnea result from ventilation–perfusion mismatches and alveolar hypoventilation. As COPD progresses, neurochemical and proprioceptive ventilatory responses become aberrant. Pulmonary arterial hypertension develops leading to right ventricular hypertrophy and cor pulmonale. Clinically, compensated patients present with exertional dyspnea, chronic productive cough (frequently with minor hemoptysis), and expiratory wheezing. Coarse crackles are heard in patients with primarily bronchitic disease. An expanded thorax, impeded diaphragmatic motion, and diminished breath sounds are noted in those with emphysema.

Acute exacerbations of asthma/COPD are usually due to increased bronchospasm, smoking and exposure to other noxious stimuli, adverse response to medications (antihistamines decongestants, β-blockers, hypnotics tranquilizers), allergic reactions, and noncompliance with prescribed therapies. Respiratory infection, pneumothorax, myocardial infarction, dysrhythmias, pulmonary edema, chest trauma, metabolic disorders, and abdominal processes are triggers and complications of asthma/COPD. Patients with exacerbations of asthma/COPD present complaining of dyspnea, chest tightness, wheezing, and cough. Physical examination reveals wheezing with prolonged expiration. Wheezing does not correlate with degree of airflow obstruction. A "quiet chest" indicates severe airflow restriction. Patients and physicians often underestimate the severity of attacks. Patients with severe attacks may demonstrate sitting-up-and-forward posturing, pursed-lip exhalation, accessory muscle use, paradoxical respirations, and diaphoresis. Pulsus paradoxicus of 20 mmHg or more may be noted. Hypoxia is characterized by tachypnea, cyanosis, agitation, apprehension, tachycardia, and hypertension. Signs of hypercapnea include confusion, tremor, plethora, stupor, hypopnea, and apnea.

Diagnosis and Differential

ED diagnosis of asthma/COPD usually is made clinically. The clinician should attempt to determine the severity of the attack and the presence of complications. Objective measurements of airflow obstruction, such as peak expiratory flow rate, have been shown to be more accurate than clinical judgment in determining the severity of the attack, and the response to therapy. Laboratory examinations should be used selectively. Chest x-ray is used to diagnose complications such as pneumonia and pneumothorax. Arterial blood gases should not be obtained routinely. ABGs serve primarily to evaluate hypercapnea in moderate-to-severe attacks. Hypoxia can usually be evaluated by pulse oximetry. ABG results should be interpreted in light of the total clinical picture. Compensated hypercapnea and hypoxia is common in COPD patients, therefore, comparison with previous ABGs is helpful. Normocarbia in the setting of an acute asthmatic attack is an ominous finding if the patient is doing poorly. An arterial pH below that consistent with renal compensation implies either acute hypercarbia or metabolic acidosis. ECGs are useful to identify arrhythmias or ischemic injury. Measurements of methylxanthine levels should be obtained.

The differential diagnosis of decompensated asthma/COPD includes many of the disorders listed above as complications. In addition, interstitial lung diseases, pulmonary embolism, pulmonary neoplasia, aspirated foreign bodies, pleural effusions, and exposure to asphyxiants must be considered.

Emergency Department Care

Although patients with COPD often have more underlying illnesses than asthmatics, therapy for acute bronchospasm and inflammation is similar. Treatment should precede history-taking in acutely dyspneic patients, as patients may decompensate rapidly. These patients should be placed on a cardiac monitor, noninvasive BP device, and have continuous pulse oximetry. An intravenous line should be started in patients with moderate and severe attacks. The primary goal of therapy is to correct tissue oxygenation.

1. Hypoxemia is nearly universal during asthmatic attacks. Therefore, empiric supplemental oxygen should be administered. The need for supplemental oxygen with COPD must be balanced against the suppression of hypoxic ventilatory drive. Arterial saturation should be corrected to above 90%.
2. Beta-adrenergic agonists produce prompt effects and are the drugs of choice to treat bronchospasm. Aerosolized or parenteral forms should be used in critical settings. Aerosol therapy minimizes systemic toxicity and is preferred. **Albuterol sulfate**, 1.25 to 5 mg, and **metaproterenol**, 10 to 15 mg, are the most β2-specific agents. **Isoetharine**, 2.5 to 5 mg, or **bitolterol mesylate**, 0.5 to 1.5 mg, can also be delivered by nebulizer. Delivering doses in rapid succession maximizes results. Frequency of dosing depends on clinical response and signs of drug toxicity. Metered dose inhalers with spacer devices may be reasonable to use in less ill patients. Subcutaneous **terbutaline sulfate** (0.25–0.5 mL) or **epinephrine** 1:1000 (0.1–0.3 mL) may also be administered. Epinephrine should be avoided in the first trimester of pregnancy and possibly in patients with underlying cardiovascular disease. β-adrenergic agonists may inhibit uterine contractions when used near term.
3. Systemic glucocorticoids elicit bronchodilatory responses, facilitate the actions of concurrently given β-agonists and methylxanthines, and have antiinflammatory effects. As onset of action may take hours, they should be given early in the course of treatment. Steroids should be given immediately to patients with severe attacks, as well as patients who are currently taking, or have recently taken, these drugs. The optimal daily dose is the equivalent of 60 to 180 mg of Prednisone day, with an initial dose being the equivalent of 60 to 80 mg of **prednisone**. The choice of steroid is not critical. If the patient is unable to take oral medication, use **methylprednisolone** 125 mg IV. Hydrocortisone should be avoided, however, because of excess mineralocorticoid effect. Inhaled steroids are extremely useful in the treatment of chronic asthma/COPD, but should not be used for the treatment of acute symptoms.
4. Anticholinergics are useful adjuvants when given with other therapies. Iprotroprium bromide has recently replaced nebulized atropine

sulfate (1–3.5 mg) and glycopyrrolate (0.2–1mg) as the agent of choice. Nebulized **iprotroprium** (500 mg = 2.5 mL) may be administered either alone or mixed with albuterol. Iprotroprium is available as a metered dose inhaler. The effects of iprotroprium peak in 1 to 2 h and last 3 to 4 h. Dosages may be repeated every 1 to 4 h. When used with β-agonist agents, effects may be additive. The use of nebulized anticholinergics has been reported to cause attacks of narrow angle glaucoma due to topical ophthalmic absorption.

5. The role of methylxanthines in the treatment of acute asthma has been seriously challenged. Theophylline produces less bronchodilation than β-adrenergic agents. In addition, studies have shown that when used in combination with inhaled β-adrenergic agents, theophylline increases toxicity but not efficacy of therapy. Although methylxanthines are no longer first-line drugs, some patients not responding to β-agonists and steroids may benefit from the addition of theophylline. Methylxanthines seem to have more of a role in the treatment of chronic, stable asthma. The efficacy of methylxanthines in COPD is still controversial. The loading dose of theophylline is 5 to 6 mg/kg ideal body weight. In patients previously medicated, a mini-load should be given. The mini-load is calculated as (target concentration − measured concentration) × (0.5 × ideal body weight in liters). The maintenance dose is 0.2 to 0.8 mg/kg ideal body weight. These dosages should be used as guidelines. Metabolism of methylxanthines is highly variable. Increased serum levels are associated with liver disease, CHF, cor pulmonale, viral respiratory infections, advanced age, cimetidine, erythromycin, oral contraceptives, and allopurinol. Decreased levels are seen with cigarette smoking, phenobarbital, phenytoin, large consumption of charcoaled beef, and factors that promote the hepatic P450 enzyme system. Toxicity can be severe and can occur at drug levels that fall within the normal range. Serum levels should be measured to guide appropriate therapy.

6. Broad spectrum antibiotics (**TMP/SMX DS** bid, or **doxycycline** 100 mg bid, or others) are indicated for treatment of bacterial respiratory infections. Preventive polyvalent pneumococcal and trivalent influenza vaccination may be administered to stable COPD patients.

7. Although some authors have reported that 1 to 2 gm of intravenous magnesium sulfate reduces bronchospasm, no consistent clinical benefit has been demonstrated.

8. Sedatives, hypnotics, and other medications which depress respiratory drive are generally contraindicated. β-blockers may exacerbate bronchospasm. Antihistamines and decongestants should also be avoided as they diminish the ability to clear respiratory secretions. Mucolytics may provoke further bronchospasm. The benefit of iodides and glyceryl guaicolate in asthma and of doxapram in COPD

TABLE 42-1. Criteria for Hospital Admission in Acute Asthma*

Emergency visit within the preceding 3 days
Failure of subjective improvement following treatment
Failure of post-treatment FEV_1 to increase by >500 mL, or absolute value <1.6 L
Failure of post-treatment PEFR to increase more than 15% above initial value, or absolute value <200 L/min
Change in mental status (lethargy, agitation, exhaustion, confusion)
Failure of hypercarbia to resolve after treatment
Presence of pneumothorax

*Presence of any of these conditions warrants admission to the hospital.

are unproven. Many asthmatics respond poorly to ultrasonic nebulization and IPPB.

Criteria for admission are presented in Table 42-1.

If Standard Treatment Fails

Assisted mechanical ventilation is indicated for inability to maintain O_1 saturation above 90%, or severe hypercarbia associated with stupor, narcosis, or acidosis. In selected patients, noninvasive, positive-pressure ventilation (Bi-PAP) may avert artificial ventilation. Oral intubation is preferred as larger endotracheal tubes can be used. Larger tubes facilitate suctioning, fiberoptic bronchoscopy, and ventilator weaning. Initially, high inspired oxygen concentrations may be used. A volume-cycled ventilator should always be used. Excessive tidal volumes (over 15 mL/kg ideal body weight) and air trapping (due to bronchospasm) can cause barotrauma and hypotension. Utilizing high flow rates at a reduced respiratory frequency allows for adequate expiration. The goal of this approach, referred to as controlled mechanical hypoventilation, is to maintain adequate oxygenation with little regard to hypercarbia. Therapy should be guided by pulse oximetry and ABG results. Sedation and continued therapy for bronchospasm should continue after the patient has been placed on artificial ventilation.

For further reading in *Emergency Medicine, A Comprehensive Study Guide*, see Chapter 71, Acute Asthma in Adults, by Stanley Sherman; and Chapter 72, Chronic Obstructive Pulmonary Disease, by Joel C. Seidman.

7 | THE DIGESTIVE SYSTEM

Cary C. McDonald

BLEEDING ESOPHAGUS

Although most esophageal conditions are relatively infrequent and benign, both esophageal hemorrhage and perforation carry a high morbidity and mortality if not recognized and treated promptly.

Clinical Features

Patients with esophageal bleeding can present with life-threatening hematemesis, coffee-ground emesis, melena, hematest-positive stools, or anemia of chronic, occult blood loss, depending on the rate and duration of bleeding.

Diagnosis and Differential

Mild blood loss (less than 10%) is due to capillary bleeding or to sudden, nonrecurring arterial bleeding caused by inflammation, infection, or injury. Moderate blood loss (10%–20%) is due to laceration of an artery or nondistended vein. Major blood loss (20%–40%) and massive blood loss (>40%) are due to a ruptured varix or an artery eroded by a peptic ulcer. Vital signs are abnormal.

Emergency Department Care

Patients with self-limited mild bleeding, normal vital signs, and normal blood counts may require elective endoscopy, but not necessarily admission. Patients with moderate blood loss that is not self-limited usually require intravenous crystalloid infusion and possibly 1 to 2 units of blood to restore blood volume. Hospital admission for monitoring and diagnostic evaluation is required. Patients with major blood loss should receive fluids and blood plus undergo prompt fiberoptic endoscopy and admission to a critical care unit. Patients with massive blood loss require more than 4 units of blood, and coagulation abnormalities should be sought and corrected with fresh frozen plasma. Endoscopic confirmation of the bleeding source should be performed in the ED, and surgical consultation is mandatory.

If Standard Treatment Fails

If bleeding is from esophageal varices, initiate a vasopressin drip, 20 units in 200 mL of saline at 0.25 to 0.5 units per min. Sclerotherapy or Gelfoam embolization of the left gastric vein may be considered if bleeding continues. Blakemore-tube intubation is indicated in massive, uncontrolled lower esophageal bleeding not caused by esophageal laceration or peptic ulcer with stricture. The site of bleeding must be confirmed by endoscopy and the airway must be protected by endotracheal intubation prior to Blakemore-tube placement. The endotracheal tube cuff pressure must be released when passing the esophageal tube.

ESOPHAGEAL TRAUMA

Esophageal injury, which may be partial- or full-thickness, is infrequent and is usually iatrogenic or self-induced.

Clinical Features

Partial-thickness tears, which usually heal spontaneously, occur as a result of a swallowed sharp object and can cause symptoms such as dysphagia, odynophagia, and mild upper gastrointestinal bleeding (GI). Full-thickness injury without perforation can result from ingestion of caustic substances. Laceration of the mucosa and submucosa (Mallory–Weiss syndrome) and perforation of the full-thickness of the thoracic and abdominal esophageal wall (Boerhaave's syndrome) are associated with sudden, violent, and usually repeated increase in the intra-abdominal pressure against a weakened esophageal wall. The cause is a Valsalva movement occurring during violent emesis, hiccuping, defecation, seizure, or lifting a heavy weight. Lacerations cause usually moderate and self-limited bleeding of the submucosal plexus of veins and arteries. Perforation can occur from penetrating trauma, foreign bodies, or instrumentation and can lead to mediastinitis. Perforation associated with Boerhaave's syndrome causes the most malignant type of mediastinitis, because of the forced expulsion of acid into the mediastinal tissues and rapid spread of virulent bacteria. Patients complain of severe abdominal and chest pain radiating to the neck and rapidly develop shock and septicemia over 48 h.

Diagnosis and Differential

Patients with hematemesis or who develop chest or abdominal pain after vomiting are suspect for a lacerated or perforated esophagus. Patients with penetrating wounds of the chest or neck and with crushing chest wounds should also be suspect, as well as those patients with a history of swallowed foreign body. Radiologic signs of perforation on chest x-ray include pneumomediastinum, pneumothorax, pleural effusion, and subdiaphragmatic free air.

Emergency Department Care

Confirmation of esophageal perforation can be evaluated by a water-soluble contrast swallow study. Esophagoscopy should only be performed if a perforation cannot be confirmed by contrast studies or in an unconscious patient who cannot undergo a contrast study. Intravenous antibiotics, **cefoxitin** (1–2 g q6–8h) and **clindamycin** (300–600 mg q8h or 900–1200 mg q12h), should be given immediately and surgical consultation should be obtained. Mortality from perforation is 5% if surgical repair is made in under 24 h, and mortality can increase to 75% if surgical treatment is delayed.

FOOD BOLUS

Dysphagia, an awareness of difficulty swallowing, is associated with a foreign body sensation in patients with an esophageal food bolus.

Clinical Features

Patients tend to drool, are often hoarse, and have a bad cough with laryngeal involvement. Patients can usually localize the area of the food bolus.

Diagnosis and Differential

Mechanical causes of esophageal body dysphagia in the young include congenital stricture, vascular ring anomalies of the aortic arch, and swallowed foreign bodies. In older patients the most common causes include hiatal hernia, reflux esophagitis, webs, rings, and cancer of the throat, neck, or esophagus. Immunocompromised patients can have infectious causes, such as herpes virus, cytomegalovirus, and *Candida albicans*. Neuromuscular causes include achalasia, diffuse spasm, scleroderma, cerebrovascular accidents, dermatomyositis, polymyositis, and bulbar palsies. Rare causes in younger patients include myasthenia gravis, thyrotoxic myopathy, and lead poisoning.

Emergency Department Care

Indirect laryngosopy of the pharynx and hypopharynx may reveal abrasions or lacerations that may be responsible for some of the patient's symptoms. Swallowed bones may be identified on chest and lateral soft tissue cervical spine x-rays.

1. Parenteral **glucagon**, 0.5 to 2.0 mg, lowers smooth-muscle tone of the lower esophageal sphincter without inhibiting peristalsis. Patients with complete relief of symptoms can be discharged with a gastroenterology referral to rule out serious causes of obstruction.
2. If relief has not occurred with 2 doses of glucagon over 1 h, food bolus or radiolucent foreign body can be identified by a water-soluble contrast study. Balloon catheter retrieval should be avoided because of potential aspiration of the foreign body. The use of papain for proteolytic enzyme degradation of food bolus can result in perforation and mediastinitis.

If Standard Treatment Fails

Esophagoscopy must be performed to relieve food bolus obstruction or to retrieve a foreign body.

HEARTBURN AND ESOPHAGEAL COLIC

Esophageal disease must be considered with respect to more common emergency complaints, including chest pain and dysphagia.

Clinical Features

Heartburn or pyrosis is the most common symptom of esophageal disease and is caused by esophageal reflux of acid or alkaline gastric contents causing inflammation or ulceration. Heartburn is perceived as a substernal burning discomfort occurring after meals and is worse in recumbency and with exertion. Esophageal colic is an acute, agonizing, spasmodic, or crescendolike pain that can mimic cardiac ischemia. Substernal pain radiates directly through to the back into the interscapular area lasting seconds to hours and usually is indistinguishable from angina pectoris in terms of intensity, radiation, and relation to exertion.

Diagnosis and Differential

Pain arising from the esophagus is the most alarming esophageal symptom since it most often mimics chest pain due to cardiac ischemia or mediastinitis. Pain of esophageal origin may be the most common cause of noncardiac chest pain. It is often associated with other esophageal symptoms, such as dysphagia or reflux, but there are no classic clinical features to distinguish esophageal pain from cardiac pain. Both cardiac and esophageal patients can have ECG ST abnormalities.

Emergency Department Care

Relief of chest pain by antacids or repeated swallowing suggests esophageal origin. Esophageal colic may improve with sublingual **nitroglycerin**, but it usually takes 7 to 10 min for relief, instead of 2 to 3 min for relief of angina pectoris. Pain due to a myocardial infarction may not improve at all with nitroglycerin. Patients with abnormal ECGs should be approached as having cardiac disease. Any patient with cardiac risk factors and pain of unclear origin should be strongly considered for cardiologic consultation and admission.

If Standard Treatment Fails

Nonsteroidal anti-inflammatory medications (NSAIDs) should be avoided; narcotic analgesics can be considered for treatment of pain.

For further reading in *Emergency Medicine, A Comprehensive Study Guide*, see Chapter 74, Esophageal Emergencies, by Richard E. Burney and James R. Mackenzie.

Peggy E. Goodman

Foreign-body ingestion occurs in all age groups. Most cases occur in children, who swallow coins, toys, crayons, and other small objects. The remaining cases tend to occur in edentulous adults, psychiatric patients, or prisoners. Adults generally ingest meat or bones, and psychiatric and prison inmates ingest atypical foreign bodies, such as toothbrushes, spoons, and razor blades. Objects lodge in areas of physiologic narrowing where they can cause airway obstruction, stricture, or perforation, with infection, abscess, and fistula. Once an object has passed through the pylorus, it will generally pass without difficulty.

Clinical Features

Objects lodged in the esophagus can produce anxiety, retrosternal discomfort, retching, vomiting, dysphagia, coughing, choking, or aspiration, and the patient may be unable to swallow secretions. The adult patient can usually provide an accurate history as to the nature of the foreign body and the time of its impaction. In the pediatric patient it may be necessary to rely on clues such as refusal to eat, vomiting, gagging, choking, stridor, neck or throat pain, dysphagia, and increased salivation.

Diagnosis and Differential

Physical examination includes evaluation of the entire upper airway, including the neck and subcutaneous tissues. Direct or indirect laryngoscopy should be performed; in the absence of a foreign body, findings consistent with foreign-body ingestion, particularly in the pediatric age group, consist of red throat, palatal abrasion, temperature elevation, and peritoneal signs. Radio-opaque objects can be visualized on standard x-rays of the neck, chest, or abdomen, or by laryngoscopy or endoscopy. Esophagogram can be performed for localization but interferes with endoscopy.

Emergency Department Care

General care. Aspiration of the foreign body or builtup secretions should be prevented. If necessary, a tube should be placed proximal to the foreign body to remove unswallowed fluids or secretions. Serial abdominal examinations should be performed to detect early signs of developing peritonitis secondary to perforation. The progression of the foreign body through the GI tract can be monitored with the use of serial x-ray films or handheld metal detectors.

Food impaction. If the patient is able to manage secretions, conservative treatment is appropriate. If the food does not pass within 12 h, or the patient is unable to swallow fluids, intervention is necessary. These include administration of sublingual nitroglycerin (0.3–0.4 mg) or sublingual nifedipine (10 mg), monitoring carefully for hypotension, or glucagon, 1 mg IV, after test dose. Since 97% of adults with meat impaction have pathologic esophageal conditions, followup evaluation is indicated.

Coin ingestion. Approximately one third of children with coins lodged in the esophagus will be asymptomatic. Radiographs should be performed on all children suspected of swallowing coins to determine the presence and location of the object. Coins in the esophagus lie in the frontal plane; coins in the trachea lie in the sagittal plane. Coins usually pass spontaneously.

Button battery ingestion. Button battery ingestion is a true emergency because of potentially rapid caustic action. Esophageal burns have occurred within 4 h with perforation within 6 h. Outcome is affected by battery composition; lithium cells have a high incidence of adverse outcomes, and mercuric oxide cells fragment more frequently than other cells, although heavy metal poisoning does not appear to be a significant complication. Blood and mercury levels should be monitored if a mercury containing cell has opened while in the GI tract. If a button battery is in the esophagus, location should be documented by radiograph followed by emergent endoscopy. Button batteries that have passed the esophagus in an asymptomatic patient may be treated conservatively, unless the battery has not passed the pylorus after 48 h of observation (Most batteries pass through the body within 48 to 72 hours.) Battery identification assistance is available from the National Button Battery Ingestion Hotline at (202) 625-3333.

Ingestion of sharp objects. Management is controversial. Objects longer than 5 cm and wider than 2 cm rarely pass the stomach, and objects with extremely pointed edges, such as open safety pins or razor blades, may cause intestinal perforation, most commonly at the ileocecal valve. For children who have swallowed sharp objects, initial radiograph and examination should be performed. Asymptomatic children can be managed conservatively with serial radiographs.

Cocaine ingestion. Cocaine packet ingestion is used for drug concealment. Multiple small packets of cocaine may be contained within a condom. Conservative treatment and full bowel irrigation have been used.

If Standard Treatment Fails

Endoscopy is the procedure of choice for foreign-body retrieval, except for cocaine, due to risks of packet rupture. Endoscopy should be performed for objects lodged in the esophagus, heavy objects, sharp objects, coins and batteries that don't pass through the pylorus within 48 h, open batteries, and for other symptomatic patients. Fewer than 1% of ingested foreign bodies require surgical treatment.

Surgical intervention is necessary in cases of gastrointestinal obstruction or perforation, when objects fail to pass through the GI tract, and when endoscopic retrieval is not successful. It is also considered the safest method of cocaine packet recovery.

For further reading in *Emergency Medicine, A Comprehensive Study Guide,* see Chapter 75, Swallowed Foreign Bodies, by Wade R. Gaasch & Robert A. Barish.

45 | Peptic Ulcer Disease

Christian A. Tomaszewski

Peptic ulcers are mucosal defects in the gastroduodenal mucosa whose regenerative properties have been overcome by increased hydrochloric acid production or prostaglandin depletion by NSAIDs. Risk factors include: cigarette use, ethanol use, NSAID use, familial history, gastric outlet obstruction, infection with *Helicobacter pylori*, CPD, hepatic cirrhosis, and renal failure.

Clinical Features

Peptic ulcer disease classically presents with burning epigastric pain 1 to 3 h after meals, often awakening the patient at night. Although the patient may relate relief with food, more classic is relief with antacids or vomiting. Elderly patients or people using NSAIDs tend to have less pain associated with their ulcers. History may provide confirming clues, such as tobacco use, NSAID or alcohol ingestion, or familial predisposition to ulcers.

A history of frequent vomiting, weight loss, early satiety, or nausea should suggest gastric outlet obstruction. Hemodynamic instability, hematemesis or melena all confirm hemorrhagic complications. Although bleeding is not common, a perforation will usually present with severe pain or peritoneal signs.

Diagnosis and Differential Diagnosis

Typically the diagnosis of peptic ulcer disease is based on history and examination. The patient may have very mild epigastric tenderness. A succussion splash in the presence of excessive vomiting suggests gastric outlet obstruction. Directed laboratory work may confirm associated illness and can include cell blood count, creatinine, and calcium. Rectal exam and possible nasogastric aspiration may aid in diagnosing bleeding complications. In the presence of bleeding, one should consider clotting studies and, perhaps, liver function tests. A nasogastric tube may aid in the diagnosis of perforation by allowing the instillation of 250 ml air prior to an upright chest radiograph, specifically checking for air under the diaphragm. Definitive diagnosis of peptic ulcer disease can only be made with an upper GI series using barium or by direct endoscopic visualization. Such tests can be reserved for patients with severe pain or bleeding. Serologic tests for *H. pylori* and a serum gastrin may be useful in cases of persistent or recurrent peptic ulcer disease.

Many disorders can mimic peptic ulcer disease in pattern and location of pain. Pancreatitis is usually associated with worse pain and more commonly radiates to the back. With gastroesophageal reflux the patient may relate positional pain originating substernally. Clues to biliary colic include a history of fatty food intolerance (rather than relief of pain with food) in a middle-aged obese female. The most serious diagnosis confused with peptic disease is myocardial ischemia or infarction, which should be considered in any patient over 40 or with cardiac risk factors.

Emergency Department Care

Treatment is primarily done on an outpatient basis unless complications exist.

1. Pain can be relieved with liquid antacids (e.g., aluminum hydroxide gel, 30–60 ml) to be continued 1 and 3 h after each meal, and at bedtime.
2. Peptic ulcers are most conveniently treated with H_2 receptor antagonists, **cimetidine**, 300 mg IV or 400 mg po bid; **ranitidine**, 50 mg IV or 150 mg po bid; **famotidine**, 20 mg IV or 20 to 40 mg po qhs; and **nizatidine**, 150 to 300 mg po qhs.
3. Dietary modification should be encouraged, with avoidance of caffeine, alcohol, and NSAIDs.
4. In cases of resistant ulcers, one can consider omeprazole, a proton pump inhibitor. Sucralfate and misoprostol are secondary drugs that may be useful.

Patients who demonstrate any complication of peptic ulcer disease should be stabilized and admitted to the hospital. For hemorrhage, this includes intravenous fluids (RL or NS) with packed red blood cells (PRBCs) and fresh frozen plasma (FFP) as dictated clinically. Gastric lavage with room temperature water will help assess extent of bleeding and prepare the patient for both diagnostic and therapeutic endoscopy (see Chap. 14). Perforation requires nasogastric suction, broad-spectrum antibiotics, and surgical consultation (see Chap. 46). Pyloric stenosis requires correction of fluid and electrolyte abnormalities, with referral for surgical correction.

For further reading in *Emergency Medicine, A Comprehensive Study Guide*, see Chapter 76, Peptic Ulcer Disease, by John T. Sessions.

Acute Appendicitis and Perforated Viscus

Peggy E. Goodman

Classically appendicitis is a disease of people 10 to 30 years old, although it can affect all ages, often with atypical presentation. In 20% to 30% of cases, the appendix has ruptured by the time of diagnosis. Morbidity and mortality are directly related to delay between onset of symptoms and definitive treatment. The common, immediate complications include soft-tissue wound infection, intra-abdominal abscess, ileus, and prolonged hospitalization. Delayed morbidities include small-bowel obstruction, adhesions, and in females infertility can result.

Clinical Features

Classic presentation of (1) anorexia, (2) periumbilical pain associated with nausea or emesis, and (3) the development of steady periumbilical pain shifting to the right lower quadrant developing over a 24-h period occurs in approximately 60% of cases. Anorexia and pain are the more frequent symptoms, with nausea, emesis, diarrhea, and localized abdominal tenderness usually present. Left lower quadrant abdominal palpation with referred pain to the right lower quadrant is known as Rovsing's sign. The psoas sign, characterized by right lower quadrant pain on thigh extension, and the obturator sign (right lower quadrant pain on internal rotation of the flexed right thigh) are often helpful in the diagnosis of inflamed appendices that are posterior. Rebound tenderness supports the diagnosis but may be subtle. Severe colicky pain associated with acute appendiceal luminal obstruction is less common. Recurrent diarrhea associated with the pelvic location of the inflamed appendix is often misdiagnosed as acute gastroenteritis. This may be differentiated by localized tenderness on rectal exam. Rectal and pelvic exams are essential and may show localizing tenderness within the pelvis. Cutaneous hyperesthesia of the T10, T11, and T12 dermatomes may be present. In patients less than 2 years old, appendicitis is associated with a high degree of perforation and associated mortality. It may be manifested only as irritability, emesis, and abdominal distension. Clinical presentation in young children is similar to that in adults, however, in children the incidence of mesenteric adenitis and acute gastroenteritis is higher than in adults. Appendicitis in the elderly is associated with high percentage of rupture, but leukocytosis is less pronounced. Appendicitis during pregnancy often presents with pain at a higher location than usual, but is consistent with migration of the cecum from the right lower quadrant to the subcostal position. Perforating appendicitis during pregnancy carries an increased risk to the fetus and mother from septic complications and is associated with an increased risk of abortion.

Diagnosis and Differential

Due to its atypical nature, diagnosis of appendicitis is often difficult. Other diagnoses to consider are Crohn's disease, diverticulitis, pin worms, neoplasms, intussusception, torsion, mesenteric lymphadenitis, pelvic inflammatory disease, mittelschmerz, and acute gastroenteritis. An elevated leukocyte count is present in 86% of appendicitis cases, and an elevated absolute neutrophil count is present in 89%, although the magnitude of leukocytosis does not correlate with the severity of the appendicitis. If the inflammatory process lies close to the ureter, urinalysis will often reveal microscopic hematuria. Abdominal radiographs are neither sensitive nor specific for the diagnosis of appendicitis. Barium enema is useful with an equivocal diagnosis. If the appendix shows gas collection at the tip, extra-luminal gas in an abscess, extravasation of barium, or a sharp cutoff sign, suspect appendicitis. Visualization of a normal appendix does not exclude the diagnosis of appendicitis, however, barium enema may help to rule out terminal ileitis, diverticulitis, and neoplasm. Ultrasound examination has been shown to have a 75% to 90% sensitivity and an 86% to 100% specificity for appendicitis, if the appendix is an immobile, tender, noncompressible structure. Computed tomography is not effective in detecting early appendicitis, but can diagnose perforation, abscess, carcinoma, appendiceal mucocele, or pseudomyxoma peritonei.

Emergency Department Care

Surgical intervention is the treatment of choice for appendicitis.

1. The patient should have nothing by mouth. Intravenous fluids should be administered to maintain current needs and to correct any deficits.
2. A nasogastric tube may be inserted to diminish gastric distension.
3. Antibiotics are indicated after surgical intervention to decrease wound infection.

If Standard Treatment Fails

If the diagnosis is not clearcut, patients with mild symptoms and good followup may be discharged with careful instructions to return if symptoms worsen. If follow up is suboptimal, admission and observation with serial abdominal examinations is recommended.

PERFORATED VISCUS

Visceral perforation can be an early or late manifestation of underlying disease. Main causes of nontraumatic perforation of the gastrointestinal tract are increased intraluminal pressure, visceral wall abnormalities, iatrogenic causes, or ingested foreign bodies. Most perforations of the GI tract occur freely into the peritoneal cavity but may be localized by other structures or occur into a restricted space. Symptoms and signs are determined by (1) the viscus involved, (2) the location of the perforation, (3) the volume and chemical composition of the leaking fluids, (4) the underlying disease, (5) the host response mechanism, and (6) the elapsed time since perforation.

Spillage of intestinal contents into the peritoneal cavity produces a sudden increase in capillary permeability, with significant fluid shifts into the bowel lumen, bowel wall, and the mesentery. Bacterial contamination with release of endotoxin and exotoxins increase cell permeability and compound fluid losses into the third space. Initially, bowel irritability and hypermotility occur, followed by adynamic ileus and distension. Vascular compromise with hypovolemia and shock occur and can progress to septic shock with full cardiopulmonary collapse.

Perforated Ulcer

Chemical peritonitis due to acid and pepsin develops within the first 6 to 8 h. Posterior duodenal ulcers penetrate into the pancreas, where they are contained and result in pancreatitis. Anterior ulcers generally perforate into the peritoneal cavity, although the omentum or adjacent structures may be adherent and limit signs and symptoms. An antecedent history of ulcer disease is not always present and perforation may be the first manifestation. The pain of ulcer perforation is usually sudden and severe and is usually localized to the epigastrium but may radiate straight through to the back. Significant upper GI bleeding does not accompany perforation, although chronic blood loss may occur if the ulcer has been present for a long time.

Gallbladder Perforation

Obstruction of the cystic or common bile duct by stones produces distension of the gallbladder with vascular compromise, gangrene, and perforation. Gangrene can occur in acalculous cholecystitis, in diabetics, particularly postoperative, posttrauma, or burn patients, or in patients with hemolytic transfusion reactions or narcotic use. Others at risk are the elderly, patients with a history of stones or repeated cholecystitis, and patients with sickle-cell disease. Infection is often associated with a cystic or common bile-duct obstruction and stone formation, and there is a male predominance of two or three to one. Gallbladder perforation should be suspected in elderly patients with right upper-quadrant mass, fever, and leukocytosis who are deteriorating clinically or who develop signs of peritonitis. The bilirubin level and amylase level may be elevated. On routine x-ray, a stone may be seen free in the abdomen.

Perforation of the Small Bowel

Nontraumatic perforations of the mid-GI tract are uncommon. Jejunal rupture may result from drugs, infections, tumors, strangulated hernias, or regional enteritis. Jejunal rupture produces severe peritonitis. Perforations of the jejunum and ileum, especially if due to regional enteritis, may become walled off, and signs of generalized peritonitis may be delayed. Tachycardia and fever are common. The abdomen may be distended with hypoactive bowel sounds. Tenderness, rebound, guarding, and rigidity usually associated with peritonitis may be absent, especially in the elderly.

Perforation of the Large Bowel

Nontraumatic perforations of the lower GI tract are most commonly due to diverticulitis, carcinoma, colitis, and foreign bodies. Colon perforation produces signs and symptoms of sepsis rather than chemical irritation and, therefore, may be more subtle. If there is no obstruction, the more proximal the perforation, the more serious the clinical picture because the fecal stream is more liquid and disseminates rapidly. An antecedent history of partial or complete obstruction, change in bowel habits, or other findings consistent with carcinoma should be sought. Perforation secondary to obstruction, as in carcinoma or acute diverticulitis, may be associated with a temporary improvement of symptoms because the local distension has been relieved. Perforation from carcinoma is a result of erosion, not rupture, and is quickly followed by peritonitis, hypovolemia, and sepsis. Perforation secondary to diverticulitis usually results in abscess formation so that signs and symptoms of the abscess and mass may predominate.

Clinical Features

The hallmark of perforated viscus is abdominal pain. The severity, location, and acuity of onset help localize the site. Patients may be in acute distress and initially prefer a sitting or rocking position, although later they avoid movement, usually lying on one side with hips flexed to minimize peritoneal tension. Vomiting is usually present and follows the onset of pain. Bile in the vomitus indicates that the pylorus is open; coffee ground vomitus may be present in patients with duodenal or gastric ulcer. Feculent drainage from the nasogastric tube or feculent vomiting may indicate the presence of a long-standing small bowel obstruction, or the presence of dead bowel. Abdominal distension, the inability to pass gas, and constipation are all signs and symptoms of ileus or bowel obstruction. Marked tenderness on abdominal examination, with percussion tenderness over the area of inflammation, is frequently detected. Rigidity is often present if generalized peritonitis has developed. Immunocompromised patients, including those receiving glucocorticoids or chemotherapy, or AIDS patients, often have delayed recognition as well as increased risk of perforated viscus. Fever, tachycardia, narrowed pulse pressure, oliguria, and tachypnea are signs of hypovolemia and sepsis.

Diagnosis and Differential

The WBC count is generally elevated with a shift to the left, and the serum amylase level may also be elevated, although nonspecific. Metabolic acidosis may be present. An upright chest x-ray, or left lateral decubitus film of the abdomen are helpful in detecting free air, but may be falsely negative in early perforation. Pneumoperitoneum is pathognomonic for perforated viscus but is present in only 60% to 70% of perforated ulcer patients. Most patients will have clinical findings suggesting the diagnosis. If the diagnosis is equivocal, insufflation of 400 to 500 ml of air into the nasogastric tube, followed by tube clamping and an upright chest x-ray, may help confirm the diagnosis. Psoas shadows may be obscured by presence of fluid in the abdomen or in the retroperitoneal space. If there is no gas in the intestine, dead bowel may be present. Other findings on abdominal radiographs include: air-fluid levels in a stepladder pattern, indicating the presence of mechanical obstruction; dilated loops of bowel, indicating adynamic ileus; air along the biliary tract, if a gallstone has eroded into the bowel; intestinal wall edema; and free stones. Ultrasonography may be necessary to rule out the presence of cystic or common duct stones and to detect free intraperitoneal fluid. Abdominal CT scan may also be useful in identifying perforation and abscess formation. Radionuclide hepatobiliary scans for gallbladder perforation are not universally available. Diagnostic peritoneal lavage can be performed in cases of obscure diagnosis. If gas, food, bowel content, bile, turbid or bloody fluid is detected on initial aspiration, lavage is not necessary.

Emergency Department Care

1. Vigorous intravenous fluid resuscitation with balanced electrolyte solution is mandatory. Central venous pressure and hourly urinary output should be monitored, in addition to the pulse and pressure.
2. Intravenous, broad-spectrum antibiotics are indicated when the diagnosis of perforation is suspected, using agents active against both aerobic or facultative gram-negative bacteria and anaerobes. Antibiotic treatment protocols should be determined in conjunction with the surgeon.
3. Nasogastric tube insertion should be done early, even if the diagnosis is uncertain.
4. Short acting, reversible analgesics, such as fentanyl, may be used judiciously for pain relief.
5. Early surgical intervention is indicated at the time of diagnosis to minimize contamination, unless the patient has a specific contraindication.

For further reading in *Emergency Medicine, A Comprehensive Study Guide,* see Chapter 77, Perforated Viscus, by W. Kendall McNabney; and Chapter 78, Acute Appendicitis, by James A. Catto.

N. Heramba Prasad

Intestinal obstruction can either be due to mechanical factors or to the loss of normal peristalsis. The latter, known as adynamic or paralytic ileus, is more common but is usually self-limiting. Mechanical bowel obstruction is caused by various intrinsic or extrinsic factors. Commonly, mechanical small bowel obstruction (SBO) occurs from adhesions resulting from previous surgical procedures or inflammatory diseases. Incarcerated inguinal hernia is the second most common cause of SBO. Occasionally, hernias at other sites such as the umbilicus, the femoral canal, or the obturator foramen may cause incarceration and obstruction. Intraluminal causes such as polyps, lymphomas, and adenocarcinomas are some rare causes of SBO. Inflammatory bowel diseases such as regional enteritis, granulomatous colitis, ulcerative colitis, and diverticulitis may also affect the intestines at various levels. Congenital causes, such as atresia and stenosis, and foreign bodies such as bezoars, worms, gallstones, and hematomas should be considered in appropriate circumstances. Fecal impaction is a common problem in the elderly. Finally, intussusception in children and volvulus in the elderly should be kept in mind. Adynamic ileus is usually due to electrolyte abnormalities, peristaltic defects, infections, or retroperitoneal injuries.

Clinical Features

Crampy, intermittent abdominal pain is the main feature of intestinal obstruction. Vomiting, bilious in early stages and feculent in late stages, is usually present. Inability to have a bowel movement or to pass flatus is often a presenting complaint. Physical signs vary, ranging from abdominal distension, localized or general tenderness, to obvious signs of peritonitis. Localization of pain may provide clues as to the site of obstruction. Although most small intestinal disorders tend to cause periumbilical pain initially, colonic diseases localize in the hypogastric region. Active high pitched bowel sounds are usually heard in mechanical SBO. Organomegaly, if present, may suggest the cause for the obstruction. Presence of abdominal surgical scars, hernias, and other mass lesions should be noted. Systemic symptoms and signs will depend upon the extent of dehydration and the presence of bowel necrosis or infection. The patient may be septic and acutely dehydrated. Rectal examination may reveal fecal impaction, rectal carcinoma, or occult blood. Empty rectal ampulla may be strongly suggestive of intestinal obstruction. Presence of preexisting stool in the rectum, does not rule out obstruction. Pelvic examination may reveal any gynecologic infectious or neoplastic processes.

Diagnosis and Differential

Intestinal obstruction should be suspected in any patient with abdominal pain, distension, and vomiting, especially in those with previous abdominal surgery or groin hernias. Flat and upright abdominal radiographs and an upright chest x-ray should be obtained. In severely ill patients who cannot be upright, a left lateral decubitus film will be helpful. Distended intestines in the flat plate and step-ladder pattern of air-fluid levels in the upright or decubitus film will confirm the diagnosis. X-rays are helpful in localizing the site of obstruction to large or small bowel. Films should be closely examined for the presence of free air from perforation, pneumonitis, pleural effusion, of presence of gall stones and mass lesions such as enlarged viscera or phlegmon from inflammatory processes. Laboratory tests should include a complete blood count, electrolytes, BUN and creatinine, serum amylase, lipase, and a urinalysis. Liver function tests and typing and cross-matching for blood products may be required. Extreme dehydration from vomiting and fluid sequestration in the bowel may cause hematocrit and BUN to be elevated. Leukocytosis with left shift may suggest abscesses, gangrene, or peritonitis. High WBC count may suggest mesenteric vascular occlusion. High urine specific gravity, ketonuria, and metabolic acidosis may indicate the severity of the obstruction. Sigmoidoscopy and barium enema may be necessary to determine site and etiology of obstruction.

Emergency Department Care

Once the diagnosis of mechanical obstruction is established, surgical intervention is usually necessary.

1. Surgical consultation should be obtained without delay. In the ED, the bowel should be decompressed with a nasogastric tube.
2. Intravenous crystalloid replacement should be initiated. The patient's response to fluid therapy should be monitored closely with the BP, pulse, and urine output. Impending shock should be recognized, and the patient should be vigorously resuscitated.
3. Most patients will need broad-spectrum antibiotic coverage (such as **cefoxitin** 2 gm IV). When the diagnosis is uncertain, or if adynamic ileus is suspected, conservative measures, such as nasogastric decompression, IV fluids, and observation without surgical intervention, may be appropriate.

Pseudo-obstruction

Pseudo-obstruction commonly occurs in the low-colonic region. Depression of intestinal motility from medications such as anticholinergic agents or tricyclic antidepressants will cause large amounts of gas to be retained in the large intestine. Colonoscopy will be diagnostic as well as therapeutic. Surgery is not indicated.

If Standard Treatment Fails

Intestinal obstruction requires surgical intervention. Failure to adequately resuscitate may occur in patients at extremes of age, those who are septic and severely dehydrated, or when the diagnosis is unclear. Extra-abdominal causes of abdominal pain and distension such as metabolic diseases and pulmonary problems should be kept in mind.

For further reading in *Emergency Medicine, A Comprehensive Study Guide*, see Chapter 79, Intestinal Obstruction, by Salvator J. Vicario and John L. Glover.

Hernia in Adults and Children

Angelique Fontenette

A hernia is an external or internal protrusion of a body part from its natural cavity. Predisposing factors include family history, lack of developmental maturity of anatomic structures, undescended testes, genitourinary abnormalities, and conditions that increase abdominal pressure (i.e., ascites, peritoneal dialysis, VP shunt, cystic fibrosis, COPD). Potential locations for hernias include the inguinal, umbilical, femoral, epigastric, pelvic, lumbar areas, surgical incision sites, and after trauma in various organs.

Clinical Features

The majority of hernias are detected on routine physical exam or inadvertently by the patient. A hernia that can be returned to its normal cavity by manipulation is defined as reducible. On examination, patients exhibit abnormal swelling and may have a history of heavy lifting. Inguinal-hernia swelling extends to the scrotum. Examine the inguinal canal by inverting the scrotal skin. Pass a digit through the external ring and have the patient cough or bear down, which detects most inguinal hernias in men. The external ring in females is more difficult to assess. An indirect inguinal hernia is herniation through the internal ring lateral to the inferior epigastric vessels and may extend through the more medial ring defect in the external oblique aponeurosis. Internal inguinal hernias are congenital failure of obliteration of the process vaginalis. They are more common on the right and do not frequently incarcerate, particularly in the first year of life or in females. Direct inguinal hernias protrude medial to the epigastric vessels through the transversalis fascia and the external ring. Direct hernias are acquired defects that rarely incarcerate or strangulate. An irreducible or incarcerated hernia cannot be returned to its natural cavity and is the second leading cause of bowel obstruction (the leading cause is postoperative adhesions). Patients frequently have a history of a reducible hernia. Sudden swelling and tenderness develop if the incarceration is acute. If bowel is contained in the hernia, bowel sounds or peristalsis may be detected. Nausea and vomiting may develop if partial or complete obstruction occurs. In infants the presenting complaint may be irritability. Strangulation of a hernia occurs when an incarcerated hernia develops vascular compromise. Patients develop signs and symptoms of bowel obstruction. Gangrene and perforation can ensue along with abscess formation, peritonitis, and septic shock.

Diagnosis and Differential

Patients may exhibit a slightly elevated WBC count with a left shift. Toxic patients exhibit electrolyte and BUN abnormalities. In elderly patients these may not be reliable indicators. Obtain an upright CXR to detect free air secondary to perforation or dead bowel. To evaluate for bowel obstruction obtain upright and flat abdominal films. Spigelian hernias (located at the site of the semilunar line, lateral to the rectus muscle) or pelvic hernias are frequently interparietal, best evaluated by abdominal ultrasound or CT.

The differential diagnosis of groin hernias includes testicular torsion or tumor, tender lymph nodes, and hydroceles. Lymph nodes are movable, firm, and multiple. Hydroceles may transilluminate and are nontender. Incarcerated hernias do not transilluminate and are tender. In children, retractable or undescended testes may be mistaken for inguinal hernias.

Emergency Department Care

If there is a history of recent incarceration, attempt to reduce the hernia. If there is a question of the duration of incarceration, no attempt should be made. Do not introduce dead bowel into the abdomen. To reduce a hernia:

1. Place patient in Trendelenburg position.
2. Give mild sedation and place a warm compress on area.
3. Gently compress the hernia. Do not use excessive force for a prolonged time.

In children, inguinal hernias have a high risk of incarceration, particularly in the first year of life. Infants with inguinal hernias reduced in the ED should generally have repair within 24 h. Umbilical hernias in children rarely incarcerate. For children with hernias less than 2 cm in diameter and who are less than 4 years old, care includes discharge and primary-care observation. Referral for surgical evaluation is appropriate for children older than 4 or with hernias greater than 2 cm in diameter. In adults with reducible hernias, discharge patient and refer for surgical evaluation and repair. Discharge instructions should include avoiding increased intra-abdominal pressure, such as lifting, and to return to the ED if unable to reduce promptly.

Surgery is the treatment of choice for incarcerated hernias that are tender and unable to reduce or are strangulated. Patients should have noninvasive BP and cardiac monitoring. The patient should not be fed by mouth with fluids replenished with intravenous fluids. Insert a nasogastric tube. Broad-spectrum antibiotics and vigorous fluid resuscitation may be necessary, but only as a prelude to surgery.

For further reading in *Emergency Medicine*, *A Comprehensive Study Guide*, see Chapter 80, Hernia in Adults and Children, by Frank W. Lavoie.

Cary C. McDonald

CROHN DISEASE

Crohn disease, also described as regional enteritis, terminal ileitis, and granulomatous ileocolitis, is an idiopathic GI tract disease. Segmental involvement of any part of the GI tract from the mouth to the anus by a nonspecific granulomatous process characterizes the disease. There is a 3.5-fold risk of developing the disease in first-degree relatives of patients with Crohn disease.

Clinical Features

Abdominal pain, anorexia, diarrhea, and weight loss are present in up to 80% of cases, although the clinical course is variable and unpredictable. Patients commonly experience an insidious onset of recurring fever, abdominal pain, and diarrhea over several years without a definitive diagnosis. The 1 year recurrence rate is 25% to 50%, and the majority of patients develop perianal fissures or fistulas, abscesses, or rectal prolapse. Fistulas occur between the ileum and sigmoid colon, the cecum, another ileal segment, or the skin. Abscesses are characterized as intraperitoneal, retroperitoneal, interloop, or intramesenteric. Obstruction, hemorrhage, and toxic megacolon also occur. Half of all cases of toxic megacolon, frequently associated with massive GI bleeding, occur in patients with Crohn disease. Mortality from toxic megacolon is 50%.

Up to 20% of patients initially present with extraintestinal manifestations of arthritis, uveitis, or liver disease. Common hepatobiliary complications include gallstones, pericholangitis, and chronic active hepatitis. Some patients develop thromboembolic disease and have a 25% mortality rate. Malabsorption, malnutrition, and chronic anemia develop in longstanding disease, and the incidence of GI tract malignant neoplasm is triple that of the general population.

Diagnosis and Differential

The definitive diagnosis of Crohn disease is usually established months or years after the onset of symptoms. Common misdiagnoses are appendicitis and pelvic inflammatory disease. A careful and detailed history for bowel symptoms that preceded acute presentation may provide clues for correct diagnosis. The absence of true guarding or rebound is noted. Peritonitis and leukocytosis can be masked in patients taking glucocorticoids.

The differential diagnosis of Crohn disease include lymphoma, ileocecal amebiasis, tuberculosis, Kaposi sarcoma, *Campylobacter* enteritis, and yersinial ileocolitis. Most of these are uncommon and the latter two can be differentiated by stool cultures. A definitive diagnosis is confirmed by an upper GI series, an air-contrast barium enema, and colonoscopy. Plain abdominal radiography will identify obstruction and toxic megacolon, which may appear as a long, continuous segment of air-filled colon greater than 6 cm in diameter. Computerized tomography or ultrasound of the abdomen best identifies abscesses and fistulas.

Emergency Department Care

The aim of therapy includes relief of symptoms, suppression of the inflammatory disease, avoidance or management of complications, and maintenance of hydration and nutrition. Available pharmacologic agents are as follows:

1. **Sulfasalazine** (Azulfidine) (4 g/day) is effective for mild to moderate active Crohn disease but has multiple toxic side-effects, including GI and hypersensitivity reactions.
2. **Prednisone** (40 to 60 mg/day) is reserved for severe disease involving the small intestine and those patients with ileocolitis.
3. Immunosuppressive drugs, **6-mercaptopurine** (1 to 1.5 mg/kg/day) and **azathioprine** (2 mg/kg/day) are used as steroid-sparing agents, in healing fistulas, and in patients with surgical contraindications.
4. **Metronidazole** (Flagyl) (10 to 20 mg/kg/day) is useful in patients with perianal complications and fistulous disease.
5. Diarrhea can be controlled by **loperamide** (Imodium) (4 to 16 mg/day), **diphenoxylate** (Lomotil) (5 to 20 mg/day), and **cholestyramine** (4 g 1 to 3 times/day).

If Standard Treatment Fails

If patients experience toxic side-effects of sulfasalazine, alternate agents include: mesalamine (Pentasa and Asacol) in a 4-g/day, slow, time-dependent release form and a 2.4-g/day pH-dependent release form; and olsalazine (Dipentum), 1 g/day. These topical 5-aminosalicylic-acid derivative preparations have limited usefulness and should be used only when the disease involves the rectum and no more than 40 cm of distal rectosigmoid colon. Cyclosporine, methotrexate, broad-spectrum antibiotics, lipoxygenase inhibitors and immunoglobin therapy are current experimental agents.

Surgical intervention is indicated in patients who fail medical therapy and in those with intestinal obstruction or hemorrhage, perforation, abscess or fistula formation, toxic megacolon, or perianal disease. More than three out of four Crohn disease patients require surgery within 20 years of onset. The recurrence rate after surgery is nearly 100%.

ULCERATIVE COLITIS

Ulcerative colitis is an idiopathic chronic inflammatory and ulcerative disease of the colon and rectum characterized most often clinically by bloody diarrhea. There is a 15-fold risk of developing the disease in first-degree relatives of patients with ulcerative colitis.

Clinical Features

Ulcerative colitis is commonly characterized by intermittent attacks of acute disease with complete remission between bouts. Patients with mild disease (60%) may present with constipation and rectal bleeding, fewer than four bowel movements per day, no systemic symptoms, and few extraintestinal manifestations. The disease is limited to the rectum in 80% of cases and progresses to pancolitis in 10% to 15% of patients. Severe disease (15%) is associated with more than six bowel movements per day, weight loss, fever, tachycardia, anemia, and more frequent extraintestinal manifestations. Extraintestinal manifestations include peripheral arthritis, ankylosing spondylitis, episcleritis, posterior uveitis, pyoderma gangrenosum, and erythema nodosum. Virtually all patients with severe disease have pancolitis. Ninety percent of mortality from ulcerative colitis is in patients with severe disease.

The most common complications of the disease are blood loss from hemorrhage and toxic megacolon. Abscess and fistula formation, which is much more common in patients with Crohn disease, occur in 20% of patients with ulcerative colitis. There is a 10- to 30-fold risk of developing colon carcinoma. Other complications are similar to those of Crohn disease.

Diagnosis and Differential

Ulcerative colitis may be considered with a history of abdominal cramps, diarrhea, and mucoid stools. Laboratory findings are nonspecific and may include leukocytosis, anemia, thrombocytosis, decreased serum albumin, abnormal liver function tests, and negative stool studies for ova, parasites, and enteric pathogens. Rectal biopsy can exclude amebiasis and metaplasia. Barium enema can confirm the diagnosis and defines the extent of colonic involvement, but colonoscopy is the most sensitive method. These procedures should not be performed in moderately or severely ill patients. Rigid or fiberoptic proctosigmoidoscopic examination is abnormal in 95% of patients with ulcerative colitis and can be used in severely ill patients.

The differential diagnosis includes infectious, ischemic, irradiation, pseudomembranous, and Crohn colitis as well as irradiation. When the disease is limited to the rectum, consider sexually acquired diseases such as rectal syphilis, gonococcal proctitis, lymphogranuloma venerum, and inflammation caused by herpes simplex virus, *Entamoeba histolytica*, *Shigella*, and *Campylobacter*.

Emergency Department Care

The majority of patients with mild and moderate disease can be treated as outpatients. In addition to gastroenterology referral, treatment includes:

1. **Prednisone** (40 to 60 mg/day) is the mainstay of therapy in acute attacks. Steroids should be tapered once clinical remission is achieved. Topical steroid preparations, such as beclomethasone, hydrocortisone, tixocortol, and budesonide can be used to maintain remission.
2. **Sulfasalazine** (Azulfidine) (1.5 to 2 g/day) is most useful in maintenance therapy and reduces the recurrence rate.
3. The 5-aminosalicylic acid derivatives, mesalamine and olsalazine (see above) orally are quite effective in inducing remission. These drugs can be successful in topical enema preparations to treat active proctitis, left-sided colitis, and proctosigmoiditis.
4. Supportive measures include replenishment of iron stores, dietary elimination of lactose, and addition of bulking agents, such as psyllium (Metamucil). Antidiarrheal agents can precipitate toxic megacolon and should be avoided.

Patients with severe disease should be admitted for intravenous fluid replacement and electrolyte abnormality correction as well as the following treatment:

1. Intravenous steroids or ACTH.
2. Broad-spectrum antibiotics, such as ampicillin and clindamycin or metronidazole, active against coliforms and anaerobes.
3. Hyperalimentation should be considered.

If Standard Treatment Fails

A combination of glucocorticoids and immunomodulators (see Crohn disease above) should be considered, but beneficial effects may not be seen for 8 to 12 wks. Surgical consultation is indicated with toxic megacolon, massive lower GI bleeding, perforation, and disease that is refractory to medical therapy. Surgical treatment of choice is total proctocolectomy with ileostomy. Unlike Crohn disease, surgical intervention in ulcerative colitis is curative.

PSEUDOMEMBRANOUS COLITIS

Pseudomembranous colitis is an inflammatory bowel disorder in which membrane-like yellowish plaques of exudate overlay and replace necrotic intestinal mucosa. The incidence is increasing and three different syndromes have been described: pseudomembranous enterocolitis, postoperative pseudomembranous enterocolitis, and antibiotic-associated pseudomembranous colitis.

Clinical Features

Clinical manifestations can vary from frequent watery mucoid stools to a toxic picture including profuse diarrhea, crampy abdominal pain, fever, leukocytosis, and dehydration. Toxic megacolon or colonic perforation occurs rarely.

Diagnosis and Differential

Any antibiotic, but most commonly broad-spectrum antibiotics such as clindamycin, cephalosporins, and ampicillin alter the gut flora to allow toxin-producing *Clostridium difficile* to flourish within the colon. The diagnosis is made by a history of antibiotic use and by endoscopy. The disease typically begins 7 to 10 days after the institution of antibiotics, but the range is between a few days to 6 weeks. The diagnosis is confirmed by the presence of stool *C. difficile* toxin.

Emergency Department Care

The treatment of pseudomembranous colitis includes discontinuing antibiotic therapy and initiating intravenous fluid replacement and electrolyte abnormality correction. This is effective without additional treatment in 25% of patients.

1. **Metronidazole**, 250 mg, or **vancomycin**, 125 to 250 mg 4 times/day, orally is the treatment of choice in patients with mild to moderate disease who do not respond to supportive measures.
2. Severely ill patients must be hospitalized and should receive vancomycin, 500 mg 4/day for 7 to 10 days. Symptoms usually resolve within a few days.
3. Antidiarrheal agents may prolong or worsen symptoms and should be avoided.

If Standard Treatment Fails

Relapses occur in 10% to 20% of patients, necessitating a second course of treatment with vancomycin or with bacitracin 1 g/day orally for 7 to 10 days. Steroids and surgical intervention are rarely needed.

For further reading in *Emergency Medicine, A Comprehensive Study Guide*, see Chapter 81, Ileitis and Colitis, by Howard A. Werman, Hagop S. Mekhjian, and Douglas A. Rund.

| Colonic Diverticular Disease
Cary C. McDonald

Diverticular disease of the colon continues to increase in prevalence in industrialized nations. One third of the population will have acquired the disease by age 45 and two thirds by age 85. Clinical diverticulitis occurs in 10% to 25% of patients with diverticulosis. Diverticulitis in the younger age group tends to be a more virulent form of the disease, with frequent complications requiring earlier surgical intervention.

Clinical Features

The most common symptom is a steady, deep discomfort in the left lower quadrant of the abdomen. Right lower quadrant pain can occur with ascending colonic involvement and in patients with redundant right-sided sigmoid colon. Other symptoms include tenesmus and changes in bowel habits, such as diarrhea or increasing constipation. The involved diverticulum can irritate the urinary tract and cause frequency, dysuria, or pyuria. If a fistula develops between the colon and the bladder, the patient may present with recurrent urinary tract infections or pneumaturia. Paralytic ileus with abdominal distension, nausea and vomiting may develop secondary to intra-abdominal irritation and peritonitis. Small-bowel obstruction and perforation also can occur. Diverticular bleeding, which can be massive but is usually self-limited, occurs in 5% to 15% of patients with diverticulosis.

Diagnosis and Differential

Patients frequently present with a low-grade fever, but the temperature may be more elevated in patients with generalized peritonitis or in those with an abscess. Abdominal examination reveals localized tenderness, often with voluntary guarding and localized rebound tenderness. Right lower quadrant pain can be indistinguishable from acute appendicitis. With careful palpation, a fullness or mass may be appreciated over the involved segment of the colon. Rectal examination may reveal tenderness on the involved side. A pelvic exam should always be performed in female patients to exclude a gynecologic source of symptoms. Differential diagnosis is listed in Table 50-1.

Laboratory studies should include routine screening blood tests, urinalysis, and abdominal x-ray series. Leukocytosis is present in less than one third of patients with diverticulitis. The abdominal series may be normal or may demonstrate an associated ileus, partial small-bowel obstruction, colonic obstruction, free air indicating bowel perforation, or extraluminal collections of air suggesting a walled-off abscess. Ultrasonography or CT of the abdomen and pelvis may demonstrate bowel-wall thickening, mesenteric inflammation, or abdominal fluid

TABLE 50-1. Differential Diagnosis for Diverticulitis

Acute appendicitis
Abdominal aortic aneurysm
Irritable bowel syndrome
Inflammatory bowel disease
Carcinoma of the colon
Ischemic colitis
Pelvic inflammatory disease
Renal calculus
Other colonic diseases
   Amebiasis
   Lymphogranuloma venerum
   Gonorrheal proctitis
   Fecal impaction
   Foreign-body granuloma
   Endometriosis
   Collagen disease
   Postirradiation proctosigmoiditis
   Hytic tuberculosis
   Syphilis
   Actinomycosis

collections suggestive of abscess. Performing sigmoidoscopy or contrast radiographic studies during the acute inflammatory state is controversial.

Emergency Department Care

Localized pain without signs and symptoms of local peritonitis or systemic infection may be treated on an outpatient basis.

1. Treatment consists of bowel rest and broad-spectrum oral antibiotic therapy, including **ampicillin** (500 mg q6h), **trimethoprim–sulfamethoxazole** (2 tablets q12h), **ciprofloxacin** (500 mg q12h), or **cephalexin** (500 mg q6h) *and* **metronidazole** (500 mg q8h), or **clindamycin** (300 mg q6h) to cover both aerobic and anaerobic organisms.
2. Patients should limit activity and maintain a liquid diet for 48 h. If symptoms improve, low-residue foods are added to the diet.
3. Patients are advised to contact their physician or return to the ED if they develop increasing abdominal pain, fever, or malaise.
4. Admission is indicated in patients with systemic signs and symptoms of infection or localized peritonitis.
5. Nasogastric suction may be indicated in patients with bowel obstruction or adynamic ileus; surgical consultation should be obtained. Intravenous antibiotics, usually **ampicillin** (2 g q6h), an aminoglycoside, such as **gentamicin** or tobramycin (2 mg/kg loading dose, then 1.0 mg/kg q8h), and **metronidazole** (1 g q12h), or **clindamycin**

(300–600 mg q8h or 900–1200 mg q12h) are given for aerobic and anaerobic organism coverage.

For further reading in *Emergency Medicine, A Comprehensive Study Guide,* see Chapter 82, Colonic Diverticular Disease, by Stephen G. Priest and Steven N. Klein.

Anorectal disorders may be due to local disease processes or underlying serious systemic disorders. Whenever a patient presents with rectal bleeding or pain, disorders discussed below should be considered.

ANATOMY

The endodermal intestine joins with the ectodermal anal canal at the dentate line, at approximately 1 to 2 cm from the anal verge. The rectal ampulla narrows proximal to the dentate line, causing the mucosa to form pleated columns of Morgagni. At the dentate line, the columns form small anal crypts. These crypts may sometimes contain small anal glands that extend through the internal sphincter. The submucosa of the rectum contains blood vessels that thicken at the dentate line, forming the internal hemorrhoidal plexus. The inner circular muscle layer of the rectum forms the internal sphincter. Voluntary muscles of the pelvic floor, levator ani, and puborectalis form the external sphincter. (See Fig. 51-1.)

Examination

After a detailed history of the complaints, a digital examination of the rectum, followed by anoscopy or rectosigmoidoscopy, must be performed. The patient should be placed in one of three positions:

1. Left lateral or Sim's position, with the left leg extended and the right leg flexed at the knee and hip. This is probably the most common position used in the ED.
2. Supine or lithotomy position for debilitated patients.
3. Knee–chest position in patients who are cooperative provides for a thorough examination.

HEMORRHOIDS

The internal hemorrhoidal veins are part of the portal system whereas the external hemorrhoidal veins drain into the systemic circulation through the iliac and pudendal veins. Engorgement, prolapse, or thrombosis of these veins is termed hemorrhoids. Internal hemorrhoids are not readily palpable and are best visualized through an anoscope. They are constant in location and are found at 2, 5 and 9 o'clock positions when the patient is prone. Constipation and straining at stool, pregnancy, and increased portal venous pressure are some of the common causes of hemorrhoids. Tumors of the rectum and sigmoid colon should be considered in patients over 40 years old.

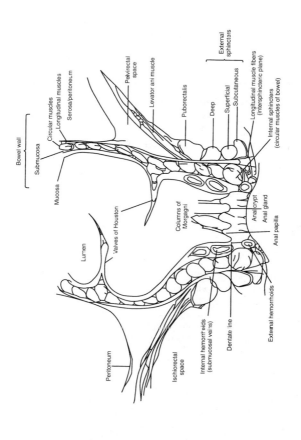

FIG. 51-1. Coronal section of the anorectum.

Clinical Features

Painless, self-limited, bright-red rectal bleeding is the usual symptom in uncomplicated hemorrhoids. Pain is usually associated with thrombosed hemorrhoids. Large hemorrhoids may result in prolapse that may spontaneously reduce or require periodic reduction by the patient. They may become incarcerated and gangrenous, necessitating surgical intervention. Prolapse may cause mucous discharge and pruritus. Strangulation, severe bleeding, and thrombosis are common complications.

Emergency Department Care

Unless complication is present, management is usually nonsurgical.

1. Hot sitz baths for at least 15 min 3 times/day and after each bowel movement will ameliorate pain and swelling. Following the sitz baths, the anus should be gently but thoroughly dried. Use of topical steroids, antibiotics, and analgesics are usually of no value and, in fact, may cause harm.
2. Bulk laxatives, such as psyllium seed compounds or stool softeners, should be used after the acute phase has subsided. Laxatives causing liquid stool are best avoided as they may result in cryptitis and sepsis.
3. Surgical treatment for hemorrhoids is indicated for severe, intractable pain, continued bleeding, incarceration, or strangulation.
4. Thrombosed external hemorrhoids may need surgical decompression and excision of the clots. If they have been present for less than 48 h and the pain is tolerable, sitz baths and bulk laxatives may be tried initially. Acute and recently thrombosed, painful hemorrhoids should be treated with excision of the clots. After analgesia with appropriate conscious sedation and local infiltration, an elliptical skin incision is made over the hemorrhoids and the thrombosed vein is removed along with the elliptical skin (Fig. 51-2). Packing and a pressure dressing will usually control the bleeding. The pressure dressing may be removed after about 6 h, when the patient takes the first sitz bath.

CRYPTITIS

Sphincter spasm and repeated trauma from large hard stools cause breakdown of the mucosa over the crypts. This may lead to inflamed anal glands and abscess formation, fissures, and fistulae.

Clinical Features

Anal pain, especially with bowel movements, and itching, with or without bleeding, are the usual symptoms of cryptitis. Diagnosis is confirmed by palpation of tender, swollen crypt with associated hyper-

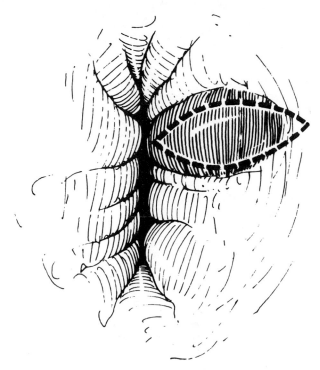

FIG. 51-2. Elliptical excision of thrombosed external hemorrhoid. (From Goldberg SM et al: *Essentials of Anorectal Surgery*. Philadelphia, Lippincott, 1980. Used by permission.)

trophied papillae. Anoscope provides definitive diagnosis. The crypts commonly involved are in the posterior midline of the anal ring.

Emergency Department Care

Bulk laxatives, additional roughage, hot sitz baths, and warm rectal irrigations will enhance healing. Surgical treatment may be needed in refractory cases.

FISSURE IN ANO

Anal fissures are the most common cause of painful rectal bleeding. Swelling of the surrounding tissues produces hypertrophied papillae proximally and sentinel pile distally. Most anal fissures occur in the midline posteriorly. A fissure not in the midline should alert the physician for other potentially life-threatening causes, such as Crohn disease, ulcerative colitis, carcinomas, lymphomas, syphilis, and tuberculosis.

Clinical Features

Sharp cutting pain occurs with defecation and subsides between bowel movements, which distinguishes fissures from other anorectal disorders. Bleeding is bright and in small quantities. Rectal examination is very painful and often not possible without application of topical anesthetic agents. In many instances, sentinel pile and the distal end of the fissure can be seen after gently retracting the buttocks, and further rectal examination may be deferred.

Emergency Department Care

Treatment is aimed at relieving sphincter spasm, pain, and at preventing stricture formation. Hot sitz baths and the addition of bran (fiber) to the diet are helpful. Use of topical anesthetics, while temporarily helpful, may cause hypersensitivity reaction. Topical steroids are not recommended, as they may retard wound healing. Surgical excision of the fissure may be required if the area does not heal after adequate treatment.

ANORECTAL ABSCESSES

Abscesses start from the anal crypts and spread to involve the perianal, intersphincteric, ischiorectal, or the deep perianal space. Perianal abscess is the most common form seen at the anal verge. When not associated with any other perirectal infection or systemic symptoms, perianal abscess is the only one that can be safely incised in the ED.

Clinical Features

Pain can be dull, aching, or throbbing and becomes worse before defecation, but persists between bowel movements. Fever and leukocytosis may be present.

Emergency Department Care

Most abscesses should be drained in the operating room. Simple perianal abscesses may be drained in the ED, if surgical consultation is not readily available. After adequate local analgesia with conscious sedation, a cruciate incision is made over the abscess, and the dog ears excised. Packing is usually not required. Sitz baths should be started the next day.

FISTULA IN ANO

Fistulae commonly result from perianal or ischiorectal abscess. Crohn disease, ulcerative colitis, tuberculosis, gonococcal proctitis, and carcinomas should be considered in the etiology. Persistent bloody, malodorous discharge occurs as long as the fistula remains open. Blockage of the tract causes recurrent bouts of abscess formation.

Emergency Department Care

Surgical excision is the definitive treatment. Sitz baths and local cleansing will temporize the condition until surgery.

VENEREAL PROCTITIS

Clinical Features and Emergency Department Care

Most sexually transmitted diseases (STDs) of the anorectum manifest with itching, discharge, and mild pain or irritation. Condyloma acuminata (common warts) are caused by papilloma virus. They are discrete, soft fleshy growths associated with pruritus and pain. Other STDs and carcinomas should be ruled out. Multiple biopsies to rule out associated squamous cell carcinoma will be necessary. Gonococcal proctitis occurs mostly in homosexual men and is characterized by severe rectal pain and profuse discharge. Anoscopy will reveal diffuse inflammation and discharge from the anal crypts. Venereal cryptitis is not confined to the posterior crypts. *Chlamydia trachomatis* infections may cause abscesses, rectal scarring, fistulae and strictures. Syphilitic lesions may be primary chancre or condylomata lata, a manifestation of secondary syphilis. Condylomata lata are characterized by flat, smooth, confluent, firm, and raised lesions. Herpes simplex virus (HSV-2) infections cause discrete vesicles that coalesce to form tender aphthous ulcers. AIDS-related disorders of the anorectal region include infections by herpes simplex virus, cytomegalovirus, *Salmonella, Shigella, Mycobacterium ovium, Campylobacter*, and *Giardia*. History, anoscopy and cultures, gram stain and serological tests, will help confirm the diagnosis of venereal proctitis. Appropriate antibiotic therapy should be instituted without delay (Chapter 82, Sexually Transmitted Diseases).

RECTAL PROLAPSE

Prolapse (procidentia) may involve either just the mucosa or all the layers of the rectum. In addition, intussusception of the rectum may present as a prolapse.

Clinical Features

Most patients will complain of protruding mass, mucous discharge, associated bleeding, and pruritus may be present.

Emergency Department Care

In children under proper analgesia and sedation the prolapse can be gently reduced. Every effort should be made to prevent the child from being constipated. Surgical correction is usually necessary in all other age groups.

RECTAL FOREIGN BODIES

Emergency Department Care

Most rectal foreign bodies are low lying and can be removed in the ED. If the size and shape are such that perforation is suspected, a followup proctoscopy or x-rays may be required. Adequate sphincter relaxation is essential for removal of foreign bodies. Local infiltration anesthesia injected through a 30-gauge needle into the internal sphincter muscle circumferentially will provide good relaxation. The examiner's finger in the rectum will help guide the needle into the sphincter. Large bulbar objects may create a vacuum-like effect proximally, making removal by simple traction impossible. In these cases, the vacuum can be overcome by passing a catheter around the foreign body into the ampulla and injecting air. Occasionally, passing a Foley catheter proximal to the foreign body, inflating the balloon and applying gentle traction may help maneuver the foreign body into a more desirable position for ease of removal.

PILONIDAL SINUS

Clinical Features

Pilonidal sinus and cyst occur in the midline over the lower sacrum and coccyx. Abscesses may form from ingrown hair. The sinus may present with persistent discharge; cyst or abscess may present with pain and swelling. Infected pilonidal cysts are sometimes mistakenly diagnosed as perirectal abscesses.

Emergency Department Care

Surgery is indicated in almost all cases. Acute abscesses may be drained in the ED, but a definitive elective excision in the operating room still may be necessary. Drainage in the ED should be undertaken, when indicated, under proper conscious sedation and local infiltration analgesia. The abscess should be drained and the sinus tract should be exposed with the aid of a groove-director probe. All loculations must be released. Wound should be packed and analgesics prescribed.

PRURITUS ANI

Clinical Features and Emergency Department Care

Although primary or idiopathic pruritus does occur, other causes should be ruled out. These include: fissures, fistulae, hemorrhoids, and prolapse;

dietary factors, such as caffeine, milk, chocolate, tomatoes, and citrus fruits; infections, pinworms, *Candida, Trichophyton*, and local irritants. Treatment will depend upon the underlying condition.

If Standard Treatment Fails

Failure of therapy usually indicates unrecognized underlying problems such as inflammatory diseases, carcinomas, or infections. Surgical consultation should be obtained in refractory cases. Inadequately drained abscesses that recur are commonly seen by emergency physicians. One should remember that drainage of anorectal abscesses should be undertaken in the operating room whenever possible. Drainage in the ED will only serve as a temporizing measure, and prompt surgical followup is mandatory.

For further reading in *Emergency Medicine, A Comprehensive Study Guide*, see Chapter 83, Anorectal Disorders, by James K. Bouzoukis.

Christian A. Tomaszewski

Diarrhea is a prevalent disease that kills up to 10 million people a year in developing countries and is the third most common cause of pediatric hospitalization in the United States. Causes of severe acute diarrhea include food poisoning and infectious diseases. Other etiologies include antibiotic enterocolitis, inflammatory bowel disease, cystic fibrosis, lactose/milk intolerance, malignancy, obstruction, or endocrinopathies. Although diarrhea may result from a variety of toxic contaminants, this section will concentrate on infectious etiologies.

Clinical Features

Diarrhea is defined as any increase in frequency or liquidity of stool output. It can be divided into two gross types based on the presence of an inflammatory response to an invasion of the gastrointestinal mucosa. *Noninflammatory* diarrhea is usually due to loss of absorptive surface from viral or protozoal infection. Alternatively, enterotoxins from *Vibrio cholerae* or strains of *E. coli* can stimulate a secretory type diarrhea. All these diarrheas are watery and are not associated with fecal leukocytes. *Inflammatory* diarrhea, also known as dysentery, is due to mucosal penetration. Accompanied by fever and abdominal pain, this is a diarrhea that has fecal leukocytes or even blood present. This type of diarrhea is caused by invasive organisms such as *Shigella, Campylobacter, Salmonella, Yersinia*, and invasive *E. coli. Clostridium difficile, Vibrio*, and *Aeromonas* intermittently present with fecal leukocytes. *Yersinia, Campylobacter*, and *Salmonella* can progress to enteric fever with penetration of intestinal cells and systemic infection. The former two organisms have been known to mimic appendicitis.

The biggest complication of diarrheal illness is dehydration and electrolyte imbalance, especially in the prone young and old. Improper fluid replacement, without salt, improper antibiotics, and antimotility agents may further complicate the illness.

The etiologies of diarrhea can be divided into three broad categories:

Viruses. This is the most common cause of acute diarrhea. The most common viruses are rotavirus, adenovirus, enterovirus, calcivirus, astrovirus, and Norwalk agent. The first three can cause upper respiratory symptoms as well. Rotavirus, adenovirus, and Norwalk are associated with severe vomiting. Rotavirus is notorious for causing severe dehydration in infants less than 12 mo.

Bacterial. Bacterial causes of diarrhea can be divided into invasive and noninvasive. The invasive organisms usually require a day or two of incubation before causing a severe diarrhea accompanied by abdominal cramps, fever, and often fecal leukocytes. The noninvasive organisms cause diarrhea through a toxin, either preformed or formed after gastrointestinal colonization.

Escherichia coli, the main cause of traveler's diarrhea, can be either toxigenic (noninflammatory) or invasive (inflammatory). Abdominal cramps and watery diarrhea occur 2 to 4 days after ingesting contaminated food or water. *E. coli* serotype O157:H7 can produce a toxin-mediated hemorrhagic colitis after the ingestion of improperly cooked beef. Children are especially prone to complications, including hemolytic uremic syndrome and, occasionally, TTP.

Shigella causes a fulminant invasive diarrhea 36 to 72 h after ingestion of as little as 100 organisms through fecal, oral, or food contamination. In children this infection is associated with high temperatures and febrile seizures. Although rare, bacteremia can occur.

Salmonella enteritis occurs 8 to 48 h after ingestion of contaminated eggs or poultry, or it can come from pet turtles. An invasive form of illness can occur from *S. typhi*, with fever, abdominal pain, occasional rose spots, and meningismus. Patients with sickle cell, AIDS, or splenectomies are especially prone to bacteremia.

Yersinia can be ingested in food and water through fecal–oral transmission from domestic animals, including pets. Special features of this infection include bloody diarrhea in 25% of cases; less common features include mesenteric adenitis, or pseudoappendicitis, and erythema nodosum in women.

Campylobacter, through both an enterotoxin and tissue invasion, causes fever and bloody diarrhea, with abdominal pain in two-thirds of cases, and vomiting in one-third. Contaminated food, especially poultry, and water are the sources of this infection.

Clostridium perfringens is caused by an enterotoxin from heat-resistant stains. This leads to abdominal cramps and diarrhea 6 to 24 h after ingestion of contaminated meat products.

Clostridium difficile can overgrow to cause pseudomembranous enterocolitis after a short course of antibiotics. The cytotoxic diarrhea caused by this organism can occasionally lead to mucosal damage with leukocytes in the stool.

Staphylococcus aureus can cause vomiting and diarrhea 2 to 24 h after ingestion of the preformed toxin in meats, poultry, or dairy products.

Bacillus cereus enterotoxins can cause an early vomiting illness 1 to 6 h after ingestion of fried rice. Later, 6 to 24 h after eating contaminated food, an enteritis may develop with diarrhea.

Vibrio cholerae infection results in enterotoxin production that initially begins with vomiting followed by copious rice water stools. More invasive is *Vibrio parahemolyticus*, which can result in either mild diarrhea or full-blown dysentery after a 12-h incubation, from ingestion of raw shellfish. *Vibrio vulnificus*, also from contaminated raw oysters and shellfish, is associated with mortality in patients with pre-existing liver disease.

Aeromonas and *Plesiomonas* can cause mild diarrhea with fever but can be extremely invasive with dysenteric stools. The former organism results from contaminated fresh water; the latter from contaminated shellfish as well as domestic animals.

Parasites. Although a variety of protozoans and helminths can produce diarrhea, only a few are important causes of acute diarrheal illness:

Entamoeba histolytica is present in up to 5% of Americans as asymptomatic cyst carriers. Infection from contaminated food or anal sex can cause colitis, or in more severe cases, acute amebic dysentery, with profuse bloody diarrhea. Five percent of these patients can have extraintestinal infections, most commonly as liver abscess.

Giardia lamblia is a very common intestinal parasite in the United States, most typically from drinking waters infested by beavers or from fecal-oral transmission in day care centers. Symptoms include excessive bloating, cramps, flatus, and frothy, floating foul-smelling diarrheal stools.

Cryptosporidium has been seen in day care centers, travelers, and even in contaminated city water supplies in the U.S. Although it typically results in self-limited, profuse, watery diarrhea, patients with AIDS may have chronic unremitting infection. *Isospora belli* can cause a similar illness.

Diagnosis and Differential

History should include mention of travel—foreign or wilderness—and particular foods, such as meat or fish. Duration of diarrhea, especially if 2 wks or longer, may suggest parasitic illnesses. History of antibiotic use may explain simple diarrheal illness or portend more serious pseudomembranous colitis. A history of blood may imply invasive inflammatory diarrhea. The physical exam should include attention to signs of dehydration: mucous membranes, skin turgor, orthostatics, level of consciousness, and the anterior fontanel in infants. Abdominal tenderness can be problematic because of its implications for surgical disease.

The most important laboratory study in the workup of diarrheal illness is direct examination of the stool. Methylene blue preparation will reveal the presence of leukocytes, a fairly reliable indicator of invasive/inflammatory diarrhea. A positive hemoccult can indicate invasive diarrhea as well. Electrolytes and urine specific gravity can confirm dehydration and its complications. Stool cultures can be reserved for cases of suspected *Salmonella, Shigella, Campylobacter,* or *Vibrio,* which includes: (1) patients with severe dysentery; (2) presence of white cells on smear; or (3) patients that work in the health, food, or day care industries. Ova and parasite exams can be done with chronic diarrhea that persists beyond 2 wks. An acid-fast stool stain may reveal *Crypto-sporidium* or *Cyclospora*.

The most disastrous misdiagnosis in the differential of diarrhea is a missed surgical disorder. Up to 20% of appendicitis cases may present with diarrhea. In addition, intussusception in the young and ischemic bowel in the elderly may present with loose blood-tinged stools. Gross bloody diarrhea may be the result of increased transit time from gastro-intestinal bleeding. Many toxins, including iron, arsenic, and organo-phosphates can cause diarrhea. Among potential food toxins, consider poisonous mushrooms or fish, such as ciguatoxin, which may be accom-panied by burning paresthesias.

Emergency Department Care

Treatment of diarrhea consists of correcting fluid and electrolyte prob-lems and rarely requires specific antibiotic therapy.

1. Replacement of fluids can be intravenous with normal saline in seriously ill patients. Most patients will tolerate any pediatric oral rehydrating solution containing at least 45 mEq/L of sodium, as well as glucose, to enhance fluid absorption. Commercial sports rehydrating drinks contain less sodium but are adequate in older children and adults.
2. Nutritional supplementation should be started as soon as nausea and vomiting subside. Clear liquids can be quickly advanced to solids such as rice and bread. Because lactase deficiency is not a clinical problem, the American Academy of Pediatrics recommends an early, first day return to breastfeeding or formula in infants. By reinstituting regular feeds, the diarrhea and fluid and electrolyte problems tend to abate sooner.
3. Antibiotics are generally reserved for patients with fever and toxicity from invasive diarrhea (Table 52-1). Almost all invasive diarrhea responds to quinolones (**ciprofloxacin**, 500 mg po bid, or **norfloxa-cin**, 400 mg po bid). In children, trimethoprim/sulfamethoxazole can be used instead, especially for recalcitrant cases of *Salmonella* or *Shigella*. Most normal hosts will clear the infection if they can maintain a good fluid and electrolyte balance. Antibiotics are espe-cially indicated in patients who appear toxic, immunocompromised, or are involved in sensitive areas (e.g., food handling, day care, health care).
4. Antidiarrheal agents are controversial and should be avoided in invasive diarrhea unless the cause is being treated as well. Both loperamide and diphenoxylate/atropine are available, the former hav-ing a better safety profile in children.

If Standard Treatment Fails

Consider admission to the hospital for fluid and electrolyte correction. Remember antibiotic-associated diarrhea, because treatment will usually

TABLE 52-1. Common Infectious Diarrheas and Antibiotic Treatment

Type	Organism	Treatment
Bacteria	*Campylobacter**	Erythromycin, 20–50 mg/kg/day divided qid
		or
		Eythromycin, 250–500 of sustained release formulations bid in adults
	*Escherichia coli**	TMP/SMX (DS bid in adults, 6–12 mg TMP + 30–60 mg/ SMX per kg/day divided bid in children)
	*Salmonella**	TMP/SMX as above
		or
		Ampicillin, 50–100 mg/kg/day divided qid, up to 500 mg/dose
	*Shigella**	TMP/SMX as above
	*Yersinia**	TMP/SMX as above
		or
		Tetracycline, 1–2 gm/day divided qid, adults only
	Clostridium difficile	Metronidazole, 500 mg po tid x 7 days
		or
		Vancomycin, 125 mg po qid
Parasites	Entamoeba histolytica asymptomatic	Iodoquinol, 650 mg/ po tid x 20 days
	symptomatic	Iodoquinol + metronidazole, 750 mg po tid X 10 days
	Giardia lamblia	Quinacrine, 100 mg po tid x 5 days
		or
		Metronidazole, 250 mg po tid x 5 days

*Quinolones are indicated for severe or persistent cases (adults only).

respond to discontinuing the antibiotic. If severe *Clostridium difficile* infection exists, metronidazole can be used orally. Parasites are usually treated, based on confirmation, with such drugs as quinacrine (or metronidazole) for *Giardia* and tetracycline for amebic dysentery. Remember other possible causes of diarrhea, especially surgical, in the young and elderly.

For further reading in *Emergency Medicine, A Comprehensive Study Guide*, see Chapter 84, Diarrhea and Food Poisoning, by James S. Seidel.

Gregory S. Hall

Emergencies pertaining to the biliary tract generally result from obstruction of the gallbladder or biliary ducts by gallstones. Among the four prominent biliary tract emergencies caused by gallstones—symptomatic cholelithiasis, acute cholecystitis, gallstone pancreatitis, and ascending cholangitis—the first two are most frequently encountered in the ED. Risk factors associated with the formation of biliary calculi include: increased age, female sex and parity, obesity, familial tendency, Asian descent, chronic biliary tract infection or liver disease, sickle cell anemia, and hereditary spherocytosis.

Clinical Features

Biliary colic is the most common presenting symptom of cholelithiasis and typically presents with right upper quadrant or epigastric abdominal pain, which may be referred to the right shoulder. Pain may range from mild to severe, is usually intermittent, often begins suddenly 30 to 60 min following a meal, and is usually accompanied by nausea and vomiting. Examination commonly reveals right upper quadrant tenderness without findings of peritonitis along with volume depletion due to emesis. Acute episodes typically last for 1 to 6 h, followed by a gradual or sudden resolution of symptoms. Many patients may experience mild residual abdominal aching or soreness for another 24 to 48 h. The patient may give a history of similar past episodes, with a recent increase in frequency or severity of the attacks prompting the ED visit.

Acute cholecystitis presents with pain similar to biliary colic that has lasted longer than the typical 6 h. Fever or chills, nausea, vomiting, and anorexia are often found. The initial dull, poorly localized upper abdominal pain may have become sharp and localized to the right upper quadrant (RUQ). The patient may be in moderate to severe distress with systemic toxicity (fever and tachycardia). Abdominal exam reveals tenderness in the RUQ, sometimes with signs of localized peritonitis, distension, and hypoactive bowel sounds. Abdominal rigidity (generalized peritonitis), though rare, suggests perforation. Murphy's sign—increased pain or inspiratory arrest during deep subcostal palpation of the RUQ on inspiration—may be found. Volume depletion is often present, but jaundice is unusual.

Of all patients with gallstones, 15% to 20% may develop pancreatitis due to obstruction of the ampulla of Vater by a stone. Findings will be similar to other forms of pancreatitis, including epigastric or diffuse abdominal pain radiating to the back, nausea, vomiting, and fever. Ascending cholangitis, a life-threatening emergency caused by complete biliary obstruction (usually by a common duct stone) will often present with a patient in extremis. Mental confusion, shock, and Charcot's triad of fever, jaundice, and RUQ pain (all 3 present in only 25%) are suggestive.

Acalculous cholecystitis (5–10% of cases) occurs more frequently in the elderly and patients with diabetes mellitus. Other risk factors include multiple trauma or burns, prolonged labor, major surgery, and systemic vasculitic states. Clinical features are similar to the calculous form, but the course tends to be more rapid and malignant.

Diagnosis and Differential

Suspicion of gallbladder/biliary tract obstruction must be maintained in any patient at risk with suggestive clinical features. Appropriate laboratory studies that may help diagnosis include serum alkaline phosphatase, bilirubin, transaminase, electrolytes, BUN, creatinine, amylase, lipase, and a CBC. Urinalysis-with-sediment exam may help exclude urinary tract infection (UTI) and all females of childbearing potential should have a serum or urine pregnancy test to rule out obstetrical causes of abdominal pain. Patients having only symptomatic cholelithiasis usually have normal labs. A leukocytosis, possibly with a left shift, is more consistent with acute cholecystitis, but a normal WBC count does not exclude the diagnosis. With either cholelithiasis or cholecystitis serum bilirubin and alkaline phosphatase may be normal or mildly elevated. Plain x-ray films of the abdomen may reveal other causes of upper abdominal pain, but gallstones will be radiopaque in only 10% to 20% of patients. A chest x-ray may be useful to exclude right lower lobe pneumonia or pleural effusion. A 12-lead EKG should be obtained in all patients to rule out myocardial infarction or ischemia.

Ultrasound scan of the hepatobiliary system is considered by most the procedure of choice for diagnosis of cholelithiasis and biliary obstruction, and it accurately demonstrates 95% of gallstones, if present. Additional findings of a thickened gallbladder wall, gallbladder distention, pericholecystic fluid, and a positive sonographic Murphy's sign have a reported positive predictive value of >90% for acute cholecystitis. Oral cholecystography may be a useful adjunct for patients suspected of symptomatic cholelithiasis who have an unsatisfactory ultrasound scan. Radionuclide cholescinitigraphy (HIDA or DISIDA scans) offers sensitivity approaching 100% for the detection of acute cholecystitis. A reasonable ED approach to patients suspected of acute cholecystitis would be to initially obtain an ultrasound exam followed by radionuclide scan if ultrasound fails to establish the diagnosis.

The differential diagnosis of patients with upper abdominal pain includes hepatitis, hepatic abscess, pancreatitis, gastritis, peptic ulcer, appendicitis, Fitz-Hugh-Curtis syndrome, PID with or without tubo-ovarian abscess, pyelonephritis, and pleurisy.

Emergency Department Care

The ED management of patients who present with biliary colic always begins with the ABCs of resuscitation and supportive therapy alone will usually suffice for those without infection. Acute cholecystitis will require surgical consultation for definitive management.

1. Isotonic crystalloid IV fluids should be given to correct volume deficits and electrolyte imbalances. Patients in septic shock should be aggressively resuscitated, and IV vasopressors may be required to support perfusion.
2. Symptomatic treatment for emesis is best achieved with antispasmodic agents (glycopyrrolate 0.1 mg IV) and antiemetics (**promethazine** 12.5–25 mg IV). Gastric decompression with NG tube suctioning may be needed if vomiting is intractable.
3. Pain relief is best achieved with **meperidine**, 0.5 to 1 mg/kg IV or IM (preferred over other narcotics since it causes less spasm of the sphincter of Oddi). **Ketorolac tromethamine** (15–30 mg IV or 30–60 mg IM), an injectable NSAID, may help relieve the pain of gallbladder distension in patients without cholecystitis. Narcotics should be used judiciously when the diagnosis is in doubt.
4. Early antibiotic therapy should be initiated in any patient suspected of cholecystitis. Single-agent therapy with a parenteral third-generation cephalosporin (**cefotaxime** 1–2 gm q8 hr IV, **ceftazidime** 1–2 gm q 8 hr IV, **ceftizoxime** 1–2 gm q 8–12 hr IV, or **ceftriaxone** 1–2 gm q 24 hr IV in a single dose or divided q 12 hr) is adequate for patients without sepsis. Those with sepsis or obvious peritonitis are best managed with triple coverage, using **ampicillin** (500–1000 mg q 6 hr IV), **gentamicin** (3 mg/kg/day IV in divided doses q 8 hr), and **clindamycin** (1200–2700 mg/kg/day IV) divided in 2, 3, or 4 equal doses, or the equivalent.
5. Patients suspected of acute cholecystitis or its complications should have immediate surgical consultation and require hospital admission. Signs of systemic toxicity or sepsis should warrant ICU admission pending surgical treatment.
6. Patients accurately diagnosed with uncomplicated cholelithiasis whose symptoms resolve with supportive therapy within 4 to 6 hours of onset may be discharged home if they are able to maintain oral hydration. Oral narcotic–acetaminophen analgesics may be given for common residual aching for the next 24 to 48 h. Fatty meals should be avoided if they seem to incite symptoms. Timely outpatient followup should be arranged with a surgical consultant or the patient's primary care physician, and the patient should be instructed to return to the ED if fever develops or another significant attack occurs prior to followup.

If Standard Treatment Fails

If the patient with uncomplicated biliary colic fails to improve in 4 to 6 h with rehydration, antiemetics, and analgesics, reconsider the diagnosis. If ultrasound exam fails to demonstrate gallstones or findings of cholecystitis, but clinical suspicion remains high for biliary infection, initiate antibiotic therapy and obtain a radionuclide scan.

For further reading in *Emergency Medicine, A Comprehensive Study Guide*, see Chapter 85, Cholecystitis and Biliary Colic, by Tom P. Aufderheide and William J. Brady.

Acute Jaundice and Hepatitis

Gregory S. Hall

JAUNDICE AND VIRAL HEPATITIS

Jaundice, a yellowish discoloration of the skin, sclerae, and mucous membranes, is caused by hyperbilirubinemia, which may have many etiologies (Table 54-1). Hyperbilirubinemia may be divided into two types. The *unconjugated* form results from increased bilirubin production or a liver defect in its uptake or conjugation. The *conjugated* form is seen with intra- or extrahepatic cholestasis resulting in decreased excretion of conjugated bilirubin. The serum total bilirubin level should be elevated in a patient with jaundice. An indirect fraction of 85% or higher is consistent with the unconjugated type, whereas a direct fraction of 30% or higher suggests the conjugated form. Conjugated bilirubin is water soluble and may be detected in the urine at even low serum levels. Hepatitis is defined by inflammation of the liver with necrosis of hepatocytes. In the United States it is most commonly the result of viral infection, but it may also be seen in association with ethanol and other hepatotoxins (see chapters on toxicology). Risk factors for viral hepatitis include male homosexuals, hemodialysis, intravenous drug abuse, raw seafood ingestion, blood transfusion, ear piercing, tattoos, needle puncture, foreign travel, or close contact with an infected patient.

TABLE 54-1. Causes of Jaundice

Unconjugated	Conjugated
Hemolytic anemia	Intraheptic
Hemoglobinopathy	Infections
Transfusion reaction	Viral hepatitis
Gilbert disease	Leptospirosis
Crigler–Najjar syndrome	Infectious mononucleosis
Premature neonates	Toxic (drugs/chemicals)
Congestive heart failure	Familial
	Rotor syndrome
	Dubin–Johnson syndrome
	Alcoholic liver disease
	Other
	Sarcoidosis
	Lymphoma
	Liver metastasis
	Cirrhosis
	Biliary cirrhosis
	Amyloidosis
	Extrahepatic
	Gallstones
	Pancreatic tumors/cysts
	Cholangiosarcoma
	Bile-duct stricture
	Sclerosing cholangitis

Clinical Features

Viral hepatitis ranges in severity from asymptomatic infection to fulminant hepatic failure. Symptomatic patients usually report sudden or insidious onset of a constitutional prodrome of nausea, vomiting, fatigue, malaise, and alterations in taste. Low-grade fever with pharyngitis, coryza, and headache may mislead the clinician leading to an initial misdiagnosis of upper respiratory infection or flulike illness. Most patients do not become jaundiced and recover gradually in a couple of months. When jaundice develops it usually begins 1 to 2 wks after the prodrome. A few days of generalized pruritis and dark urine may precede the jaundice and GI symptoms, and malaise will often persist while the other prodromal symptoms resolve. Right upper quadrant pain with an enlarged liver or spleen may be noted. Most patients clinically recover gradually over the ensuing 3 to 4 mo. Rarely, fulminant hepatic failure develops with a clinical picture consisting of encephalopathy, coagulopathy, and rapidly worsening jaundice.

Five different viral agents have been causally linked to hepatitis. Hepatitis A (infectious hepatitis) is caused by a small RNA picornavirus (HAV) with predominantly fecal–oral transmission. Children and adolescents are more commonly affected, but often subclinically, whereas adult cases typically are symptomatic with jaundice and a longer, more severe course. Symptom onset is usually more abrupt than with other viruses. Epidemic outbreaks have been associated with children in day care centers, institutionalized patients, and those exposed to a common source case through contaminated food or water. Hepatitis B (serum hepatitis) is caused by a double stranded DNA hepadnavirus (HBV) and is contracted primarily by a percutaneous route. Most cases are anicteric and subclinical. Symptom onset is often insidious and in 5% to 10% may be preceded by a serum-sickness-like syndrome with polyarthritis, proteinuria, and angioneurotic edema. Symptomatic patients usually have a more severe and protracted illness than those with HAV. Hepatitis C is caused by a linear, single stranded RNA virus (HCV) and may be obtained by parenteral, sexual, and perinatal contact. Most patients are asymptomatic or have milder symptoms than is seen with HBV. Unfortunately, many patients with HCV develop chronic hepatitis with a predisposition to cirrhosis and hepatocellular carcinoma. Hepatitis D is a defective single-stranded RNA virus, which can only replicate in the setting of acute or chronic HBV infection. Acute HDV superinfection of an HBV carrier may lead to acute hepatic failure.

Hepatitis E is caused by a small RNA virus and is seen in sporadic waterborne outbreaks in Asia, Africa, Mexico, and the former Soviet Union. So far, only imported cases have been reported in the United States. The clinical course is comparable to that of HAV but results in a higher incidence of acute hepatic failure and death, particularly in gravid females. Non-A, Non-B hepatitis is a waste-basket term used to describe clinical illnesses resembling viral hepatitis for which no known viral agents or other causes may be found, hence it is a diagnosis of exclusion.

Diagnosis and Differential

Establishing the diagnosis of acute viral hepatitis depends primarily on liver function laboratory abnormalities in the proper clinical setting. Serum transaminases (GGT, AST, ALT) should be checked, as marked elevations are most consistent with viral hepatitis. A serum alkaline phosphatase level should also be determined. If it is elevated more than threefold above normal, suspect cholestasis. Insight into the type of hyperbilirubinemia can be obtained by determining total serum bilirubin levels along with indirect and direct fractions. A conjugated (direct) fraction of 30% or higher is consistent with viral hepatitis. The magnitude of transaminase elevation is not a reliable marker of disease severity, but a persistent total bilirubin >20 mg/dL, or a prothrombin time prolonged by more than a few seconds, indicates a poor prognosis. Serum electrolytes, BUN, and creatinine should be checked if there is clinical suspicion of volume depletion or electrolyte imbalance, such as from protracted emesis. Abnormal mental status should prompt an immediate determination of a serum glucose level which may be depressed because of poor intake or hepatic failure. Other causes of abnormal mentation, such as hypoxia, sepsis, intoxication, or structural intracranial process, must also be considered. Lastly, a CBC may be useful, as an early transient neutropenia followed by a relative lymphocytosis with atypical forms is often seen with viral hepatitis. Anemia, if present, may be more indicative of alcoholic hepatitis, decompensated cirrhosis, or a hemolytic process. Serologic studies to determine the particular viral etiology responsible may be ordered in the ED to facilitate the final diagnosis, but these results are rarely immediately available and hence play no significant role in ED management. Important differential diagnoses include alcoholic or toxin-induced hepatitis, infectious mononucleosis, cholecystitis, ascending cholangitis, sarcoidosis, lymphoma, liver metastasis, and pancreatic or biliary tumors.

Emergency Department Care

Supportive care is the mainstay of therapy for patients with acute viral hepatitis.

1. The majority of patients can be successfully managed as outpatients with emphasis on rest, adequate oral intake, strict personal hygiene, and avoidance of hepatotoxins (ethanol). Patients discharged from the ED must have access to early outpatient followup and should be given instructions to return for any worsening of symptoms, particularly vomiting, fever, or jaundice.

2. Patients with one or more of the following should be admitted to the hospital: encephalopathy, prothrombin time prolonged >3 times normal, intractable vomiting, hypoglycemia, bilirubin >20 mg/dL, age >45 years, orimmunosuppression.
3. Volume depletion and electrolyte imbalances should be corrected with IV crystalloid. Hypoglycemia, if present, should be initially treated with 1 amp of 50% dextrose in water IV followed by the addition of dextrose to IV fluids.
4. Fulminant hepatic failure should warrant ICU admission with aggressive support of circulation and respiration, treatment of increased intracranial pressure, correction of hypoglycemia and coagulopathy, administration of oral lactulose or neomycin, and a protein-restricted diet. (See Alcoholic Cirrhosis below.)
5. Glucocorticoid therapy has no value in acute viral hepatitis, even with fulminant hepatic failure, and should be avoided.

If Standard Treatment Fails

Carefully review the patient's history and clinical and laboratory findings to reconsider the diagnosis accuracy. Consider additional diagnostic maneuvers such as hepatobiliary imaging by ultrasound, radionuclide, or CT scanning to be certain that cholecystitis, biliary calculi, or extrinsic compression on the common bile duct are not present. In cases of fulminant hepatitis, consider the possibility of toxic liver injury such as might occur with occult or accidental overdose of acetaminophen or other hepatotoxins.

ALCOHOLIC LIVER DISEASE AND CIRRHOSIS

Liver injury secondary to ethanol takes the form of three clinical syndromes: hepatic steatosis (fatty liver), alcoholic hepatitis, and alcoholic cirrhosis. The enlarged, nontender liver of steatosis is most often encountered in a relatively asymptomatic patient. Alcoholic hepatitis may present as a very mild or severe acute illness in a chronic alcohol abuser, whereas alcoholic cirrhosis is a chronic process with intermittent exacerbations triggering most ED visits.

Clinical Features

Alcoholic hepatitis is typically seen in the chronic alcoholic who reports a gradual onset of anorexia, nausea, weight loss, abdominal pain, and generalized weakness. Dark urine, jaundice, and fever are frequent complaints. Examination reveals a tender, enlarged liver, low-grade fever, and jaundice. Other stigmata of chronic alcohol use may also be present. Patients suffering from alcoholic cirrhosis will report a gradual deterioration in health with anorexia, muscle loss (often masked by edema/ascites), easy fatigability, nausea, vomiting, diarrhea, and increasing abdominal girth if ascites is present. Low-grade and continuous fever may also be present, while hypothermia may be seen at end-stage disease. Palpation of the abdomen may reveal hepatosplenomegaly or a small firm liver. Jaundice, pedal edema, ascites, palmar erythema, spider angiomata, and gynecomastia are also common. Hepatic encephalopathy, characterized by a fluctuating level of consciousness and possibly hyperreflexia, spasticity, and generalized seizures, may also be present. Asterixis (liver flap) is characteristic, but not specific, for hepatic encephalopathy. Cirrhotics often present to the ED because of worsening ascites or edema, complications such as GI bleeding or encephalopathy, spontaneous bacterial peritonitis, and other types of concurrent infections.

Diagnosis and Differential

Alcoholic hepatitis and cirrhosis should be recognized by their clinical features and laboratory findings. Labs which should be obtained include: serum transaminase (GGT, AST, ALT), alkaline phosphatase, total bilirubin (with fractions), albumin, CBC, serum glucose, and electrolytes, including magnesium, BUN, creatinine, and prothrombin time. With alcoholic hepatitis, serum transaminase levels are usually elevated to a range 2 to 10 times normal with a ratio of AST to ALT >1.5. With cirrhosis, transaminases are usually only mildly elevated. Alkaline phosphatase and bilirubin levels are often only mildly elevated with both cirrhosis and alcoholic hepatitis. Anemia, leukopenia, and thrombocytopenia are common to all chronic alcohol abusers. Serum amylase and lipase will help evaluate the possibility of pancreatitis. Fever with or without leukocytosis in an alcoholic patient mandates a chest x-ray to rule out pneumonia, cultures of blood, urine, and ascitic fluid, and a thorough search for other sources of sepsis, such as meningitis. Spontaneous bacterial peritonitis (SBP) should be suspected in any cirrhotic with fever, worsening ascites or hepatic failure, or abdominal pain or tenderness. Other subtle clues to SBP include deteriorating renal function, hypothermia, diarrhea, or encephalopathy. Diagnostic paracentesis may be performed, and ascitic fluid should be tested for total protein, glucose, LDH, and WBC count with differential. A polymorpholeukocyte count >500/mm^3 is highly specific for SBP. A total WBC count >10,000/mm^3, total protein >1 gm/dL, glucose <50 mg/dL, or elevated LDH point to the possibility of peritonitis secondary to a localized focus of infection. Altered mental status in an alcoholic should prompt consideration of hypoglycemia, encephalopathy, hypoxemia, and occult head trauma. The differential for alcoholic cirrhosis is usually limited to other causes of cirrhosis whereas alcoholic hepatitis may share features with viral and other forms of hepatitis as well as other causes of upper abdominal pain (see differential for viral hepatitis above).

Emergency Department Care

Alcoholic Hepatitis

1. Hospitalization is required for all but the mildest cases of alcoholic hepatitis.
2. Fluid therapy with dextrose containing IV fluids should be started with the goal of maintaining adequate intravascular volume while avoiding fluid overload in the edematous or ascitic patient. Central venous pressure monitoring may be needed to guide fluid resuscitation. Thiamine (100 mg) should be given with IV fluids. Correction of electrolyte abnormalities should be initiated (most patients will require supplemental potassium and magnesium).
3. Concurrent identified infections should be treated with appropriate parenteral antibiotics and broad-spectrum coverage (e.g., cefotaxime 2.0 gm IV) should be started in any alcoholic with suspected sepsis pending culture results.

Alcoholic Cirrhosis

1. Abstinence from alcohol is the mainstay of outpatient management. Adjunctive measures include salt and water restriction, cautious diuretic use (i.e., spironolactone), and a protein-restricted diet.
2. Emergency management often includes changing diuretic dosage, correction of fluid and electrolyte abnormalities, and blood transfusion for symptomatic anemia.
3. Encephalopathy must be aggressively managed with supplemental oxygen, support of respiration and perfusion, treatment of increased intracranial pressure, if present (hyperventilation and mannitol 0.5–1.0 gm/kg IV), and supplemental dextrose in IV fluids. Precipitating factors such as concurrent infection or GI bleeding require aggressive intervention (see Chap. 43, on Esophageal Emergencies, for treatment of variceal bleeding). **Lactulose** (30 ml) may be given orally, by NG tube, or by enema. Neomycin may also be given to help clear the gut of bacteria and nitrogenous products.
4. **Cefotaxime** parenterally in a dose of 1 to 2 grams every 6 h is the current drug of choice for spontaneous bacterial peritonitis. It should be given early if the clinical picture suggests SBP, even if laboratory results are equivocal.
5. The ED physician should consider admission for a cirrhotic patient whose clinical stability is in question. All patients with clearly decompensated cirrhosis (i.e., worsening hepatic function), fever, hypothermia, or complications such as concurrent infection, SBP, GI or variceal bleeding, or encephalopathy, should be admitted. Discharged patients should have timely followup arranged with their primary care provider.

If Standard Treatment Fails

In patients with alcoholic hepatitis with liver failure, reconsider the diagnosis and consider the possibility of concurrent acute pancreatitis, toxic liver injury, cholecystitis, appendicitis, spontaneous bacterial peritonitis, and other occult sources of sepsis. If a patient with alcoholic cirrhosis seems to be deteriorating, search for precipitating factors, such as infection, GI bleeding, excessive diuresis, occult intracranial hematoma, and myocardial infarction.

For further reading in *Emergency Medicine, A Comprehensive Study Guide*, see Chapter 86, Acute Jaundice and Hepatitis, by Richard Owen Shields, Jr.

Acute Pancreatitis

Michael E. Chansky

Acute pancreatitis (AP) is a common disorder the diagnosis of which rests primarily on clinical grounds. The severity of the disease may range from mild pancreatic edema to frank necrosis and hemorrhage and is most often related to alcohol abuse, gallstones, and trauma (Table 55-1).

Clinical Features

Presenting symptoms are dependent on the amount of glandular destruction. In the mildest form, patients present with epigastric pain, abdominal distension, nausea, vomiting, and hyperamylasemia. Refractory hypotensive shock, blood loss, hypocalcium, prerenal azotemia, and respiratory failure may accompany the most severe forms. Patients may only have one or a constellation of signs and symptoms.

Diagnosis and Differential

Since no clinical features are pathognomonic for AP, the diagnosis must be suspected by the history and exam and presence of abnormal laboratory tests, most often elevated serum amylase and lipase levels. The isoenzymes of amylase are produced by the fallopian tubes, ovaries, lungs, salivary glands, and lacrimal glands, in addition to the pancreas. These multiple organ sources of amylase have resulted in less reliance on the simple measurement of serum amylase as an indicator of pancreatic disease. Differentiating isoamylases is time-consuming, and utilizing the amylase–creatinine clearance ratio is unreliable. Serum lipase is nearly always elevated in AP. Lipase level is a more sensitive sign of AP than amylase, but it also lacks specificity. Lipase elevation more closely follows the clinical course than serum amylase. As with most inflammatory conditions, leukocytosis is usually present, but rarely exceeds 20,000/ml in complicated AP. Elevated BUN is common secondary to third spacing, and an elevated alkaline phosphatase supports biliary disease. Persistent hypocalcemia ($<7mg/100$ ml), hypoxia, and metabolic acidosis are associated with poor prognosis.

Plain radiographs play little role in the diagnosis of AP, although calcification, when present, suggests pre-existing pancreatic disease. More often their role is to exclude other diseases in the differential. Patients with AP may have a partial ileus or gaseous distension of the colon with a distally collapsed colon. Neither of these signs are truly diagnostic. The hypoxic patient may show signs of adult respiratory distress syndrome (ARDS). Although ultrasound or CT may reveal edema indicative of acute pancreatic inflammation, routine early use of these tests is unnecessary.

TABLE 55-1. More Common Etiologic or Contributing Factors in Acute Pancreatitis

Ethanol ingestion
Biliary tract disease
Trauma, penetrating or blunt
Penetrating peptic ulcer
Following endoscopic retrograde cholangiopancreatography
Obstruction secondary to neoplasms, diverticula, round worms, polyps
Perisphincteric fibrosis
Metabolic disturbances
  Hyperlipemia (Frederickson types I, IV, V)
  Hypercalcemia
  Diabetes mellitus, DKA
  Uremia
Viral Infections
  Viral hepatitis
  Infectious mononucleosis
  Coxsackie group B
Pregnancy—any trimester, postpartum
Collagen vascular disease
Liver disease
Generalized infections
Drugs
  Oral contraceptives
  Azathioprine
  Glucocorticoids
  Tetracyclines
  Isoniazid
  Thiazides
  Salicylates
  Calcium
  Warfarin

The differential diagnosis of AP includes left lower lobe pneumonia, rupture of a pseudocyst, gallbladder disease (cholecystitis, choledocholithiasis), peritonitis (appendicitis, diverticulitis, perforated viscus), peptic ulcer disease (gastritis, gastric outlet obstruction), small bowel obstruction, renal colic, dissecting aortic aneurysm, diabetic ketoacidosis, and gastroenteritis. AP may be a difficult diagnosis to establish, and repeated observation and surgical consultation is often necessary.

Emergency Department Care

Treatment of AP revolves around fluid resuscitation, prevention of vomiting, pain control, and pancreatic rest (nothing per oral) (NPO).

1. Crystalloid IV fluids are the mainstay of treatment. Bolus normal saline to maintain BP and adequate urine output. A CVP or Swan–Ganz catheter should be considered if the patient is hypoxic with

ARDS on the chest film or has hypotension unresponsive to aggressive fluid resuscitation.

2. Administer oxygen to maintain a pulse oximetry reading of 95% O_2 saturation. Respiratory failure is rare, but is known.

3. Consider a NG tube to low suction if the patient is distended or actively vomiting. The NG tube theoretically reduces pancreatic stimulation and prevents vomiting, although no controlled trial has shown its value.

4. Parenteral analgesia is often necessary for patient comfort. IV or IM narcotics should be used short-term.

5. Prophylaxis for alcohol withdrawal in the appropriate setting is indicated. Most patients can be admitted to a floor bed on the surgical or medical service. Patients who demonstrate poor prognostic signs (dropping hemoglobin, poor urine output, persistent hypotension, hypoxia, acidosis, hypocalcemia) despite aggressive early treatment should be admitted to the ICU with surgical consultation.

If Standard Treatment Fails

Patients with severe systemic disease will require intubation, intensive monitoring, Foley catheter, and transfusion of blood and blood products as needed. Peritoneal lavage should be considered for ill patients who fail to respond to initial supportive measures. Patients with gallstones, pancreatitis, and choledocholithiasis may benefit from biliary tract decompression.

For further reading in *Emergency Medicine, A Comprehensive Study Guide*, see Chapter 87, Acute Pancreatitis, by Donald Weaver.

Complications of General and Urologic Surgical Procedures

N. Heramba Prasad

Outpatient surgical procedures are becoming increasingly common. Emergency physicians, therefore, will see more and more postoperative complications. Fever, respiratory complications, genitourinary complaints, wound infections, vascular problems, and complications of drug therapy are some common postoperative disorders seen in the ED. Most of these are discussed elsewhere in this book, certain specific problems will be mentioned here. The causes of postoperative fever are listed as the five Ws: Wind (respiratory), Water (UTI), Wound, Walking (DVT), and Wonder drugs (pseudomembranous colitis).

Clinical Features

Fever in the first 24 hours is usually due to atelectasis, necrotizing fasciitis, or clostridial infections. In the 24 to 72 h period, pneumonia, atelectasis, IV-catheter-related thrombophlebitis, and infections are the major causes. Urinary tract infections (UTI) are seen 3 to 5 days postoperatively. Deep venous thrombosis (DVT) typically occurs 5 days after the procedure, and wound infections generally manifest 7 to 10 days after surgery. Antibiotic-induced pseudomembranous colitis (PMC) is seen 6 wks after surgery.

Respiratory Complications

Postoperative pain and inadequate clearance of secretions contribute to the development of atelectasis. Fever, tachypnea, tachycardia, and mild hypoxia are usually seen. Hypoxia, ECG changes, widened A–a gradient and respiratory distress should point to the diagnosis of pulmonary embolism.

Genitourinary Complications

UTIs are more common after instrumentation of the urinary tract. Urinary retention occurs in 4% of all surgical patients and in 60% of patients after urethral surgery. It is more common in elderly males, especially after excessive fluid administration and after spinal anesthesia. Lower abdominal pain, urgency, and inability to void should alert the clinician to suspect urinary retention.

Oliguria or anuria commonly results from volume depletion. Intrinsic factors such as acute tubular necrosis (ATN), drug nephrotoxicity, and postrenal obstructive uropathy also may lead to acute renal failure.

Wound Complications

Hematomas result from inadequate hemostasis. Careful evaluation to rule out infections must be undertaken. Seromas are collections of clear fluid under the wound.

Extremes of age, diabetes, poor nutrition, necrotic tissue, poor perfusion, foreign bodies, and wound hematomas contribute to the development of wound infections.

Necrotizing fasciitis is characterized by extremely painful, erythematous, swollen, and warm areas without sharp margins. This staphylococcal infection spreads rapidly; the patient will exhibit marked systemic toxicity; crepitance and bullae may be present.

Wound dehiscence can occur due to diabetes, poor nutrition, chronic steroid use, and inadequate or improper closure of the wound. Dehiscence of abdominal wound may result in evisceration of abdominal organs.

Vascular Complications

Superficial thrombophlebitis usually occurs in the upper extremities after IV catheter insertion or in the lower extremities because of stasis and varicosity of veins. Deep venous thrombosis (DVT) commonly occurs in the lower extremities. Swelling and pain of the calf are commonly encountered.

Drug Therapy Complications

Many drugs are known to cause fever and antibiotic-induced diarrhea. Pseudomembranous colitis (PMC), a dreaded complication, is caused by *C. difficile* toxin. Bloody, watery diarrhea, fever, and crampy abdominal pain are the usual complaints.

Diagnosis and Differential

Patients with suspected respiratory complications should have chest x-rays. They may reveal plate-like or discoid atelectases, pneumonia, or pneumothorax. Pneumothorax occurs early after certain surgical procedures or catheter insertion, and chest x-ray with expiratory view will help confirm the diagnosis of pneumothorax.

Diagnosis of pulmonary embolism can be established by ventilation perfusion scan or angiography, supplemented by Doppler ultrasonography of the extremities.

The patient with oliguria or anuria should be evaluated for signs of hypovolemia or urinary retention. Treatment consists of Foley catheter insertion and fluid bolus for hypotension. Suspected DVT can be confirmed by Doppler ultrasonography. Diagnosis of PMC is established by demonstrating *C.difficile* cytotoxin in the stool. In 27% of the cases, however, the assay can be negative.

Emergency Department Care

Always discuss the patient and proposed treatment with the surgeon who initially cared for the patient. Although debilitated patients may need hospitalization, many patients with atelectasis can be treated as outpatients. Postoperative pneumonia is polymicrobial, and an antipseudomonas antibiotic with an aminoglycoside is usually recommended. Most patients with UTI can be managed as outpatients with oral antibiotic therapy.

Insertion of a Foley catheter and prompt drainage will alleviate urinary retention. There is no need for clamping the catheter periodically. Prophylactic antibiotics are reserved for patients who have had urinary tract instrumentation, those with prolonged retention, and those at risk for infection.

Wound hematomas may require removal of some sutures and evacuation of the hematoma. Surgical consultation before to treatment is appropriate. Seromas can be treated with needle aspiration and wound cultures. Admission may not always be necessary.

Most wound infections can be treated with oral antibiotics (usually the surgeon's choice) unless the patient manifests systemic symptoms and signs. Perineal infections usually require admission and parenteral antibiotics. Surgical debridement and parenteral antibiotics are indicated for necrotizing fasciitis.

Most patients with superficial thrombophlebitis can be treated with local heat and elevation of the affected area if there is no evidence of cellulitis or lymphangitis. Patients with suppurative thrombophlebitis, characterized by erythema, lymphangitis, fever, and severe pain, should be hospitalized and treated with excision of the affected vein.

Fluid resuscitation, oral vancomycin, metronidazole, orally or intravenously, are currently available treatment modalities for drug-induced PMC (see Chap. 52, Diarrhea and Food Poisoning)

SPECIFIC CONSIDERATIONS

Complications of Breast Surgery

Wound infections, hematomas, pneumothorax, necrosis of the skin flaps, and lymphedema of the arms after mastectomy are common problems seen after breast surgery. Lymphedema of the arm occurs in 5% to 10% of patients. Nighttime elevation and minor activity restriction help reduce swelling.

Complications of GI Surgery

Intestinal Obstruction. Neuronal disfunction following any surgery where peritoneum is entered causes paralytic ileus. Following GI surgery, small bowel tone returns within 24 h, gastric function within 2 days, and colonic function within 3 days.

Prolonged ileus should alert the clinician to peritonitis, abscesses, hemoperitoneum, pneumonia, sepsis, and electrolyte imbalance. Clinical features include nausea, vomiting, obstipation, constipation, abdominal distension, and pain.

Abdominal x-rays, complete blood count, electrolytes, BUN, creatinine, and urinalysis should be obtained. Treatment of adynamic ileus consists of NG suction, bowel rest, and hydration. Mechanical obstruction is usually due to adhesions and may require surgical intervention.

Intraabdominal abscesses are caused by preoperative contamination or postoperative anastomotic leaks. Diagnosis can be confirmed by CT scan or ultrasonography. Surgical exploration, evacuation, and parenteral antibiotics will be required.

Pancreatitis occurs especially after direct manipulation of the pancreatic duct. Patients typically present with nausea, vomiting, abdominal pain, leukocytosis, and left pleural effusion. Lumbar pain, Turner's sign (discoloration of the flank), and Cullen's sign (periumbilical ecchymosis) may be present. Serum amylase and lipase are elevated. Treatment consists of hospitalization, IV hydration, and NG decompression.

Fistulas, either internal or external, may result from direct bowel injury and require surgical consultation and hospitalization.

Anastomotic leaks are especially devastating after esophageal or colon surgery. Esophageal leaks occur 10 days after the procedure. Dramatic presentation with shock, pneumothorax, and pleural effusion is usually seen.

Dumping syndrome is noticed in gastric bypass procedures. It is due to the sudden influx of hyperosmolar chyle into the small intestine resulting in fluid sequestration and hypovolemia. Patients experience nausea, vomiting, epigastric discomfort, palpitations, dizziness, and sometimes syncope.

Alkaline reflux gastritis is caused by the reflux of bile into the stomach. Endoscopic evaluation will establish the diagnosis. Postvagotomy diarrhea and afferent loop syndrome are seen in some patients.

Complications of percutaneous endoscopic gastrostomy (PEG) tubes include infections, hemorrhage, peritonitis, aspiration, wound dehiscence, sepsis, and obstruction of the tube.

Complications arising from stomas are due to technical errors or from underlying disease such as Crohn disease and cancer. Ischemia, necrosis, bleeding, hernia, and prolapse are sometimes seen.

Colonoscopy may cause hemorrhage, perforation, retroperitoneal abscesses, pneumoscrotum, pneumothorax, volvulus, and infection.

Rectal surgery complications include urinary retention, constipation, prolapse, bleeding, and infections.

Complications of Urologic Surgery

Epididymitis, scrotal swelling, and hemorrhage are sometimes seen following vasectomies.

Following extracorporeal shock wave lithotripsy, pain, and hematuria persist for some time. Suspected perineal hematomas from subscapular renal hemorrhage can be confirmed by CT or ultrasonography. Ureteric reobstruction from stone fragments can be diagnosed by IVP. Urinary tract infections occur infrequently.

For further reading in *Emergency Medicine, A Comprehensive Study Guide*, see Chapter 88, Complications of General and Urological Procedures, by Edmond A. Hooker.

8 | RENAL AND GENITOURINARY DISORDERS

57 | Emergency Renal Problems

Marc D. Squillante

Renal dysfunction and acute renal failure present with a wide variety of manifestations, depending on the underlying etiology. Although the initial symptoms may be those of the primary cause, ultimately patients will develop deterioration of renal function. Risk factors include cardiac disease, hypovolemia from any cause, vascular/thrombotic disorders, glomerular diseases, diseases affecting the renal tubules, and a variety of anatomic problems of the genital urinary tract (Table 57-1).

Clinical Features

Deterioration in renal function leads to excessive accumulation of nitrogenous waste products in the serum. Acute renal failure can be classified as *oliguric* (<500 mL urine/24 h) and *nonoliguric* (>500 mL/24 hrs). Patients will usually have signs and symptoms of their underlying causative disorder, but eventually develop stigmata of renal failure. Volume overload, hypertension, pulmonary edema, mental status changes or neurologic symptoms, nausea and vomiting, bone and joint problems, anemia and increased susceptibility to infection can occur, as patients develop more chronic uremia.

Diagnosis and Differential

History and physical examination usually provide clues to etiology. Physical exam should assess volume status, establish urinary tract patency, and search for signs of chemical intoxication, drug usage, muscle damage, or associated systemic diseases. Diagnostic studies include urinalysis, BUN and creatinine, serum electrolytes, urinary sodium and creatinine, and urinary osmolality. Analysis of these tests allows most patients to be placed in either the prerenal, renal, or postrenal group. Fractional excretion of sodium and renal failure index can also be calculated to help in this categorization (Table 57-2).

Emergency Department Care

Prerenal failure. Restore effective intravascular volume with isotonic fluids (normal saline, lactated Ringer's) at a rapid rate in appropriate patients. If cardiac failure is causing prerenal azotemia, intravascular volume should be reduced (i.e., with diuretics) to improve cardiac performance.

Postrenal failure. Establish appropriate urinary drainage. The exact procedure will vary depending on the level of obstruction. A Foley catheter should be placed to relieve obstruction caused by prostatic hypertrophy. A percutaneous nephrostomy tube may be required for ureteral occlusion until definitive surgery to correct the obstruction can

315

TABLE 57-1 Common Causes of Acute Renal Failure

Prerenal	Renal	Postrenal
Reduction in cardiac output	Vascular/ischemia	Penile lesions
Cardiac disease of any etiology	Renal vasculature thrombosis, TIP, DIC, NSAIDs, severe hypertension	Phimosis
Hypovolemia	Glomerular	Meatal stenosis
Fluid/blood loss or redistribution of intravascular fluids (sepsis)	Primary glomerular diseases or systemic disease with glomerular involvement (SLE, vasculitis, endocarditis)	Urethral stricture
		Prostatic enlargement
	Tubulointerstitial	Upper urinary tract (requires bilateral involvement)
	Ischemic, or toxin-induced tubular damage (aminoglycosides, solvents, heavy metals, ethylene glycol, myoglobin/hemoglobin)	Calculi, tumors

TABLE 57-2. Laboratory Studies Aiding in the Differential Diagnosis of Acute Renal Failure

Test Employed	Prerenal	Renal	Postrenal[#]
Urine sodium (mEq/L)	<20	>40	>40
FE_{Na} (%)[*]	<1	>1	>1
Renal failure index (RFI)[+]	<1	>1	>1
Urine osmolality (mosm/L)	>500	<350	<350
Urine/serum creatinine ratio	>40:1	<20:1	<20:1
Serum urea nitrogen/ creatinine ratio	>20:1	=10·1	>10:1

[*]Fractional excretion of sodium (%) $= \dfrac{\text{Urine sodium/serum sodium}}{\text{urine creatinine/serum creatinine}} \times 100$

[+]$RFI = \dfrac{\text{serum sodium}}{\text{urine creatinine/serum creatinine}} \times 100$

[#]Can see indices similar to prerenal early in course of obstruction. With continued obstruction, tubular function is impaired and indices mimic those of renal causes.

take place when the patient's status is stabilized. For the acutely anuric patient, obstruction is the major consideration. If no urine is obtained on initial bladder catheterization, emergency urologic consultation should be considered.

Renal failure. Acute tubular necrosis (ATN) from ischemia or nephrotoxic agents is the most common cause of intrinsic acute renal failure. History, physical exam, and baseline laboratory tests should provide clues to the diagnosis. Nephrotoxic agents (drugs, IV contrast) should be avoided. Diuretics (i.e., furosemide 20–80 mg IV) occasionally can augment diuresis and convert oliguric into nonoliguric renal failure. Low dose dopamine (1–3 µg/kg/min) may improve renal blood flow and can be used in early stages. Renally excreted drugs (digoxin, magnesium, sedatives, narcotics) should be used with caution since therapeutic doses may accumulate to excess and cause serious side effects. Fluid restriction (500 mL + daily urine output) may be required. Patients with new-onset acute renal failure should be admitted to the hospital. Consider transferring patients to another institution if nephrology consultation and dialysis facilities are not available.

If Standard Treatment Fails

If treatment of the underlying cause fails to improve renal function, hemodialysis or peritoneal dialysis should be considered. Decisions about dialysis are usually made by the nephrology consultant. Dialysis is often initiated when the BUN is >100 mg/dL or serum creatinine level is >10 mg/dL. Cardiac instability frequently results from metabolic acidosis and hyperkalemia. Patients with intractable volume overload and hyperkalemia not easily corrected by other measures should be considered for emergency dialysis.

For further reading in *Emergency Medicine, A Comprehensive Study Guide*, see Chapter 90, Emergency Renal Problems, by K. Venkateswara Rao.

Stephen H. Thomas

Urinary tract infection (UTI) is defined as significant bacteriuria in the presence of symptoms. It is a frequently occurring condition accounting for a significant number of ED visits, with acuity ranging from commonplace cystitis to life-threatening gram-negative urosepsis.

Clinical Features

The diagnosis of UTI should be considered in patients presenting with dysuria, urinary frequency, and lower abdominal pain and suprapubic tenderness. Fever, chills, malaise, flank pain, and costovertebral angle tenderness (upper tract signs) may occur with lower tract infections, but are more likely associated with pyelonephritis. Although pyelonephritis may sometimes be difficult to distinguish clinically from lower urinary tract infection, a history of several days of dysuria and frequency followed by upper tract signs is suggestive.

Diagnosis and Differential

The first step in establishing the diagnosis of UTI is collection of an adequate urine specimen for analysis and culture. A properly performed midstream urine collection enables reliable urinalysis while avoiding discomfort and potential complications (i.e., iatrogenic UTI) of urethral catheterization. Women should be instructed to spread the labia with one hand and wipe the urethral meatus with povidone–iodine swabs front to back with the other; the urine specimen is collected into the cup only after voiding the initial urine into the toilet. Men should be instructed to similarly cleanse the urethral meatus, retracting foreskin when present, prior to obtaining a midstream sample. In patients who are unable to provide a midstream sample, urethral catheterization is indicated. Inspection and smell of the urine sample provide little useful information. Laboratory analysis of the specimen will provide information on pyuria, bacteriuria, hematuria, and nitrate and leukocyte esterase tests. A urine culture should be obtained in the following settings: pyelonephritis, patients requiring hospitalization, patients with chronic indwelling urinary catheter, and all children and adult males. Significant pyuria corresponds to 2 to 5 leukocytes per high-power field (HPF) in a centrifuged specimen. In males, in whom urethritis and prostatitis are the most common causes of pyuria, 1 to 2 leukocytes/HPF may be significant. False-negative tests can result from large urine volumes, self-medication, or obstructed kidneys.

The presence of any bacteria on gram stain of uncentrifuged urine is significant; significance also is attached to the presence of more than 15 bacteria/HPF in a centrifuged sample. False positives may occur with vaginal or fecal contamination. False negatives are common in patients with *Chlamydia* or low colony count UTI.

Hematuria may accompany urolithiasis but is also seen in (hemorrhagic) cystitis. The nitrate test is a specific, but insensitive, indicator of UTI. Similarly, the leukocyte esterase test suffers from relatively low sensitivity. Thus, the information provided by these tests can be helpful, but their function as screening tests is limited.

Differential diagnosis for UTI includes mechanical or chemical urethritis, urolithiasis, vulvovaginitis, cervicitis, and salpingitis.

Emergency Department Care

Primary decisions to be considered in treatment of patients with UTI are whether patients have pyelonephritis and whether patients with pyelonephritis require hospital admission. The majority of patients with UTI have lower tract disease and are treated as outpatients. Indications for culture have been discussed.

1. Initial oral antibiotic should be a 10-day course of 1 of the following: **trimethoprim/sulfamethoxazole**, 1 double-strength tablet bid; **trimethoprim**, 200 mg bid; **nitrofurantoin**, 50 to 100 mg qid; **cefadroxil**, 500 to 1000 mg bid; **amoxicillin**, 250 to 500 mg tid.
2. In cases of treatment failure or in hosts with structural or immunologic compromise, consider **amoxicillin/clavulanic** acid (250–500 mg tid) or a quinolone (**ciprofloxacin** 250–500 mg bid or **ofloxacin** 200–400 mg bid).
3. Shorter courses of therapy may be appropriate for certain patient populations.
4. Patients with new sexual partners, sexual partners with urethritis, signs or symptoms of cervicitis, or pyuria without bacteriuria should be treated with **doxycycline** (100 mg bid for 10 days) and cultured for gonococcus.
5. Bacteriuria and symptoms should dissipate within 24 to 48 h. A short course of a urinary tract anesthetic (**phenazopyridine** 200 mg tid) should be considered when patients have significant dysuria.
6. The decision to admit patients with pyelonephritis is based on age, host factors, and response to initial ED interventions. Unremitting fever and loss of vasomotor tone are indications for admission, as are intractable nausea and vomiting. Intravenous antibiotic choices for these patients are: **trimethoprim/sulfamethoxazole** (160/800 mg TMP/SMX q12h), **ceftriaxone** (1 g q12h), or **gentamicin** (2 mg/kg load, then 1.0 mg/kg q8h). Patients with factors associated with poor outcome should also be admitted: old age and general debility, renal calculi or obstruction, recent hospitalization or instrumentation, diabetes mellitus, evidence of chronic nephropathy, sickle cell disease, underlying carcinoma, or intercurrent cancer chemotherapy. These patients must be admitted and covered with broad-

spectrum antibiotics (including anti-*Pseudomonal* agents). All admitted patients must have adequate hydration instituted in the ED.

If Standard Treatment Fails

Patients not responding to appropriate antibiotics should first be confirmed to have UTI with a urine culture, and organism-specific therapy should be started. Patients with UTI who have failed standard therapy may respond to a change in antibiotics, or may have hitherto undetected structural or immunologic compromise.

For further reading in *Emergency Medicine, A Comprehensive Study Guide*, see Chapter 91, Urinary Tract Infections, by David S. Howes.

Stephen H. Thomas

Few problems encountered in the ED match the anxiety of a male with acute genital pain. In addition to the psychological impact, symptoms are severe because of extensive sensory innervation.

TESTES AND EPIDIDYMIS

Testes

Testicular torsion must be the primary consideration in any male (of all age groups) complaining of testicular pain. Pain usually occurs suddenly, is severe, and is felt in either the lower abdominal quadrant, the inguinal canal, or the testis. The pain may be either constant or intermittent but is not positional, as torsion is primarily an ischemic event. Once the diagnosis is considered, urologic consultation is indicated for exploration, as radionuclide imaging tests are often too time-consuming. The ED physician can attempt manual detorsion. Most testes torse in a lateral to medial direction, so detorsion is performed in a medial to lateral direction, similar to opening a book. The endpoint for successful detorsion is pain relief; urologic referral is still indicated.

Torsion of the appendages is more common than testicular torsion but is not dangerous as the appendix testis and appendix epididymis have no known function. If the patient is seen early, diagnosis can be supported by the following: pain is most intense near the head of the epididymis or testis; there is an isolated tender nodule; the pathognomonic *blue dot* appearance of a cyanotic appendage is illuminated through thin prepubertal scrotal skin. If normal intratesticular blood flow can be demonstrated with color Doppler, immediate surgery is not necessary since most appendages calcify or degenerate over 10 to 14 days and cause no harm. If the diagnosis cannot be assured, urologic exploration is needed to rule out testicular torsion.

Epididymitis

Epididymitis is characterized by gradual onset of pain due to its inflammatory etiology. Bacterial infection is the most common etiology; infecting agents are dependent on patient age. In patients younger than 40 years old, epididymitis is primarily due to sexually transmitted diseases (STD). Common urinary pathogens predominate in older men. Epididymitis causes lower abdominal, inguinal canal, scrotal, or testicular pain, alone or in combination. Due to the inflammatory nature of the pain, patients with epididymitis may note transient pain relief when elevating the scrotal contents while recumbent. Initially, tenderness is well-localized to the epididymis, but progression of inflammation results in the physical-exam finding of a single, large testicular mass (epididymo-orchitis), difficult to differentiate from testicular torsion or carcinoma. At this stage the patient may appear toxic and require admission for intravenous antibiotics (e.g., ceftriaxone, 1–2 gm q12h; trimethoprim/sulfamethoxazole, 5 mg/kg, based on trimethoprim q6h), scrotal elevation and ice application, NSAIDs, narcotics for analgesia, and stool softeners. Outpatient treatment is an option in patients who do not appear toxic; urologic followup within a week is indicated. Oral antibiotic regimen should include 10 days of therapy with one of the following: doxycycline, 100 mg bid, or azithromycin, 500 mg bid for patients under 40; or, for age 40 or older, use trimethoprim/sulfamethoxazole, one double-strength tablet bid, or ciprofloxacin, 500 mg bid.

Orchitis in isolation is rare, usually occurs with viral or syphilitic disease, and is treated with disease-specific therapy, symptomatic support, and urologic follow-up.

Testicular malignancy should be suspected in patients presenting with asymptomatic testicular mass, firmness, or induration. Ten% of tumors present with pain due to hemorrhage within the tumor. Urgent urologic followup is indicated.

SCROTUM

Scrotal abscesses may be localized to the scrotal wall or may arise from extensions of infections of intrascrotal contents (testis, epididymis, bulbous urethra). A simple hair-follicle scrotal-wall abscess can be managed by incision and drainage; no antibiotics are required in immunocompetent males. Suspicion that a scrotal wall abscess is coming from an intrascrotal infection, ultrasound and retrograde urethrography demonstrate testis/epididymis and urethral pathology, respectively. Definitive care of any complex abscess calls for a urology consultant.

Fournier gangrene is a polymicrobial infection of the perineal subcutaneous tissues. Diabetic males are at highest risk. Prompt diagnosis is essential to prevent extensive tissue loss. Early surgical consultation is recommended for at-risk patients who present with scrotal, rectal, or genital pain. Aggressive fluid resuscitation with normal saline, broad-spectrum (gram-positive, gram-negative, anaerobic) antibiotic coverage, surgical debridement, and hyperbaric oxygen therapy are treatment mainstays.

PENIS

Balanoposthitis is inflammation of the glans (balanitis) and foreskin (posthitis). Upon foreskin retraction, the glans and prepuce appear purulent, excoriated, malodorous, and tender. Treatment consists of cleansing with mild soap, assuring adequate dryness, application of antifungal creams (nystatin qid or clotrimazole bid), and urologic referral for followup and possible circumcision. An oral cephalosporin (i.e., **cepha-**

lexin, 500 mg po qid) should be prescribed in cases of secondary bacterial infection.

Phimosis is the inability to retract the foreskin proximally. Hemostatic dilation of the preputial ostium relieves the urinary retention until definitive dorsal slit or circumcision can be performed.

Paraphimosis is the inability to reduce the proximal edematous foreskin distally over the glans. Paraphimosis is a true urologic emergency, as resulting glans edema and venous engorgement can progress to arterial compromise and gangrene. If surrounding tissue edema can be successfully compressed, the foreskin may be reduced. If arterial compromise is suspected or has occurred, local infiltration of the constricting band with 1% plain lidocaine followed by superficial vertical incision of the band will decompress the glans and allow foreskin reduction.

Entrapment injuries occur when various objects are wrapped around the penis. Such objects should be removed and urethral integrity (retrograde urethrogram) and distal penile arterial blood supply (Doppler) should be confirmed when indicated. Penile fracture occurs when there is an acute tear of the penile tunica albuginea. The penis is acutely swollen, discolored, and tender in a patient with history of trauma during intercourse accompanied by a snapping sound. Urologic consultation is indicated.

Peyronie disease presents with patients noting sudden or gradual onset of dorsal penile curvature with erections. Examination reveals a thickened plaque on the dorsal penile shaft. Assurance and urologic followup are indicated.

Priapism is a painful pathologic erection, which may be associated with urinary retention. Infection and impotence are other complications. Regardless of etiology, initial therapy for priapism is terbutaline, 0.25 to 0.5 mg, subcutaneously in the deltoid area. Urologic consultation is indicated in all cases.

URETHRA

Urethral stricture is becoming more common due to rising incidence of STDs. If a patient's bladder cannot be cannulated with a 14F or 16F Foley or Coudé catheter, the differential diagnosis includes urethral stricture, voluntary external sphincter spasm, bladder-neck contracture, or benign prostatic hypertrophy. Retrograde urethrography can be performed to delineate the location and extent of urethral stricture. Endoscopy is necessary to confirm bladder-neck contracture or define the extent of an obstructing prostate gland. Suspected voluntary external sphincter spasm can be overcome by holding the patient's penis upright and encouraging him to relax his perineum and breathe slowly during the procedure. After no more than three gentle attempts to pass a 12F-Coudé into a urethra prepared with anesthetic lubricant, urology should be consulted. In an emergency situation, suprapubic cystotomy can be performed. The infraumbilical and suprapubic area is prepped with povidone–iodine solution. A 25- to 27-gauge spinal needle is used to locate the bladder, followed by placement of the cystotomy using a Cook kit and Seldinger technique. Urologic followup should occur within 48 h.

Urethral foreign bodies are associated with bloody urine and slow, painful urination. X-ray of the bladder and urethral areas may disclose a foreign body. Removal of the foreign body may be achieved with a gentle milking action; retrograde urethrography or endoscopy is required in these cases to confirm an intact urethra. Often, urologic consultation for endoscopy or open cystotomy is required for foreign body removal.

Urinary retention syndromes can range from overt retention to insidious overflow incontinence. A detailed history, including over-the-counter cold and diet aids, may reveal the cause of urinary retention. Men do not void as completely when sitting down, and infrequent ejaculation may lead to secondary prostatic congestion and symptoms of outlet obstruction. An intact sensory examination, anal sphincter, and bulbocavernosus reflex differentiate chronic outlet obstruction from the sensory or motor neurogenic bladder and spinal-cord compression.

Physical examination should include search for meatal stenosis, palpation of urethral length for masses or fistulae consistent with urethral stricture disease or abscess formation, lower abdominal examination for palpation of suprapubic mass, and rectal examination to evaluate anal sphincter tone and prostate size and consistency. Most patients with bladder outlet obstruction are in distress and passage of a urethral catheter alleviates their pain and their urinary retention. Copious intraurethral lubrication including a topical anesthetic should be used, and a 16F-Coudé catheter is recommended if straight catheters fail. Be certain to pass the catheter to its fullest extent, obtaining free urine flow, before inflating the balloon. The catheter should be left indwelling and connected to a leg drainage bag. Belladonna and opium (B & O) suppositories (one every 4–6h) can be prescribed to alleviate the constant urge to void secondary to bladder spasm, which frequently accompanies an indwelling catheter. In patients whose bladder catheter will be left in longer than 5 to 7 days, prophylactic antibiotics (trimethoprim, 100 mg daily) should be instituted. Otherwise, antibiotics are indicated only if urinalysis is consistent with UTI. If urinary retention has been chronic, postobstructive diuresis may occur even in the presence of normal BUN and creatinine. In such patients, close monitoring of urinary output is indicated; they should be observed for 4 to 6 h after catheterization.

In all cases of urinary retention, urologic followup is indicated for a complete genitourinary evaluation.

For further reading in *Emergency Medicine, A Comprehensive Study Guide,* see Chapter 92, Male Genital Problems, by Robert E. Schneider.

David M. Cline

UREMIC PERICARDITIS

The classic symptom is chest pain, which is partially relieved by sitting up and leaning forward. A pericardial friction rub may not be heard or may be heard intermittently. Low-grade fever and atrial arrhythmias (paroxysmal atrial tachycardia, atrial flutter–atrial fibrillation) are common as well. Echocardiography often demonstrates a pericardial effusion. The pericardial fluid may impede venous return, leading to congestive heart failure and hypotension. Tamponade is relieved by pericardiocentesis.

CARDIAC ARRHYTHMIAS AND CARDIAC ARREST

The most common cause of cardiac arrest in uremic patients is hyperkalemia. The treatment should include administration of calcium gluconate (10 mL of 10% solution), followed by infusion of 50 mL of 50% glucose, along with 20 units of regular insulin, and infusion of 50 to 100 mEq IV sodium bicarbonate. Hemo- or peritoneal dialysis, using a lower concentration of $K+$ in the dialysate, is the most effective way to reduce the potassium level and should be employed as soon as possible.

HYPOTENSION

A sudden drop in blood pressure is a common complication during dialysis and, if not promptly treated, can lead to cardiac arrest. Subjective symptoms, such as muscle cramps, nausea, yawning, and mental confusion may precede actual hypotension in most patients, but not in all. Treatment is rapid infusion of isotonic saline. In rare instances, the use of vasopressors may be required.

DIALYSIS DISEQUILIBRIUM

Symptoms of increased intracranial pressure, manifested by nausea, vomiting, headache, and mental confusion, can develop soon after or within a few h of a dialysis treatment. It is common after first dialysis but also can occur on rare occasion, even in patients treated with chronic dialysis. The raised intracranial pressure is the result of osmotic shift of fluid from the bloodstream into cerebrospinal fluid (CSF) because of higher CSF urea content relative to plasma.

Diagnosis is based on the history and measurement of BUN levels both before and after first dialysis. It should be differentiated from other causes of raised intracranial pressure, such as subdural hematoma, cerebrovascular accident, and brain tumor. Therapy is purely symptomatic.

GASTROINTESTINAL (GI) DISORDERS

Upper GI bleeding may result from uremic gastritis, peptic ulcer disease, or excess anticoagulation. Management does not differ from that of nonuremic patients. Caution should be exercised, however, in using large doses of magnesium-containing antacids. Since magnesium is normally excreted by the kidney, abnormal levels could accumulate in the plasma of the uremic patient, leading to mental obtundation and respiratory depression.

PROBLEMS PECULIAR TO PERITONEAL DIALYSIS

Infection of the peritoneal membrane is the most frequent and critical complication in patients receiving chronic peritoneal dialysis. The symptoms may be subtle and include abdominal discomfort, pain during inflow, and fever. Physical examination may reveal abdominal tenderness, particularly around the catheter site, and decreased bowel sounds. Laboratory evaluation should include CBC and analysis of peritoneal fluid for cell count, gram-stain, protein, culture, and sensitivity. A bag of drained dialysate should be used for culture and analysis. A variety of micro-organisms (bacterial, fungal, and parasitic) have been found after culturing the fluid from the peritoneal cavity of dialysis patients. The mainstay of therapy is the infusion of an appropriate antimicrobial agent into the peritoneal cavity. Depending upon the results of gram stain, usually **vancomycin** (2 gm) plus **gentamicin** (30 to 40 mg) or **tobramycin** (30 to 40 mg) are given. To avoid fibrin formation, 1000 units of heparin are added to the infusion.

If a patient experiences recurrent bouts of peritonitis, tunnel infection, or intra-abdominal abscess, the catheter should be changed. Appropriate surgical drainage of intra-abdominal abscess is also warranted to prevent relapse.

PROBLEMS RELATED TO VASCULAR ACCESS

The most frequent complications associated with the external shunts are clotting and infection. When the shunt is acutely clotted, the vascular surgeon must be notified immediately. Declotting procedures using a Fogarty balloon catheter are normally accomplished by the surgeon in the operating suite. In some instances, however, instillation of urokinase, 5000 to 10,000 units, into the arterial and venous parts of the clotted shunt may dissolve the clot and prevent the need for further intervention.

Infection of the cannula site is a significant problem in the hemodialysis patient. Coagulase-positive staphylococci and *S. epidermidis* are frequently cultured from the exit site. Physical examination may reveal local inflammation, tenderness over the cannula tips, and purulent drainage at the exit sites. Soon after obtaining cultures from the exit site and blood, an antibiotic that is effective against penicillinase-resistant organisms (e.g., oxacillin, vancomycin, or cephalosporins should be given). The most dreaded complications associated with the external shunt infection are septic pulmonary embolism and brisk hemorrhage resulting from dislodgement of the cannula tip.

For further reading in *Emergency Medicine, A Comprehensive Study Guide*, see Chapter 94, Emergencies in Chronic Dialysis Patients, by K. Venkateswara Rao.

| Urologic Stone Disease

Elicia A. Sinor

Urologic stones can form anywhere in the urinary tract, although primary bladder stones are rare. The most common clinical presentation occurs when the stones migrate down the ureter, causing some degree of obstruction.

Clinical Features

Both adults and children present with kidney stones. In adults, the frequency is three times more common in males than females and usually occurs in the third to fifth decade of life. Children constitute 7% of cases seen, with the distribution being equal between the sexes. Patients usually present with an acute onset of severe pain that can be associated with nausea, vomiting, and diaphoresis. The pain is sharp and episodic in nature due to the intermittent obstruction and is relieved after the stone passes. Pain typically originates in either flank, radiating around the abdomen toward the groin, however, as the stone passes distally it may become anterior, abdominal, or suprapubic in nature.

Vesicular stones may present with intermittent dysuria and terminal hematuria. Patients are frequently anxious, pacing, or writhing, and are unable to hold still or converse. Children may present in a similar fashion, but up to 30% have only painless hematuria. Physical findings can include tachycardia and elevated BP, secondary to pain. Patients are usually afebrile unless a urinary-tract infection is concurrent. Examination may reveal costovertebral tenderness or abdominal tenderness over the site of the impacted stone.

Diagnosis and Differential

On clinical suspicion of a kidney stone, a urinalysis for initial dipstick and complete urinalysis expedites differential diagnosis and rules out infection. Microscopic hematuria is present 90% of the time, although there is no correlation between the quantity of blood present and the degree of obstruction. A kidneys, ureters, bladder (KUB) x-ray can be helpful in excluding other pathologies and in visualizing stones, as 90% are radiopaque. The gold standard for diagnosis of renal stone and colic is the IVP that gives both functional and anatomic information. Prior to obtaining an IVP, the patient should be questioned regarding allergy to radiocontrast media and appropriate materials for managing allergic reactions should be readily available. A pregnancy test should be obtained for any patient at risk. Pregnant patients and children are preferentially evaluated with ultrasound to decrease radiation exposure. BUN and creatinine should be obtained prior to the IVP on any patient at risk for radiocontrast agent nephrotoxicity. This is most likely in patients with pre-existing renal insufficiency, diabetes mellitus, dehydration, hypovolemia, hypotension, advanced age (>70 years), multiple myeloma, hypertension, hyperuricemia, a history of radiocontrast media within 72 h, and those with cardiovascular disease taking a diuretic.

Maintaining adequate urinary output with administration of intravenous fluids also decreases risk of renal injury. After contrast dye is administered, a scout film is obtained followed by films at 5-, 10-, and 20-min intervals. Positive findings include distention of the renal pelvis, calyceal distortion, dye extravasation, hydronephrosis, ureteral column dye cutoff, and a delay in appearance of a nephrogram. Post-void films are useful in distal stones. False-negative IVP can occur in the radiolucent, partially obstructing stone. Ultrasound, an anatomic rather than functional test, is useful in patients that are not candidates for IVP. It detects hydronephrosis and larger stones, although it is not sensitive for midureteral stones or small stones (<5 mm). Differential diagnosis of renal stones includes rupturing aortic abdominal aneurysm, pyelonephritis, renal infarction, papillary necrosis, ectopic pregnancy, appendicitis, biliary colic and acute muscle strain. Patients receiving outpatient extracorporeal shock wave lithotripsy for urolithiasis may present to the ED with renal colic as the resulting sludge is passed in the urine.

Emergency Department Care

In most cases, the diagnosis of urologic stones and renal colic is clinical. Management consists of excluding infection and other diagnoses, supportive care, analgesia, and appropriate referral. Patients should be monitored, if possible, and an intravenous line established for hydration and pain medication administration.

1. Crystalloid IV fluids should be given to maintain adequate urinary output in the event an IVP is ordered.
2. Administer adequate analgesia that may require large doses of titrated narcotics, such as morphine or its equivalent. Narcotics may be accompanied by NSAIDs but should not be replaced by them, as NSAIDs' onset of pain relief is much slower.
3. Perform an IVP to confirm the diagnosis and assure the presence of two anatomically normal kidneys. In patients who are not candidates for IVP, ultrasound is an appropriate diagnostic adjunct. If diagnosis is clinically evident or the diagnosis is already established, a KUB is sufficient.
4. While the patient is in the ED, collect and strain all urine for pathologic analysis of collected stones. In cases of complicating urinary tract infection, antibiotics should be started.

Discharge is appropriate in patients with small unilateral stones (<6 mm), no infection, and pain controlled by oral analgesics. Patients may be given a urinary strainer, prescriptions for oral narcotics, and urologic followup within 5 days. If the stone is passed in the ED, no treatment is necessary other than elective urologic followup. Patients should be instructed to return if they develop fever, vomiting, or uncontrolled pain. Admission is indicated in patients with infection and concurrent obstruction, solitary kidney with obstruction, uncontrolled pain or emesis, and large or proximal stones. Hospitalization should be discussed with the urologist for patients with renal insufficiency, severe underlying disease, IVP with extravasation or complete obstruction, suspected vesicular stone, or who have made multiple visits to the ED.

If Standard Treatment Fails

Urologic consultation on an emergent basis is prudent in the patient who may have classic urolithiasis and does not appear to be responding to appropriate pain medication. If the diagnosis is in question, the differential diagnosis should be reviewed. The most critical alternative diagnosis to consider is a rupturing or dissecting aortic abdominal aneurysm, which can have a similar presentation. Other diagnoses to consider are ruptured ectopic pregnancy or appendicitis, as these can be life-threatening if missed.

For further reading in *Emergency Medicine, A Comprehensive Study Guide*, see Chapter 95, Urologic Stone Disease, by W. F. Peacock, IV.

Rebecca S. Rich

PELVIC PAIN IN THE NONPREGNANT PATIENT

Although most women with pelvic pain have gynecologic problems, consider nongynecologic conditions as well, such as inflammatory bowel disease, gastroenteritis, diverticulitis, urinary-tract infection and obstruction and, particularly, appendicitis.

PELVIC INFLAMMATORY DISEASE

Pelvic inflammatory disease (PID) is the most common serious infection of reproductive-age women in the United States. PID is polymicrobial, involving *Neisseria gonorrhoeae* and *Chlamydia*, as well as anaerobes and *E. coli*. Bacteria spread from the lower genital tract to the normally sterile endometrium and adnexae. Risk factors for PID include prior gonoccoccal salpingitis, sex with multiple partners, adolescence, and presence of an IUD. Most cases of PID are sexually transmitted.

Clinical Features and Diagnosis

Symptoms include abdominal and pelvic pain, fever, and vaginal discharge. Anorexia, nausea, and vomiting are common, mimicking appendicitis or gastroenteritis. Onset often occurs after menstruation. (Diagnostic criteria are listed in Table 62-1.) Associated right upper quadrant pain suggests Fitz–Hugh–Curtis syndrome, a localized form of peritonitis due to purulent discharge from the tubes around the liver. Labs should include pregnancy test and gonococcal and *Chlamydia* cultures. A cervical gram-stain and a CBC should be considered.

Emergency Department Care

The CDC publishes treatment guidelines for PID (Table 62-2). Consider inpatient parenteral treatment in the following cases: uncertain diagno-

---

TABLE 62-1. Criteria for Clinical Diagnosis of PID

All three of these conditions must be present
  Abdominal direct tenderness without rebound tenderness
  Tenderness with motion of cervix and uterus
  Adnexal tenderness
One of these conditions must be present
  Gram-stain of endocervix—positive for gram-negative, intracellular
  diplococci
  Temperature greater than 38°C (100.4°F)
  Leukocytosis greater than 10,000/mm³ (μL)
  White blood cells and bacteria in peritoneal fluid collected by culdo-
  centesis or laparoscopy
  Inflammatory mass documented by pelvic examination or sonogram

Adapted from Hager WD et al: Criteria for diagnosis and grading of salpingitis. *Obstet Gynecol* 61:113, 1983.

TABLE 62-2. CDC Recommended Treatment for Acute PID

Outpatients
Regimen A
  Cefoxitin, 2 g IM, plus probenicid, 1 g po, or ceftriaxone, 250 mg IM, followed by
  Doxycycline, 100 mg po bid for 14 days
Regimen B
  Ofloxacin, 400 mg po bid for 14 days plus
  Clindamycin, 450 mg po qid, or metronidazole, 500 mg po bid for 14 days
Inpatients
Regimen A
  Cefoxitin, 2 g IV q6 h, or cefotetan, 2 g IV q12 h, plus
  Doxycycline, 100 mg q12 h IV, or po for 48 h
  After discharge doxycycline 100 mg po bid for 10–14 days
Regimen B
  Clindamycin, 900 mg IV q8 h, plus
  Gentamicin, load IV or IM (2 mg/kg), then maintenance dose (1.5 mg/kg) q8 h for at least 48 h
  After discharge, doxycycline, 100 mg po bid for 10–14 days, or clindamycin, 450 mg po qid for 10–14 days

sis, suspected or diagnosed pelvic abscess, pregnancy, adolescence, underlying HIV infection, severe illness with systemic toxicity or peritoneal signs, nausea and vomiting precluding use of oral antibiotics, unreliable patient, presence of IUD, or failure to respond to outpatient oral therapy. Instruct discharged patients to be rechecked within 72 h. Treat male contacts to prevent reinfection.

ADNEXAL ACCIDENTS

The most common noninfectious causes of pelvic pain are rupture or torsion of a cyst or solid ovarian, tubal, or uterine mass. With the exception of persistent corpus luteum cyst, these occur in women with normal menstrual cycles. Ovarian enlargement is initially asymptomatic or causes poorly defined visceral pain due to poor afferent innervation. When leakage or rupture occurs, acute pain results from irritation of the parietal peritoneum from contents of the cyst or mass. In the case of a dermoid tumor, serious chemical peritonitis can occur.

Clinical Features

Rupture of a corpus luteum cyst is a common cause of acute pelvic pain. Normally, the corpus luteum lyses 2 weeks after ovulation if pregnancy does not occur. Sometimes corpus luteum persists. The patient is amenorrheic for an additional 1 to 3 wks after which luteolysis occurs and then heavy menstrual flow occurs. If the corpus luteum persists and ruptures, the patient presents with vaginal bleeding and pelvic pain.

Diagnosis and Emergency Department Care

Once pregnancy is excluded, ultrasound is the most useful test for adnexal pathology and for detection of free fluid. Patients with unruptured cysts should be referred for gynocologic followup. If a cyst has ruptured and the patient is hemodynamically stable without evidence of hemorrhage, she may be discharged with analgesics and followup. Rupture of a persistent corpus luteum cyst may result in hemoperitoneum, which requires surgical intervention.

OVARIAN TORSION

Clinical Features

Ovarian torsion is rare. It often occurs in an enlarged or abnormal ovary. The ovary twists on its pedicle and the blood supply is compromised, which may lead to necrosis. Torsion of tubal masses and pedunculated fibroids also occurs, with similar clinical presentation.

Diagnosis

Patients describe sudden onset of severe unilateral lower abdominal and pelvic pain. Many patients have nausea and vomiting, suggesting appendicitis. There may be a prior history of similar painful episodes. On pelvic exam, patients haveunilateral adnexal pain, tenderness, and often a mass. Ultrasound may be helpful, although the diagnosis is often established at surgery.

Emergency Department Care

Immediate gynecologic referral is warranted. Laparoscopic ovarian or adnexal detorsion or removal is the treatment of choice.

MITTELSCHMERTZ

Clinical Features

Mittelschmertz (middle pain) is midcycle pain from ovulation, occurring around days 14 to 16 of the typical menstrual cycle. The pain is typically unilateral, mild to moderate, and often lasts a day or less. There may be light vaginal spotting.

Diagnosis and Emergency Department Care

Diagnosis is clinical, and more serious causes of adnexal pain should be ruled out. The pelvic exam may show mild adnexal tenderness without mass. Treatment is symptomatic using analgesics. Mittelschmertz is self-limited and resolves spontaneously. Advise patients to keep a menstrual calendar to confirm the diagnosis.

ENDOMETRIOSIS

With endometriosis, normal endometrium occurs in ectopic locations. All pelvic structures, as well as ligaments, cul-de-sac, gutters, and peritoneum may be affected.

Clinical Features

Symptoms include pelvic pain, dysmenorrhea, and dyspareunia. Patients may be infertile. Pelvic exam may show pain and tenderness but is often nonspecific. Rupture of an ovarian endometrioma may present with acute, severe pelvic pain with peritoneal signs.

Diagnosis and Treatment

The diagnosis may be suspected in the ED but cannot be established noninvasively. The extent of disease often correlates poorly with clinical symptoms. To confirm the diagnosis, visualization by laparoscopy or laparotomy is necessary. Barring the need for urgent operative intervention, the most appropriate ED management is analgesia and gynecologic referral.

VAGINAL BLEEDING IN THE NONPREGNANT PATIENT

Once pregnancy has been excluded, consider structural and traumatic causes of bleeding. A thorough pelvic exam will often show the source. Bleeding may arise from the cervix or uterus, including cervicitis, cervical cancer, endometrial cancer (especially in older women), cervical or endometrial polyps, or submucosal fibroids. Most of these patients can be referred for definitive care.

Trauma to the vulva and vagina may cause profuse bleeding and hypotension. In most cases, control of bleeding may require analgesia and gynecologic consultation. Consider coagulopathy in young women with heavy vaginal bleeding. In particular, platelet disorders may first present with heavy menstrual bleeding. Skin clues such as petechiae are often absent.

If the pelvic exam is normal, anovulatory dysfunctional uterine bleeding (DUB) is a likely cause. Patients present with prolonged menstrual periods or intermenstrual bleeding. Virtually all severe cases occur in adolescents shortly after onset of menarche.

Emergency Department Care

Many cases require no immediate interventions, however, bleeding may be severe enough to cause hemorrhagic shock.

1. For severe bleeding, start a large-bore IV line and give 0.9 normal saline and blood as needed.

2. Hemodynamically unstable patients, give conjugated estrogen, 20 mg IV over 15 min. IV estrogen causes vasospasm of the uterine arterioles, which reduces bleeding.
3. For stable patients, consider a combination oral contraceptive agent (such as Lo/Ovral), four pills/day for 7 days.
4. Refer to gynecologist. Patients with postmenopausal bleeding (or age >40) should be referred for possible endometrial biopsy prior to estrogens.

For further reading in *Emergency Medicine, A Comprehensive Study Guide,* see Chapter 96, Gynecologic Emergencies, by Veronica Mallett.

Rebecca S. Rich

Vulvovaginitis is a common problem whose causes include infections, irritants and allergies, foreign bodies, and atrophy. The normal vaginal flora helps maintain an acidic pH of between 3.5 and 4.1, which decreases pathogen growth.

CANDIDA VAGINITIS

Candida albicans is a normal vaginal commensal in up to 50% of women, and candidiasis is not considered an STD. Conditions that promote candida vaginitis include systemic antibiotics, diabetes, pregnancy, birth control pills, and postmenopausal.

Clinical Features

Symptoms include vaginal discharge, itching dysuria, and dyspareunia. Signs include vulvar and vaginal edema, erythema, and a thick, cottage-cheese discharge.

Diagnosis

Examine vaginal secretions microscopically in a few drops of saline or make a KOH prep. Ten% KOH dissolves vaginal epithelial cells, leaving yeast buds and pseudohyphae intact and easier to see. The sensitivity of the KOH technique is 80%.

Emergency Department Care

The imidazoles (**clotrimazole** 1% cream, **miconazole** 2% cream) are the drugs of choice, topically for 3 to 7 days. **Fluconazole**, 150 mg po, is an alternative. Treatment of sexual partners is not necessary unless candidal balanitis is present.

TRICHOMONAS VAGINITIS

Trichomoniasis, caused by a protozoan, is almost always an STD. Up to 25% of women harboring the organism, however, are asymptomatic.

Clinical Features

Most patients have vaginal discharge. Other symptoms include perineal irritation, dysuria, spotting, and pelvic pain. Discharge may be frothy and malodorous. Vaginal erythema and irritation are common. The vaginal pH is greater than 4.5.

Diagnosis

Saline wet prep shows motile, pear-shaped, flagellated trichomonads slightly larger than leukocytes. The sensitivity of this test is 50% to 70%.

Emergency Department Care

A single 2-gram oral dose of **metronidazole** is the drug of choice. For treatment failures, metronidazole, 500 mg bid, for 7 days is recommended. Concomitant alcohol use may induce an Antabuse-like reaction. Most infected men are asymptomatic; male partners need treatment to avoid retransmission of disease. Metronizadole is not recommended for use in the first trimester of pregnancy. Topical clotrimazole is less effective but safe. If symptoms persist and are severe, metronidazole can be given after the first trimester. During lactation, the single 2-gram oral dose is recommended, with no breastfeeding for 24 hours.

BACTERIAL VAGINOSIS

This infection is due to an increase in the aerobe *Gardnerella vaginalis* and anaerobes. *Gardnerella's* mere presence does not constitute infection, as it is found in 40% of asymptomatic women.

Clinical Features

If symptomatic, women have vaginal discharge and may have itching. Exam ranges from mild vaginal redness to a frothy gray-white discharge.

Diagnosis

Three of the following: (1) discharge; (2) pH greater than 4.5; (3) fishy odor when 10% KOH is added to the discharge (positive amine test); and (4) clue cells, which are epithelial cells with clusters of bacilli stuck to the surface seen on saline wet prep. Often, however, the diagnosis is suspected from a compatible presentation, along with absence of *Candida* and *Trichomonas*.

Emergency Department Care

Metronidazole, 500 mg po bid for 7 days, is standard. **Clindamycin**, 300 mg po bid for 7 days, is an alternative. Neither treatment of male partners nor asymptomatic women is recommended. Routine treatment of pregnant women with bacterial vaginosis is not recommended. If treatment is necessary, clindamycin is preferred.

GENITAL HERPES

Genital herpes is an STD caused by herpes simplex virus (HSV) and is the most common cause of genital ulcers in United States women.

Clinical Features

Symptoms begin a mean of 6 days after exposure. Initial infections are more severe and prolonged than recurrences. Painful vesicles or papules progress to shallow ulcers which then crust over. Lymphadenopathy and pelvic pain are common. Urethritis is also common, with dysuria and sometimes urinary retention requiring catheterization. Systemic symptoms include fever, malaise, myalgias, and headache. Hepatitis and aseptic meningitis can also occur. Sacral autonomic involvement is rare but can cause bowel and bladder dysfunction. Recurrent episodes are milder, shorter, and lack systemic symptoms. The average number of symptomatic recurrences is 5 to 8 per year.

Diagnosis

HSV is largely a clinical diagnosis confirmed by culture. Intact vesicles should be unroofed and the fluid cultured; the yield is about 90%. A positive Tzanck smear, showing multinucleated giant cells, occurs in about 50% of cases.

Emergency Department Care

There is no cure for HSV at this time. Pain control with narcotics may be necessary, especially for a first attack. Systemic acyclovir accelerates healing of lesions and provides some relief of symptoms. The dose is 200 mg po 5 times/day, or 400 mg tid for 10 days. For rectal disease, use 800 mg tid. Topical acyclovir is ineffective. Acyclovir is less effective for recurrences; treatment should start at the prodrome of genital tingling or within 2 days of onset to be beneficial. HIV-positive patients often have frequent and severe attacks and may benefit from higher doses, such as 400 to 800 mg 3 to 5 times/day. Although not FDA-approved, acyclovir has been safely used for genital HSV in pregnant women.

CONTACT VULVOVAGINITIS

Common causes include douches, soaps, bubble baths, deodorants, perfumes, feminine hygiene products, topical antibiotics, and tight undergarments. Patients complain of perineal burning, itching, swelling, and often dysuria. The exam shows a red and swollen vulvovaginal area. In severe cases, there may be vesicles and ulceration. Vaginal pH changes may promote overgrowth of *Candida*, obscuring the primary problem.

Try to identify the precipitating agent and rule out infectious causes. Most cases resolve spontaneously when the precipitant is withdrawn. For more severe reactions, cool sitz baths, compresses with Burrow's solution, and topical corticosteroids may help. Oral antihistamines are too drying and should be avoided.

VAGINAL FOREIGN BODIES

In younger girls, common items are toilet paper, toys, and small household objects. Later, a forgotten or unretrievable tampon or diaphragm is often the culprit. Patients present with a foul-smelling or bloody discharge. Removal of the object is usually curative without other therapy.

ATROPHIC VAGINITIS

Lack of estrogen after menopause leads to vaginal mucosal atrophy. The epithelium becomes pale, thin, and less resistant to minor trauma or infection. Bleeding can occur. The vaginal pH also increases, and subsequent changes in the vaginal flora can predispose to bacterial infection with purulent discharge. A sulfa cream should be used for secondary infection, and an estrogen cream should be applied topically for 2 to 3 weeks. Estrogen creams should not be prescribed in the ED for women with prior reproductive tract cancer, and of course, in women with postmenopausal bleeding. Carcinoma is a major concern, so a Pap smear should be taken and the patient referred to a gynecologist.

For further reading in *Emergency Medicine, A Comprehensive Study Guide*, see Chapter 97, Vulvovaginitis, by Gloria Kuhn.

Problems in Pregnancy

Sally S. Fuller

Physiology of Pregnancy

The physiologic changes of pregnancy are listed in Table 64-1.

Diagnosis of Pregnancy

The most commonly used test is the ELISA test on urine for β-HCG, with sensitivity as low as 20 mIU. ß-HCG is detectable 9 to 11 days after ovulation and usually reaches 100 mIU by the time of the first missed menses. Serum qualitative tests are only slightly more sensitive than the urine test. Quantitative serum measurements of β-HCG, when measured serially, are useful in diagnosis of ectopic pregnancy and other suspected abnormalities of the first trimester. β-HCG should increase at least 66% every 48 h in the first 6 wks of pregnancy. The level of β-HCG, which corresponds to a visible gestational sac on transvaginal ultrasound, must be established for each individual hospital lab. The sac may be visible as early as 5 wks from the LMP.

Pregnancy-Related Problems

First-trimester bleeding   First-trimester bleeding occurs in 40% of all pregnant women, half of whom proceed to a spontaneous abortion. In another 2%, bleeding is a sign of ectopic pregnancy. These women must be evaluated to rule out ectopic pregnancy and spontaneous abortion. Current recommendation is that every Rh-negative unimmunized

TABLE 64-1. Physiologic Changes in Pregnancy

Cardiac output	Elevated 30%–50%
Blood volume	Elevated 45%
Mean hemoglobin	10.2–11.6 g/dL
Heart rate	Increased 15–20 bpm
Blood pressure	Decreased 5–10 mmHg systolic; decreased 10–15 mmHg diastolic
Normal arterial blood gas	pH 7.40–7.45; PO2 95–105 mmHg; PCO2 28–32
GFR	Elevated 50%
Normal serum creatinine	0.5–0.75 mg/dL
ESR	Markedly elevated in normal pregnancy
Coagulation	Thromboembolism is the #1 cause of maternal mortality. Risk of thromboembolism increased 1.8 times normal in pregnancy and 5.5 times normal in postpartum period.
WBC count	10,000–15,000/μL
Insulin requirements in IDDM	Dramatically increased in early pregnancy

woman who presents with threatened abortion should receive an IM dose of 300 μg of **RhoGAM**.

Third-trimester bleeding Vaginal bleeding in the late second and early third trimester is often from a placenta previa or placental abruption. Other potential diagnoses are preterm labor, preterm cervical dilation, incompetent cervix, and cervicovaginal lesions. A speculum examination is a safe and appropriate first step, but digital examination is contraindicated until placenta previa is ruled out with ultrasound.

Placental abruption classically presents as vaginal bleeding with pain. The visible amount of bleeding may be large or small, and the pain may vary from mild to severe. The amount of pain or visible bleeding does not correlate with the risk to the fetus. Women with a history of smoking, hypertension, cocaine use, or trauma are at higher-than-normal risk for abruption. A patient with minimal abruption should be hospitalized for close observation. Moderate or severe abruption necessitates immediate delivery.

Placenta previa classically presents as painless bleeding, which may or may not be accompanied by uterine irritability. Digital vaginal examinations are contraindicated. The diagnosis is made by ultrasound. The bleeding patient with a previa must be admitted for close observation and cesarean-section delivery, if indicated.

ECTOPIC PREGNANCY

Two percent of all pregnancies are ectopic. Of pregnancies following tubal sterilization, 50% to 75% are ectopic. All women of reproductive age presenting with abdominal pain, regardless of birth control or tubal sterilization, should have a pregnancy test.

Clinical Presentation

Ninety percent of women with ectopic pregnancy will have abdominal or pelvic pain and vaginal bleeding; 20% will present to the ED having already ruptured.

Diagnosis

In the setting of unstable hemodynamics, culdocentesis is the most rapid means of diagnosing a hemoperitoneum. In the patient presenting with stable vital signs along with pelvic or abdominal pain, vaginal bleeding, and positive pregnancy test, the diagnosis of ectopy may be more difficult. The presence of an intrauterine gestational sac on ultrasound virtually rules out the diagnosis of ectopic pregnancy, as there is only a 1:4000 to 1:15,000 chance of coexisting intrauterine and ectopic pregnancies. In the absence of an intrauterine gestational sac, transvaginal ultrasound may be helpful in establishing the diagnosis. In the hemodynamically stable patient in whom the diagnosis of ectopic pregnancy still cannot be conclusively excluded or confirmed, serial quantitative HCG tests may be helpful in making the diagnosis.

Emergency Department Care

Immediate management consists of stabilization of vital signs.

1. Two large-bore IV lines should be placed with rapid infusion sets for infusion of crystalloid.
2. Blood should be typed and cross-matched, and packed red blood cells should be infused if needed.
3. Immediate consultation for emergent surgical intervention should be made. Special nonsurgical protocols using methotrexate may also be employed in selected cases.

SPONTANEOUS ABORTION

Clinical Presentation and Diagnosis

Spontaneous abortion occurs in 15% to 20% of all clinically recognized pregnancies. Threatened abortion refers to any uterine bleeding at less than 20 wks gestation without cervical dilatation or effacement. Inevitable abortion refers to uterine bleeding with cervical dilatation but without expulsion of tissue at less than 20 wks gestation. Incomplete abortion involves passage of some, but not all, of the fetal and placental tissue. Completed abortion occurs when there is spontaneous and complete expulsion of all products of conception. The most common time for spontaneous abortion is 8 to 12 wks gestation.

Emergency Department Care

Initial management includes stabilization of vital signs, if necessary, with crystalloid or packed red blood cells. Patients with suspected inevitable or incomplete abortion should receive evaluation by an Ob/Gyn consultant for consideration of dilatation and curettage. Suspected complete abortions may be difficult to distinguish from incomplete and should also be grounds for consultation. The consequences of incomplete abortion are continued pain, bleeding, and septic complications. All Rh-negative unsensitized women with spontaneous abortion should receive **RhoGAM**, 300 μg IM.

SEPTIC ABORTION

Any abortion accompanied by uterine infection is a septic abortion. Workup should include CBC, UA, blood cultures, chest x-ray, and coagulation studies. These patients should be admitted for IV antibiotics; a triple-antibiotic regimen of ampicillin, gentamicin, and clindamycin is often used. Operative uterine evacuation should follow institution of antibiotic therapy.

PRE-ECLAMPSIA AND HELLP SYNDROME

Seven percent of pregnancies are complicated by pre-eclampsia, which occurs most commonly in primigravidas. The clinical presentation can be variable, however, the classic case is characterized by hypertension, proteinuria, and edema. Criteria for severe preeclampsia are: BP $\geq$ 160/110, proteinuria $\geq$ 5 g/24h, oliguria $\leq$ 500 mL/24h, epigastric pain, cerebral or visual disturbances, or pulmonary edema. The HELLP syndrome (*h*emolysis, *e*levated *l*iver enzymes, *l*ow *p*latelet count) may be a related entity or variant of pre-eclampsia that usually presents with epigastric or right upper-quadrant pain, nausea, or vomiting. Laboratory data that supports the diagnosis of HELLP include hemolysis, platelet count <100,000/μL, LDH >600 IU/L, bilirubin $\geq$ 1.2 mg/dL, and SGOT >72 IU/L.

Emergency Department Care

ED care consists of seizure prevention (**MgSO4** loading dose of 4–6 g in 100 mL of fluid over 20 min, followed by maintenance infusion of 2 g in 100 mL fluid/h) and BP control (**hydralazine**, 20–40 mg IV/IM, or **labetalol**, 20 mg IV). Delivery of the fetus is indicated if gestational age is at or near term. Management of pre-eclampsia in the preterm patient remains controversial.

PRETERM LABOR

Preterm labor is defined as labor occurring prior to the end of 36 wks gestation, with cervical changes in response to regular uterine contractions, or contractions greater than 5 to 8 per h that do not resolve with bed rest and hydration. Causes of preterm labor include infection, uterine abnormalities, incompetent cervix, leiomyoma, exposure to DES, overdistension due to multiple gestations or polyhydramnios, and premature placental separation. In an individual case the reason for preterm labor may not be identifiable, but history of previous preterm birth is an identifiable risk factor. Clinical presentation of preterm labor may be nonspecific, including low-back pain or sense of intermittent pressure, lower abdominal pain, intestinal cramping with or without diarrhea, or change in vaginal discharge. The diagnosis often requires an extended period of close observation with external monitoring and serial cervical examinations. A woman for whom this diagnosis is seriously considered should be admitted to a labor and delivery unit.

Emergency Department Care

ED care of preterm labor begins with maternal hydration. Tocolytics are commonly used for idiopathic preterm labor at 34 weeks or less; and selectively at 34 to 37 wks. Magnesium sulfate IV is the tocolytic agent of choice for use in the ED. Relative contraindications to tocolysis include preeclampsia, chorioamnionitis, advanced labor, fetal maturity, fetal distress, and maternal hemodynamic instability.

PRETERM PREMATURE RUPTURE OF MEMBRANES

Premature rupture of membranes (PROM) is defined as rupture prior to the onset of labor, regardless of gestational age. Preterm PROM may be due to polyhydramnios, incompetent cervix, and placental abruption. Ninety percent of term patients and 50% of preterm patients will be in labor within 24 h, and 85% of preterm patients will be in labor within 1 wk. Clinical presentation of PROM is usually copious rush of fluid from the vagina. Sterile speculum examination may be undertaken to confirm the diagnosis, but digital cervical examination should be avoided in preterm patients to minimize risk of infection. The diagnosis of PROM may be confirmed by identifying a pool of fluid in the posterior fornix of the vagina with pH of 7.1 to 7.3 (dark blue on nitrazine paper) and ferning pattern on smear. Ultrasound may confirm abnormally low amniotic fluid. False positives with the nitrazine test may be observed with semen, blood, or certain infectious discharges. Patients with the diagnosis of PROM, or in whom the diagnosis remains unclear, should be admitted where proper neonatal support is available. Tocolytics are generally not used.

POSTPARTUM PROBLEMS

Postpartum Endometritis

Postpartum endometritis occurs in 3% of vaginal deliveries and 15% to 30% of cesarean deliveries. Most infections are polymicrobial. Clinical presentation includes fever, malaise, lower abdominal pain, and foul-smelling lochia. Diagnosis is made by physical exam revealing uterine fundus tenderness, cervical motion tenderness and, often, purulent discharge.

Emergency Department Care

Laboratory data should include CBC, urinalysis and urine culture, and cervical or uterine cultures. Blood cultures may be indicated in patients appearing septic. Broad-spectrum IV antibiotics should be initiated, and the patient should be admitted. Mild endometritis usually responds to a second- or third-generation cephalosporin, penicillin and ß-lactamase-inhibitor combination, or to clindamycin and gentamicin. More severe cases usually respond to a combination of ampicillin, gentamicin, and clindamycin.

Mastitis

Mastitis is cellulitis of the periglandular breast tissue occurring most commonly in lactating women. Clinical presentation includes pain, induration, redness, and warmth of the affected breast, with axillary adenopathy, fever, chills, and myalgias.

Emergency Department Care

ED care consists of outpatient **dicloxacillin**, 100 mg bid, or **cephalexin**, 500 mg qid, with instructions to continue nursing on the affected breast. Breast milk cultures are not useful. Abscess formation may occur rarely and require incision and drainage.

Drug Use in Pregnancy

Table 64-2 provides generalizations regarding drug use in pregnancy. Extensive reference books should be available to the ED physician for more in-depth information.

Diagnostic Imaging in Pregnancy

The threshold for teratogenesis from ionizing radiation is 10 rads, with 8 to 15 wks gestation being the most vulnerable period. No single diagnostic test exceeds this threshold, however the effects of multiple tests are cumulative and may exceed the threshold. The dose of ionizing radiation from ventilation/perfusion scanning also does not approach the threshold, however, since the isotope is excreted from the bladder with close proximity to the developing fetus, hydration and frequent voiding must be encouraged. MRI and ultrasonography have not shown any teratogenic effects.

Pregnancy and Coexisting Diseases

Pneumonia Alteration in maternal immune response in the second and third trimesters increases susceptibility to pneumonias of all sorts. Complications of pneumonia include fetal injury due to hypoxemia and fever, preterm labor, thought to be the result of bacterial enzymes and prostaglandins. *H. Influenzae* and *Streptococcus pneumoniae* are the most common primary pathogens, with *Staphylococcus aureus* being a frequent secondary pathogen following influenza. Primary influenza pneumonia also occurs and may be treated with amantadine and inhaled ribavirin. Varicella pneumonia is more severe in the pregnant population, with mortality rates reported from 11% to 35%. Pregnant women with varicella pneumonia should be hospitalized for aggressive management, including IV acyclovir.

Cystitis The most common pathogens encountered in uncomplicated lower urinary tract infections are *E. coli, K. pneumoniae, P. mirabilis,* and group B *streptococci*. Ampicillin, nitrofurantoin, or sulfamethoxazole may be used for a 7- to 10-day course. Sulfamethoxazole should not be used at or near term. Efficacy of shorter treatment protocols has not been proven.

TABLE 64-2 Drugs Use During Pregnancy

Antibiotics

Cephalosporins	May use throughout pregnancy.
Penicillins	May use throughout pregnancy.
Erythromycin	Estolate salt (Ilosone) contraindicated due to hepatotoxicity, otherwise may use throughout pregnancy.
Nitrofurantoin	May use throughout pregnancy.
Clindamycin	May use throughout pregnancy.
Azithromycin	May use throughout pregnancy.
Gentamicin	No reports of fetal toxicity, but other drugs of this class are contraindicated.
Kanamycin	Contraindicated
Streptomycin	Contraindicated
Metronidazole	Use in pregnancy is controversial.
Sulfonamides	May be used in pregnancy except near-term, because of potential harm to newborn.
Trimethoprim/ sulfamethoxazole	Contraindicated
Tetracyclines	Contraindicated because of damage to developing teeth and bones.
Quinolones	Contraindicated due to abnormality in cartilage formation.
INH	May be used throughout pregnancy.
PAS	May be used throughout pregnancy.
Ethambutol	May be used throughout pregnancy.

Antivirals

Acyclovir	May be used for life-threatening maternal illness.

Antihypertensive Agents

Alpha methyldopa	May be used throughout pregnancy.
ß-blockers	May be used throughout pregnancy.
Calcium channel blockers	May be used throughout pregnancy.
Prazosin	May be used throughout pregnancy.
Hydralazine	May be used throughout pregnancy.
Diuretics	Generally not recommended, but may be continued if patient has been on long-term diuretic therapy. Contraindicated in pre-eclampsia.
ACE inhibitors	Contraindicated
Ganglionic blockers	Contraindicated

Anticonvulsants

All	Congenital malformations have been reported with all anticonvulsants, however, seizures present higher risk, so use of anticonvulsants is indicated if needed. Use of folic acid supplementation (1 mg/day) may be beneficial in preventing teratogenesis.

Table continues

TABLE 64-2 Continued

Glucocorticoids

	May be used for control of serious maternal diseases such as asthma, lupus, and other serious dermatologic conditions.

Anticoagulants

Heparin	Drug of choice for pregnant women requiring anticoagulation.
Warfarin (Coumadin)	Contraindicated

Analgesics

Acetaminophen	May be used throughout pregnancy.
Propoxyphene	May be used, but caution advised when used close to term. Neonatal withdrawal may occur.
Opiates (codeine, morphine, meperidine)	May be used, but caution advised when used close to term. Neonatal withdrawal may occur.
NSAIDs	May be used for short duration (48–72 h) and not after 32 weeks gestation.

Antiemetics

Meclizine	May be used throughout pregnancy.
Dimenhydrinate (Dramamine)	May be used throughout pregnancy.
Diphenhydramine (Benadryl)	May be used throughout pregnancy.
Trimethobenzamide (Tigan)	May be used throughout pregnancy.
Phenothiazines (Phenergan, Compazine)	May be used throughout pregnancy.

OTC Cold Medications

Pseudoephedrine	Contraindicated
Phenylpropanolamine	May be used; topical nasal sprays are preferable.

Vaccines

Live vaccines (MMR, et al)	Should not be given during pregnancy
Inactivated viral vaccines (rabies, hepatitis B, flu)	May be given when indicated.
Pneumococcal vaccine	May be given when indicated.
Tetanus and Diphtheria	May be given when indicated.

Pyelonephritis Pyelonephritis in pregnancy necessitates admission. Urine cultures should be obtained routinely, and blood cultures are recommended since 10% of patients will be bacteremic. IV antibiotics should be instituted immediately. Cephalosporins are the first choice for treatment, with gentamicin added for signs of sepsis. Admission to labor and delivery is warranted to rule out preterm labor. The recurrence rate after treatment is 10% to 20%: suppression with a low dose antibiotic for the remainder of pregnancy is often recommended. Adult respiratory distress syndrome has been reported in pregnant patients with pyelonephritis, which necessitates aggressive management in an intensive care unit.

Asthma   Inhaled ß-agonists, inhaled glucocorticoids, and short courses of high-dose systemic steroids may be safely used in pregnant patients with asthma. Because of the increased susceptibility to pneumonia, chest x-ray should be considered. Patients should be assessed frequently for signs of maternal hypoxia, and oxygen should be administered to keep the maternal saturation above 95%. Arterial pCO_2 in pregnancy is normally 28 to 32, so a finding of normal pCO_2 of 40 represents significant CO_2 retention in the pregnant patient with asthma.

Thromboembolism   Thromboembolism is 5.5 times more frequent in pregnant and postpartum patients than in nonpregnant women. The clinical presentation of deep venous thrombosis includes calf or thigh pain, palpable cord, tenderness, swelling, positive Homan's sign, and dilated superficial veins. Doppler ultrasound is the diagnostic study of choice. Blood tests for fibrinopeptide A, fibrin degradation products, and D-dimer will rule out DVT if the tests are negative. Positive results may occur with hematomas or inflammatory exudates, as well as DVT. Admission and anticoagulation with heparin is the treatment of choice.

Pulmonary embolism is the primary cause of maternal mortality. The clinical presentation includes tachypnea, dyspnea, pleuritic pain, anxiety, cough, tachycardia, and low-grade fever. EKG, ABG, chest x-ray, and ventilation/perfusion scan should be obtained.

Acute abdominal pain in pregnancy   The differential diagnosis of acute abdominal pain in pregnancy includes ectopic pregnancy, preterm labor, placental abruption, chorioamnionitis, pre-eclampsia, degenerating leiomyomata, and adnexal torsion, in addition to the usual causes seen in nonpregnant women.

Appendicitis in pregnancy can be especially difficult to diagnose due to the displacement of the appendix from the usual McBurney's location and the natural leukocytosis that occurs in pregnancy. When other potential causes for pain are excluded and the findings for appendicitis are equivocal, the patient should be admitted to the hospital for serial examinations and leukocyte counts. The risk of premature birth or abortion following appendiceal rupture and peritonitis is greater than the risk of preterm labor following laparotomy, which can usually be controlled with tocolytic agents.

Cholecystitis, characterized by right upper-quadrant pain, nausea, vomiting, fever with leukocytosis, may be differentiated from HELLP syndrome by use of right upper-quadrant ultrasonography. The patient should be managed medically with IV hydration, antibiotics, analgesics, and NPO status. Recurrent episodes of cholecystitis are common. The ideal time for planned surgery is the second trimester, as there is a decreased chance of preterm birth, and the enlarged uterus has not yet displaced the liver.

For further reading in *Emergency Medicine, A Comprehensive Study Guide*, see Chapter 98, Problems in Pregnancy, by Wendy F. Hansen and Alfred R. Hansen.

65 | Blunt Abdominal Trauma During Pregnancy

Gary D. Wright

Trauma is a frequent cause of maternal death, the major causes of which are vehicular accidents, falls, and penetrating objects. Generally, there are few differences in the treatment of the pregnant trauma victim and the nonpregnant victim. Divergence of treatment in the pregnant patient can be accounted for by the major physiologic changes that occur during pregnancy.

Clinical Features

Maternal death is the leading cause of fetal death in trauma. Seatbelts in autobobiles protect the mother from death, thereby protecting the fetus. Two-point restraints increase the risk of abruptio placentae over that of the three-point restraint systems.

As with the nonpregnant trauma victim, pelvic fractures remain associated with life-threatening intra-abdominal retroperitoneal hemorrhage. Bleeding may exceed 4 l and may be manifested as refractory hypovolemic shock. Recent pelvic fracture does not necessarily preclude vaginal delivery.

The gravid uterus has been shown to be protective to intra-abdominal organs. Most commonly, hemorrhage will be retroperitoneal, however, spleen, kidney, and liver remain the most commonly injured organs.

The uterus is protected until the 12th week by the bony pelvis, at which time it becomes an abdominal organ. Uterine rupture accounts for <1% of traumatic injuries to the pregnant patient. The uterus is a highly resilient organ and can withstand pressures up to 10 times that of normal labor. Rapid deceleration injuries are the cause of uterine rupture.

Abruptio placentae represents a major cause of fetal loss from trauma. This condition is manifested by vaginal bleeding (78%), abdominal pain (66%), uterine irritability (17%), tetanic uterine contractions (17%), and fetal death (15%). Abruptio placentae is involved in 1% to 5% of minor trauma and 20% to 50% of major trauma. Abruptio placentae has been associated with subsequent deseminated intravascular coagulopathy (DIC).

Fetomaternal hemorrhage (FMH) is of significant concern in the Rh-negative pregnant trauma victim. FMH occurs in 8% to 30% of traumatized pregnant patients. This condition is caused by breakdown of the fetomaternal barrier, with exposure of the maternal circulation to fetal blood.

Diagnosis and Emergency Department Care

Maternal stabilization is the primary concern in the pregnant trauma victim, since maternal shock is associated with up to 80% fetal mortality.

1. Rapid resuscitation and stabilization should proceed as with the non-pregnant patient, with the following exceptions: (1) positioning the uterus to the left; and (2) aggressive fluid resuscitation (often up to 50% more than the nonpregnant patient).
2. Obstetric physical examination must be included in the secondary survey. Uterine tenderness, contractions, or vaginal bleeding may be indicative of abruptio placentae. Determination of fundal height with implied fetal age should be accomplished early to determine fetal viability. Pelvic examination should be performed early to determine cervical competence and presence of amniotic fluid (nitrazine-blue).
3. Radiographic evaluation, including CT scanning, should be performed as necessary. Diagnostic peritoneal lavage may also be performed, using a supra-umbilical approach. Standard trauma lab testing, with particular attention to clotting studies and Kleihauer–Betke assay (in the Rh-negative patient), is indicated.
4. In the Rh-negative patient, administration of RhoGAM is indicated in the presence of FMH. Standard dose RhoGAM (300 μg) may be inadequate in massive hemorrhage.

The use of vasopressors may lead to restriction of uterine blood flow, and should be used with caution. High levels of oxygen should be administered as in the nonpregnant patient.

Disposition After appropriate ED evaluation and stabilization are complete, all pregnant women >20 wks gestation with evidence of direct or indirect abdominal trauma, 4 hours of cardiotocographic monitoring is indicated. The liberal use of obstetrical consultation is recommended *after* initial evaluation and stabilization are completed.

If Standard Treatment Fails

In the absence of maternal response to vigorous resuscitation, emergency cesarean section should be considered. Successful postmortem cesarean section has been well described. Rapid laparotomy with a vertical uterine incision should be used to extract the fetus. The most important factors associated in predicting fetal outcome are: (1) fetal age >28 weeks; (2) interval between maternal death and delivery; (3) absence of prolonged hypoxia, and (4) quality of maternal resuscitation.

For further reading in *Emergency Medicine, A Comprehensive Study Guide*, see Chapter 99, Blunt Abdominal Trauma During Pregnancy, by Mark D. Pearlman.

David M. Cline

PREPARATION FOR EMERGENCY DELIVERY

Any pregnant woman arriving in ED who is beyond 20 weeks' gestation and appears to be actively contracting should be rapidly evaluated with a bimanual pelvic examination to assess cervical dilatation. Maternal vital signs and fetal heart rate also should be checked. The gravida with active vaginal bleeding, however, should be evaluated with ultrasound to rule out placenta previa before pelvic exam is attempted. Also, if there is suspicion of ruptured membranes, the patient should be evaluated with sterile speculum and with Nitrazine paper and ferning tests to confirm ruptured membranes unless delivery appears imminent. The speculum exam will show the cervix to estimate dilatation.

If the cervix is 6 cm or more dilated in a woman experiencing active contractions, further transport, even short distances, may be hazardous. Preparations should be made for emergency delivery. An intravenous line should be established with lactated Ringer's solution, if there is time before delivery, to be prepared for the administration of medications, fluids, or blood products immediately postpartum, if this becomes necessary. Minimal blood testing should include hemoglobin or hematocrit measurement (or a complete blood-cell count), hepatitis-B surface antigen (HBsAG), blood typing (if unknown), and a clotted tube of blood should be made available for emergency crossmatching, if necessary. If possible, urine should be tested for protein and glucose.

Emergency Delivery Procedure

As the baby's head descends, imminent delivery can be anticipated by bulging of the perineum and the appearance of the fetal scalp at the introitus. At this point, no attempt should be made to delay delivery, but a controlled delivery is important in preventing both fetal and maternal injury.

1. If the dorsal lithotomy position is chosen, the mother should be tilted slightly to one side to lessen vena caval compression and should be brought to the edge of the bed or stretcher, or the buttocks raised on pillows, to allow room for delivery of the baby's head and shoulders. The mother's legs should be widely separated and supported with her knees flexed.
2. With each contraction the vaginal outlet bulges to accommodate a greater portion of the fetal head; this process may be aided by gentle digital stretching of the perineum. Episiotomy may be performed at this time if necessary to allow delivery without spontaneous lacerations. A local anesthetic should be injected just prior to episiotomy with 5 to 10 mL of 1% lidocaine in a syringe with

a small-gauge needle. A midline perineal incision should be made, taking care not to extend into the rectum.

3. As the head emerges, the palm of one hand should be placed over the head to assist with the normal extension of the head and at the same time prevent the head from suddenly popping out of the vagina. At this point the mother is asked not to push in order to minimize the trauma associated with uncontrolled expulsive efforts. The best method to inhibit the overwhelmingly strong desire to bear down when the fetal head is distending the perineum is generally reassurance and asking the mother to pant or breathe through her nose.

4. With expulsive efforts under control, and one hand on the infant's crowning head, the second hand, draped with a sterile cloth, can be used to gently lift the infant's chin posterior to the maternal anus. This facilitates further extension and a slow, controlled emergence of the baby's head (modified Ritgen's maneuver; Fig. 66-1). As the head is delivered, usually with the face down, it tends to restitute to one or the other lateral positions.

5. The baby's neck region should be palpated immediately after delivery of the head to check for a nuchal cord, which may be found about 25% of the time. If the cord is relatively loose, it can be

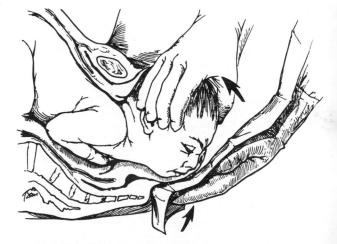

FIG. 66-1. Modified Ritgen maneuver. Palm of hand on infant's head while second hand, draped with sterile cloth, gently lifts the infant's chin. (From Cunningham et al. William's Obstetrics, Norwalk CT, Appleton and Lange, 1993, p. 382. Used by permission.)

slipped out of the way over the baby's head. If the cord is tight, two clamps should be placed close together on the most accessible portion of the cord (usually anteriorly) and the cord cut in between. The cord can then be unwound if there are multiple loops.

6. Before the delivery of the shoulders and thorax is continued, the baby's face should be wiped off and the mouth and nose aspirated with a soft rubber bulb syringe to clear the airway. This is especially important to prevent meconium aspiration if there has been meconium staining of the amniotic fluid. If no bulb syringe is available, the mouth should be scooped out with the finger as well as possible. Squeezing the nose between the fingers and stroking the upper neck from the larynx toward the mandible may also be helpful.

7. Attention should now be turned to delivery of the shoulders. This can be facilitated by placing a hand on either side of the baby's head; a gentle downward traction will ease the anterior shoulder under the pubic symphysis (Fig. 66-2). Care should be taken not to use undue force, as this may result in brachial plexus injury. If there is resistance, an assistant should be asked to use suprapubic pressure (not fundal pressure) to avoid impaction of the shoulder behind the symphysis.

8. When the anterior shoulder is visible, gentle upward traction will deliver the posterior shoulder. The posterior shoulder should not pop out uncontrolled, as this may result in a laceration of the anal sphincter, into the rectum (third-degree perineal laceration).

9. The baby will be very slippery, especially if there is thick vernix (white, cheesy, desquamated skin). The posterior hand should slide down onto the posterior shoulder as it is delivered and then behind the back of the neck to support the baby's head. The anterior hand should then be brought along the baby's back as the body delivers spontaneously. Placing the index finger between the lower legs, and the third finger and thumb around each leg, ensures a safe grip.

10. If the baby is breathing spontaneously and is close to term, there is no need to rush cutting the cord. The baby can be dried off, wrapped in a warm blanket, and placed on the mother's abdomen to help minimize heat loss.

11. The cord should be doubly clamped before cutting with a sterile scissors. If sterile scissors are unavailable, it is better to leave the cord uncut until sterile instruments can be found. (See Chap 3 for details of neonatal resuscitation.)

Management of Shoulder Dystocia

The first step in dealing with shoulder dystocia is to position the mother for maximum room and maneuverability. The maternal perineum should be at the end of the examining table and the maternal legs should not be in stirrups but sharply flexed toward the abdomen in the McRoberts

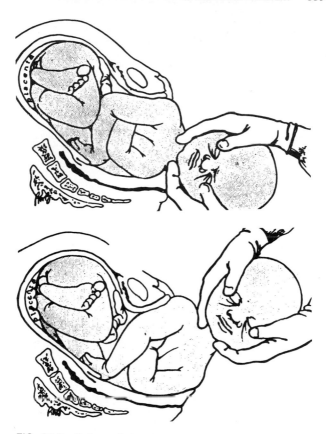

FIG. 66-2. Delivery of shoulders. **Top:** Gentle downward traction to ease anterior shoulder under pubic symphysis. **Bottom:** Delivery of anterior shoulder completed; gentle upward traction to deliver posterior shoulder. (From Cunningham et al. William's Obstetrics, Norwalk CT, Appleton and Lange, 1993, p. 384. Used by permission.)

maneuver. A generous episiotomy, extending through the anal sphincter if necessary, should be cut, preferably with adequate local anesthesia. At this time suprapubic, not fundal, pressure should be applied by an assistant. Shoulder dystocia is likely to be further aggravated by fundal pressure, but suprapubic pressure can help dislodge the anterior shoulder impacted behind the pubic symphysis. If these measures fail, manual rotation of one or both shoulders toward the anterior surface of the fetal chest should be attempted to try to produce a smaller shoulder-to-shoulder diameter and displace the anterior shoulder from behind the pubic symphysis. A variation of this, the Woods corkscrew maneuver, consists of progressively rotating the posterior shoulder 180° in a corkscrew fashion, resulting in the release of the impacted anterior shoulder. Of course, any maneuvering in the birth canal may be difficult with a large, macrosomic infant filling it. At the same time, suprapubic pressure may be applied, but at a 45° lateral angle in the direction of the attempted rotation of the anterior shoulder.

Management Immediately Postpartum

The placenta should be allowed to separate spontaneously, unless there is considerable active bleeding. Pulling on the cord risks cord rupture or the possible catastrophe of inversion of the uterus. The usual signs of placental separation are a gush of blood and lengthening of the cord. As the placenta is expelled, the membranes may be teased out by rotating the placenta and twisting the membranes.

After the placenta is out, the uterus should be massaged to help it to contract and remain firm. Oxytocin, 10 units, may be given slowly intravenously (or mixed in the intravenous bag), or by intramuscular injection if no intravenous line is available, to help maintain uterine contraction. Uterine atony often results after precipitous labor (total labor less than 3 h). Excessive bleeding calls for vigorous uterine massage, increased amount of intravenous crystalloid solutions, and additional oxytocin or methylergonovine (Methergine) (Table 66-1). Bleeding sites for lacerations should also be identified and controlled with clamps or direct pressure. Episiotomy or laceration repair should await the availability of an experienced practitioner or obstetrician.

TABLE 66-1. Medications for Emergency Delivery

Oxytocin, 10 units/mL	Epinephrine, 1:1000
Methylergonovine (Methergine), 0.2 mg/mL	Diazepam, 10 mg
	Lidocaine (Xylocaine), 1%
Magnesium sulfate, 50% (5 g/10 mL)	Sodium bicarbonate, 50 mEq
	Prochlorperazine (Compazine), 10 mg/2 mL
Magnesium sulfate, 10% (2 g/20 mL)	Diphenhydramine (Benadryl) 50 mg/mL
Calcium gluconate, 10 mL	Naloxone (Narcan), 0.4 mg/mL
Hydralazine, 20 mg/mL	Dimenhydrinate (Dramamine), 50 mg
Ephedrine sulfate, 0.05	
Sodium amytal, 250 mg	
Terbutaline sulfate, 1 mg/mL	Sterile water for injection

For further reading in *Emergency Medicine, A Comprehensive Study Guide*, see Chapter 100, Emergency Delivery, by Paul T. von Oeyen.

Common Complications
of Gynecologic Procedures

David M. Cline

With the advent of same-day surgery and the increasing necessity to discharge patients within 3 days of a major procedure, postsurgical gynecologic patients are presenting to EDs with increasing frequency. (Complications common to gynecologic and general surgery are covered in Chap. 56.)

COMMON COMPLICATIONS OF ENDOSCOPIC PROCEDURES

Laparoscopy

The major complications associated with the use of the laparoscope are (1) thermal injuries to the bowel; (2) bleeding at the site of tubal interruption or sharp dissection; and (3) rarely, ureteral or bladder injury, large bowel injury, and pelvic hematoma or abscess. Of these complications, the most serious and dreaded is that of thermal injury to the bowel. These patients generally appear 3 to 7 days postoperatively, depending upon the degree of necrosis, with signs and symptoms of peritonitis, including bilateral lower abdominal pain, fever, elevated white cell count, and direct and rebound tenderness. X-rays may show an ileus or free air under the diaphragm. Although gas has been used to insufflate the abdomen, it should be absorbed totally within 3 postoperative days. Patients who have increasing pain after laparoscopy, either early or late, have a bowel injury until proved otherwise. If thermal injury is a serious consideration and cannot be distinguished from other causes of peritonitis, it is best to err on the side of early laparotomy.

Hysteroscopy

Complications of hysteroscopy fortunately are rare but include: (1) reaction to the distending media, (2) uterine perforation, (3) cervical laceration, (4) anesthesia reaction, (5) intra-abdominal organ injury, (6) infection, and (7) postoperative bleeding. Postoperative bleeding will be the most likely cause of hospital revisit. After hemodynamic stabilization of the patient, an intrauterine tampon, such as a pediatric Foley, generally can control this problem. Infection as a result of the hysteroscopic procedure is uncommon. Treatment should be commensurate with presentation and symptoms. Uterine perforations are mentioned only because they are relatively common complications associated with the procedure but seldom require more than observation.

MISCELLANEOUS COMPLICATIONS OF MAJOR GYNECOLOGIC PROCEDURES

Cuff Cellulitis

Clinical Features

Cuff cellulitis refers to infections of the contiguous retroperitoneal space immediately above the vaginal apex and including the surrounding soft tissue. It is a common complication following both abdominal and vaginal hysterectomy. It usually produces a fever between postoperative days 3 to 5. These women present with a complaint of fever and lower quadrant pain. Pelvic tenderness and induration are prominent during the bimanual examination. A vaginal cuff abscess may be palpable.

Emergency Department Care

The treatment of choice is readmission, drainage, and intravenous antibiotics as determined by the gynecologist.

Postconization Bleeding

Clinical Features

The most common complication associated with these procedures is bleeding. If delayed hemorrhage occurs, it usually occurs 7 days postoperatively. Bleeding following this procedure can be rapid and excessive.

Emergency Department Care

Visualization of the cervix is the key to controlling such bleeding. Application of Monsel's solution is a reasonable first step if it is easily available. Usually, however, suturing of the bleeding arteriole is necessary. Quite often, the patient must be taken to the operating room for repair secondary to poor visualization.

Induced Abortion

Clinical Features

Retained products of conception and a resulting endometritis are the most common complications. The patient will usually present 3 to 5 days posttermination with complaints of excessive bleeding, fever, and abdominal pain. She may not present for up to 2 wks. Pelvic examination reveals a subinvoluted tender uterus with foul-smelling blood vaginally. An elevated WBC count is common.

Emergency Department Care

Treatment must include evacuation of intrauterine contents and intravenous antibiotic therapy. Triple antibiotic therapy is the standard, however, there is increasing evidence that ampicillin with sulbactam (Unasyn) is equally effective. If the patient has pain, bleeding, or both—but unaccompanied by fever—ectopic pregnancy must be ruled out. The presence of villi on the pathology report (if available) confirms the presence of an intrauterine gestation but cannot rule out the rare occurrences of ectopic and intrauterine gestations.

For further reading in *Emergency Medicine, A Comprehensive Study Guide,* see Chapter 101, Common Complications of Gynecologic Procedures, by Veronica T. Mallett.

Assessment of the Child in the Emergency Department: A Practical Approach to Normal Child Development

Debra G. Perina

Recognition of the critically ill child is one of the most challenging aspects of emergency medicine practice. Significant illness in children is frequently indicated by altered mental status, which can only be detected if normal is known by the examiner. The key to recognizing the ill child is applying a thorough working knowledge of child development to the child's behavior in the ED.

Clinical Features

A few assessment principles are applicable to children of all ages. These are observation, communication with the child, communication with the caregivers, and obtaining vital signs. Observing the child's behavior from a distance can be revealing. A child's baseline behavior, however, can be affected by fever or hunger. Thus antipyretic therapy or feeding may be crucial to achieving optimal observation.

Next, begin by communicating with the child, as the first impression sets the tone for the whole encounter. Look at the child at eye level and be honest regarding what the child can expect. This establishes trust. Whenever possible, isolate the child from the sights and sounds of other patient-care experiences, as they can heighten the child's anxiety. Nonemergent, uncomfortable parts of the exam should be performed last. Assess the child with his family, trying not to separate the child, whenever possible. Address caregiver concerns, as children of all ages watch their parents for cues of how to respond to the medical staff. Parents are intimately familiar with their child's behavior, and their concerns that the child is not behaving normally should be heeded. When evaluating vital signs of children, remember that anxiety, pain, fever, and crying will increase all values. Also remember that weight is a pediatric vital sign. Weight estimates are frequently inaccurate for resuscitation purposes, and length-based resources such as the Broselow tapes are recommended.

Diagnosis and Differential

Diagnosis and differential can only be accomplished by being familiar with age-specific growth and developmental stages. Developmental stages are generally described for associated age ranges, but individual variations abound. Two developmental aspects of each age that are particularly important when assessing the child in the ED are physical aspects (growth and physiological parameters) and neurological aspects (motor, language, and social milestones). An awareness of these developmental stages is very important as it impacts patient assessment and therapeutic response. Growth and developmental stages are discussed below, with emphasis on physical, neurologic, and age-specific aspects.

Growth and Developmental Stages

Early infancy (0 to 6 mo)—physical aspects: Young infants have high surface-to-body mass ratio with a proportionally large head, resulting in a high rate of heat loss and hypothermia. Young infants are obligate nose breathers, and normal neonates exhibit periodic breathing. A heart rate greater than 180 or less than 60 should be considered abnormal. Due to excellent compensatory mechanisms, hypotension is a late finding. The pulmonary vascular bed dilates over the first 6 months, so congenital heart lesions may present around this age.

Neurologic aspects—Primitive reflexes, such as suck, grasp, and Moro, should be present and always symmetrical. Infants can lift their heads, follow objects, and smile by 1 mo. Head control is steady, and the child can roll over and can reach and grasp objects by 4 mo. Young infants have few motor abilities, so there is limited potential for self-inflicted accidental injury. Child abuse must be considered whenever the observed injury is developmentally inconsistent with the stated mechanism. *Age-specific approach*: Assessment begins with observation and direct interaction with the infant by smiling and using a pleasant tone of voice. Observation of muscle tone, spontaneous activity, eye contact, responsive smile, and recognition of parents is most important.

Late infancy (6 to 18 mo)—physical aspects: The normal infant triples his birth weight by 1 year. The primary teeth erupt, and the anterior fontanel closes by 18 mo. *Neurological aspects*: The child is normally able to lift his head, transfer objects from hand to hand, smile, babble, and coo by 6 mo. Stranger anxiety begins between 9 and 12 mo, along with fear of separation from parents. Failure of the older child to recognize and respond to parents suggests significant illness. *Age-specific approach:* Begin with observation while the child is in the parent's arms. Undress the child to assess respiratory effort while breathing. Approach the child gradually and engage the caregivers first to gain the child's confidence. A caregiver should remain with the child to provide reassurance during the exam.

Toddler (18–36 mo)—physical aspects: Decreasing growth rate and decreased appetite are seen. The primary teeth are present and dental caries may be seen. A high center of gravity and curiosity leads to an increased risk of orthopedic and head injuries. The toddler's open growth plates are more likely to sustain epiphyseal fractures than ligamentous injury. If there is tenderness over the growth plate following an injury, a splint should always be placed even if x-rays are negative. Traction injuries to the elbow (i.e., nursemaid's elbow) are common.

Neurologic aspects—The child becomes very mobile, running, climbing, and walking. Parents often underestimate the child's capabilities, and this age has a peak risk for falls and ingestions. Toddlers can feed themselves, follow simple commands, and speak in four- to six-word sentences. Stranger anxiety is at its peak. *Age-specific approach*: The best approach is indirect observation, followed by direct interaction with the child as he is held in his parents' arms. Older toddlers may indicate the site of pain, but many are unable to localize pain or tenderness. Talk to the child in simple language and offer to let him touch or hold examination instruments to gain his trust. The examiner should ask the parents to have the toddler walk and follow commands as an important part of the assessment.

Preschool age (3 to 5 y)—Expressive language skills develop, and children this age can identify the site of complaint. They develop progressive autonomy, mobility, and self-care. Fear of pain and anxiety remain high. Preschoolers live in the present and thus forget prior symptoms. *Age-specific approach*: Directly approach the child and always talk to the preschooler to establish rapport and confirm the complaint. Generally they may be examined in the traditional systemic fashion. Often cooperation can be elicited with explanations. Restraint may be necessary for painful procedures, and rewards should be provided afterward.

School age (5 to 12 y)—physical aspects: Rapid language growth and maturing motor skills are seen. This is the slowest period of growth in childhood. Secondary teeth erupt. *Neurologic aspects*: The child is aware of his body and develops a sense of modesty. Task-oriented behavior and concrete thinking develop. Children are eager to please and often reluctant to discuss their fears. *Age-specific approach*: The direct examination approach is preferred. Historical information should be got from both the child and the parent. A change in school performance is an indicator of chronic disease. Painful procedures are best explained to the child and parent, and the child should be given some degree of choice in how the procedure is to be accomplished to minimize the sense of loss of control.

Adolescence (12 to 17 y)—physical aspects: Secondary sexual development begins. Sexual activity and drug use are common. Alcohol abuse is particularly a problem. *Neurologic aspects*: Abstract reasoning develops paired with a self-centered world view and self-consciousness concerning appearance. Feelings of immortality and risky behavior are common. Loss of autonomy is the adolescent's greatest fear. Psychiatric and suicidal behavior increases. *Age-specific approach*: The examiner should approach the adolescent as an adult. Choices should be allowed, with limit-setting regarding cooperative behavior. The parent's concerns must be individually addressed, possibly in private. Confidentiality should be stressed, particularly with respect to pregnancy and STD.

Again, familiarity with the normal growth and developmental milestones presented above is important to assessment and recognition of the critically ill child in the ED. The abnormal can only be detected if the normal is known.

For further reading in *Emergency Medicine, A Comprehensive Study Guide*, see Chapter 102, Assessment of the Child in the Emergency Department: A Practical Approach to Normal Child Development, by Peter Mellis.

David M. Cline

NORMAL VEGETATIVE FUNCTIONS

Most bottle-fed infants will want 6 to 9 feedings per 24 h by the first week of life, whereas breastfed infants may require feeding every 2 to 4 h. Intake is satisfactory if infants are no longer losing weight by 5 to 7 days and gaining 10 to 30 g/kg per day by 12 to 14 days of age. Stool frequency may vary from 1 to 7 times per day, with loose stools frequent in breastfed infants. Breastfed infants may occasionally go 5 to 7 days without a bowel movement. Stool color is of no significance unless blood is present.

CRYING, IRRITABILITY, LETHARGY

Infants who present with an episode of acute inconsolable crying should be observed closely for an underlying cause (Table 69-1).

TABLE 69-1. Conditions Associated with Uncontrollable Crying or Irritability or Lethargy in Neonates

Intestinal colic
Traumatic conditions
Battered child syndrome (fractures, burns, etc.)
Falls (skull or extremity fractures)
Open diaper pin
Strangulation of digit or penis
Corneal abrasion or foreign body
Infections
Meningitis
Generalized sepsis
Otitis media
Urinary tract infection
Gastroenteritis
Surgical
Incarcerated hernia (umbilical or inguinal)
Testicular torsion
Anal fissure
Improper feeding practices

Intestinal Colic

The most common cause of crying is intestinal colic. This usually occurs in normal, healthy, thriving babies in the second or third week of life and persists until 3 mo of age. Episodes commonly occur in the late afternoon or evening and begin with screaming episodes with drawing up of knees, as if the infant is in pain, and usually passage of flatus.

Diagnosis is usually made when there is no evidence of physical illness and if the bouts of crying are episodic in nature. A careful history, physical examination, and appropriate laboratory investigations will enable the emergency physician to diagnose colic and exclude the serious conditions listed in Table 69-1.

Emergency Department Care

1. Suggest changes in caretaking styles, such as increased carrying and rocking, decreased interfeed intervals, and use of pacifier.
2. Suggest changes in environment (e.g., background music, rides in car and stroller).
3. Suggest a trial of feeding change in refractory cases. Changes in feeds are helpful if the infant has other manifestations, such as visible peristalsis, persistent regurgitation, and symptoms following cow's milk protein. Removal of cow's milk from the diet of the mother of a breastfed baby may be tried. A switch to formula or change of formula is not indicated.

ABUSE AND TRAUMA

An inconsistent or implausible history may lead the physician to suspect a diagnosis of child abuse, and physical examination may reveal unexplained injuries (bruises at varying stages, skull fractures, extremity fractures, cigarette burns, etc.). If a diagnosis of abuse suspected, the child should be admitted for protection and further investigations. An examination of the eye, though difficult, is essential since the presence of retinal hemorrhage, especially in the absence of external signs of trauma, suggest whiplash injury due to severe shaking. Examination of the eye is also useful to rule out an eyelash in the eye or a corneal abrasion as reasons for the infant's symptoms.

INFECTIONS

Infections in the neonate manifest as a variety of symptoms and signs, such as feeding difficulties, fever, jaundice, or respiratory distress. A septic neonate may present with a normal or subnormal temperature rather than fever. Urinary tract infections in neonates are often associated with nonspecific signs, such as irritability, diarrhea, or poor feeding, and diagnosis is established by urine culture rather than urinalysis. All neonates with possible sepsis should be hospitalized and started on broad-spectrum antibiotic therapy pending results of appropriate cultures (urine, blood, cerebrospinal fluid, etc.).

Surgical Lesions

The most common signs are irritability and crying, followed by poor feeding, vomiting, constipation, and abdominal distension. Physical examination may reveal a red, edematous, tender lump at the site of the hernia or testicular torsion. Anal fissures may also present at this age and may be difficult to diagnose.

IMPROPER FEEDING PRACTICES

Improper feeding practices may result in an irritable infant with periods of inconsolable crying. This usually results from overfeeding, with inadequate burping during feeds.

GASTROINTESTINAL (GI) TRACT SYMPTOMS

Feeding Difficulties

Most visits for feeding difficulties are due to parental perception that the infant's food intake is inadequate. If weight gain is satisfactory and the infant is satisfied after feeds, intake is adequate. Rarely, anatomic abnormalities can cause difficulty in feeding and swallowing. A careful history usually pinpoints these difficulties as occurring from birth. These infants appear malnourished and dehydrated. Infants with a recent decrease in intake, who were feeding normally previously, have an acute disease, usually an infection.

Regurgitation

Regurgitation of small amounts is common in the neonate and is due to reduced lower-esophageal sphincter pressure and relatively increased intragastric pressure. Parents may confuse regurgitation with vomiting. Vomiting results from forceful contraction of the diaphragm and abdominal muscles, whereas regurgitation is independent of any effort and probably represents the ultimate degree of gastrointestinal reflux. If the neonate is thriving, parents can be reassured that regurgitation is of no clinical significance and will decrease as the infant grows. Infants who are not thriving or having respiratory symptoms should be investigated for anatomical causes of regurgitation or chronic aspiration.

Vomiting

Acute vomiting may be part of the symptom complex of some diseases (Table 69-1), especially increased intracranial pressure, and infections (sepsis, urinary tract infections, gastroenteritis).

Projectile vomiting is usually seen in infants with pyloric stenosis and usually assumes its characteristic pattern after the second and third week of life. This condition usually occurs in firstborn males and is characterized by projectile vomiting at the end of feeding or shortly thereafter. The vomitus does not contain bile or blood. Examination of these infants should be done with the infant relaxed and the stomach empty. Prominent gastric waves may be seen going from left to right as well as a firm olive mass felt by palpating up and down under the liver edge. Malnutrition and dehydration may be evident. Hospitalization is necessary for rehydration and surgical referral.

In any infant who is vomiting, signs of dehydration and candidiasis of the mouth should be sought. Signs and symptoms of hepatobiliary disease (e.g., jaundice), urinary tract, and central nervous system disease should be sought. Vomiting may also be due to inborn errors of metabolism and may present with nonspecific signs, as well as metabolic abnormalities such as hypoglycemia and metabolic acidosis. Infants who are vomiting should be admitted for evaluation and therapy.

Diarrhea

Diarrhea is associated with the excessive loss of fluid and electrolytes in stools. Where the infant is feeling well and gaining weight appropriately, the only treatment necessary is to reassure parents that all is well. Infectious diarrhea is usually associated with fever and is mostly of viral etiology, with rota and enteroviruses being most common. Bacterial and parasitic causes (*Giardia, Entamoeba histolytica*) are rare in neonates. Causes of bloody diarrhea in the neonate include necrotizing enterocolitis, bacterial enteritis, antibiotic-associated diarrhea, milk allergy and, rarely, intussusception. Infants who are moderately or severely dehydrated should be admitted for treatment.

Necrotizing enterocolitis usually presents with other signs of sepsis (jaundice, lethargy, fever, poor feeding, abdominal distension, and discoloration). Abdominal radiography may demonstrate pneumatosis intestinalis. True milk allergy presents with abdominal distension, explosive bloody diarrhea and, in severe cases, shock.

ABDOMINAL DISTENSION

Abdominal distension is normal in the neonate and is usually due to lax abdominal musculature and relatively large intra-abdominal organs. In the majority of cases, if the infant is comfortable and feeding well and the abdomen is soft, there is no need for concern.

CONSTIPATION

Infrequent bowel movements in neonates do not necessarily mean that the infant is constipated. The breastfed infant may on occasion go without a bowel movement for 5 to 7 days and then pass a normal stool. If the infant has never passed stools, however, the possibility of intestinal stenosis or atresia, Hirschsprung's disease, and meconium ileus or plug should be considered. Constipation occurring after birth but within the first month of life suggests Hirschsprung's disease, hypothyroidism, or anal stenosis.

TABLE 69-2. Causes of Rapid Breathing in the Neonate

Pneumonia
  Bacterial
  Viral
  Chlamydia
  Aspiration
Bronchiolitis
Illness to other organ systems
  Septicemia
  Central nervous system (e.g., meningitis)
  Abdomen (e.g., distension, gastroenteritis)
  Metabolic acidosis
Congenital diseases
  Respiratory disease
    Delayed presentation of diaphragmatic hernia
    Tracheoesophageal fistula
    Lobar emphysema
    Tracheal stenosis, webs
  Heart disease
    Cardiac failure (e.g., hypoplastic left heart, critical coarctation of
    aorta, aortic stenosis, patent ductus arteriosus)
    Cyanotic disease (e.g., transposition of great arteries)
    Vascular ring
  Neuromuscular disease
    Infantile botulism
    Muscle weakness

CARDIORESPIRATORY SYMPTOMS

Cardiorespiratory symptoms in neonates are nonspecific and may be due to primary organ failure (cardiovascular or respiratory) and secondary to a variety of systemic diseases, such as sepsis and metabolic acidosis, abdominal pathology, and severe meningitis. Regardless of etiology, the concern is, first, the assessment and stabilization of airway, breathing and circulation; and second, establishing the diagnosis. (Causes of rapid breathing are listed in Table 69-2; pneumonia is discussed in Chap. 72; bronchiolitis is discussed in Chap. 76.)

CONGENITAL DISEASES

Occasionally, H-type tracheoesophageal fistula may present in the first month of life or later with recurrent pneumonia, respiratory distress after feeds, and problems handling mucus.

Rapid breathing due to cardiac disease is usually not associated with significant retractions and use of accessory muscles. As a general rule, the well-developed neonate who presents with unexplained cyanosis and tachypnea should be suspected of having congenital cardiac disease.

COUGH AND NASAL CONGESTION

Cough may be a prominent feature of most of the primary respiratory conditions listed in Table 69-2. Treatment of the underlying condition is the therapy of choice. Cough suppressants should be used with extreme caution in neonates. Nasal congestion is best treated with instillation of saline drops when necessary.

NOISY BREATHING AND STRIDOR

Noisy breathing is a common presenting complaint in the neonate and is usually benign. Stridor is usually due to congenital anomalies (webs, cysts, atresia, stenosis, clefts, hemangiomas) extending anywhere from the nose to the trachea and bronchi. Infants who were intubated in the neonatal period are prone to develop subglottic stenosis. Infection (croup, epiglottitis, abscess) as a cause of stridor in the neonate is rare.

APNEA AND PERIODIC BREATHING

Periodic breathing, which may occur in normal neonates, should be differentiated from apnea. Apnea is defined as a cessation of respiration for 10 to 20 s with or without bradycardia and cyanosis. Apnea may be precipitated by any of the disease conditions listed in Table 69-2 and usually indicates respiratory muscle fatigue and impending respiratory arrest.

CYANOSIS AND BLUE SPELLS

If breathing is rapid but not labored, the most likely cause is cyanotic congenital heart disease with right-to-left shunting. If breathing is labored (grunting, indrawing), pulmonary disease (pneumonia, bronchiolitis) is likely. Infants with cyanosis should be admitted for monitoring and further investigation.

JAUNDICE

The most common causes of jaundice seen in the ED are physiologic (seen at 2–3 days of age), secondary to sepsis, breast-milk jaundice and, occasionally, hemolysis due to autoimmune congenital causes.

A proper history and physical examination will provide clues to the causes of jaundice. The well-looking child who is gaining weight and feeding well is unlikely to be septic. Laboratory evaluation should include full blood count for anemia, smear for hemolysis, direct and total bilirubin, a reticulocyte count, and Coombs' test. In addition, admission, appropriate cultures, and antibiotics are appropriate for neonates who are unwell and have any of the signs and symptoms listed in Table 69-3. In all cases, arrangements should be made for monitoring of bilirubin and hemoglobin levels. Although most well infants can be

TABLE 69-3. Signs and Symptoms of Neonatal Sepsis

Temperature	Fever, hypothermia
CNS dysfunction	Lethargy, irritability, seizures
Respiratory distress	Apnea, tachypnea, grunting
Feeding disturbance	Vomiting, poor feeding, gastric distension, diarrhea
Jaundice	
Rashes	

monitored out of hospital, infants who are anemic or those with bilirubin levels approaching transfusion levels (approximately 20 mg/dL) should be admitted.

DIAPER RASH AND ORAL THRUSH

Candida diaper dermatitis is an erythematous plaque with a scalloped border, sharply demarcated edge, and studded by satellite lesions. An oral course of treatment is usually warranted to prevent colonization of the gut.

Oral lesions are white, flaky plaques covering the tongue, lips, gingiva, and mucous membranes. Treatment of ill infants consists of treating the underlying pathology, oral antifungal therapy, and an anesthetic gel prior to feeding.

FEVER AND SEPSIS

Fever (Table 69-3) is most commonly due to infectious causes. Most infections occurring in the first 5 days of life are acquired by vertical transmission from the mother. Bacterial infections are usually caused by group B streptococci (30%), *E. coli* (30%–40%), other gram-negative enteric organisms (15%–20%), and gram-positive cocci (10%). Neonates with presumed sepsis should be admitted and started on broad-spectrum antibiotics after a full sepsis workup.

SUDDEN INFANT DEATH

Although sudden infant death syndrome should be considered, catastrophic deterioration is most likely due to infectious causes (septicemia, meningitis), trauma (intracranial bleed, child abuse), and inborn errors of metabolism (medium-chain acyldehydrogenase deficiency).

When the cause of death is not known, physicians should obtain appropriate samples (blood, urine, skin biopsy, etc.) and obtain permission for an autopsy.

For further reading in *Emergency Medicine, A Comprehensive Study Guide*, see Chapter 103, Common Neonatal Problems, by Niranjan Kissoon.

Heart Disease

David M. Cline

There are six common clinical presentations of pediatric heart disease: cyanosis, congestive heart failure, pathologic murmur in an asymptomatic patient, abnormal pulses, hypertension, and syncope. Table 70-1 lists the most common lesions in each category. Evaluation of a murmur is an elective diagnostic workup that can be done on an outpatient basis. This chapter will focus on conditions producing cardiovascular symptomatology presenting in the ED. These conditions require immediate recognition, therapeutic intervention, and prompt referral to a pediatric cardiologist.

TABLE 70-1. Clinical Presentation of Pediatric Heart Disease

Cyanosis	TGA, TOF, TA, TAt, TAVR
Congestive heart failure	See Table 70-2
Murmur/asymptomatic pt.	Shunts: VSD, PDA, ASD
	Obstructions
	Valvular incompetence
Abnormal pulses	
Bounding	PDA, AI, AVM
Decreased	Coarctation, HPLV
Hypertension	Coarctation
Syncope	
Cyanotic	TOF
Acyanotic	Critical AS

Note: AI, aortic insufficiency; AS, aortic stenosis; ASD, atrial septal defect; AVM, arteriovenous malformation; HPLV, hypopoastic left ventricle; PDA, patent ductus arteriosus; TA, truncus arteriosus; TAt, tricuspid atresia; TAVR, total anomalous venous return; TGA, transposition of the great arteries; TOF, tetralogy of Fallot; VSD, ventricular septal defect.

CONGESTIVE HEART FAILURE

Clinical Features

The distinction between pneumonia and congestive heart failure in infants requires a high index of clinical suspicion and is a difficult one to make. Pneumonia can cause a previously stable cardiac condition to decompensate, so that both problems can present simultaneously. The common symptoms and signs of an infant presenting in congestive heart failure are outlined in Table 70-2.

Cardiomegaly evident on chest x-ray is universally present except in constrictive pericarditis. A cardiothoracic index greater than 0.6 is abnormal. The primary radiographic signs of cardiomegaly on the lateral chest x-ray are an abnormal cardiothoracic index and lack of retrosternal airspace due to the heart's directly abutting against the sternum.

TABLE 70-2. Recognition of Congestive Heart Failure in Infants

	Right-Sided Failure	Left-Sided Failure	Both
Cardinal signs	Hepatomegaly	Tachypnea Dyspnea and sweating on feeding Rales	Cardiomegaly Failure to thrive Tachycardia
Unusual signs	Jugular venous distension Peripheral edema		

Differential Diagnosis

Once congestive heart failure (CHF) is recognized, age-related categories simplify further differential diagnosis (Table 70-3). In contrast to the gradual onset of failure with a ventricular septal defect (VSD), coarctation of the aorta can present with abrupt onset of CHF precipitated by a delayed closure of the ductus arteriosus during the second week of life. Onset of congestive heart failure after 3 mo of age usually signifies acquired heart disease, as opposed to congenital heart disease.

TABLE 70-3. Differential Diagnosis of Congestive Heart Failure Based on Age of Presentation

Age	Spectrum	
1 min	Noncardiac origin: anemia, acidosis, hyposia, hypoglycemia, hypocalcemia, sepsis	Acquired
1 h		
1 day		
	PDA in premature infants	
1 wk	HPLV	
2 wks	Coarctation	Congenital
1 mo		
	VSD	
	SVT	
3 mo	Myocarditis	
1 y	Myocardiopathy	Acquired
	Severe anemias	
10 y	Rheumatic fever	

For meaning of acronyms, refer to Table 70-1.

Myocarditis is often preceded by a viral respiratory illness and needs to be differentiated from pneumonia. As with pneumonia, the infant often presents in distress with fever, tachypnea, and tachycardia. Chest x-ray shows a cloudy lung field, either from inflammation or pulmonary edema. Cardiomegaly with poor distal pulses and prolonged capillary refill, however, distinguish it from common pneumonia. Once cardiomegaly is discovered, admission and an echocardiogram are indicated.

Usually pericarditis presents as cardiomegaly discovered on a chest x-ray. Clinical signs, such as chest pain, muffled heart sounds, and a rub may be present. An echocardiogram is performed urgently to distinguish a pericardial effusion from a dilated myocardiopathy (myocarditis) or a hypertrophied one.

If an infant presents in pure right-sided congestive failure, the primary problem is most likely to be pulmonary. In early stages lid edema is often the first noticeable sign.

Emergency Department Care

1. The infant who presents with mild tachypnea, hepatomegaly, and cardiomegaly needs to be seated upright in a comfortable position, oxygen should be given and the child should be kept in a neutral thermal environment to avoid metabolic stresses imposed by either hypothermia or hyperthermia.
2. If the work of breathing is appreciably increased by an increased pulmonary blood flow, 1 to 2 mg/kg of **furosemide** parenterally is indicated.
3. If pulmonary edema is present, then the hypoxemia can usually be corrected by fluid restriction, diuresis, and an increased FIO_2, although continuous positive airway pressure is sometimes necessary.
4. Stabilization and improvement of left ventricular function can often first be accomplished with inotropic agents. **Digoxin** is used in milder forms of congestive failure. The appropriate first digitalizing dose to be given in the ED would be 0.02 mg/kg.
5. At some point, congestive heart failure progresses to cardiogenic shock, in which distal pulses are absent and end-organ perfusion is threatened. In such situations, continuous infusions of inotropic agents such as **dopamine** or **dobutamine** are indicated instead of digoxin. The initial starting range is 5 to 10 µg/kg per min.
6. Aggressive management is often necessary for secondary derangements, including respiratory insufficiency, acute renal failure, lactic acidosis, disseminated intravascular coagulation, hypoglycemia, and hypocalcemia.
7. For definitive diagnosis and treatment of congenital lesions presenting in congestive failure, cardiac catheterization followed by surgical intervention is often necessary.

SUPRAVENTRICULAR TACHYCARDIA

Clinical Features

With the exception of supraventricular tachycardia (SVT), arrhythmias are uncommon in the pediatric age group. In infants, SVT presents with a 4– to 24–h history of poor feeding, tachypnea, pallor, and lethargy. In the older child, palpitations and chest pain can be prominent in the symptomatology. Physical examination reveals thready pulses and tachycardia too rapid to be counted accurately. Depending on the time since onset of SVT, other physical signs can vary from CHF to cardiogenic shock with pending arrest. Low cardiac output is secondary to inadequate ventricular diastolic filling time.

An ECG rhythm strip shows an unvarying ventricular rate between 220 and 360, as opposed to a range of 150 to 200 in adults with SVT. The QRS complexes are narrow and regular. P-waves are absent or abnormal.

SVT must be distinguished from sinus tachycardia, which is the most common tachyarrhythmia in children. In sinus tachycardia, P-waves are present. The normal range for heart rate in newborns is 120 to 200. Under age 5, it is not unusual to find a sinus tachycardia up to a rate of 200, due to fever, stress, or hypovolemia. The latter requires prompt recognition and adequate volume expansion.

1. Intravenous **adenosine** (0.1 mg/kg) is now the standard treatment in most pediatric cardiology centers.
2. Digoxin has been the time-honored standard of medical management of SVT in infants. Since it takes 4 to 6 h before the rhythm converts, however, it is used more for chronic management than acute conversion. Dosage is the same as for congestive heart failure listed above.
3. Vagal maneuvers to convert SVT can be attempted but are usually not successful until after the first dose of digoxin. The diver's reflex, which is elicited by submersing the face in ice water, usually produces the greatest vagal tone. An alternative to submersion is to place the ice water in a plastic bag lowered briefly on the infant's face.
4. Cardioversion with 0.25 to 1 Ws per kg is indicated in infants and children presenting in profound cardiogenic shock with pending arrest.

TETRALOGY OF FALLOT

Clinical Features

Tetralogy of Fallot is a common cyanotic lesion that may escape detection in the nursery. The degree of cyanosis is directly proportional to the severity of the pulmonary stenosis. In fact, cyanosis may be subtle or absent at rest and clinically obvious only when the infant is active or crying.

The other cardinal features on physical examination are the holosystolic ventricular septal defect (VSD) murmur in the third intercostal space at the left sternal border and the diamond-shaped systolic murmur of pulmonary stenosis in the second intercostal space at the left sternal border. History may reveal exercise intolerance relieved by squatting.

Main radiographic findings are a boot-shaped heart with decreased pulmonary vascular markings. A right-side aortic arch is present in 25% of tetralogies. Right ventricular hypertrophy with right axis deviation are the primary ECG abnormalities.

Dynamic obstruction below the pulmonary valve can lead to an acute increase in the right-to-left shunt and produce a hypercyanotic spell or syncope with cyanosis. Prolonged or recurrent syncope due to tetralogy of Fallot can be a life-threatening emergency, so that referral after initial stabilization is indicated for further diagnostic evaluation and possible urgent surgical intervention.

Emergency Department Care

1. Initial medical management of a hypercyanotic spell includes placing the infant in the knee–chest position, maximizing the FIO_2 and administering intravenous morphine. Direct manipulation of the infant is limited to establishing an intravenous line for medications.
2. **Morphine** in the dosage of 0.1 mg/kg can relieve the hyperdynamic spell. If the syncope does not respond to this therapy, the dose of morphine can be repeated.
3. Because of the high mortality and CNS morbidity associated with hypercyanotic spells, surgical intervention is indicated.

For further reading in *Emergency Medicine, A Comprehensive Study Guide,* see Chapter 106, Heart Disease, by James H. McCreary.

Marilyn P. Hicks

OTITIS MEDIA

Otitis media (OM) infection of the middle ear commonly affects infants and young children because of relative immaturity of the upper respiratory tract, especially the eustachian tube. Common pathogens include *Streptococcus pneumoniae, Haemophilus influenzae* and *Moraxella catarrhalis*, which account for 65% to 70% of all infections.

Clinical Features

Peak age is 3 to 24 mo. Symptoms include fever, poor feeding, irritability, vomiting, earpulling, and earache. Signs include dull, bulging, immobile tympanic membrane (TM), loss of visualization of bony landmarks within the middle ear, air fluid levels or bubbles within the middle ear, and bullae on the TM.

Diagnosis and Differential

Diagnosis is based on presenting symptoms and changes of the TM and middle ear. A red TM alone does not indicate the presence of an ear infection. Fever, prolonged crying, and viral infections can cause hyperemia of the TM. Pneumatic otoscopy can be a helpful diagnostic tool, however, a retracted drum for whatever reason will demonstrate decreased mobility.

Emergency Department Care

Treatment begins with antibiotics listed in Table 71-1. If improvement has not occurred within 48 to 72 h, re-evaluation should be sought; otherwise followup in 10 to 14 days is acceptable.

If Standard Treatment Fails

Consider medication noncompliance, the presence of resistant organisms, underlying immunoincompetence, or structural abnormality of the upper respiratory tract. Recurrent or persistent otitis media can result in serious hearing and speech deficits or may extend to intracranial infections such as meningitis or brain abscess.

OTITIS EXTERNA

Otitis externa (OE) is an inflammatory process involving the auricle, external auditory canal (EAC), and surface of the TM. It is commonly

383

TABLE 71-1. Drug Treatment for Otitis Media

1st Line antibiotics	Amoxicillin	60 mg/kg/day tid × 10d
	Septra/Bactrim	8–10 mg trimethoprim/kg/day bid × 10d
	Pediazole	50 mg erythromycin/kg/day qid × 10d
2nd Line antibiotics	Augmentin	40 mg/kg/day tid × 10d
	Suprax	8 mg/kg/day bid × 10d
	Ceclor	40 mg/kg/day bid × 10d
	Ceftin	40 mg/kg/day bid × 10d
	Clarithromycin	15 mg/kg/day bid × 10d
Analgesics	Auralgan otic solution	3–4 ggts q4 h
	Tylenol with codeine elixir	0.5–1.0 mg codeine per kg/dose q4–6 h
	Pediaprofin	10 mg/kg/dose q4 h

caused by gram-negative enteric organisms, *Staphylococcus*, *Pseudomonas*, or fungi.

Clinical Features

Peak seasons are spring and summer. Peak age is older children and adolescents. Symptoms include earache, itching, and fever. Signs include erythema, edema of EAC, white exudate on EAC and TM, pain with motion of tragus or auricle, and periauricular or cervical adenopathy.

Diagnosis and Differential

Diagnosis is based on clinical signs and symptoms. Foreign body within the external canal should be excluded by carefully removing any debris that may be present.

Emergency Department Care

Place an earwick if significant edema obstructs the EAC. Use Cortisporin Otic solution, Otic Domeboro, or propylene glycol solution (Vosol, Orlex). Oral antibiotics are indicated if otitis media or auricular cellulitis is present. Analgesics, including narcotics may be necessary initially. Followup should be advised if improvement does not occur within 48 h, otherwise re-evaluation at end of treatment is sufficient.

If Standard Treatment Fails

Cultures of the EAC may identify unusual or resistant organisms. Patients with diabetes or other forms of immune-incompetence can develop malignant otitis externa. Malignant OE is characterized by systemic symptoms and auricular cellulitis. This condition can result in serious complications and requires hospitalization with IV antibiotics.

PHARYNGITIS

Etiologies include multiple viruses and bacteria, but only group A streptococcus (GAS), Epstein–Barr virus, and *Neisseria gonorrhea* require accurate diagnosis. The identification and treatment of GAS pharyngitis is important in order to prevent the suppurative complications and sequelae of acute rheumatic fever.

Clinical Features—GAS

Peak seasons are late winter or early spring. Peak age is 5 to 11 years. Symptoms (sudden onset) include sore throat, fever, headache, abdominal pain, enlarged anterior cervical nodes, palatal petechiae, and tonsillar hypertrophy. With GAS expect absence of cough, coryza, laryngitis, stridor, conjunctivitis, and diarrhea. A scarlatina-form rash associated with pharyngitis almost always is GAS and is commonly referred to as scarlet fever.

Diagnosis and Differential

Definitive diagnosis is made with the throat culture; however, this may not always be practical in the ED because of time involved and potential problems with followup. Rapid antigen detection tests, if properly performed, achieve sensitivity and specificity close to that of the throat culture. A negative rapid strep does not exclude GAS and should be verified with a throat culture. Other etiologies of pharyngitis to recognize are Epstein–Barr virus (infectious mononucleosis) and N. gonorrhea.

Epstein–Barr virus (EBV) is a herpes virus and often presents much like streptococcal pharyngitis. Common symptoms are fever, sore throat, and malaise. Cervical adenopathy may be prominent and often is posterior as well as anterior. Hepatosplenomegaly may be present. EBV should be suspected in the child with pharyngitis nonresponsive to antibiotics, in the presence of a negative throat culture. Typically the WBC will show lymphocytosis with a preponderance of atypical lymphocytes. Diagnosis is confirmed with a positive heterophil antibody (mono spot). EBV is usually self-limited and requires only supportive treatment of antipyretics, fluids, and bedrest. Occasionally EBV is complicated by airway obstruction and can be effectively treated with Prednisone, 2.5 mg/kg/day tapered over 5 days, or dexamethasone, 1 mg/kg to a maximum of 10 mg, then 0.5 mg/kg every 6 h. Gonococcal (GC) pharyngitis in children and nonsexually active adolescents should alert one to the possibility of child abuse. GC pharyngitis tends to have a more benign clinical presentation than GAS pharyngitis. Diagnosis is made by culture on Thayer–Martin medium. Vaginal, cervical, and rectal cultures should also be obtained if GC pharyngitis is suspected.

Emergency Department Care

Antipyretics and sometimes analgesics will be necessary during the first 48 to 72 h of treatment (Table 71-2). Appropriate followup should be encouraged for treatment failure and symptomatic contacts. Followup for suspected GC pharyngitis should include child sexual abuse and social service investigations.

TABLE 71-2. ED Treatment of GAS and GC Pharyngitis

GAS Pharyngitis	PenVeeK	125–250 mg tid x 10d
	Amoxicillin	60 mg/kg/day tid x 10d
	Bicillin L-A	1.2 million units IM >27 kg; 600,000 units IM <27 kg
	Erythromycin	E. estolate 20–40 mg/kg/ day tid x 10d E. ethylsuccinate 40–50 mg/ kg/ day tid x 10d
	Keflex	25–50 mg/kg/day bid x 10d (500 bid adolescent)
	Duricef	30 mg/kg/day bid x 10d
	Velosef	25–50 mg/kg/day bid x 10d (500 mg bid adolescent)
	Ceclor	40 mg/kg/day bid x 10d
	Zithromax	(>16 y) 5–12 mg/kg qd x 5d
Gonococcal Pharyngitis	Ceftriaxone	125 mg IM < 45 kg
	Ceftriaxone	250 mg IM > 45 kg
	Spectinomycin (PCN allergy) And	40 mg/kg/ IM x 7d
	Erythromycin	40 mg/kg/day (< 8 y old)
	Doxycycline	100 mg bid (>8 y old) x 7d

For further reading in *Emergency Medicine, A Comprehensive Study Guide,* see Chapter 107, Otitis and Pharyngitis in Children, by Kimberly S. Quayle, Susan Fuchs, and David M. Jaffe.

Marilyn P. Hicks

In children, pneumonia is an age-related disease with a much higher frequency of serious illness in infants and young children (Table 72-1).

Risk factors include the presence of chronic or debilitating disease, attendance at day care, and young age of the patient, especially prematurity.

Clinical Features

The clinical presentation is also age-based. Symptomatology in the infant may be nonspecific, characterized by fever, poor feeding, vomiting, irritability, or lethargy. Auscultation of the chest in the infant or young child does not often yield localized rales due to the small chest size; however, one may hear decreased breath sounds, wheezing, or rhonchi. Cough, retractions, grunting, and hypoxia are more reliable signs of pulmonary pathology. Older children may complain of chest pain or dyspnea, and auscultatory findings are more reliable. Occasionally fever, abdominal pain, and distension may be the presenting symptoms with respiratory signs absent or minimal. Impending respiratory failure is heralded by hypoxia, cyanosis, altered mental status, or shock.

TABLE 72-1. Common Organisms Causing Pediatric Pneumonia

Age Group	Organism(s)*
Newborn	Group B streptococci
	Gram-negative bacilli
	Listeria monocytogenes
	Herpes simplex
	Cytomegalovirus
	Rubella
0.5 to 4 mo	Viruses
	Chlamydia trachomatis
	Streptococcus pneumoniae
	Haemophilus influenzae
	Staphylococcal aureus
4 mo to 4 y	Viruses
	Streptococcus pneumoniae
	Haemophilus influenzae
	Staphylococcal aureus
5 y to 17 y	*Mycoplasma*
	Viruses
	Streptococcus pneumoniae

*Listed from top to bottom by greatest to lowest frequency of occurrence.

Diagnosis and Differential

Radiographic findings in viral pneumonia are interstitial infiltrates, atelectasis, peribronchial infiltrates, and cuffing. Bacterial pneumonias typically present as lobar or segmental consolidation. Pneumatoceles, empyema, or pneumothorax suggest *Staphylococcal aureus* infection. *Mycoplasma* pneumonia may appear as streaky interstitial infiltrates or lobar consolidation; the presence of upper respiratory symptoms and benign clinical course help differentiate *Mycoplasma* from bacterial etiologies. WBC is usually elevated with a shift to the left in bacterial pneumonias. Blood cultures are positive in 10% to 30% of bacterial pneumonias and should be performed on all toxic appearing children. All patients with pneumonia need pulse oximetry and hypoxic children need admission. Other indications for admission include vomiting, dehydration, or signs of impending respiratory failure or sepsis. All infants <3 mo of age should be considered for admission.

Emergency Department Care

1. During the newborn period, **ampicillin**, 200 to 400 mg/kg/d IV q4 to 6h, and **gentamicin**, 5 mg/kg/d IV q12h, during the first week or gentamicin, 7.5 mg/kg/d q8h, after the first week of life are the drugs of choice. The third generation cephalosporin **cefotaxime**, 75 to 200 mg/kg/d IV q8h, may also be used. Ceftriaxone should be avoided during the immediate newborn period due to its interference with bilirubin metabolism.
2. In hospitalized patients >3 mo of age, a cephalosporin alone is acceptable; **cefotaxime**, 75 to 200 mg/kg/d q8h, or **ceftriaxone**, 75 to 200 mg/kg/d q8h. If staphylococcal pneumonia is considered, **nafcillin**, 100 to 200 mg/kg/d q4 to 6h, should be added to the regimen. **Erythromycin**, 15 to 50 mg/kg/d IV q4 to 6h, is the drug of choice for *Mycoplasma* and *Chlamydia*. Children should be monitored for hypoxia and O_2 should be administered when appropriate.
3. Outpatient treatment of uncomplicated pneumonia in children >3 mo and <4 y is **amoxicillin**, 60 mg/kg/day divided tid; **Augmentin**, 40 mg/kg/day tid, or **Pediazole**, 50 mg/kg/day tid, of the erythromycin component are acceptable alternatives. **Erythromycin**, 50 mg/kg/day, is the drug of choice in children >4 y of age and in PCN allergic children.
4. If bronchospasm is a prominent symptom, aerosolized or oral ß agonist (Albuterol) therapy may be tried.
5. Attention should be paid to fever control and adequate hydration; followup should occur within 1 to 2 days. Specific instructions concerning complications should be given to the caregiver.

If Standard Therapy Fails

Admission and administration of IV antibiotics should be considered.

For further reading in *Emergency Medicine, A Comprehensive Study Guide*, see Chapter 110, Viral and Bacterial Pneumonia in Children, by Kathleen Connors and Thomas E. Terndrup.

C. James Corrall

This chapter discusses several common skin and soft-tissue infections of childhood, including conjunctivitis, impetigo, sinusitis, and cellulitis. Because of its particular severity, orbital and periorbital cellulitis will be highlighted in a separate section.

CONJUNCTIVITIS

Conjunctivitis is an inflammation of the membranes that line the surface of the eye; it may be secondary to infection, allergy, or mechanical or chemical irritation. Keratoconjunctivitis involves the cornea, as well as the conjunctivae. Conjunctivitis is the most common ocular infection of childhood and is usually a sporadic disease, but epidemics of viral illness may occur particularly in the summer months. *Neisseria gonorrhoeae* poses the greatest threat to the integrity of the eye in the neonate. Later in childhood, the respiratory tract pathogens predominate, particularly *Haemophilus* species. Other agents more specific to certain geographic areas are discussed fully elsewhere.

Clinical Features

Older children with conjunctivitis may complain of photophobia, ocular pain, or a sensation of a foreign body in the eye associated with crusting of the eyelids or conjunctival injection. A thorough examination of the structure and function of both eyes should be performed, including visual acuity, extraocular muscle function, slit-lamp examination if age-appropriate, and fluorescein staining of the cornea with lid eversion. Erythema and increased secretions characterize conjunctivitis, with intense redness and purulence being more common with infectious rather than allergic causes. Fever and other systemic manifestations do not occur with isolated conjunctivitis. The duration of symptoms with infectious causes is often 2 to 4 days.

Diagnosis and Differential

The diagnosis of infectious conjunctivitis depends on the clinical examination. A gram stain should be performed in neonates or in particularly confusing cases and will usually show more than five white blood cells per field and, in many cases, bacteria. The finding of gram-negative intracellular diplococci is particularly important in identifying *N. gonorrhoeae* in the first weeks of life and should be considered in any child with severe purulent conjunctivitis. Conjunctival scrapings or cultures may be performed to diagnose *C. trachomatis* or other viral or bacterial pathogens. Conjunctivitis may be a manifestation of a systemic disorder, such as measles or Kawasaki disease.

TABLE 73-1. Differential Diagnosis of Allergic and Infectious Conjunctivitis

	Allergic	Infectious
History		
Pruritis	Yes	No
Chronic	Yes	No
Recurrent	Yes	No
Seasonal	Yes	No
Sneezing, rhinorrhea	Yes	Variable
Exam		
Discharge	Watery	Watery or purulent
Chemosis	Present	Usually absent
Fluorescein	Negative	Negative, except keratitis
Lab		
Gram stain	Negative	White cells, bacteria

Diagnosis of red eye includes conjunctivitis, orbital and periorbital infection, retained foreign body, corneal abrasion, uveitis, and glaucoma. Lack of limitation of ocular motility, absent foreign body, or corneal abrasion with fluorescein staining, and clarity of the anterior chamber limit the differential considerably. Normal intraocular pressure, lack of perilimbal erythema, corneal edema, and other than clear tearing discharge reduces the diagnostic possibility of glaucoma further.

Emergency Department Care

Bacterial and other viral conjunctivitides are the most common cause for red eye in childhood and are generally self-limited, with the notable exception of *Herpes simplex* and *N. gonorrhoeae*, which are complicated by corneal ulceration and scar formation. Allergic conjunctivitis is often confused with bacterial causes but is distinguished by seasonality, chronicity, pruritis, and associated allergic rhinitis. Fluorescein staining and gram stain should be done if in doubt but are usually not necessary in children beyond 1 month of age (Table 73-1).

Treatment is directed at the most common causes of conjunctivitis based on the age of the patient and the findings on examination, fluorescein staining, and gram staining, if needed, as outlined in Figure 73-1.

1. Antibiotics—For infants under 3 mo of age, treatment with **erythromycin** (50 mg/kg/day) is instituted to treat *C. trachomatis* and to prevent later development of the associated pneumonia syndrome. Older children require only topical antibiotic instillation into the conjunctival sac. **Sulfacetamide** 10% drops (2 drops q2h when awake) or **gentamicin** 0.3% solution (2–4 drops q2h when awake) are useful agents initially. Ciprofloxacin 0.3% and Tobramycin 0.3% solution are seldom indicated initially. Followup care should be performed in 48 h and, if not improved, patients should be prescribed

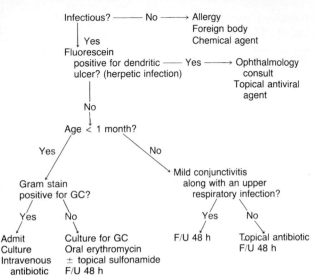

FIG. 73-1. Approach to the child with isolated infections conjunctivitis. F/U: followup; GC: gonorrhea culture.

an alternative agent or referred for ophthalmologic consultation. Infants under 1 mo old with exceptionally purulent conjunctivitis or gram-stain positive for *N. gonorrhoeae* should receive a single dose of **ceftriaxone** (125 mg IM), hospital admission, close followup care, with possible additional doses of ceftriaxone. Public health reporting and investigation are mandatory.

2. Antiviral agents—Consultation with an ophthalmologist is required. Topical, oral, or parenteral therapy may be indicated and is beyond the scope of this text.

3. Corticosteroids—Of most value in the treatment of allergic conjunctivitis under the direction of an ophthalmologist.

4. Antihistamines—The administration of **diphenhydramine** (5 mg/kg/24h divided q4–6h PO) or **hydroxyzine** (2 mg/kg/24h divided qid PO) may be useful for allergic conjunctivitis along with eradication of exposure to the offending allergen.

5. Vasoconstrictor—Topical application of a vasoconstrictor such as Vasocon A (2–4 drops q4–6h when awake) may provide relief from vernal conjunctivitis.

6. Supportive therapy—Cool compresses will lessen edema and loosen crusting that may be present in the mornings early in the course of treatment.

If Standard Treatment Fails

All children with conjunctivitis should be reevaluated within 48 h of treatment, and no child should be treated for longer than 5 days with topical antibiotic solutions or ointments without improvement. Failure to improve warrants further investigation and ophthalmologic consultation.

IMPETIGO

Impetigo is the most common skin infection seen in the ED and is a superficial bacterial infection of the skin confined to the epidermis. Two variants of the illness exist: impetigo contagiosa (strep or staph) and bullous impetigo (staph). Impetigo may spread locally, lead to remote, nonsuppurative sequelae, or may progress to cellulitis or lymphadenitis.

Clinical Features

The chief complaint of children with impetigo is sores on the body. There are no associated systemic symptoms such as fever or malaise. Regional lymph nodes may be minimally enlarged. The typical lesions of impetigo contagiosa begin as erythematous papules but rapidly progress to crusted lesions that are initially honey-colored and fine in consistency. Lesions may appear in any area of the body but are often localized to the upper lip and nose. The lesions enlarge over days to weeks and thicken. Erythema is mild and no induration is present. Bullous impetigo is characterized by superficial bullae filled with purulent material. The bullae range in size from 0.5 to 3 cm and have minimal surrounding erythema.

Diagnosis and Differential

The diagnosis of impetigo rests with the visual appearance of the lesions. Laboratory testing is rarely needed. In cases where the diagnosis is in doubt, a gram-stain of the lesions is helpful and will reveal the typical gram-positive bacteria and associated polymorphonuclear response. Lesion culture may be obtained from patients who do not respond to standard therapy. Several dermatologic disorders may mimic both types of impetigo. These include tinea corporis, nummular eczema, burns, allergic contact dermatitis, eczema herpeticum, and scalded skin syndrome.

Emergency Department Care

The treatment of impetigo is oral antibiotic therapy or an appropriate topical antibiotic for limited eruptions.

1. Oral antibiotics—A first-generation cephalosporin such as **cepha-lexin** (50–100 mg/kg/day q6h), **erythromycin** (50 mg/kg/day q8h), or **dicloxacillin** (25–50 mg/kg/day q6h) provides effective therapy when used for 7 days.
2. Topical antibiotics—Mupirocin ointment is the only topical agent with proven efficacy, but it is currently unavailable.
3. Local care—Vigorous scrubbing with antibacterial soaps, alcohol, or hydrogen peroxide offer no advantage.

If Standard Treatment Fails

It is unlikely that the clinical diagnosis of impetigo will be missed due to its characteristic appearance. Failure to respond implies either poor compliance or a more unusual diagnosis that warrants appropriate culture, skin scraping, or dermatologic referral for biopsy.

SINUSITIS

Sinusitis is an inflammation of the paranasal sinuses—maxillary, ethmoid, frontal, or sphenoid. Inflammation may be secondary to infection or allergy and may be acute, subacute, or chronic. The major pathogens in acute bacterial sinusitis in childhood are *Streptococcus pneumoniae* and *Haemophilus influenzae* (60%–70% of cases).

Clinical Findings

Two major types of sinusitis may be distinguished on clinical grounds—acute, severe sinusitis, and mild, subacute sinusitis (Table 73-2). Acute, severe sinusitis is associated with elevated temperature, headache, and localized swelling and tenderness or erythema in facial areas corresponding to the sinuses. It is most often seen in adults. Mild, subacute sinusitis is most often manifested in children as a protracted cold. Rather than improve in 3 to 7 days, these children persist with symptoms of upper respiratory infection beyond 2 wks. Fever is infrequent. This type of sinusitis may be confused with congestion of brief duration found in association with some upper respiratory infection and does not constitute a purulent infection.

TABLE 73-2. Signs and Symptoms in Children with Sinusitis

	Acute, Severe Disease	Mild, Subacute Disease
Headache	+ + +	+ +
Fever	+ + +	+
Facial tenderness	+ +	—
Facial swelling	+ +	—
Nasal discharge	+ + +	+ + + +

Diagnosis and Differential

The diagnosis is made on clinical grounds without laboratory or radiographic studies. Transillumination of the maxillary or frontal sinuses seldom helps. Standard sinus radiographs should be obtained in patients with uncertain clinical diagnosis and in cases of severe sinusitis. The most diagnostic findings for purulence are an air-fluid level or complete opacification. A normal radiograph suggests, but does not prove, that a sinus is free of disease. CT is an excellent diagnostic tool but is cost-prohibitive. Confirmation of infection is obtained by transnasal aspiration with culture and gram stain of secretions. Aspiration is indicated for life-threatening complications, immunosuppressive conditions, clinical unresponsiveness, and unusually severe disease. Few other conditions masquerade as sinusitis, and the differential is limited, particularly in children.

Emergency Department Care

The first step in management is to differentiate bacterial sinusitis from nasal congestion of an upper respiratory infection. The former mandates antibiotic therapy for resolution, and the latter resolves spontaneously. Treatment is outlined in Table 73-3 for acute, severe, and mild forms of the illness. Acute, severe sinusitis mandates intravenous antibiotic therapy to prevent life-threatening complications.

If Standard Treatment Fails

Untreated or inadequately treated infection may spread from the sinuses to surrounding structures and can be life-threatening. Complications include epidural, subdural or brain abscess, meningitis and cavernous

TABLE 73-3. Antibiotic Therapy for Sinusitis

	Acute, Severe Sinusitis	Mild, Subacute Sinusitis
Initial	Cefuroxime, 100 mg/kg per day IV divided q8h or Ceftriaxone, 75 mg/kg per day IV or Ampicillin/sulbactam, 200 mg/kg of Ampicillin per day IV divided q8h	Amoxicillin, 40 mg/kg per day PO divided tid
Persistent	Antibiotics, as above, plus surgical drainage	Cefprozil, 30 mg/kg per day PO or Erythromycin/sulfisoxazole; 40 mg/kg per day of erythromycin PO

sinus thrombosis or, more commonly, periorbital and orbital cellulitis. These complications necessitate immediate surgical consultation for drainage procedures and culture to direct antibiotic therapy.

CELLULITIS

Cellulitis is an infection of the skin and subcutaneous tissues that extends below the dermis, differentiating it from impetigo. It is a frequent infection in warm weather. Under normal circumstances, *Staphylococcus aureus, Streptococcus pyogenes*, and *Haemophilus influenzae* are the most commonly isolated organisms, as shown in Table 73-4. Since the advent of effective conjugated vaccines against *H. influenzae*, such infections have fallen dramatically and are rare in appropriately immunized children.

TABLE 73-4. Etiology of Cellulitis

	Most Likely	Less Likely
Immunocompetent Host		
Trunk/extremity	*Staphylococcus aureus* *Streptococcus pyogenes*	*Haemophilus influenzae*
Face* (periorbital/ buccal); unimmunized	*H. influenzae*	*S. aureus* *S. pneumoniae*
Face* (periorbital/ buccal); immunized	*S. aureus* *S. pneumoniae*	*H. influenzae*
Any site/animal bite	*S. aureus*	*Pasteurella multocida*
Any site/human bite	Anaerobic organisms	*S. aureus*
Immunocompromised Host		
Any site	*S. aureus*, gram-negative rods	Anaerobic organisms

*Definitive epidemiology awaits further studies since the advent of widespread immunization against *H. influenzae* type B.

Clinical Features

Cellulitis manifests a local inflammatory response at the site of infection with erythema, warmth and tenderness. Fever is unusual, except in cellulitis caused by *H. influenzae*. Usual clinical features are outlined in Table 73-5.

Diagnosis and Differential

The diagnosis of cellulitis is made by inspection. Cellulitis must be differentiated from other causes of erythema and edema including trauma, allergic reaction, and cold-induced lesions. Laboratory studies, including WBC concentration, blood culture, and aspirate culture are

TABLE 73-5. Usual Clinical and Laboratory Features
of Children with Cellulitis

Characteristic	H. influenzae	S. aureus
Age	<3 yrs	Any
Fever	Yes	No
Color of lesion	Violaceous	Erythematous
Location	Cheek, periorbital	Trunk, extremity
Preceding wound	No	Yes
WBC count	>15,000/mm³	<15,000/mm³
Bacteremia	Yes	No

obtained in specific circumstances, to include immunocompromise, fever, severe local infection, facial involvement, and failure to respond
to standard therapy.

Emergency Department Care

The treatment of cellulitis is the administration of systemic antibiotic
therapy. Most patients respond to conservative treatment with oral
antibiotics as outlined in Figure 73-2, however, the clinician must
identify patients who require broad-spectrum or intravenous antibiotics
and are at risk for bacteremia. Patients at risk for infection with

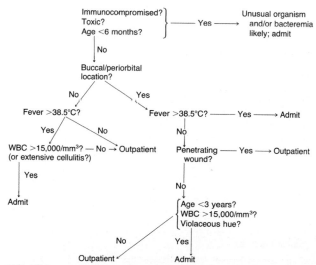

FIG. 73-2. Approach to the child with cellulitis.

TABLE 73-6. Initial Antibiotic Therapy for Cellulitis

Presumptive	Drug/Dose/Route
Immunocompetent	
Extremity	
Afebrile	Dicloxacillin 50–100 mg/kg per day PO
	or
	Cephalexin 50–100 mg/kg per day PO
Febrile/leukocytosis	Ampicillin/sulbactam 200 mg/kg as ampicillin per day IV
	or
	Cefuroxime 100 mg/kg per day IV
	or
	Ceftriaxone 75 mg/kg per day IV
Buccal/periorbital	As above
Immunocompromised	
Any site	Oxacillin 150 mg/kg per day IV
	or
	Cefazolin 100 mg/kg per day IV
	and
	Gentamicin 5–7.5 mg/kg per day IV
	or
	Tobramycin 5–7.5 mg/kg per day IV

H. influenzae should be admitted for IV therapy. Antibiotic choices are outlined in Table 73-6.

If Standard Treatment Fails

Patients must be followed carefully and should have improvement in erythema and induration within 72 h of institution of therapy. Patients who fail to respond to reasonable outpatient antibiotic therapy must be further evaluated and considered for admission and intravenous antibiotic therapy. Other underlying conditions, such as diabetes or underlying immune compromise, must be sought.

PERIORBITAL/ORBITAL CELLULITIS

Periorbital celluliis is an inflammatory process of the tissues anterior to the orbital septum or within the orbit (orbital cellulitis). *S. aureus* and *S. pneumoniae* are the principal etiologic agents. Orbital infections are most often due to *S. aureus*, particularly when puncture wounds are involved. Children under 3 years old are more likely to be bacteremic, thus experiencing the highest incidence of periorbital cellulitis. Orbital cellulitis can occur at any age but is usually seen in children less than 6 years old.

Clinical Findings

Orbital and periorbital cellulitis cause the periorbital area to appear red and swollen. Periorbital edema is usually more pronounced with preseptal infections. Proptosis or limitation of extraocular muscle function indicates orbital involvement. The eye is usually painful to touch and nonpruritic.

Diagnosis and Differential

Periorbital and orbital cellulitis are distinguished from noninfectious disorders on the basis of clinical findings and the WBC concentration. As with cellulitis at other locations, allergic and traumatic causes for edema must be considered. Tumors and metabolic disease may cause swelling and discoloration, particularly thyrotoxicosis in adolescents and neuroblastoma in the young child. Leukocytosis occurs frequently with cellulitis and more often with bacteremic preseptal infections. Blood cultures in patients with leukocytosis are often positive. CT is performed when orbital involvement is suspected and may easily demonstrate an inflammatory mass or tumor.

Emergency Department Care

Admission and treatment with intravenous antibiotics is mandatory to prevent complications of meningitis and subperiosteal abscess. Such antibiotic therapy is outlined in Table 73-6.

If Standard Treatment Fails

Children initially treated with intravenous antibiotics should have rapid defervescence and improvement in clinical status within 48 to 72 h of therapy. Continued worsening or the development of proptosis or ophthalmologia should prompt CT of the orbit and consideration of an etiology other than infectious causes or a severe complication of infection such as retro-orbital abscess or orbital cellulitis. Changing antibiotic therapy should be made only on the basis of culture and consultation. Surgical drainage may be necessary with abscess formation.

For further reading in *Emergency Medicine, A Comprehensive Study Guide*, see Chapter 108, Skin and Soft Tissue Infections, by Richard Malley and Gary R. Fleischer.

BACTEREMIA

Children aged 3 mo to 3 y are at increased risk of occult bacteremia (OB), occurring in approximately 5% with rectal temperatures of 39°C or higher. *Streptococcus pneumoniae* accounts for 85% of OB, with *H. influenzae, N. meningitidis*, group A streptococcus, and *Salmonella* responsible for the remainder. As many as 10% of children with OB risk progression to a major infection.

Clinical Features

The hallmark symptom of OB is fever, with the incidence of positive blood culture rising incrementally with rectal temps >39°C. The child may appear relatively well, exhibiting fever alone or in combination with signs of minor infection, such as URI, vomiting, or diarrhea. Because children with OB typically do not appear toxic, clinical signs are not reliable indicators of the presence of bacteremia.

Diagnosis and Differential

Definitive diagnosis of OB is made by blood culture. A WBC >15,000 has been shown repeatedly to correlate with an increased risk of bacteremia. Erythrocyte sedimentation rate and C-reactive protein also correlate well with OB, but are not particularly practical in the ED setting.

Emergency Department Care

Children between 2 and 36 mo old with temperature >39°C who do not have clinical signs and symptoms of major infection should have a WBC. If the WBC exceeds 15,000, the blood should be cultured. **Ceftriaxone**, 50 mg/kg IM, effectively reduces the progression of OB to major complications and should be considered for all children who meet the above criteria. Follow up within 24 h is mandatory and clear instructions should be given regarding potential deterioration of the child's condition. Repeat daily doses of ceftriaxone may be given until the blood culture proves negative or the child is afebrile and well.

If Standard Treatment Fails

Admission and septic workup should occur if the clinical condition of the child deteriorates or if the blood culture is positive for *H. influenzae* or *N. meningitidis*. Positive blood cultures for *S. pneumoniae* in the presence of a well-appearing child indicate repeat blood culture and close followup, but not necessarily admission.

SEPSIS

Sepsis in bacteremia with evidence of systemic infection can rapidly progress to multiorgan failure and death. Risk factors include prematurity, immuno-incompetence, recent invasive procedures, and indwelling foreign objects such as catheters. Sepsis tends to have age-related etiologies in children with common organisms causing sepsis and meningitis in children (Table 74-1).

Clinical Features

Clinical signs may be vague and subtle in the young infant and include lethargy, poor feeding, irritability, or hypotonia. Hyperpyrexia is common, however, very young infants may be hypothermic. Tachypnea and tachycardia are usually present as a result of fever, but they may also be due to hypoxia and metabolic acidosis. Sepsis can rapidly progress to shock, manifested as prolonged capillary refill, diminished peripheral pulses, altered mental status, and hypotension. Bradycardia and respiratory failure indicate a grave prognosis.

Diagnosis and Differential

Diagnosis is based on clinical findings and confirmed by positive blood culture. Young infants <1 mo old who are ill-appearing or febrile should be considered septic and should be admitted. The workup of a child with presumed sepsis should include a CBC, blood culture, catheterized urinalysis with culture, lumbar puncture, and chest x-ray. The critically ill child should also have coagulation studies, including fibrin split products and fibrinogen level, as well as arterial blood gas analysis.

Emergency Department Care

Treatment should begin with the ABCs of resuscitation to ensure adequate oxygenation and perfusion.

TABLE 74-1. Common Organisms Causing Sepsis and Meningitis in Children

Age	Organisms
0–1 mo	Group B Streptococcus
	E. coli
3 mo–5 y	H. influenzae
	N. meningitidis
	S. pneumoniae
>5 y	N. meningitidis
	ß-hemolytic streptococcus

1. Administration of high-flow oxygen, cardiac monitoring, and securing IV access are first steps. Endotracheal intubation should be performed in the presence of respiratory failure.
2. Shock is treated with 20 mL/kg boluses of normal saline with serial assessments of perfusion.
3. If fluid resuscitation fails, **dopamine**, 5 to 10 μg/kg/min, or **epinephrine**, 0.1 μg/kg/min, may be necessary.
4. Hypoglycemia is corrected with 0.5 gram/kg boluses of 25% dextrose.
5. Antibiotic therapy should begin as soon as IV access is achieved and should not be delayed due to difficulty with procedures such as lumbar puncture. Empiric antibiotic coverage is chosen based on the age of the patient (Table 74-2).

If Standard Treatment Fails

Consider the presence of drug-resistant organisms or immunoincompetence and infection with unusual or opportunistic organisms.

MENINGITIS

Meningitis is usually a complication of a primary bacteremia and has a peak incidence in children between birth and 2 y of age. Prematurity and immunoincompetence put children at higher risk. Organisms responsible for meningitis are essentially the same as those causing sepsis (see Table 74-1).

Clinical Features

Meningitis may present with the subtle signs that accompany less serious infections, such as otitis or sinusitis. Typical of these are irritability, inconsolability, hypotonia, and lethargy. In young infants suspicion should be especially high due to the often nonspecific presentation of the illness. Older children may complain of headache, photophobia, nausea and vomiting, and exhibit the classic signs of meningismus and

TABLE 74-2. Antibiotic Therapy for Sepsis and Meningitis

Age	Antibiotic	Dose
<1 mo	Ampicillin and gentamicin	200–400 mg/kd/day q4–6h 5 mg/kg/day q12h 1st wk of life 7.5 mg/kg/day q8h >1st wk of life
1–2 mo	Ampicillin and gentamicin or ceftriaxone or cefotaxime	200–400 mg/kg/day q4 6h 7.5 mg/kg/day q8h 100 mg/kg/day q12 24h 200 mg/kg/day q6–8h
>2 mo	Ceftriaxone or Cefotaxime	100 mg/kg/day q12–24h 200 mg/kg/day q6–8h

neck pain. Occasionally meningitis presents as a rapidly progressive, fulminant disease characterized by shock, seizures, or coma.

Diagnosis and Differential

Diagnosis is made by lumbar puncture and analysis of the CSF. The spinal fluid should be examined for white cells, glucose, protein, gram stain, and culture. If white cells are present or previous antibiotic therapy has occurred, the CSF should be screened for bacterial antigens. In the presence of immuno-incompetence, also consider infections with opportunistic or unusual viral organisms. Contraindications to performing lumbar puncture are cardiorespiratory compromise, increased intracranial pressure, and coagulopathy. Cranial CT should be performed prior to lumbar puncture in the presence of focal neurologic signs or increased intracranial pressure.

Emergency Department Care and Disposition

Treatment should always begin with the ABCs and restoration of oxygenation and perfusion (see specific treatment recommendations in Sepsis, above). Empiric antibiotics are based on the patient's age (see Table 74-2). Antibiotic administration should not be deferred when meningitis is strongly suspected. **Dexamethasone** 0.6 mg/kg/d q6h x 4 days, should be considered in children >6 wks of age who have *H. influenzae*, pneumococcal, or meningococcal meningitis. If given, it should be given at the time or shortly after the first antibiotic dose to be most effective.

If Standard Treatment Fails

Consider the presence of resistant organisms, CNS structural abnormalities, or complications such as brain abscess.

For further reading in *Emergency Medicine, A Comprehensive Study Guide*, see Chapter 109, Bacteremia, Sepsis, and Meningitis in Children, by Peter Mellis.

Rebecca S. Rich

URINARY TRACT INFECTION

Bacteria enter the urinary tract after colonizing the perineum. In infants, urinary tract infection (UTI) can also occur during bacteremia. Gram-negative enterics, most commonly *Escherichia coli,* predominate. *Enterococci, Proteus,* and *Pseudomonas* are seen more often with recurrent infections or in children on antibiotic suppression. Under 3 mo, the rate of bacteriuria is 1%. In febrile infants, bacteriuria occurs in 7% to 17%. At this age, sepsis accompanies UTI in 10% to 35% of cases. In infancy, boys have more UTIs, but after age 3 mo and into adulthood girls are at much higher risk.

Clinical Features

Infants and young children usually present with nonspecific symptoms such as fever, vomiting, diarrhea, and irritability. Older children may have dysuria, urinary frequency, enuresis, or abdominal pain. In older children there may be flank or suprapubic pain on exam. Differentiation of upper versus lower UTI can be difficult clinically, although fever, vomiting, and back pain suggest pyelonephritis.

Diagnosis

Urine culture is necessary; urinalysis alone is not adequate. Although pyuria is suggestive of urinary tract infection (UTI), it is nonspecific and is absent in half of infants with culture-proven UTI. Bag-urine cultures are the least invasive, and a negative culture from bag urine does exclude UTI. But positive bag-urine cultures are unreliable, so bladder catheterization or suprapubic aspiration are preferred. Older children can often get an adequate clean-catch specimen with good cleansing and coaching.

Differential Diagnosis

Vulvovaginitis is a more common cause of dysuria than UTI and must be specifically sought on physical exam. STDs, such as gonorrhea, chlamydia, and trichomonas, often present with dysuria as well.

Emergency Department Care

1. Hospitalization for parenteral therapy is preferred for infants under 3 mo or for children who appear toxic or are vomiting. **Ampicillin** (200–400 mg/kg/day q6h) with gentamicin (5–7.5 mg/kg/day q8h) is a standard empiric regimen.
2. The less ill child can be treated as an outpatient with oral agents; **TMP/SMX** (6–8 mg/kg/day TMP; 30–40 mg/kg/day SMX divided

bid) is a good first choice. **Amoxicillin** (50 mg/kg/day divided tid) is an alternative, but there is increasing resistance. Fluoroquinones are not recommended in children. Children with suspected pyelonephritis should be treated for 10 days; 3 to 5 days is probably adequate for most bladder infections in children with normal urinary tract anatomy. Patients should be reassessed within 48 h. Most children with UTI should undergo radiologic imaging of the urinary tract after recovery from the acute infection to look for structural abnormalities, scarring, and vesicoureteral reflux (VUR), which are preventable causes of renal insufficiency. Almost half of children under 1 y with UTI will have VUR or a structural abnormality.

PEDIATRIC VULVOVAGINITIS

The Prepubertal Girl

A vaginal discharge may occur in girls in the first 2 wks of life due to intrauterine estrogen. It can become bloody due to maternal estrogen withdrawal. The infant's vagina is also susceptible to *Candida* and *Trichomonas* acquired during vaginal delivery. *Trichomonas* may cause a persistent urethritis or vaginitis even after estrogen levels fall. *Chlamydia trachomatis* may also be acquired perinatally, although most children are culture negative by 18 mo. Maternally acquired condyloma may appear up to 1 y and generally resolves without treatment. The prepubertal girl's vulva is vulnerable to trauma, contact irritants, and bacterial contamination due to location and typical childhood hygiene. Infections are less common at this age than in older girls.

Clinical Features

Children may complain of vaginal and perineal pain, itching, burning, and dysuria. Squirming and an awkward walk may be seen in younger girls.

Differential Diagnosis and Management

Nonspecific vulvovaginitis is the most common cause in the prepubertal age group. There is no specific cause. The vulva and distal vagina are red and swollen. Discharge is scanty. Excoriations and ulcerations occur in severe cases. Cultures, if performed, grow normal enteric and vaginal flora. Treatment includes elimination of chemical irritants and improvement of hygiene with loose cotton underpants, mild soaps, handwashing, and front-to-rear wiping. Cool sitz baths and moist compresses are also recommended. **Amoxicillin** may help in persistent cases.

Pinworms (*enterobius vermicularis*) should be a consideration in this age group, since 20% of infestations have an associated vulvovaginitis with prominent nocturnal itching. Treatment is one 100-mg dose of

mebendazole for the child and for all household members, repeated in 2 wks.

Candidiasis is less common at this age than nonspecific vaginitis. Itching is prominent. Topical **imidazoles** are the treatment of choice, as in women (see Chap. 63, Vulvovaginitis).

Vaginal foreign bodies, most often bits of toilet paper, can cause a foul bloody discharge. Removal of the object is usually curative.

Respiratory and enteric pathogens (i.e., *Streptococcus, Escherichia coli, Hemophilus influenzae, Yersinia*) may spread by autoinoculation from the primary site. A bloody discharge should suggest *Shigella* or group A *streptococcus*. Diagnosis is by culture; treatment is for the primary pathogen.

Sexually Transmitted Diseases. Prepubertal gonorrhea presents as a vaginitis. Symptoms include dysuria, purulent discharge and, less often, abdominal pain. Culture is mandatory as nongonoccocal *Neisseria* can also cause infection. Asymptomatic infection is common and has been found in a third of household members of an infected child. In culture-proven gonorrhea, all household members should have cultures of the vagina (urethra in boys), rectum, and pharynx.

The presence of *Trichomonas, Chlamydia*, HSV, and condyloma usually indicates sexual contact. *Gardnerella* can be found in asymptomatic children without sexual contact, but symptomatic infection is more common in sexually abused girls. *Trichomonas* and *Gardnerella* are otherwise unusual in prepubertal girls because their unestrogenized vaginas are relatively resistant to them. The occurrence of STD should clearly prompt investigation into sexual abuse. STDs should be treated according to CDC guidelines. Patients weighing over 40 kg are treated with adult regimens. Children under age 8 should not be treated with tetracyclines due to dental staining.

Peripubertal Girl

With puberty, a physiologic discharge of mucus and epithelial cells without leukocytes often occurs. This discharge is odorless, gray–white, and nonirritating. If copious, it may be irritating, especially if the child wears nonabsorbent panties. Yellow staining of underwear is due to protein, which changes color when heated in the wash; reassurance and changing underwear to absorbent cotton is helpful.

Pubertal girls are more likely than younger patients to have an infectious cause of vaginitis. A speculum exam, which can be omitted in the younger virginal girl, should be part of the exam here. (See Chap. 63 for further discussion of Vulvovaginitis and STD.)

For further reading in *Emergency Medicine, A Comprehensive Study Guide*, see Chapter 111, Pediatric Urinary Tract Infections and Vulvovaginitis, by Denise J. Fligner.

Marilyn P. Hicks

ASTHMA

Asthma affects approximately 10% of the pediatric population and is the most common chronic disease of childhood. The rate of incidence, as well as the death rate, has increased significantly in past years. Factors that put children at risk for death are listed in Table 76-1.

Several factors contribute to exacerbation of asthma, the most common being infection. Allergens, exercise, and irritants, especially cigarette smoke, also often trigger asthma.

TABLE 76-1. Risk Factors Associated with Asthma Death

Intubation for asthma
Two or more hospitalizations, three or more ED visits in past year
Hospitalization or ED visit in past month
Syncope or hypoxic seizure with asthma
Recent steroid use or dependence
Increased use of β_2-agonists
Poor access to health care or psychosocial problems

Clinical Features

Wheezing is the most common symptom of asthma, however, if there is severe bronchoconstriction one may only hear decreased breath sounds. Also, persistent nonproductive cough or exercise-induced cough may be the result of bronchospasm. Occasionally rales or rhonchi may be present in conjunction with wheezing. Tachypnea and tachycardia almost always accompany wheezing. Retractions, nasal flaring, and accessory muscle breathing usually reflect the severity of the attack. Cyanosis, altered mental status, and somnolence often indicate respiratory failure. Bradycardia and shock herald impending cardiac arrest.

Diagnosis and Differential

Chest x-rays usually reveal hyperinflation and flattening of the diaphragm and are not useful in the treatment of uncomplicated, chronic asthma. Children experiencing a first episode of wheezing should have a chest x-ray. Other indications for x-ray include unilateral wheezing or rales, productive cough, or fever. Measurement of peak flow is useful in older children; PEFR < 50% predicted indicates severe obstruction. All children should have initial pulse oximetry on room air and if <93%, continuous monitoring should occur. Arterial blood gases are indicated if the oxygen saturation is < 88%, remains < 90% in spite of therapy or at any time the child exhibits signs of fatigue or impending respiratory failure. Hypercarbia, not hypoxia, is often the initial sign

407

of respiratory failure. A P_{CO_2} of 40 or greater is usually an early indication of impending respiratory failure.

The most common cause of wheezing in infants and young children is bronchiolitis, especially during fall and winter, when respiratory syncytial virus is prevalent. Infants with bronchopulmonary dysplasia often exhibit wheezing as a manifestation of chronic lung disease or secondary infections. These children also may develop wheezing as a symptom of CHF, as will children with sickle cell disease or congenital heart disease. Recurrent aspiration resulting from gastroesophageal reflux may cause wheezing in young children. Structural abnormalities, such as vascular rings, bronchial stenosis, or mediastinal cysts, can cause wheezing. Often early cystic fibrosis will present with wheezing and may mimic asthma. Pneumonia in young children may also be accompanied by wheezing. Aspiration of a foreign body may manifest as unilateral wheezing and should be considered in association with sudden onset of respiratory distress preceded by choking.

Emergency Department Care

Nebulized β_2-agonist therapy, specifically albuterol, is the mainstay of acute asthma therapy, along with the administration of supplemental O_2 and early use of corticosteroids.

1. Oxygen should be administered when O_2 sats are $< 93\%$.
2. **Albuterol** can be administered as episodic treatments at 0.15 mg/kg every 20 min or as continuous nebulization up to 0.5 mg/kg/hr, depending on the severity of the patient.
3. Steroids used early can prevent progression of an attack, decrease incidence of ED visits and hospitalization, and reduce morbidity. Indications for use are children: with mild asthma who do not respond to 3 albuterol nebs at 20-min intervals; with moderately severe asthma who do not respond to the first neb; with severe asthma; with frequent attacks in recent past (1 wk to 1 mo); who are steroid dependent; and with a history of respiratory failure or intubation. Steroids may be given as **prednisone** or **prednisolone** 1 to 2 mg/kg/day and, if given for 5 days or less, need not be tapered. Steroids are contraindicated in varicella-susceptible patients who have had known exposure or might have potential exposure to varicella.
4. **Atrovent** is an effective bronchodilator, especially when used in combination with nebulized albuterol. It can be administered at a dose of 250 μg in 2 cc of saline and should be reserved for patients with severe distress or those who do not respond readily to albuterol alone. It should be used with caution in children < 5 y old.
5. Terbutaline, also a β_2-agonist, may be given as an aerosol, as well as subcutaneously and intravenously. The nebulized dose is 1 mg of a 0.1% solution in 2 mL of saline for children < 1 y of age and 2 mg for children > 1 year of age every 15 to 20 min (max dose,

3 mg). Terbutaline may also be given subcutaneously at a dose of 0.01 mL/kg every 15 to 20 min (max dose, 0.25 mL).

6. Subcutaneous injection of epinephrine is rarely used anymore but is an acceptable alternative when nebulized therapy is delayed or unavailable or as initial therapy for the child with severe hypoventilation or apnea. It is given at doses of 0.01 mL/kg SQ every 15 to 20 min (max dose, 0.3 mL).

7. Theophylline is no longer recommended for ED treatment of asthma except for children who are already receiving theophylline or hospitalized children who have failed therapy with β_2-agonists and steroids. If used, an appropriate loading dose of 5 to 7 mg/kg of aminophylline is infused over 20 min to achieve a therapeutic serum level of 10 to 15 mg/mL. For patients currently receiving theophylline, a serum theophylline level should be obtained prior to aminophylline administration and an age-appropriate continuous infusion (Table 76-2) should be given while awaiting the results. A bolus is necessary only if the level is subtherapeutic. For each 1 mg/kg of aminophylline delivered as a bolus, the theophylline level will rise by 2 mg/mL. Patients receiving aminophylline should be cautiously monitored for side-effects such as arrhythmias, vomiting, and headache. It should not be given concomitantly with erythromycin or cimetidine, as these drugs alter the metabolism and decrease the clearance of aminophylline/theophylline. Febrile illnesses also decrease clearance, and doses should be lowered 30% to 50% in these circumstances.

Children who have not returned to baseline after 5 to 6 β_2-agonist treatments will require admission. Children in status asthmaticus rapidly become dehydrated due to decreased oral intake and increased insensible water loss. IV fluids should be administered as maintenance therapy. Treatment of children with respiratory failure includes continuous β_2-agonist nebulization, intravenous β_2-agonist therapy, or mechanical ventilation. Children who fail continuous albuterol therapy may benefit from intravenous terbutaline, given as a loading dose of 10 µg/min of a 0.1% solution over 10 min, followed by an initial infusion of 0.4 µg/kg/min and titrated in 0.2 µg/kg/min increments. The usual effective range is 3 to 6 µg/kg/min. Children should be monitored for unacceptable tachycardia and the infusion should be adjusted accordingly.

If mechanical ventilation is required, volume ventilation is the method of choice, using larger than average tidal volumes (18–24 mL/kg), age-

TABLE 76-2. Aminophylline Infusion

1–6 mo	0.5 mg/kg/h
6 mo–9 y	0.8–1.5 mg/kg/h
10–16 y.	0.8–1.2 mg/kg/h
>16 y	0.6 mg/kg/h

appropriate rates, and long expiratory times. Ketamine (1–2 mg/kg/IV) is a useful induction agent for intubation due to its bronchodilating effects. Morphine, Demerol and atracurium should be avoided because of increased bronchospasm from histamine release.

Children who are discharged should be given either oral albuterol (0.1–0.15 mg/kg/dose every 8 h) or a metered dose inhaler (MDI) and spacer if they are 5 years old or older (2 puffs every 4–6 h). If oral steroids are prescribed, they should be continued for no longer than 5 days at a dose of 1 to 2 mg/kg/day. Timely follow up within 24 to 48 h should be arranged prior to discharge. Parents and children should be given clear instructions as to signs of worsening problems and to return to the ED if needed.

BRONCHIOLITIS

Bronchiolitis occurs typically during fall to early spring, affects infants less than 2 y old, and is primarily characterized by tachypnea and wheezing. Respiratory syncytial virus accounts for the majority of infections; however, other respiratory viruses have been isolated. Young infants (< 2 mo of age), those with history of prematurity, bronchopulmonary dysplasia, congenital heart disease, or immunosuppression are at particular risk.

Clinical Features

Although wheezing is the prominent clinical manifestation, symptoms of URI will precede the respiratory distress. Most infants will exhibit fever, and apnea can occur with those 6 mo of age or less. Other signs of respiratory distress, such as tachypnea, retractions, nasal flaring, and grunting, may be present. Rales may be present as well, either alone or in conjunction with wheezing. Decreased or absent breath sounds signifies severe bronchoconstriction. Cyanosis and altered mental status are ominous signs of respiratory failure.

Diagnosis and Differential

All children should have a chest x-ray with the first episode of wheezing. The chest x-ray in bronchiolitis shows hyperinflation and peribronchial cuffing. Occasionally small areas of atelectasis may mimic pneumonic infiltrates. True consolidation is indicative of primary pneumonia or bronchiolitis with superinfection.

Identification of RSV can be made from nasal washings using fluorescent monoclonal antibody testing. This is particularly useful in identifying children at risk for severe disease and in identifying hospitalized children who require respiratory isolation. All children with respiratory distress should have initial pulse oximetry on room air and if the SaO_2 is $< 93\%$; pulse oximetry should be continuous. Arterial blood gases are indicated for children exhibiting signs of respiratory failure or shock and those whose SaO_2 remains low in spite of adequate β_2-agonist therapy. WBC and blood culture are not useful unless a superimposed bacterial infection is suspected.

Emergency Department Care

1. Many children with bronchiolitis respond to inhaled β_2 agonists and should be given a trial of nebulized **albuterol** at 0.15 mg/kg/dose q20 min for 3 treatments or administered continuously if needed.
2. Dehydration may complicate bronchiolitis because the increased respiratory effort prevents adequate oral intake, as well as increases insensible fluid loss. IV fluids should be administered to children requiring hospitalization and close attention should be paid to the hydration state of discharged children.

Other complications include respiratory failure and bacterial superinfection. Corticosteroids and theophylline are not indicated in the treatment of bronchiolitis. Infants who have apnea, fail to improve with nebulized β_2-agonist therapy, or who are vomiting and unable to maintain hydration should be hospitalized. Recurrent apnea or respiratory failure mandate endotracheal intubation and mechanical ventilation. Ribavirin, an antiviral agent, is recommended for hospitalized children at high risk and those on ventilators.

Infants not hypoxic, who are well-hydrated, and who respond to nebulized albuterol may be discharged from the ED on oral albuterol (0.1–0.15 mg/kg/dose every 8 h). Infants who continue to be tachypneic (RR >60) in the absence of wheezing should be observed and considered for admission. Clear instructions should be given to the caregiver regarding signs of dehydration and worsening respiratory distress. All infants should have follow up within 24 to 36 h.

If Standard Treatment Fails

Consider the presence of bacterial superinfection or other etiologies of wheezing, such as foreign-body aspiration or structural abnormalities.

For further reading in *Emergency Medicine, A Comprehensive Study Guide*, see Chapter 112, Asthma and Bronchiolitis, by Stanley H. Inkelis.

| Seizures in Children

Michael C. Plewa

There are numerous causes and manifestations of seizure activity, ranging from benign to life-threatening disorders. Although the majority of seizures are idiopathic in nature (epilepsy), several risk factors include encephalitis, disorders of amino-acid metabolism, structural abnormalities (hydrocephalus, microcephaly, arteriovenous malformations), congenital infections, or neurocutaneous syndromes (tuberous sclerosis, neurofibromatosis, Sturge–Weber syndrome). Precipitants of seizures can include fever, sepsis, hypoglycemia, hypocalcemia, hypoxemia, hyper- or hyponatremia, hypotension, toxin or medication exposure, and head injury.

Clinical Features

Symptoms of seizure may include any of the following: loss of or alteration in consciousness, including behavioral changes and auditory or olfactory hallucinations; involuntary motor activity, including tonic or clonic contractions, spasms, or choreoathetoid movements; and incontinence. Signs could include: alteration in consciousness; motor activity; autonomic dysfunction, such as mydriasis, diaphoresis, hypertension, tachycardia, and salivation, and postictal somnolence.

Diagnosis and Differential

The diagnosis of seizure disorder is based primarily on history and physical examination with laboratory studies (other than a bedside assay for glucose) obtained in a problem-focused rather than routine manner. Serum antiepileptic drug levels (Table 77-1) should be assayed in patients with breakthrough seizures or status epilepticus. Serum chemistries (electrolytes, magnesium, calcium, creatinine, BUN) are usually not indicated except in neonatal seizures, febrile seizures that are complex in nature (with duration >15 min, focal involvement, or several recurrences in 24 h), status epilepticus, or suspected metabolic or gastrointestinal disorder. Cardiac monitoring is useful to assess the PR and QT intervals and the possibility of cardiac dysrhythmia as the precipitant

TABLE 77-1. Therapeutic Antiepileptic Drug Levels

Drug	Level (μg/ml)
Phenytoin	10–20 (free level 1.2–2.1)
Phenobarbital	15–20
Carbamazepine	6–2
Primidone	5–12
Valproic acid	50–130 (free level 10–25)
Ethosuximide	50–100

of seizure. Although outpatient neuroimaging (contrast-enhanced CT or MRI) will be obtained for most cases of new-onset seizures, immediate imaging with noncontrast CT or MRI (or echoencephalogram in neonates) is indicated in cases of nonfebrile status epilepticus, head trauma and focal seizures, focal neurologic signs, or focal electroencephalogram (EEG) abnormalities. Lumbar puncture should be performed in neonatal seizure patients, and those with febrile seizures at age below 18 mo or with prior physician visit within 48 h, complex seizure, second seizure in the ED, or suspicious physical or neurologic examination. The only indication for emergent EEG monitoring is status epilepticus.

It is important to differentiate true seizure activity from one of several nonepileptic paroxysmal disorders, such as neonatal jitteriness, hyperekplexia (startle disease), near-miss sudden death syndrome, breath-holding spells (of cyanotic or pallid types), hyperventilation, syncope, migraine, hysterical pseudoseizures, narcolepsy, cataplexy, night terrors, vertigo, Tourette syndrome, chorea, or paroxysmal choreoathetosis, which are characterized by normal EEGs and are unresponsive to antiepileptic drugs.

Emergency Department Care

1. Airway maintenance (supplemental oxygen, suctioning, airway opening, or intubation, when necessary)
2. Seizure termination
3. Correction of reversible causes
4. Initiation of appropriate diagnostic studies
5. Arrangement of followup or admission, as appropriate

Termination of seizure activity is important to prevent irreversible pathologic changes and risk of persistent seizure disorder, especially in the setting of status epilepticus, defined as one seizure >20 min in duration, or a series of seizures >30 min without interictal awakening. Intravenous access is essential in cases of neonatal seizures, status epilepticus, and recurrent seizures.

First seizure Patients with an uncomplicated simple seizure may not require antiepileptic drugs. Patients considered high-risk for seizure recurrence (such as prolonged or recurrent seizures or neurologic insult) can be started on antiepileptic drugs according to seizure type. **Phenobarbital** (3–8 mg/kg/day in 1–2 daily doses), **phenytoin** (4–8 mg/kg/day in 2–3 daily doses), or **carbamazepine** (10–40 mg/kg/day in 2–4 daily doses) are used for tonic, tonic–clonic, clonic, or partial seizures. **Felbamate** (45 mg/kg/day in 3 daily doses) or **gabapentin** (20–30 mg/kg/day in 3 daily doses) are used for complex partial seizures. **Ethosuximide** (20–30 mg/kg/day in 2–3 daily doses), **valproate** (20–60 mg/kg/day in 2–4 daily doses), or **acetazolamide** (10 mg/kg/day in 1–2 daily doses) are used for absence seizures. Discharged patients should have close followup arranged.

Febrile seizure Identification and treatment of the cause of fever is the primary goal of therapy for febrile seizures. Fever can be controlled by acetaminophen or ibuprofen and tepid water baths. Antiepileptic drug therapy with oral **phenobarbital** (15 mg/kg loading dose, followed by 4–6 mg/kg/day) should be considered in patients at high risk of recurrence, such as age <12 mo, neurologic deficit (i.e., mental retardation or cerebral palsy), repeated seizures in the same febrile illness, history or family history of epilepsy, or more than three febrile seizures in 6 mo. Admit patients with suspected sepsis or meningitis, as well as those with recurrent seizures. Discuss antiepileptic drug administration or EEG monitoring and arrange close followup with the primary care physician for discharged patients.

Neonatal seizures The cause of neonatal seizures should be investigated and treated aggressively in an intensive care setting. Therapy includes empiric 25% glucose solution (2 ml/kg IV) and **pyridoxine** (50 mg IV). Hypocalcemia should be treated with **calcium gluconate** (4 ml/kg or 200 mg/kg of 5% solution IV) and **magnesium sulfate** (0.2 ml/kg of 2% solution IV or 0.2 ml/kg of 50% solution IM). **Diazepam** (0.2 mg/kg IV) or **lorazepam** (0.05 mg/kg IV) are first-line agents (both may be repeated twice) and should be followed by IV **phenobarbital** (20 mg/kg for premature, or 15 mg/kg for full-term infant) or **phenytoin** (15 mg/kg) loading. **Clonazepam** (0.1 mg/kg NG) may be used if high therapeutic levels of phenobarbital and phenytoin are ineffective.

Infantile spasms Prompt recognition of infantile spasms is essential to optimal outcome. Therapy with adrenocorticotropic hormone (ACTH), or prednisone or valproic acid, is often started in the inpatient setting after specialty consultation.

Head trauma and seizures Immediate seizures following head trauma may require short-term treatment with phenytoin, especially following severe head injury. Early and late posttraumatic seizures may require long-term antiepileptic therapy with phenytoin, carbamazepine, or phenobarbital, depending on incidence of recurrent seizures.

Breakthrough seizures in the known epileptic Patients with a single breakthrough seizure should have antiepileptic drug levels measured (see Table 77-1), since low levels (secondary to noncompliance or altered metabolism), or occasionally toxic levels, may be the cause. The daily dose of phenobarbital or phenytoin is often administered orally, assuming the levels are low. Those with recurrent or frequent tonic, tonic–clonic, or clonic seizures and low antiepileptic drug levels should receive intravenous loading of antiepileptic drug and consideration of a second antiepileptic agent if levels are high therapeutic. Admission should be considered for patients with frequent or recurrent seizures despite therapeutic drug levels and those with serious medical illness or toxic drug levels. Close outpatient followup should be arranged for discharged patients.

Status epilepticus. Airway maintenance is of primary importance in status epilepticus because all therapeutic agents can result in respiratory depression. With IV access, **lorazepam** (0.05 mg/kg), **diazepam** (0.2 mg/kg to a total of 2.6 mg/kg), or **midazolam** (0.1 mg/kg) are the primary agents of choice. Without IV access, alternatives include **midazolam** (0.1–0.2 mg/kg IM), rectal **diazepam** (0.5 mg/kg pr), or **valproic acid** (60 mg/kg pr), or intraosseous (IO) infusion of lorazepam, diazepam, or midazolam (in similar dosages as IV). Phenytoin (20–25 mg/kg IV or IO) should be started immediately after the primary agent. Hypoglycemia should be treated with 25% glucose (2 ml/kg IV or IO). If seizures persist beyond 25 min, administer **phenobarbital** (20–30 mg/kg IV or IO, and repeated 10 mg/kg every 20 min to levels of 60 μg/ml). If seizures persist beyond another 25 min, general anesthesia should be induced (along with continuous EEG monitoring) with pentobarbital (2 mg/kg bolus followed by 1–2 mg/kg/hr IV infusion), or inhalational agents such as isoflourane (0.25–1.5%), halothane (1.25%), or nitrous oxide (60%). Oral clonazepam (0.3 mg/kg/day per NG tube) can be used for noncontinuous status epilepticus.

If Standard Treatment Fails

For refractory status epilepticus, or when general anesthesia is not immediately available, several options have been described, including: continuous infusion of lorazepam (0.05–0.1 mg/kg/hr), diazepam (0.5 mg/kg/hr), lidocaine (2 mg/kg bolus, then 5–10 mg/kg/hr), propofol (1–4 mg/kg/hr), or rectal chloral hydrate (30 mg/kg pr). Consider treatable causes, such as hypoglycemia, hyponatremia, toxin exposure (iron, lead, carbon monoxide, salicylates, stimulants, etc.), or infections (meningoencephalitis or brain abscess). Specific toxicologic therapy (i.e., activated charcoal, hyperbaric oxygen, or chelation therapy) should be used for suspected toxin exposure when appropriate.

For further reading in *Emergency Medicine, A Comprehensive Study Guide*, see Chapter 113, Seizures and Status Epilepticus in Children, by Michael A. Nigro

Gastroenteritis and Pediatric
Abdominal Emergencies

Debra G. Perina

GASTROENTERITIS

Gastroenteritis is a major public health problem accounting for up to one fifth of all acute care outpatient visits to hospitals by families. Most enteric infections are self-limited, but clinical dehydration may be seen in 10% of cases and may be life-threatening in 1%.

Clinical Features

Gastroenteritis may be caused by viral, bacterial, or other infectious organisms, and spread occurs by the fecal–oral route. Acute diarrhea is the most prominent symptom in infants and children. The causative agent may be isolated from nearly 50% of children with diarrhea with laboratory testing.

Viral gastroenteritis is the most common etiology. Viral pathogens cause acute gastroenteritis through tissue invasion, which produces villous damage and decreased intestinal absorption of water resulting in diarrhea. Rotavirus is the most common viral pathogen in children. It typically occurs in the cooler months and is associated with concurrent respiratory symptoms. Norwalk virus has been implicated in epidemic outbreaks and produces nausea, vomiting, diarrhea, abdominal cramps, headache, fever, chills, and myalgias. In Norwalk virus infections, vomiting is more common in children, and diarrhea is more common in adults. Watery diarrhea is usually a sign of viral gastroenteritis, but it may also be seen with certain enterotoxigenic bacteria such as *E. coli* and *Vibrio cholerae*.

Bacterial pathogens can be isolated in up to 4% of all cases of gastroenteritis. Bacteria cause diarrhea by a variety of mechanisms, including enterotoxin production, cytotoxins, and damage to the intestinal mucosal absorptive surface. The major bacterial enteropathogens in the United States are *Campylobacter jejuni, Shigella, Salmonella, Yersinia enterocolitica, C. difficile,* and *E. coli.* Other agents that produce enteric infections include the parasite *Giardia lamblia,* which is particularly problematic in day-care centers. *Cryptosporidium,* once thought only to be an opportunistic infection, is now known to be a cause of protracted watery diarrhea in otherwise healthy children.

Diagnosis and Differential

The most important aspect of diagnosis is a thorough history and physical exam with particular attention to the child's state of hydration and the presence of other disease processes. Vomiting and diarrhea may be a nonspecific presentation for other disease processes, such as otitis media, urinary tract infections, metabolic acidosis, intussusception, increased intracranial pressure, drug or toxin ingestions, and malrotation.

Specific components of the history may suggest certain pathogens. *Yersinia* may produce signs and symptoms suggesting appendicitis or mesenteric adenitis. There may also be a history of exposure to a sick pet with diarrhea. *Shigella* is more likely in the setting of persistent or recurrent diarrhea, especially with weight loss, day care center exposure, or in immunocompromised children. *Shigella* is a fastidious pathogen and is more likely to be recovered from a rectal swab than from a stool specimen. Its clinical presentation includes watery or bloody diarrhea, encephalopathy, fever, or convulsions.

Specific food-borne pathogens produce toxins that may be ingested directly in food. *Staphylococcus aureus* produces five distinct heat-stable toxins present in improperly stored meats, poultry, and dairy products. *Bacillus cereus* also produces a heat-stable toxin most often found in boiled or fried rice. *E. coli* enteritis has been associated with undercooked ground meat and unpasteurized milk.

If clinical signs of dehydration are present, serum electrolytes should be measured. An elevated BUN does not correlate with the degree of dehydration. Significantly dehydrated children will be acidotic often with a pH less than 7.35 and a reduced serum CO_2 content.

Selective laboratory studies may be warranted. Microscopic evaluation for fecal leukocytes and routine stool cultures for common enteric bacterial pathogens are available in most hospital settings. Enzyme immunoassays are also available to test the stool for the presence of common enteric pathogenic viruses. Most children present with a nonspecific gastroenteritis. Under these circumstances, the physician must weigh the cost-effectiveness of obtaining cultures against the likelihood of determining the presence of a treatable etiology.

If the patient is febrile, has abrupt onset of diarrhea with more than four stools a day, or has blood in the stool, the illness is most likely bacterial in origin. The likelihood of isolation of the bacteria is increased if there are positive fecal leukocytes detected by methylene blue stain. This has a 90% correlation with bacterial enterocolitis. The presence of anal fissures or skin lesions, however, could result in contamination of the stool sample with blood, resulting in a false-positive test. Stool cultures should be obtained if there is a history of seafood ingestion, day-care-center exposure, ingestion of poorly cooked ground meat, or prior antibiotic treatment, even if fecal leukocytes are not seen. Also, any child presenting with a dysentery-like illness should have a stool culture performed.

Emergency Department Care

As most cases are self-limited, oral rehydration is generally all that is necessary.

1. The majority of children can be treated with an oral glucose–electrolyte solution. Commercial rehydration solutions contain 310 mOsm/L, and maintenance solutions contain 40 to 60 mEq of sodium per l with 2 to 2.5% glucose. Table 78-1 presents a guide to using oral solutions.
2. If the patient is moderately to severely dehydrated (see Chap. 17), rapid IV hydration with 30 to 50 mL/kg of Ringer's lactate may be given over 3 h.
3. Antibiotics do not affect the clinical course in most cases, however, infants less than 6 mo are generally treated with antibiotics because of overall risk of bacteremia. **Ampicillin** (50–200 mg/kg/day divided q6h), **chloramphenicol** (50–100 mg/kg/day divided q6h), or **trimethoprim/sulfamethoxazole** (6–12 mg TMP + 30–60 mg SMX per kg/day divided bid) are the most commonly used agents. Antibiotics are also employed with shigellosis, as the usual clinical course is shortened and the period of shedding is reduced.
4. Antimotility agents are contraindicated.
5. Any child who has had diarrhea for more than 10 to 14 days, significant fever, or systemic complaints should also be treated empirically with antibiotic agents after a stool culture is obtained. Ampicillin (50–100 mg/kg/day divided qid) or trimethoprim/sulfamethoxazole (6–12 mg TMP + 30–60 mg SMX per kg/day divided bid) are the most likely choices.

Any child who is not dehydrated or who has responded well to oral or intravenous hydration may be discharged on an oral maintenance solution for at least 4 to 6 h. Breastfeeding should be routinely continued or, if on formula, the child may resume his usual diet within 24 h. In general, the regular diet should be resumed after a 4- to 6-h rehydration period and should never be delayed beyond 24 h. There is no evidence of the efficacy of dilute or lactose-free feedings.

The family should be counseled to return or contact their pediatrician if the child is unable to drink the rehydration solution, continues to vomit, shows signs of dehydration, decreased urine output or tearing, or a decrease in alertness or level of activity. Infants and small children should be re-evaluated within 24 h by telephone contact with their primary care provider to determine if a followup visit is necessary.

TABLE 78-1. Oral Treatment of Acute Dehydration

Rehydration solution
  Give volume equal to estimated fluid deficit (e.g., 5% dehydration = 50 mL/kg deficit)
  Usually 40–50 mL/kg over 4 h
Maintenance solution
  Daily volume should not exceed 150 mL/kg per day
  Supplement with water, breast milk, or lactose-free formula
  Do not delay refeeding more than 24 h

A child who presents with any of the following should be admitted: toxic appearance, circulatory compromise, 10% to 15% dehydration, inability to drink, altered level of consciousness, bloody diarrhea, laboratory evidence of hemolytic anemia, thrombocytopenia, azotemia, elevated creatinine, or intractable vomiting.

If Standard Treatment Fails

Remember to assess the child for other sites of infection. Small frequent feedings (2 oz or less) may lessen stomach distension in a child who has been vomiting, promoting retention of oral rehydration solutions.

PEDIATRIC ABDOMINAL EMERGENCIES

Abdominal pain in children is a diagnostic challenge to the ED physician. To be effective in treating these patients, the physician must recognize clinical manifestations of the more common diseases, be able to develop a differential diagnosis, and know how to approach a child. Obtaining a thorough history is very important. If possible, this should be done from both the child and parent, with attention to chronology of events, fever, quality and location of pain, feeding, bowel habits, weight changes, and blood in vomitus and stools.

Clinical Features

The child's age influences the presenting signs and symptoms. The most important gastrointestinal signs and symptoms are pain, vomiting, diarrhea, constipation, bleeding, jaundice, and abdominal masses. There are two types of abdominal pain: peritonitic and obstructive. Peritonitic pain is exacerbated by motion, whereas obstructive pain is spasmodic and associated with restlessness. Patients with peritonitic pain tend to lie still; those with obstructive pain tend to be unable to remain still. In a child up to 2 y old the pain is usually described by the parent as fussiness and irritability. Abdominal pain in those over 2 y tends to be referred to the periumbilical area. Associated symptoms, or the presence of illness in other family members, may be helpful in arriving at a diagnosis.

Vomiting may be the result of a minor disease process or may herald something more severe. Bilious vomiting is always significant. Diarrhea may be osmotic, secretory, or transient in nature, caused by viral or bacterial pathogens. Quantitate the number, volume, consistency, and presence of blood in the stool.

Constipation may be due to a pathological or functional process. The shape and girth of the abdomen, presence of bowel sounds or masses and abnormalities in the anal area should be noted. Bleeding may be a sign of GI tract duplication, inflammation, foreign body, infection, or systemic illness. Causes of GI bleeding vary with age, and the cause for minimal to moderate amounts of blood in the stool frequently is never identified. Jaundice is usually an ominous sign, as it represents hepatic dysfunction. Also, the presence of an abdominal mass is worrisome and may be the first sign of a tumor, pyloric stenosis, or intussusception.

Diagnosis and Differential

It is helpful to split the causes of GI emergencies in the first year of life from those in children 2 y or older. Table 78-2 indicates the most common causes of abdominal pain occurring in each age group.

The most common GI emergencies in the first year of life include malrotation of the gut, incarcerated hernia, intestinal obstruction, pyloric stenosis, and intussusception. Malrotation of the gut, although a relatively uncommon entity, can present with a volvulus which can be life-threatening. Presenting symptoms are bilious vomiting, abdominal distention, and streaks of blood in the stool. The infant will appear pale with grunting respirations. One third of these children will appear jaundiced. The majority of cases occur in the first mo of life. Abdominal x-rays, although nondiagnostic, may reveal the presence of a loop of bowel overriding the liver. Intussusception, duodenal stenosis, or atresia can produce a similar clinical picture.

TABLE 78-2. Etiology of Pediatric Abdominal Pain

Common to All Ages	Over 11 Y
Appendicitis	Appendicitis
Gastroenteritis	Cholecystitis
Sickle-cell crisis	Dysmenorrhea
Toxins	Ectopic pregnancy
Urinary tract infection	Diabetic, ketoacidosis
	Henoch–Schönlein purpura
Infant to 10 Y	Incarcerated hernia
	Inflammatory bowel disease
Diabetic ketoacidosis	Peptic ulcer disease
Colic	Pneumonia
Hemolytic uremic syndrome	Pancreatitis
Incarcerated hernia	Pregnancy
Congenital abnormalities	Obstruction
Henoch–Schönlein purpura	Renal stones
Intussusception	Streptococcal pharyngitis
Malrotation	Torsion of ovary or testicle
Malabsorption	
Metabolic acidosis	
Obstruction	
Pyloric stenosis	
Pneumonia	
Volvulus	

Pyloric stenosis presents with a history of nonbilious projectile vomiting that occurs just after feeding. It usually manifests itself in the second or third week of life. It is male predominant and particularly common in first-born males. Palpation of the pyloric mass, or olive, may be felt in the left upper quadrant and is diagnostic. Intussusception occurs when one portion of the gut telescopes into another. GI edema and bleeding in the involved area give rise to bloody mucous-containing stools, producing classic currant jelly stools. The greatest incidence is between 3 mo and 6 y of age. Ileocolic intussusceptions are the most common. The classic presentation is sudden epigastric pain with pain-free intervals during which the examination may reveal the classic sausage-shaped mass in the right side of the abdomen. This mass is present in up to two thirds of patients. Vomiting is rare in the first 6 h.

The most common GI emergencies in children over age 2 include appendicitis, Meckel's diverticulum, colonic polyps, GI bleeding, and foreign bodies. Appendicitis can occur in those under age 2, but diagnosis is often delayed and the presentation is usually one of peritonitis or sepsis. In children over 2 y the classic progression of symptoms is seen beginning with anorexia, followed by mild to moderate periumbilical pain, then vomiting and pain movement to the right lower quadrant. The child may have a low-grade fever and mildly elevated white count in the range of 11,000 to 20,000. An x-ray may reveal an appendicolith. It is wise to remember that one or more of the classic signs and symptoms may not be present, so a high index of suspicion must be maintained. Meckel's diverticulum may simulate some of the same symptomatology as appendicitis, but the presence of gastric mucosa in the diverticulum can cause ulcer formation and bleeding. This bleeding presents as painless rectal bleeding and is usually bright red and brisk. Colonic polyps may be single, multiple, or represent classic familial polyposis. All give rise to painless lower GI bleeding which is rarely life-threatening. Single polyps are usually benign and often easily palpated on rectal exam. Familial polyposis is premalignant, and these children should always be referred to a pediatric surgeon.

GI bleeding in otherwise healthy children is usually due to an anal fissure or related to food substances that have a red or melanotic coloration. If the child appears ill, stress ulceration, sepsis, peptic-ulcer disease, inflammatory bowel disease, severe gastroenteritis, Henoch–Schönlein purpura, or hemolytic–uremic syndrome may be the cause. If an abdominal mass is palpated, Wilms' tumor, neuroblastomas, and rhabdomyosarcoma should be considered. Children with Wilms' tumor also may have hematuria.

The most important laboratory studies include urinalysis, complete blood count and differential, and stool for occult blood. Other tests, such as electrolytes, amylase, pregnancy test, and chest and abdominal x-rays, may be helpful in selected cases.

Emergency Department Care

Remove all of the child's clothing when doing the assessment and never omit the rectal exam or stool test for occult blood. If the child is critically ill, resuscitation and evaluation must be done simultaneously. Search for the causative disease process must be rapidly done so as to begin definitive treatment as soon as possible. The most important life-threatening causes of abdominal pain are presented in Table 78-3.

It is helpful to split the management of children in the first year of life from those 2 y or older. Those with malrotation of the gut, intestinal obstruction, pyloric stenosis, or intussusception should have prompt surgical consultation, NG tube, intravenous fluids, and type and cross-match. Those children with incarcerated hernias should undergo attempted manual reduction in the ED. This can usually be accomplished without sedation, however, intramuscular meperidine may be needed in some cases. If the hernia can be reduced, elective surgical referral is needed. If the reduction is difficult, the child should be admitted for 6 to 12 h of observation.

Children with suspected intussusception or obstruction should have a barium enema. Barium enema is curative in intussusception up to 80% of the time, however, there is a 5% to 10% recurrence rate. Ultrasonography may be useful in children suspected of having pyloric stenosis. Surgery is the treatment of choice when the diagnosis is confirmed.

In children over 2 y, if appendicitis is suspected, the patient should be made NPO, intravenous fluids should be initiated, rectal acetaminophen may be given, and surgical consultation should be obtained. A coagulation profile should be done if the child presents with rectal bleeding along with a shock-like state. If an abdominal mass is palpated, ultrasonography or CT scan may be indicated.

Most ingested foreign bodies will pass spontaneously, and no specific treatment is necessary. The only exceptions are if it is caught in the

TABLE 78-3. Life-Threatening Causes of Pain

Appendicitis
Metabolic acidosis
Congenital abnormalities
Diabetic ketoacidosis
Volvulus
Peptic–ulcer disease
Sepsis
Ectopic pregnancy
Incarcerated hernia
Intussusception
Hemolytic–uremic syndrome
Toxins
Trauma
Pneumonia

esophagus or too big to transverse the duodenum. Referral and outpatient followup should be arranged to ensure the passage of the foreign body. Laxatives are contraindicated. Dehydration and electrolyte imbalances from prolonged vomiting or diarrhea must be corrected. Most cases of vomiting are self-limited, however, a one-time dose of antiemetic can be safely given to children over 6 mo of age if prolonged vomiting occurs. The child who has been observed for 2 h and appears clinically well may be given clear liquids followed by a rehydration solution. Stool cultures are indicated in children with bloody diarrhea, toxic appearance, suspected epidemics, or illness more than 5 days.

Acute constipation is treated with increased oral fluid intake, stool softeners, or mild laxatives. Chronic constipation requires prolonged therapy with cleanout, maintenance, and behavior modification. The cleaning out process should start in the ED with disimpaction, if needed, followed by stool softeners and mild laxatives. In young infants with no systemic cause, dark thick molasses or corn syrup can be added to the diet to help alleviate the problem.

If Standard Treatment Fails

Trauma must always be considered when a pediatric patient presents with an abdominal emergency. Remember to evaluate extra-abdominal areas, such as pharynx, neck, mucous membranes, lung fields, testis, scrotum, and femoral and inguinal triangles for possible sources of disease causing referred abdominal pain, as the process may not be truly abdominal in origin. Do not forget the possibility of ectopic pregnancy or STDs in females of reproductive age.

For further reading in *Emergency Medicine, A Comprehensive Study Guide*, see Chapter 114, Gastroenteritis, by Ronald D. Holmes and Allan D. Olson; and Chapter 115, Pediatric Abdominal Emergencies, by Robert W. Schafermeyer.

Leslie C. McKinney

Type I, or insulin-dependent, diabetes mellitus (IDDM) is a common disease of childhood. The diagnosis of the disease, management of diabetic ketoacidosis (DKA), and hypoglycemia are important entities for the emergency physician to recognize.

DIABETIC KETOACIDOSIS

Clinical Features

Type I diabetes is probably an autoimmune disease and is characterized by the triad of polyuria, polydipsia, and polyphagia. Other associated symptoms include weight loss, anorexia, nocturia, as well as coma or DKA. DKA is a common complication of diabetes characterized by hyperglycemia, metabolic acidosis, and ketosis.

Diagnosis and Differential

DKA should be considered clinically in patients with hyperventilation, acetone-smelling breath, lethargy, abdominal pain, vomiting and, in young children, symptoms may mimic sepsis. Laboratory tests required to manage and diagnose DKA include glucose, electrolytes, urinalysis, venous or arterial pH, BUN, creatinine, and serum ketone. When the cause of DKA is not apparent, consider an infectious etiology and obtain CBC, CXR, and specific cultures, as clinically indicated.

Emergency Department Care

The treatment of DKA consists of volume replacement, insulin therapy, correction of electrolyte abnormalities, and search for a causative factor. Patients should be placed on a cardiac monitor, noninvasive BP device, and pulse oximetry, and an intravenous line should be placed. Initially, hourly monitoring of electrolytes and pH may be necessary.

1. Volume replacement using a normal saline bolus of 10 to 20 mL/kg over 1 h should be given initially. To calculate the total fluid deficit, compare the patient's weight on presentation with recent weight. If this is not available, assume a deficit of 10%. If shock is present, characterized by tachycardia, capillary refill >2 sec, obtundation, and orthostasis, repeat the 20 mL/kg bolus until the patient is stabilized. After initial stabilization is complete, the remaining fluid deficit should be replaced over 24 to 36 h (usually 1.5 times maintenance rate). After 1 to 2 h or when the patient is stabilized, change to 0.45% NS as the maintenance fluid. Monitor glucose levels closely and use D_5 0.45% NS when the blood glucose is approximately 250 mg/dL.

2. A regular insulin infusion may be started at 0.1 unit/kg/hr as soon as a glucose level of >250 mg/dL has been identified. An initial bolus of insulin is no longer recommended as the infusion is easier to control and there are concerns that rapidly decreasing glucose levels may contribute to cerebral edema. Glucose determinations should be checked hourly, and if the patient's glucose falls below 250 mg/dL before their pH has reached 7.30, continue both the insulin infusion and D_5 0.45% NS, adjusting the insulin infusion to maintain a glucose level of 200 to 250 mg/dL.

3. Management of potassium abnormalities are critical to the care of patients in DKA. Because of the shift of potassium to the extracellular space secondary to the acidosis of DKA, you may see falsely elevated serum K^+ levels despite total body depletion. If the pH is 7.10 or less and the K^+ is normal or low, begin replacement therapy immediately by adding 40 mEq of KCL to each liter of maintenance fluid. If the K^+ level is less than 3.5 mEq/L, consider doses as high as 60 mEq/L. If the K^+ level is elevated (greater than 6.0 mEq/L) consider holding K^+ therapy until the pH is correcting and the K^+ level is normal, then begin therapy.

4. Bicarbonate therapy has not been proven to play a role in the management of DKA in children and is therefore recommended only in life-threatening situations, such as cardiac arrhythmias or dysfunction.

5. A potentially fatal complication of DKA in children is cerebral edema, usually presenting about 6 to 10 h after initiating therapy, as mental status changes progressing to coma. Although the etiology of this complication is unknown, it is felt that overly aggressive fluid therapy and correction of electrolyte abnormalities may contribute to this problem. Treatment should include intubation with hyperventilation, mannitol 1 to 2 g/kg and fluid restriction. No therapy has yielded promising results, however, as there is a 90% mortality rate associated with cerebral edema.

HYPOGLYCEMIA

Any patient presenting with altered mental status, seizures or history of diabetes should have their blood glucose determined immediately by Dextrostix and/or serum measurement. See Chap. 19 for management.

If Standard Treatment Fails

Although the therapies outlined above should provide management for either DKA or hypoglycemia, consider laboratory or medication errors when the patient is not responding appropriately.

For further reading in *Emergency Medicine, A Comprehensive Study Guide*, see Chapter 116, The Diabetic Child, by David A. Poleski.

Rebecca S. Rich

BACTERIAL INFECTIONS

Bullous Impetigo

Bullous impetigo is a staphylococcal skin infection of infants and young children (see Chap. 73). Typical skin lesions are superficial, thin-walled bullae that occur mostly on the extremities. The bullae contain clear to yellow fluid. They rupture easily, leaving a denuded base that dries to a shiny coating. Diagnosis is based on the characteristic appearance of the lesions but, if there is doubt, aspirated bullous fluid may be cultured for staphylococci. Treatment is with oral antistaphylococcal agents (such as **cephalexin**, 50 mg/kg/day divided qid, or **dicloxacillin**, 50 mg/kg/day divided qid) along with local wound care and topical agents, such as **bacitracin**.

Erysipelas

Erysipelas is cellulitis and lymphangitis of the skin due to group A hemolytic streptococci, usually associated with fever and systemic toxicity. The rash starts as a red plaque that gradually enlarges with local redness, heat, and swelling. A key feature is the raised, sharply-demarcated indurated border. The face is the most common site, with the portal of entry often a skin wound or pimple. Diagnosis is clinical. If there is clear evidence by gram-stain that this is streptococcal, then **PCN G**, 100,000 U/kg/day IV divided q6h, is adequate. Otherwise, initial therapy should be broader: **ceftriaxone** (75 mg/kg/day IV divided q12h), **cefuroxime** (100 mg/kg/day IV divided q8h), or **oxacillin** (150 mg/kg/day IV divided q4h) plus **chloramphenicol** (100 mg/kg/day IV divided q6h).

Mycoplasma Infections

Mycoplasma pneumonia is a common cause of pneumonia, bronchitis, and upper respiratory infections in children and young adults. This infection should always be considered in patients with rash and pneumonia. Common symptoms are fever, cough, sore throat, headache, and rash. The rash is typically red, maculopapular and, often, truncal. An even more frequent rash associated with mycoplasma is erythema multiforme and, sometimes, Stevens–Johnson syndrome. Effective antibiotics for mycoplasma include **erythromycin** (40 mg/kg/day po divided qid) and **tetracycline** (10–20 mg/kg/day po divided qid).

Scarlet Fever

Scarlet fever is a streptococcal infection with a distinctive toxin-mediated rash. The etiologic agent is group A beta-hemolytic streptococci, although recently group-C strep has been implicated. School age children are most commonly affected. Symptoms include fever, sore throat, headache, vomiting, and abdominal pain, followed by rash in 1 to 2 days. The pharynx and tonsils are typically red with white exudate. The tongue is bright red with a white coating (strawberry tongue). The rash starts on the neck, groin, and axillae. It is red, punctate, and blanches with pressure. The rash is often accentuated at the flexural creases (Pastia's lines). When palpated, the rash has a characteristic rough, sandpaper feel. Desquamation occurs with healing. Scarlet fever is diagnosed by the rash's appearance in the setting of fever and pharyngitis. Throat swabs yield streptococci. Treatment is as for streptococcal pharyngitis, with **penicillin VK** (50 mg/kg/day po divided qid) being the drug of choice (**erythromycin**, 40 mg/kg/day po divided qid for PCN-sensitive patients).

Staphylococcal Scalded-Skin Syndrome (SSSS)

SSSS is a febrile illness of neonates and infants characterized by generalized confluent skin exfoliation. The disease is caused by a toxin produced by *Staphylococcus aureus*, arising not in the affected skin but at a separate site, such as the nose, pharynx, wound, or abscess, and inducing separation at the epidermis's granular layer. The illness begins with fever and irritability, followed by diffuse erythroderma, which typically spares the palms, soles, and mucosa. Soon large thin-walled bullae appear, rupturing easily and leaving large areas of moist denuded skin. The skin separates readily in response to gentle stroking (Nikolsky's sign). Once again, the diagnosis is clinical. SSSS may be confused, however, with toxic epidermal necrolysis (TEN), a more serious skin disease also characterized by bullae and exfoliation. Skin biopsy shows that in SSSS the cleavage is the granular layer, whereas in TEN the separation occurs more deeply, leading to greater morbidity. Therapy includes parenteral antistaphylococcal antibiotics (see Bullous Impetigo above) and eradication of any underlying focus of infection, local wound care, prevention of hypothermia, and fluid support. The skin usually heals without scarring unless superinfection occurs.

RICKETTSIAL INFECTIONS

Rocky Mountain Spotted Fever (RMSF)

RMSF is a tick-borne systemic illness found most often in the spring and summer in the southeastern United States. Headache, fever, rash, and myalgias are the major clinical features. Many, but not all, patients recall a tick bite. The rash usually starts a day or two after fever and begins at the wrist and ankles, then spreads quickly to the rest of the body. The lesions start as small, red blanching macules that rapidly become papular and petechial. The rickettsiae multiply within the vascular endothelium, resulting in a systemic vasculitis that may terminate in shock. At present, RMSF is a clinical diagnosis since serologic confirmatory tests are not immediately available (see Chap. 88, Tick-Borne Diseases, for management).

VIRUSES

Enteroviruses

Enteroviruses are common causes of exantha in young children. They include Coxsackie and echoviruses and typically occur in summer and early fall. Clinical syndromes caused by these viruses include myo- and pericarditis, aseptic meningitis, orchitis, hepatitis, bronchitis, and pneumonia, as well as nonspecific febrile illness with vomiting and myalgias. Skin manifestations are also varied, ranging from macular, morbilliform, vesicular, petechial, purpuric, and scarlatiniform. In fact, it may be difficult to differentiate enterovirus infections with rash from more serious conditions, such as sepsis, with organisms such as meningococcus. Echovirus 9, for example, causes a febrile illness with headache, cough, vomiting, pharyngitis, and sometimes nuchal rigidity. The rash is usually maculopapular, but there may be an exanthem resembling Koplik's spots and, the rash may be petechial, raising concern for meningococcemia.

Diagnosis

There are no specific clinically available tests for enterovirus, so diagnosis is by exclusion. Once other, more serious illnesses are ruled out, therapy for enterovirus illnesses is supportive. Although many enteroviral infections are clinically indistinguishable, hand–foot and mouth disease, due to coxsackie A 16, is very commonly seen and has distinctive features. Patients become febrile and develop painful oral lesions and skin rash. The oral lesions are small vesicles that quickly ulcerate. Children are often irritable and will not eat or drink due to pain. The skin lesions start as red papules, which become greyish vesicles, occurring on the palms, soles, and buttocks. The oral and skin lesions heal without scarring in 7 to 10 days. Herpetic gingivostomatitis in toddlers may have similar oral lesions, although there is no skin rash.

Emergency Department Care

Since the oral lesions often preclude eating, IV hydration is occasionally necessary. Cool foods, such as ice cream and custards, can be helpful, as well as combinations of liquid antacids, liquid diphenhydramine, and careful use of viscous lidocaine (magic mouthwash).

Erythema Infectiosum (EI)

Also known as fifth disease, EI is an acute febrile illness with unique rash caused by parvovirus B 19. Outbreaks occur primarily in the spring, most often affecting children age 5 to 15. The abrupt appearance of the rash is usually EI's first sign. It starts as a bright red rash on the cheeks (slapped-cheek appearance). There is circumoral pallor and sparing of eyelids and chin. The facial rash fades after 4 to 5 days. About 1 to 2 days after the facial rash appears, a nonpruritic erythematous macular or maculopapular rash occurs on the trunk and limbs. This stage may last 1 wk. The rash fades with central clearing, giving a distinctive lacy or reticulated appearance. The palms and soles are rarely affected. The rash may recur intermittently over the next few weeks, sometimes after sun exposure. Associated constitutional, respiratory, and gastrointestinal symptoms are common. Arthralgias and arthritis tend to occur only in adults. There is no specific therapy for EI.

Measles

Measles used to be a common childhood illness before nationwide immunizations. It is much less common now, but there have been recent local epidemics. It is a highly contagious myxovirus infection, occurring in the winter and spring in the United States. Incubation period is 10 days, followed by a 3-day prodrome of upper respiratory symptoms, then malaise, fever, coryza, conjunctivitis, photophobia, and cough. Patients look quite ill. The rash develops at day 14 after exposure, first behind the ears and at the hairline, spreading from head to feet. It is initially red, blanching, and maculopapular, but it rapidly coalesces, especially on the face. As the rash fades, it looks coppery-brown and may desquamate with healing. The rash generally lasts about a week. Koplik's spots, an associated pathognomonic exanthem, occurs just before the onset of rash. They are tiny white spots (grains of sand), usually found on the buccal mucosa opposite the lower molars. Measles is a self-limited disease; treatment is supportive.

Infectious Mononucleosis (IM)

IM, caused by Epstein–Barr virus, affects primarily children, teens, and young adults. Symptoms include fever, malaise, and sore throat. On exam, the pharynx is inflamed, often with exudate, and may be clinically indistinguishable from strep pharyngitis. Lymphadenopathy affects both anterior and posterior cervical chains and may be generalized as well. There is a 5% to 10% incidence of maculopapular rash in IM. Nearly all patients who are treated with ampicillin or a congener, however, develop rash. The diagnosis is suggested by increased atypical lymphocytes on blood smear and is confirmed by a positive heterophil antibody (Monospot) test; the Monospot is more reliable in patients over age 5 than younger children. Treatment of IM is supportive. The main emergency complications of IM are splenic rupture and airway obstruction. Patients with IM should avoid contact sports for 4 to 6 wks. A short course of corticosteroids (such as Prednisone, 1–2 mg/kg po q day) is helpful in patients with enlarged tonsils and potential airway obstruction.

Rubella (German measles)

Rubella was also more common before immunizations but still occurs, usually in the spring. Incidence among teens is increasing. Rubella may start with a mild prodrome of fever and upper respiratory symptoms. The pink maculopapular rash begins on the face and spreads down and out, then coalescing. The rash is less marked than in measles or chicken pox and may be fleeting. Lymphadenopathy, especially in the posterior cervical and auricular chains, is characteristic. Rubella is a mild disease often hard to diagnose; it is important to recognize the disease, however, due to serious congenital malformations when contracted in pregnancy.

Varicella

Varicella (chicken pox), caused by varicella–zoster virus, is a pruritic, generalized vesicular exanthem occurring most often in the winter. It is very contagious in the prodromal and vesicular stages. Most patients are less than 10 years old, but chicken pox occurs at all ages, and is usually more severe in adults. There is a prodrome of fever and upper respiratory symptoms. The rash starts on the trunk or head as faint red macules. Within 24 h the lesions vesiculate (dewdrop on a rose petal) and, over the next 1 to 2 wks, dry and crust over. Successive fresh crops appear in the initial days, leading to the characteristic finding of lesions in all stages of development. Low-grade fever occurs, but systemic toxicity is not severe. Diagnosis is clinical, based on the rash and contact with chicken pox. Uncomplicated varicella requires no specific therapy. Aspirin should be avoided, as it may predispose to Reye's syndrome. Oral antihistamines (such as **hydroxyzine** 0.5 mg/kg q6h) can help the intense itching. Superinfection of lesions is the most common complication in normal hosts. Administration of varicella–zoster immune globulin should be considered in nonimmune immunocompromised patients exposed to varicella.

Roseola Infantum

This common childhood febrile illness is caused by human herpes virus 6. Most patients are between 6 mo and 3 y old. The illness starts with high fever that persists for 3 to 5 days. Children may be quite irritable. The rash usually occurs as the child's fever is resolving and consists of blanching macular or maculopapular rose or pink discrete lesions, most prominent on the neck, trunk, and buttocks. Mucous membranes are not involved. The rash lasts 1 to 2 days, then rapidly fades. Although roseola is ultimately benign, febrile seizures may occur and, until the rash occurs, it may be hard to differentiate from more serious febrile illness such as sepsis.

Erythema Nodosum

Currently, this inflammatory exanthem is most commonly associated with medications, especially oral contraceptives. Other common etiologies include sarcoidosis, inflammatory-bowel disease, leukemias, and vasculitis. Infectious causes such as TB, fungal diseases, and streptococcal infections are less common now than in the past. Erythema nodosum is clinically distinctive, with bilateral tender nodules developing symmetrically, particularly over the shins and extensor prominences. The nodules are 1 to 5 cm in size but may merge. The overlying skin is red, smooth, and shiny. The eruption lasts several weeks. Constitutional symptoms often occur too, including fever, arthralgias, myalgias, and fatigue. The diagnosis is usually readily made clinically. There is no known therapy, but analgesics are often indicated. Since underlying causes are often present, look for these during ED workup and refer patients promptly.

Kawasaki's Disease (Mucocutaneous Lymph-Node Syndrome)

Kawasaki's Disease (KD) is a generalized vasculitis of unknown cause, particularly involving the coronary arteries. It affects about 5000 United States children per y, with peak age of onset being 1 to 2 years. Table 80-1 lists clinical criteria for the diagnosis. The fever is high and prolonged, lasting 1 to 2 wks in untreated children. The conjunctivitis is nonexudative. The polymorphous rash is usually red raised plaques. It is most widespread on the trunk and proximal extremities and tends to affect the perineum. There may be multiple organ system involvement as well. The Erythrocyte Sedimentation Rate is often dramatically elevated. The acute febrile phase lasts 7 to 14 days. During the next, subacute phase, lasting 2 to 4 wks, there is desquamation of the hands and feet. Thrombocytosis also occurs during this phase, when the child is at greatest risk for coronary thrombosis.

TABLE 80-1. Diagnostic Criteria for Kawasaki Syndrome

Fever of at least 5 days' duration (100%)
Presence of at least four out of the following five conditions:
1. Bilateral conjunctivitis (85%)
2. Changes of the lips and oral mucosa (90%)
   Dry, red, fissured lips
   Strawberry tongue
   Oropharyngeal edema
3. Changes of the extremities (75%)
   Erythema of palms and soles
   Edema of hands and feet
   Periungual desquamation
4. Polymorphous rash (80%)
5. Cervical lymphadenopathy (70%)
Illness not explained by other known disease process

Coronary artery aneurysmal dilatation occurs in 20% of untreated patients, peaking 4 wks after onset of illness. Sudden death occurs in 1% to 2% of untreated patients.

Patients meeting diagnostic criteria are usually admitted. Intravenous immunoglobulin (IVIG) within the first 10 days of illness reduces the incidence of aneurysm. A single IVIG infusion of 2 g/kg over 10 h is recommended. Aspirin at 80 to 100 mg/kg/day is used for the first 2 wks, reduced to 3 to 5 mg/kg/day after that for its antiplatelet effect until the platelet count is normal.

Pityriasis Rosea (PR)

PR occurs mostly in patients from age 10 to 35 in the spring and fall months. The cause is not known, but the disease is not contagious. PR often starts with a herald patch, one red lesion with raised border, usually on the trunk. About 1 to 2 wks later, there is a widespread eruption of pink maculopapular oval patches, often affecting the trunk. The lesions have a dry, scaly collarette border. The classical example of PR is the shape of a Christmas tree over the patient's back. There may be mucosal involvement. The illness may last 3 to 8 wks, with new crops of skin lesions arising. PR is largely a clinical diagnosis, but it may resemble fungal diseases (KOH prep of skin scrapings may help differentiate) or viral exantha. The classic mimic of PR is secondary syphilis, so a rapid plasma reagin (RPR) should be sent. There is no specific therapy. Since the rash can be very itchy, antihistamines or oatmeal baths may be helpful.

For further reading in *Emergency Medicine, A Comprehensive Study Guide*, see Chapter 117, Pediatric Exanthems, by Michael S. Weinstock and Michael S. Catapano.

Musculoskeletal Disorders in Children

Rebecca S. Rich

CHILDHOOD PATTERNS OF INJURY

The growth plate (physis) is the weakest point in children's long bones and the frequent site of fractures. The ligaments and periosteum are stronger than the physis, tolerating mechanical forces at the expense of physeal injury. The blood supply to the physis arises from the epiphysis, so separation of the physis from the epiphysis may be disastrous for future growth. The Salter-Harris classification is widely used to describe fractures involving the growth plate (see Figure 81-1).

Type I Physeal Fracture

In this injury (6% of all physeal injuries), the epiphysis separates from the metaphysis. The reproductive cells of the physis stay with the epiphysis. There are no bony fragments. Bone growth is undisturbed. Diagnosis is suspected clinically in a child with point tenderness over a growth plate. On x-ray, the only abnormality may be an associated joint

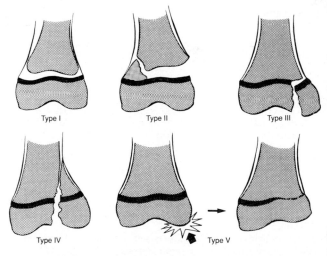

FIG. 81-1. Salter-Harris classification of physeal injuries. (Reproduced with permission from Tolo and Wood, 1994.)

Type I

Type II

Type III

Type IV

Type V

effusion. There may be epiphyseal displacement from the metaphysis. In the absence of epiphyseal displacement, the diagnosis is clinical, supported by the joint effusion. Treatment consists of splint immobilization, ice, elevation, and referral.

Type II Physeal Fracture

This is the most common (75%) physeal fracture. The fracture goes through the physis and out through the metaphysis. The periosteum remains intact over the metaphyseal fragment, but is torn on the opposite side. Growth is preserved since the physis remains with the epiphysis. Treatment is closed reduction with analgesia and sedation, followed by cast immobilization.

Type III Physeal Fracture

The hallmark here is an intra-articular fracture of the epiphysis with the cleavage plane continuing along the physis. This injury usually involves the proximal or distal tibia and accounts for 8% of physeal injuries. The prognosis for bone growth depends on the circulation to the epiphyseal bone fragment and is usually favorable. Reduction of the unstable fragment with anatomic alignment of the articular surface is critical. Open reduction is often required.

Type IV Physeal Fracture

The fracture line begins at the articular surface and extends through the epiphysis, physis, and metaphysis. This most often involves the distal humerus, accounting for 8% of physeal injuries. Open reduction is required to reduce the risk of premature bone-growth arrest.

Type V Physeal Fracture

This rare (1%) pattern usually involves the knee or ankle. The physis is essentially crushed by severe compressive forces. There is no epiphyseal displacement. The diagnosis is often difficult. An initial diagnosis of sprain or Type I injury may prove incorrect when later growth arrest occurs. X-rays may look normal or demonstrate focal narrowing of the epiphyseal plate. There is usually an associated joint effusion. Treatment consists of cast immobilization, nonweightbearing, and close orthopedic followup in anticipation of focal bone-growth arrest.

Torus Fractures

Children's long bones are more compliant than adults and tend to bow and bend under forces under which an adult's might fracture. Torus, cortical, or buckle, fractures involve a bulging or buckling of the bony cortex, usually of the metaphysis. Patients have point tenderness over the fracture site and soft-tissue swelling. Radiographs may be subtle but show cortical disruption. Torus fractures are not typically angulated, rotated, or displaced, so reduction is rarely necessary. Splinting or casting in a position of function for 3 to 4 wks, with orthopedic followup is recommended.

Greenstick Fractures

In this fracture, the cortex and periosteum are disrupted on one side of the bone but intact on the other. Treatment is closed reduction and immobilization.

Plastic Deformities

This pattern is seen in the forearm and lower leg in combination with a completed fracture in the companion bone. The diaphyseal cortex is deformed, but the periosteum is intact.

FRACTURES ASSOCIATED WITH CHILD ABUSE

Certain injury patterns are consistently seen in abused children, particularly multiple fractures in various stages of healing. Twisting injuries create spiral fractures in long bones, highly specific for abuse in nonambulatory children. In ambulatory children, spiral fractures may occur accidentally, the classic example being the spiral fracture of the lower third of the tibia (toddler's fracture), but they can also be seen with abuse. The injury pattern most closely associated with abuse is the chip fracture of the metaphysis. The tight attachment of the periosteum to the metaphysis will cause avulsion of little chips of the bone with pulling. There is exuberant callus formation and periosteal new bone formation. With direct trauma, subperiosteal hemorrhage characteristically lifts the periosteum off the bone, where it appears as opacified line. Fragmentation of the clavicle and acromion and separation of the costochondral junctions of the ribs are very suggestive of abuse. Bony injuries from shaking are similar to twisting, but also include spinal compression fractures and other vertebral injuries. Distraction injuries to the long bones cause hemorrhagic separation of the distal metaphysis, creating a lucency proximal to the physis. Squeezing injuries create rib fractures, which are highly suggestive of abuse.

Clavicle Fracture

This is the most common fracture in children. Fractures may occur in the newborn during a difficult delivery. Babies may have nonuse of the arm. If the fracture was not initially noticed, parents may notice a bony callus at 2 to 3 wks of age. In older infants and children, the usual mechanism is a fall onto the outstretched arm or shoulder. Care of the patient with a clavicle fracture is directed towards pain control.

Displaced fractures usually heal well, even if anatomic alignment is not achieved in the ED, although patients may have a residual bump at the fracture site.

Emergency Department Care

Figure-eight shoulder abduction restraints have been the traditional treatment, but many patients have more pain with this device. Many orthopedists find a sling-and-swathe or shoulder immobilizer to be equally effective and less painful. Both devices should be worn day and night for 2 wks, then during the day for another few weeks.

Supracondylar Fractures

The most common elbow fracture in childhood is the supracondylar fracture of the distal humerus. The mechanism is a fall on an outstreched arm. The close proximity of the brachial artery to the fracture predisposes the artery to injury. Subsequent arterial spasm or compression by casts may further compromise distal circulation. A forearm compartment syndrome, Volkmann's ischemic contracture, may occur; symptoms include pain in the proximal forearm upon passive finger extension, stocking-glove anesthesia of the hand, and hard forearm swelling. Pulses may remain palpable at the wrist, despite serious vascular impairment. Injuries to the ulnar, median, and radial nerves are common, too, occurring in 5% to 10% of supracondylar fractures. Children complain of pain on passive elbow flexion and maintain the forearm pronated. X-rays show the injury, but the findings may be subtle. A posterior fat-pad sign is indicative of intra-articular effusion and thus fracture. Normally, the anterior humeral line, a line drawn along the anterior distal humeral shaft, should bisect the posterior two thirds of the capitellum on the lateral view. In subtle supracondylar fractures, the line often lies more anteriorly.

Emergency Department Care

Splinting of the elbow in extension is recommended. In cases of neurovascular compromise, immediate fracture reduction is indicated. If an ischemic forearm compartment is suspected after reduction, surgical decompression or arterial exploration may be indicated. Admission is recommended for patients with displaced fractures or significant soft-tissue swelling. Open reduction is often required. Outpatient treatment is acceptable for nondisplaced fractures with minimal swelling. Such children need orthopedic reassessment within 24 h.

Lateral and medial condylar fractures, intercondylar and transcondylar fractures carry risks of neurovascular compromise, especially to the ulnar nerve. These patients present with soft-tissue swelling and tenderness, maintaining the arm in flexion. Most patients require open reduction.

Radial Head Subluxation (Nursemaid's Elbow)

This very common injury is seen most often in children between ages 1 and 4. Typical history is that the child is lifted up by an adult pulling on the hand or wrist. Sometimes there is a history of trauma, and sometimes no event at all but a child refusing to use the arm. The arm is held close to the body, flexed at the elbow with the forearm pronated. Gentle exam reveals no tenderness to direct palpation, but any attempts to supinate the forearm or move the elbow cause pain. If the history and exam is classic, radiographs are not needed, but if the history is atypical or there is point tenderness or signs of trauma, x-rays should be taken.

Emergency Department Care

To reduce the injury, hold one hand over the child's radial head and hold the child's hand with the other. Then simultaneously press down on the radial head with the thumb while fully flexing the elbow and supinating the forearm. There may be a click with reduction. (Be prepared for the child to scream and resist!) Usually the child will resume normal activity within 15 min if reduction is achieved. If the child is not better after a second reduction attempt, consider alternate diagnoses and radiographs. No specific therapy is needed after successful reduction. Remind parents to avoid linear traction on the arm, as there is risk of recurrence.

Slipped Capital Femoral Epiphysis (SCFE)

This disorder is more common in boys, with peak incidence between ages 12 to 15 in boys and ages 10 to 13 in girls. With chronic SCFE, the child complains of dull pain in the groin, anteromedial thigh, and knee, becoming worse with activity. With walking, the leg is externally rotated and the gait is antalgic. Hip flexion is restricted and is accompanied by external rotation of the thigh. Acute SCFE is due to trauma or may occur in a patient with pre-existing chronic SCFE. The patient is in great pain, with marked external rotation of the thigh and leg shortening. Do not force the hip through full range of motion, as this may displace the epiphysis further.

The differential includes septic arthritis, toxic synovitis, Legg–Calvé–Perthes disease, and other hip fractures. The child with SCFE is not febrile or toxic and has normal WBC and ESR. On x-ray, medial slips of the femoral epiphysis will be seen on AP views while frogleg views detect posterior slips. In the AP view, a line along the superior femoral neck should transect the lateral quarter of the femoral epiphysis, but not if the epiphysis is slipped.

Emergency Department Care

The management of SCFE is operative. The main long-term complication is avascular necrosis of the femoral head.

Transient Tenosynovitis of the Hip

This is the most common cause of hip pain in children less than age 10. The peak age is 3 to 6 y, with boys affected more than girls. The cause is unknown. Symptoms may be acute or gradual. The patient has pain in the hip, thigh, and knee, as well as an antalgic gait. Pain limits the hip's range of motion. There may be a low-grade fever. Patients do not appear toxic. The WBC and ESR are usually normal. Radiographs of the hip are normal or show a mild to moderate effusion. The main concern is differentiation from septic arthritis, particularly if the patient is febrile, with elevation of WBC or ESR and effusion. Diagnostic arthrocentesis is required, either with fluoroscopic or ultrasound guidance, or in the OR. The fluid in transient tenosynovitis is a sterile, clear transudate.

Emergency Department Care

Once septic arthritis and hip fracture have been ruled out, patients can be treated with crutches to avoid weightbearing, anti-inflammatory agents (such as ibuprofen, 5–10 mg/kg q6h), and close orthopedic or pediatric followup.

AVASCULAR NECROSIS SYNDROMES

Legg–Calvé–Perthes Disease

This disease is essentially avascular necrosis of the femoral head with subchondral stress fracture. Collapse and flattening of the femoral head ensues, with potential of subluxation. The result is a painful hip with limited range of motion, muscle spasm, and soft-tissue contractures. Onset of symptoms is between ages 4 and 9; the disease is bilateral in 10% of patients. Patients present with limp and chronic dull pain in the groin, thigh, and knee, worse with activity. Systemic symptoms are absent. Hip motion is restricted; there may be flexion–abduction contracture and thigh muscle atrophy. Initial radiographs (first 1–3 mo) show widening of the cartilage space in the affected hip and diminished ossific nucleus of the femoral head. The second sign is subchondral stress fracture of the femoral head. The third finding is increased femoral head opacification. Finally, deformity of the femoral head occurs, with subluxation and protrusion of the femoral head from the acetabulum. Bone scan and MRI are very helpful in making this diagnosis, showing bone abnormalities well before plain films. The differential diagnosis includes toxic tenosynovitis, tuberculous arthritis, tumors, and bone dyscrasias.

Emergency Department Care

In the ED, the most important thing is to consider this a chronic, but potentially crippling, condition. Nearly all children are hospitalized initially for traction.

Kohler's Disease of the Tarsal Navicular

This uncommon condition mostly affects boys at about age 5. It results from repeated compression of the tarsal navicular, the last foot bone to ossify. The child presents with a limp, bearing weight on the outside of the foot. There is local pain, tenderness, and sometimes induration, but no fever. On x-ray, the tarsal navicular is flattened on lateral view, with rarefaction and sclerosis.

Emergency Department Care

A short leg walking cast and nonweightbearing is initially recommended.

Frieberg's Infarction

This condition of teens is more common in girls. The usual site is the head of the second metatarsal. The patient complains of pain, and the area is tender and swollen. X-rays show flattening, sclerosis, and irregularity of the metatarsal head. Bone scan or CT may clarify the diagnosis.

Emergency Department Care

Initial treatment is a short leg walking cast for 3 to 4 wks.

Osgood–Schlatter Disease

This common syndrome affects preteen boys more than girls. Repetitive stress on the tibial tuberosity by the quadriceps muscle initiates inflammation of the tibial tuberosity, without avascular necrosis. The child has pain and tenderness over the anterior knee, which is worse with kneebending and better with rest. The patellar tendon is thick and tender, with the tibial tuberosity enlarged and indurated. X-rays show soft-tissue swelling over the tuberosity and patellar tendon thickening without knee effusion. Normally, the ossification site at the tubercle at this age will be irregular, but the prominence of the tubercle is characteristic of Osgood–Schlatter disease.

Emergency Department Care

The disorder is self-limited. Acute symptoms improve after restriction of physical activities involving knee bending for 3 mo. Crutches may be necessary, although knee immobilizer or cylinder cast are only rarely needed. Orthopedists prescibe exercises to stretch taut and hypertrophied quadriceps muscles.

Acute Suppurative Arthritis

Septic arthritis occurs in all ages, but especially in children under 3. The hip is most often affected, followed by the knee and elbow. The diagnosis is critical because, left untreated, purulent joint infection leads to total joint destruction. Bacteria access the joint hematogenously, by direct extension from adjacent osteomyelitis or from inoculation, as in arthrocentesis or femoral venipuncture. The organisms vary with the child's age; *Hemophilus influenzae* will likely diminish due to widespread vaccination. Although systemic symptoms can be subtle in the newborn, older children will appear ill, with high fever and irritability. The affected joint is very painful and shows warmth, swelling, and severe tenderness to palpation and movement. Children with hip or knee infection will limp or not walk at all. The child maintains an infected hip in flexion, abduction, and external rotation. X-rays show joint effusion, but this is nonspecific. The differential includes osteomyelitis, transient tenosynovitis, cellulitis, septic bursitis, acute pauciarticular JRA, acute rheumatic fever, hemarthrosis, and SCFE. Distinguishing septic arthritis from osteomyelitis may be quite difficult. Osteomyelitis is more tender over the metaphysis, septic arthritis over the joint line. Joint motion is much more limited in septic arthritis. Prompt arthrocentesis is the key to diagnosis, either at the bedside or, in the case of the hip, in the OR or under ultrasound. Synovial fluid shows WBC and organisms.

Emergency Department Care

Repeated joint drainage may be necessary during hospitalization. Suggested antibiotics are listed in Table 81-1. The prognosis depends on the length of time between symptoms and treatment, which joint is involved (prognosis worse for the hip), presence of associated osteomyelitis (worse), and the patient's age (worse for youngest children).

SELECTED PEDIATRIC RHEUMATOLOGIC PROBLEMS

Henoch–Schönlein Purpura (HSP)

HSP is a self-limited generalized leukocytoclastic vasculitis mediated by immune complexes. Palpable purpura, the classic vasculitic rash, appears on the trunk, buttocks, and legs. HSP also involves the glomeruli with resulting hematuria and proteinuria. Involvement of the bowel wall causes colicky abdominal pain and may proceed to melena, hematochezia, or intussusception. A polymigratory periarticulitis occurs in most children. HSP is largely a clinical diagnosis; useful lab tests include urinalysis, CBC, tests of renal function, and sometimes tests for collagen vascular disease.

Emergency Department Care

Admission is indicated when the diagnosis is in doubt, dehydration occurs, or when gastrointestinal or renal complications require close observation. Arthritis, when present as an isolated symptom, can be

TABLE 81-1. Initial Antibiotic Therapy of Acute Suppurative Arthritis in Children

Age	Suspected Organism	Antibiotics
Newborn (0–2 mo)	Staphylococcus aureus	Methicillin or nafcillin*
	Group B Streptococcus	Ampicillin or penicillin and gentamicin
	Gram-negative bacilli	Cefotaxime/ceftriaxone
	Neisseria gonorrhoeae	Cefotaxime/ceftriaxone
	Unknown	Methicillin or nafcillin* and cefotaxime/ceftriaxone
Infant (2–36 mo)	Haemophilus influenzae	Cefuroxime or cefotaxime/ceftriaxone
	Streptococcus sp.	Penicillin G
	Staph. aureus	Methicillin or nafcillin*
	Gram-negative bacilli	Cefotaxime/ceftriaxone
	Unknown	Methicillin or nafcillin* and cefotaxime/ceftriaxone
Child (>36 mo)	Staph. aureus	Methicillin or nafcillin*
	Streptococcus sp.	Penicillin G, other beta lactams, clindamycin
	Gram-negative bacilli	Cefotaxime/ceftriaxone
	N. gonorrhoeae	Ceftriaxone or penicillin G
	Unknown	Methicillin or nafcillin* and cefotaxime/ceftriaxone

*Vancomycin, if methicillinase-resistant Staph. aureus is suspected.

treated with salicylates. Chronic renal damage, sometimes requiring dialysis, occurs in 7% to 9% of children with HSP.

Acute Rheumatic Fever (ARF)

ARF is an acute, inflammatory multisystem illness affecting primarily school-age children. It is not common in the United States, but there have been recent epidemics. ARF is preceded by infection with certain strains of group A β-hemolytic streptococcus, which stimulates antibody production to host tissues. The child develops ARF 2 to 6 wks after symptomatic or asymptomatic streptococcal pharyngitis. Arthritis, which occurs in most initial attacks, is migratory and polyarticular, primarily affecting the large joints. Carditis occurs in one third of cases, and can affect valves, muscle, and pericardium. Sydenham's chorea occurs in 10% and may occur months after the initial infection. The rash, erythema marginatum, is fleeting, faint, and serpiginous, usually accompanying carditis. Subcutaneous nodules, found on the extensor surfaces of extremities, are quite rare. Carditis confers greatest mortality and morbidity. Lab tests are used to confirm prior strep infection (throat culture, strep serology) or to assess carditis (EKG, CXR, echocardiogram). The differential includes JRA, septic arthritis, Kawasaki's disease, leukemias, and other cardiomyopathies and vasculidites. In the ED, carditis is the main management issue. Most patients are admitted.

Emergency Department Care

Significant carditis is managed with **Prednisone** (1–2 mg/kg/day initially). Arthritis is treated with high-dose **aspirin** (75–100 mg/kg/day) to start. All children with ARF are treated with penicillin (or erythromycin, if allergic): **benzathine PCN** (1.2 million U IM), procaine **PCN G** (600,000 U IM daily for 10 days), or oral **PCN VK** (25,000–50,000 U/kg/day divided qid for 10 days). Long-term prophylaxis is indicated for patients with ARF. Life-long prophylaxis is recommended for patients with carditis.

Juvenile Rheumatoid Arthritis (JRA)

This group of diseases share chronic noninfectious synovitis and arthritis, with systemic manifestations. Pauciarticular disease is the most common form, usually involving a single large joint such as the knee. Permanent joint damage occurs infrequently. Polyarticular disease occurs in one third of cases. Both large and small joints are affected. There may be progressive joint damage. Systemic JRA occurs in 20% of patients. This form is associated with high fevers and chills. Extra-articular manifestations are common, including a red macular coalescent rash, hepatosplenomegaly, and serositis. The arthritis in this form may progress to permanent joint damage. In the ED, lab tests focus mostly on excluding other diagnoses. Arthrocentesis may be necessary to exclude septic arthritis, particularly in pauciarticular disease. X-rays initially show joint effusions but are nonspecific. The diagnosis of JRA will likely not be made in the ED.

Emergency Department Care

Initial therapy for patients with an established diagnosis include aspirin or an NSAID. Glucocorticoids are occasionally used, for example, for unresponsive uveitis or decompensated peri- or myocarditis.

For further reading in *Emergency Medicine, A Comprehensive Study Guide*, see Chapter 118, Musculoskeletal Disorders in Children, by Richard A. Christoph.

11 | INFECTIOUS DISEASES, ALLERGY, AND IMMUNOLOGY

Sexually Transmitted Diseases (STDs)

Rebecca S. Rich

This chapter covers the major STDs in the United States, with the exception of HIV, discussed in Chapter 84. (Pelvic inflammatory disease [PID] and vaginitis are covered separately in Chaps. 62 and 63, respectively.)

GENERAL RECOMMENDATIONS

When treating STDs in the ED, keep in mind that STDs frequently occur concurrently, that compliance and followup are often limited, and that infertility may result from lack of treatment. For these reasons:

1. Treat even when an STD is only suspected, with emphasis on single-dose therapy if possible.
2. Perform serologic testing for syphilis on patients with other STDs.
3. Perform pregnancy tests on all female patients with STDs.
4. Counsel patients about STD prevention.
5. Counsel patients about HIV testing, and propose testing outside of the ED.
6. Advise all patients that partners must be treated to prevent reinfection. If partners are present during the ED visit, treat them at that time.

CHLAMYDIAL INFECTIONS

Chlamydia trachomatis is an obligate intracellular bacterium that causes urethritis, epididymitis, and proctitis in men, and urethritis, cervicitis, PID, and infertility in women. In both sexes, asymptomatic infection is common. Patients with gonorrhea (GC) have a high incidence of concomitant *Chlamydia*. The incubation period is 1 to 3 wks, with symptoms ranging from mild urinary burning to peritonitis. Diagnostic techniques include direct immunofluorescence, ELISA assays, DNA probes, and culture. Newer assays on urine are becoming available. As shown in Table 82-1, doxycycline or azithromycin are the treatments of choice.

GONOCOCCAL INFECTIONS

Neisseria gonorrhoeae causes urethritis, epididymitis, and prostatitis in men and urethritis, cervicitis, PID, and infertility in women. Rectal infection and proctitis can occur in both sexes. The incubation period ranges from 3 to 14 days. As with *Chlamydia*, asymptomatic infection is common. Disseminated GC is a systemic infection that occurs in 2% of patients with GC, most often women, and is the most common cause of infectious arthritis in young adults. Although there is overlap,

TABLE 82-1. Antimicrobial Therapy for Sexually Transmitted Diseases

Disease	Recommended Treatment	Alternative
Chlamydial infection	Doxycycline (100 mg PO bid × 7d) or Azithromycin (1 g PO single dose)	Ofloxacin (300 mg PO × 7d) or Erythromycin (500 mg PO qid × 7d)
Gonococcal infections	Ceftriaxone (125 mg IM single dose) or Cefixime (400 mg PO single dose) or Ciprofloxacin (500 mg PO single dose) or Ofloxacin (400 mg PO single dose)	
Gonococcal, disseminated	Ceftriaxone (1 g IV daily × 7–10d, or for 2–3d) followed by cefixime (400 mg oral bid) or ciprofloxacin (500 mg oral bid to complete 7–10d total therapy)	Ceftizoxime or cefotaxime (1 g IV q8h for 2–3d or until improved), followed by cefixime (400 mg oral bid) or ciprofloxacin (500 mg oral bid) to complete 7–10d total therapy)
Trichomoniasis	Metronidazole (2 g PO single dose)	Metronidazole (500 mg PO bid × 7d)
Syphilis, 1°, 2°, early latent	Benzathine penicillin G (2.4 million units IM single dose)	Doxycycline (100 mg PO bid × 14d)
Syphilis, late latent or unknown	Benzathine penicillin G (2.4 million units IM; 3 doses 1 wk apart)	
Herpes simplex infections	Acyclovir (200 mg [400 mg for proctitis] PO 5 times a day × 7–10d)	
Chancroid	Azithromycin (1 g PO single dose) or Ceftriaxone (250 mg IM single dose) or Erythromycin base (500 mg PO qid × 7d)	Amoxicillin (500 mg plus clavulanic acid 125 mg PO tid × 7d) or Ciprofloxacin (500 mg PO bid × 3d)
Lymphogranuloma venereum	Doxycycline (100 mg PO bid × 21d)	Erythromycin (500 mg PO qid × 21d)

Source: Adapted from Centers for Disease Control and Prevention. *MMWR* 42:RR–14, 1993.

disseminated GC tends to be biphasic. An initial febrile bacteremic stage includes skin lesions (tender pustules on a red base, usually on the extremities), tenosynovitis, and myalgias. Over the next week these symptoms subside, followed by mono- or oligoarticular arthritis with purulent joint fluid. For uncomplicated GC, urethral or cervical cultures are the standard diagnostic tests. A gram-stain of urethral discharge showing intracellular gram-negative diplococci is very useful in men, but cervical smears are unreliable in women. Diagnosis of disseminated GC is often clinical, since cultures of blood, skin lesions, and joint fluid are positive in only 20% to 50% of patients. Culturing the patient's cervix, rectum, and pharynx may improve the yield. If a partner has a positive GC culture, this is also very helpful. With the emergence of penicillin resistance, **ceftriaxone** (125 mg IM in a single dose) has become the standard treatment. Oral alternatives are available (Table 82-1). Patients should be treated for *Chlamydia* as well. Disseminated GC is treated initially with parenteral ceftriaxone (1 gram daily).

TRICHOMONAS INFECTIONS

Trichomonas vaginitis is a flagellated protozoan, which causes vaginitis with discharge. Abdominal pain may also be present. In men, infection is often asymptomatic, but urethritis may be present. Diagnosis is based on finding the motile flagellated organism on saline wet prep of vaginal discharge or urine. Metronidazole (2 grams orally in a single dose) is the standard treatment for patient and partner.

GENITAL WARTS

Human papilloma virus cause genital warts and may be connected to cervical cancer. The warts appear after an incubation period of several months; although they are not painful, they tend to coalesce and may cause discomfort due to size and location. Diagnosis is clinical. Treatment is not usually undertaken acutely in the ED, but includes cryotherapy with liquid nitrogen or podophyllin. Recurrence is frequent.

SYPHILIS

Treponema pallidum, the spirochete which causes syphilis, enters the body through mucous membranes and nonintact skin. Syphilis has been on the rise lately, thought to be related to the crack epidemic. Syphilis occurs in three stages. The primary stage is characterized by the chancre, a single painless ulcer with indurated borders found on the penis, vulva, or other areas of sexual contact (Table 82-2). The incubation period is about 21 days, with the lesions disappearing after 3 to 6 wks. There are no constitutional symptoms. The secondary stage occurs several weeks after the chancre disappears. Rash and lymphadenopathy are the most common symptoms. The rash starts on the trunk, spreading to the

TABLE 82-2. Clinical Feature of Genital Ulcers*

Disease	Nature of Genital Ulcer	Incubation Period (Range)	Painful	Inguinal Adenopathy
Syphilis	Indurated, relatively not clean base; heals spontaneously	2 wk or longer	No	Firm, rubbery nodes; tender
Herpes simplex infection	Multiple, small, grouped versicles coalesce and form shallow ulcers; vulvovaginitis	2–7d	Yes	Tender bilateral adenopathy
Chancroid	Irregular, purulent; undermined edges; not indurated; multiple ulcers	2–12d	Yes	Present in 50%; usually unilocular; if fluctuant, very painful; may form crater
Lymphogranuloma venereum	Usually not observed; small and shallow; rapid spontaneous healing	5–21d	No	More common in males; nodes in matted clusters; unilateral or bilateral multiloculated

Source: Adapted from Scientific American Medicine. *Sexually Transmitted Diseases,* New York: Scientific American Medicine, December 1993.

palms and soles, and is polymorphous, most often dull red and papular. The rash is not pruritic. Other constitutional symptoms are common, including fever, malaise, headache, and sore throat. Mucous membrane involvement includes oral lesions and condyloma lata, cauliflower-resembling wartlike growths may occur in the anogenital region. This stage also resolves spontaneously. Late stage syphilis, which is much less common, occurs years after the initial infection, and affects the cardiovascular and neurologic systems. Specific manifestations include neuropathy (tabes dorsalis), meningitis, dementia, and aortitis with aortic insufficiency and thoracic aneurysm formation. Syphilis may be diagnosed in the early stages with dark-field microscopic identification of the treponemes from the primary chancre or secondary condyloma or oral lesions. Serologic tests include nontreponemal (VDRL, RPR) and treponemal (FTA-ABS). Nontreponemal tests are positive about 14 days after the chancre's appearance. There is a false-positive rate in about 1% to 2% of the population. Treponemal tests are more sensitive and specific but harder to perform. Syphilis in all stages remains sensitive to penicillin, the drug of choice. Treatment regimens are outlined in Table 82-1.

HERPES SIMPLEX INFECTIONS

Herpes simplex virus (HSV), type 2 and less often type 1, causes genital herpes, spreading through mucosal surfaces or nonintact skin. In primary infections, painful pustules, vesicles, and ulcers occur about 1 wk after contact with an infected person (see Table 82-2). Inguinal adenopathy is usually present. Patients with HSV infection may be asymptomatic and spread the virus to their partners. Systemic symptoms are common in first infections, including fever and myalgias. Dysuria is common, and urinary retention may occur. The untreated illness lasts 2 to 3 wks, healing without scarring. The virus remains latent in the body, however, and recurrences occur in most patients, but are usually briefer and milder without systemic symptoms. The diagnosis is usually clinical, based on the characteristic appearance. Viral cultures for HSV are more reliable than the Tzanck smear for intranuclear inclusions. Acyclovir is the treatment of choice for primary infections (see Table 82-1). The drug is less effective for recurrences but may be helpful if started at the onset of an attack.

CHANCROID

Caused by *Haemophilus ducreyi*, chancroid is more common in the tropics but is on the rise in the United States. After an incubation period of 3 to 10 days, a tender papule appears at the site of infection on the external genitalia, then enlarges to form a painful purulent ulcer with irregular edges. Multiple ulcers may be present. Painful inguinal adenopathy, usually unilateral, follows in half of untreated patients, and these nodes may form a mass (bubo) that drains. Systemic symptoms are minimal. Diagnosis is usually clinical, with care to exclude syphilis. Sometimes the organism may be cultured from the ulcer or bubo. The drugs of choice are erythromycin, ceftriaxone, or azithromycin (see Table 82-1). Buboes should not be excised, but may be aspirated for decompression to relieve pain.

LYMPHOGRANULOMA VENEREUM (LGV)

Several serotypes of *Chlamydia trachomatis* cause LGV, which is endemic in other parts of the world but uncommon in the United States. The primary lesion usually occurs 5 to 21 days after exposure and is a painless small papule or vesicle, which may go unnoticed and heals spontaneously in a few days (see Table 82-2). After anal intercourse, however, primary LGV may present as painful mucopurulent or bloody proctitis. Several weeks to months after the primary lesion, painful inguinal adenopathy occurs. The nodes mat together and often suppurate and form fistulae. Late sequelae include scarring, urethral, vaginal, and anal strictures and, occasionally, lymphatic obstruction. Diagnosis is through serologic testing and culture of LGV from a lesion. Doxycycline is the drug of choice (see Table 82-1).

For further reading in *Emergency Medicine, A Comprehensive Study Guide*, see Chapter 120, Sexually Transmitted Diseases, by Dexter L. Morris.

Toxic Shock Syndrome and Toxic Shock-Like Syndrome

Leslie C. McKinney

Toxic shock syndrome (TSS) is a severe life-threatening syndrome associated with colonization or infection with *Staphylococcus aureus*. Associated primarily with tampon use in the past, the overall incidence has decreased dramatically since 1979, presumably secondary to changes in tampons and education of the public and physicians.

Clinical Features

TSS is characterized by high fever, hypotension, diffuse erythroderma, mucous membrane hyperemia, and constitutional symptoms which rapidly progress to multisystem dysfunction. TSS is associated with menstruating females, who usually present between the third and fifth day of menses. Diagnostic criteria are listed in Table 83-1.

Diagnosis and Differential

Streptococcal toxic shock-like syndrome (TSLS) presents in a similar fashion to TSS, however, TSLS is caused by a severe streptococcal soft-tissue infection. Patients with TSLS lack the profound CNS changes seen with TSS, exhibit positive streptozyme assay and ASO titers, and have a rapidly progressive course. Because it is difficult to differentiate between TSS and TSLS early on, provide antimicrobial coverage for

TABLE 83-1. Criteria for Diagnosis (Must Have All)

Temperature > 38.9°C (102°F)

Systolic BP < 90 mmHg, orthostatic decrease of systolic BP by 15 mmHg, or syncope

Rash (diffuse, macular erythroderma) with subsequent desquamation, especially on palms or soles of feet

Involvement of 3 of the following organ systems clinically or by abnormal laboratory tests:

  Gastrointestinal—vomiting, profuse diarrhea

  Musculoskeletal—severe myalgias or twofold increase in CPK

  Renal—increase in BUN and creatinine two times normal; pyuria without evidence of infection

  Mucosal inflammation—vaginal, conjunctival, or pharyngeal hyperemia

  Hepatic involvement—hepatitis (twofold elevation of bilirubin, SGOT, SGPT)

  Hematologic—thrombocytopenia < 100,000 platelets/mm^3

  CNS—disorientation without focal neurologic signs

Negative serologic tests for Rocky Mountain spotted fever, leptospirosis, measles, hepatitis-B surface antigen, fluorescent antinuclear antibody, VDRL, and monospot; and negative blood, urine and throat cultures

both *S. pyogenes* and *S. aureus.* When considering TSS in a patient, evaluation should include ABG, CBC with peripheral smear, serum electrolytes including Mg^{++} and Ca^{++}, coagulation panel, urinalysis, and CXR. Cultures of all potentially infectious sites should be obtained and a tampon removed, if present.

Emergency Department Care

The treatment of TSS consists of initial management of circulatory shock, use of antistaphylococcal antimicrobial agents, and the search for a focus of infection. All patients should be placed on a cardiac monitor, noninvasive BP device, pulse oximetry monitor, oxygen, two intravenous lines started and a Foley catheter inserted.

1. Crystalloid IV fluids should be given initially for hypotension and consideration of a CVP or Swan–Ganz catheter may be necessary if there is no response to an initial fluid bolus of 1–2 l of normal saline. Large volumes of fluid may be required over the first 24 h.
2. A **dopamine** infusion may be started at 3–20 mg/kg/min if there is no response to a fluid challenge, so as to maintain a systolic BP of 90 mmHg.
3. Fresh-frozen plasma, PRBC's, or platelets may be given to correct any coagulation abnormalities.
4. Culture all potentially infected sites, including blood cultures prior to starting antibiotic therapy.
5. Institute antistaphylococcal microbial therapy. Recommend either antistaphylococcal penicillin, such as nafcillin or oxacillin in doses of 1 to 2 g IV every 4 h, or a cephalosporin with β-lactamase stability, such as **cefazolin**, 2 g IV every 6 h. In penicillin-allergic patients, clindamycin or vancomycin may be used.

If Standard Treatment Fails

Although most patients respond to the aforementioned therapy within 48 h, there are some animal studies which show improvement in TSS with the use of methylprednisolone and intravenous immunoglobulin. Other syndromes to consider include Kawasaki disease, staphylococcal scalded-skin syndrome, Rocky Mountain spotted fever, and septic shock.

For further reading in *Emergency Medicine, A Comprehensive Study Guide,* see Chapter 121, Toxic Shock Syndrome and Toxic Shock-Like Syndrome, by Ann L. Harwood–Nuss and Shawna Perry.

Arthur H. Tascone

The spectrum of disease that results from human immunodeficiency virus (HIV) infection is commonly encountered in the practice of emergency medicine. Presentation may vary from primary infection, to an asymptomatic phase, to AIDS with life-threatening complications. Commonly associated risk factors include intravenous drug use, homosexuality, heterosexuality, bisexuality, blood transfusion recipient prior to 1985, and maternal–neonatal transmissions.

Clinical Features

The spectrum of symptoms resulting from HIV infection varies greatly. Virtually any organ system can be involved, and patients often present with symptoms referable to multiorgan disease. The most common symptoms result from disease to neurologic, pulmonary, gastrointestinal, cutaneous, and ophthalmologic systems. In addition, systemic illness is often found.

Neurologic involvement occurs in 75% to 90% of AIDS patients. Seizures and altered mental status are the most commonly encountered symptoms. Dementia, meningitis, and focal neurologic deficits are also common. The most prominent symptoms of pulmonary disease in AIDS patients include cough, hemoptysis, dyspnea, chest pain, and fever. Gastrointestinal disease causes abdominal pain, rectal bleeding, and diarrhea. Systemic disease with its related opportunistic infections and malignancies lead to fever, weight loss, and weakness. From the ED point of view, the rashes of disseminated varicella zoster and herpes simplex are important to recognize.

Diagnosis and Differential

Diagnosis of AIDS is most commonly established with laboratory evidence of HIV infection, along with the presence of one or more of the opportunistic infections or malignancies in Table 84-1. Due to the complexity of HIV infection and AIDS, many specific diagnoses cannot be established in the ED setting. Emphasis should be on recognition of specific organ systems involved and severity of illness. Diagnosis is aided by review of previous records and recent CD4 counts. CD4 counts can assist in stratifying patients. CD4 counts less than 200 cells/μl are associated with considerable risk for opportunistic infection.

An AIDS patient presenting with fever may represent infection by bacterial, fungal, viral, and protozoal pathogens. The most common etiologies of an HIV-related fever are *Mycobacterium avium* complex, cytomegalovirus (CMV), Hodgkin disease, and non-Hodgkin lymphoma. *M. avium* complex and disseminated disease occur in up to

453

TABLE 84-1. AIDS-Defining Conditions

Esophageal candidiasis
Cryptococcosis
Cryptosporiditosis
Cytomegalovirus retinitis
Herpes simplex virus
Kaposi's sarcoma
Brain lymphoma
Mycobacterium avium complex
P. carinii pneumonia
Progressive multifocal leukoencephalopathy
Brain toxoplasmosis
HIV encephalopathy
HIV wasting syndrome
Disseminated histoplasmosis
Isosporiasis
Disseminated *M. tuberculosis* disease
Recurrent *Salmonella* septicemia

50% of AIDS patients. It is associated with fever, weight loss, diarrhea, malaise, and anorexia, as well as pulmonary involvement. CMV also causes systemic illness. It commonly causes retinitis and gastrointestinal symptoms.

Appropriate laboratory investigation of systemic systems, especially fever, include electrolytes, complete blood count, blood cultures (aerobic, anaerobic, fungal), urinalysis, liver functions, chest radiography, VDRL, cryptococcal antigen, serologies for *Toxoplasma* and *Coccidioides*. Lumbar puncture should be considered if no source of infection is found.

The most common etiologies of pulmonary abnormalities include PCP, *Mycobacterium tuberculosis* (MTB), CMV, *Cryptococcus neoformans*, *Histoplasma capsulatum*, and neoplasm. Chest radiography patterns, along with etiology, are listed in Table 84-2.

PCP is the most common opportunistic infection among AIDS patients. Typically patients complain of a nonproductive cough and shortness of breath. The chest radiograph reveals diffuse infiltrates, although it may be falsely negative in 5% to 10%. Hypoxia and increased alveolar-arterial gradient (>35) are found in pulse oximetry and blood gas analysis. Bronchoscopy is often needed for the diagnosis. The incidence of MTB among AIDS patients is increasing. Chest radiography usually does not reveal the typical upper-lobe infiltrate pattern. Diagnosis is by sputum analysis and bronchoscopy.

Evaluation for CNS symptoms should include CT scan of brain and lumbar puncture if there is no contraindication. CSF studies should include opening and closing pressures, cell count, glucose, protein, gram stain, india ink stain, bacterial culture, viral culture, fungal culture, toxoplasma and cryptococcal antigen, and coccidiomycosis titer. The

TABLE 84-2. Chest Radiographic Abnormalities: Differential Diagnosis in the AIDS Patient

Finding	Etiologies
Diffuse interstitial infiltration	PCP
	CMV
	MTB
	MAI
	Histoplasmosis
	Coccidioidomycosis
	Lymphoid interstitial pneumonitis
Focal consolidation	Bacterial pneumonia
	M. pneumoniae
	P. carinii
	MTB
	MAI
Nodular lesions	Kaposi's sarcoma
	MTB
	MAI
	Fungal lesions
	Toxoplasmosis
Cavitary lesions	PCP
	MTB
	Bacterial infection
	Fungal infection
Adenopathy	Kaposi's sarcoma
	Lymphoma
	MTB
	Cryotococcosis

most common etiologies of neurologic symptoms in AIDS include AIDS dementia, *Toxoplasma gondii*, and *Cryptococcus neoformans*.

Toxoplasmosis is the most common cause of focal encephalitis in the AIDS population. CT scan and MRI of brain reveal a ring-enhancing lesion. Lymphoma, fungal infection, and tuberculosis can also cause ring-enhancing lesions on brain scan and MRI. Cryptococcal CNS infection is seen in up to 10% of AIDS patients and may present with focal abnormalities or diffuse meningeal symptoms. Diagnosis can be established by india ink stain, fungal culture, and cryptococcal antigen studies of cerebrospinal fluid.

Emergency Department Care

The initial treatment of HIV-infected and AIDS patients begins with a heightened awareness of universal precautions. Since HIV-infected patients often present asymptomatically, health care providers should consider all blood and body fluid exposures as potentially infective.

1. Control the airway as needed, place on oxygen, pulse oximetry, cardiac monitor, and start an IV line. Replace volume deficits with normal saline as needed. In the absence of volume deficits, support

perfusion with vasopressors as needed. (See Chapters 8 and 9 on the treatment of shock.)

2. Treat seizures, altered mental status, and GI bleeding with the usual first-line agents. See specific chapters for management guidelines.
3. Treat specific opportunistic infections with agents, as listed in Table 84-3.
4. Admission is indicated for all unstable, hypoxic, or febrile patients with CD4 counts below 200.

TABLE 84-3. Treatment Recommendations for Common HIV-Related Infections

Organ System	Infection	Therapy
Systemic	MAI	No known effective therapy
	CMV	Ganciclovir, 7.5–15 mg/kg/d; maintenance therapy required
Pulmonary	P. carinii	TMP-SMX, 15–20 mg TMP/kg/d and 75–100 mg SMX/kg/d, PO or IV, for 3 wks
		or
		Pentamidine, 4 mg/kg/d, IV or IM, for 3 wks
	M. tuberculosis	Isoniazid, 5–10 mg/kg/d PO
		plus
		Rifampin, 9 mg/kg/d
		plus
		Pyrazinamide, 25 mg/kg/d PO or streptomycin, 0.75–1.0 mg/kg/d IM
CNS	Toxoplasmosis	Pyrimethamine, 25–50 mg/d PO
		plus
		Sulfadiazine, 100 mg/kg/d, for 3–6 mo
	Cryptococcosis	Amphotericin B, 0.4–0.6 mg/kg/d; maintenance therapy required
Ophthalmo-logic	CMV	Ganciclovir, 5 mg/kg bid for 2 wks; maintenance therapy required
GI	Candidiasis	Clotrimazole, 30–50 mg/d
		or
		Ketoconazole, 200–400 mg/d; maintenance therapy required
		or
		Fluconazole, 100 mg/d
	Salmonellosis	TMP-SMX, 10 mg TMP/kg/d and 50 mg SMX/kg/d, IV or PO
		or
		Ampicillin, 12 g/d IV; maintenance therapy required
	Cryptosporidosis	No known effective therapy

Table continues

TABLE 84-3. Continued

Organ System	Infection	Therapy
Cutaneous	HSV	Acyclovir, 1000 mg/d PO or Acyclovir, 15 mg/kg/d IV
	Herpes zoster	Acyclovir, 25–30 mg/kg/d IV
	Candida, tricophyton	Clotrimazole, miconazole, or ketoconazole, topical therapy bid-tid for 3 wks

Admission should be considered for patients with new-onset pulmonary symptoms and for hypoxic patients. Leukocytosis, productive cough, and presence of a focal infiltrate are suggestive, but not exclusive, to bacterial pneumonia. Standard antibacterial antibiotics can be used if gram stain confirms clinical suspicions. Diffuse interstitial infiltration, nonproductive cough, and dyspnea suggest PCP. Oral steroid therapy should be considered for patients with PaO_2 <70 mmHg or alveolar–arterial gradient >35, in addition to intravenous TMP–SMX or pentamidine. AIDS patients with new or changing neurologic involvement should be admitted. A thorough investigation of mental-status changes, meningitis, focal neurologic deficits, and seizures should be undertaken. CNS infections and respective treatment is based on laboratory test results. The evaluation of coma and altered mental status is standard and is referenced in other chapters. Seizures and status epilepticus should be treated with standard medications. Neurologic and infectious disease consultation early is appropriate. Cryptococcal CNS infection is treated with IV amphotericin.

Disseminated varicella zoster and herpes complex require intravenous antiviral medications. Many HIV infected patients can be treated as outpatients if the source of fever does not dictate admission and CD4 counts are above 200. The patients can be discharged if adequate followup exists and the patient can adequately care for themselves. Patients with suspected recent HIV infection should be referred for testing and counseling.

If Standard Treatment Fails

Due to the complexity of opportunistic infections and malignancies inherent to HIV infection, the physician should seek early consultation with pulmonologists, neurologists, gastroenterologists, and infectious disease experts.

For further reading in *Emergency Medicine, A Comprehensive Study Guide*, see Chapter 122, HIV Infection and AIDS, by Catherine A. Marco.

C. James Corrall

Tetanus is an acute, frequently fatal spasmodic disease that results from a wound infected with the organism *Clostridium tetani*. The clinical manifestations of tetanus are all secondary to an exotoxin elaborated at the wound site with resultant generalized muscular rigidity and muscular contractions.

Clinical Features

Despite safe and effective immunization, the prevention of tetanus is still a major health problem worldwide and an important cause of infant mortality in developing countries. Approximately 60 cases are reported in the United States each year, the majority of cases occur in patients over 50 years old who are inadequately immunized.

Tetanus occurs most frequently following an acute unreported injury, most commonly a puncture wound, but it can also develop after minor trauma, surgical procedures, abortions or in neonates, because of inadequate umbilical cord care. The majority of cases in the United States occur in rural southern states, predominantly in California, Texas, and Florida.

The incubation period of tetanus can range from less than 24 h to over 30 days. The shorter incubation is associated with more severe disease and worse prognosis for recovery. Clinically, tetanus can be categorized into four forms based upon site of inoculation and incubation period: local, generalized, cephalic, and neonatal.

Local tetanus is manifested by persistent rigidity of muscles in close proximity to the injury site and usually resolves without sequelae. Rarely, local tetanus may progress to the generalized form of the disease. Generalized tetanus is the most common form of the disease and most frequently presents with pain and stiffness in the jaw and trunk muscles. Later, the rigidity leads to the development of trismus and the characteristic facial expression, *risus sardonicus* (devil's smile). Reflex spasms and tonic contractions of all muscle groups are responsible for the other symptoms of the disease, which include dysphagia, opisthotonos, flexing of the arms, fist clenching, and extension of the lower extremities. Patients are conscious and alert throughout these spasms unless laryngospasm and tetanic contraction of respiratory muscles causes respiratory compromise.

Autonomic nervous system dysfunction resulting in a hypersympathetic state occurs in the second week of the illness and is manifested as tachycardia, labile hypertension, profuse sweating, and hyperpyrexia. Such autonomic dysfunction contributes to morbidity and mortality and are difficult to manage.

Cephalic tetanus follows injuries to the head and neck area and occasionally results in dysfunction of cranial nerves, most often the seventh nerve. This form of tetanus has a particularly poor prognosis.

Neonatal tetanus carries an extremely high mortality rate and is uniformly associated with inadequate maternal immunization and poor umbilical cord care. It is an important cause of mortality in developing countries and in some areas of the United States.

Diagnosis and Differential

Tetanus is diagnosed solely on the basis of the clinical exam. A history of active immunization with a booster dose within the previous 10 y eliminates tetanus as a diagnostic possibility. There are no confirmatory laboratory or microbiological tests. The differential diagnosis includes strychnine poisoning, dystonic reaction to phenothiazines, hypocalcemic tetany, rabies, and temporomandibular joint disease.

Emergency Department Care

The patient with tetanus should be managed in an ICU due to the potential for respiratory compromise. Environmental stimuli must be minimized in order to prevent precipitation of reflex convulsive spasms. Identification and debridement of the inciting wound, if present, is necessary to minimize further toxin production.

1. Tetanus immune globulin—Human tetanus immune globulin (TIG) neutralizes circulating toxin in the wound but not that which is fixed in the nervous system. A commonly recommended intramuscular dosage of **TIG** of 500 U has been shown to be as effective as higher doses and is given in a single injection.
2. Antibiotics—Antibiotics are of questionable value in the treatment of tetanus. If warranted, parenteral **metronidazole** (500 mg IV q6h) is the antibiotic of choice.
3. Muscle relaxants—The benzodiazepines, and in particular **diazepam** (5 mg IV q3h to effect), have been extensively used and result in sedation as well as amnesia, but **lorazepam** (2 mg IV to effect), because of its long duration of action, may be superior and the benzodiazepine of choice. Intravenous benzodiazepines may precipitate metabolic acidosis and can be avoided by an oral benzodiazepine such as midazolam. Other agents may be helpful as well and are discussed fully elsewhere.
4. Neuromuscular blockade—Neuromuscular blockade may be required to control ventilation and muscular spasm and to prevent fractures and rhabdomyolysis. In such cases, **vecuronium** (6–8 mg/hr IV) is the agent of choice because of its minimal cardiovascular side-effects. Sedation during neuromuscular blockade is mandatory.
5. Treatment of autonomic dysfunction—Combined alpha- and beta-adrenergic blocking agent, **labetalol** (0.25–1 mg/min continuous IV

infusion), has been used to treat the manifestations of sympathetic hyperactivity, but may precipitate myocardial depression. **Magnesium sulfate** (1–4 gm/h) has been advocated as a treatment for this condition as well. Continuous epidural block may be useful in the generalized form of the disease. **Morphine sulfate** (0.5–1 mg/kg/h) is also useful and provides sympathetic control without compromising cardiac output. **Clonidine** (300 µg q8h NG), an alpha-receptor agonist, may also be helpful in managing the cardiovascular instability.

6. Active immunization—Patients who recover from clinical tetanus *MUST* undergo active immunization because of lack of conference of immunity. Adsorbed tetanus toxoid should be administered intramuscularly at time of injury, at 6 wks and 6 mo post-injury. Tetanus–diphtheria (Td) should be administered to patients >7 years of age and diphtheria–pertussis–tetanus (DPT) to patients <7 years of age. A summary of guidelines for active immunization is presented in Table 85-1.

If Standard Treatment Fails

Few entities masquerade as clinical tetanus, and the initial management consists of recognition of the entity and treatment of the immediate

TABLE 85-1. Summary Guide to Tetanus Prophylaxis in Wound Management

History of Adsorbed Tetanus Toxoid (Doses)	Clean, Minor Wounds		All Other Wounds[a]	
	Td[b], 0.5 mL IM	TIG, 250 U IM	Td[b], 0.5 mL IM	TIG, 250 U IM
Unknown or <Three	Yes[c]	No	Yes	Yes
≥Three[d]	No[e]	No	Yes[f]	No

[a]For example, wounds <6 h old, contaminated with soil, saliva, feces, or dirt; puncture or crush wounds; avulsions; wounds from missiles, burns, or frostbite.
[b]DPT for children <7 y old (DT if pertussis vaccine is contraindicated); Td for persons >7 y old.
[c]The primary immunization series should be completed. Three doses total are required, with the second dose given at least 4 wks after the first, and the third dose 6 months later.
[d]If only three doses of fluid toxoid have been received, then a fourth dose of absorbed toxoid should be given.
[e]Yes, if routine immunization schedule has lapsed in a child <7 y of age or if >10 years since last dose.
[f]Yes, if routine immunization schedule has lapsed in a child <7 y of age or if >5 y since last dose. Boosters more frequent than every 5 y may predispose to side-effects.

lifethreatening events, in particular, respiratory compromise with appropriate airway management, minimization of muscular spasms with muscle relaxants, and management of autonomic dysfunction as outlined in Table 85-2.

RABIES

Rabies is a near only always fatal disease and represents the most serious potential complication of an animal bite. The disease is caused by an RNA-containing rhabdovirus and is transmitted by inoculation with infectious saliva or by salivary contact with a break in the skin or mucous membranes. The disease exists primarily in wildlife, which serves as the viral reservoir in endemic areas, but its prevalence in wild carnivores varies in different geographic areas, which accounts for differences in prevalence of rabies in domestic animal populations.

In developing countries where rabies is endemic, dogs are the primary reservoir of disease and the principle source of human exposure. In developed countries, such as the United States, dog and cat bites are the most common reason for implementation of postexposure prophylaxis, but the most important source of active rabies is wildlife transmis-

TABLE 85-2. Treatment of Tetanus

Respiratory management	Succinylcholine, 80 mg for emergency oral intubation; tracheostomy except in localized or mild tetanus
Immunotherapy	TIG 500 U IM as a single dose
	and
	Tetanus toxoid (DPT or Td depending on age), 0.5 mL IM at presentation, and 6 wks and 6 mo after presentation
Antibiotic therapy	Metronidazole, 500 mg IV every 6 h
	or
	Erythromycin 2 g/day
Muscle relaxation	Lorazepam, 2 mg IV to effect
	or
	Diazepam, 5 mg IV every 1–3 h to effect
	or
	Midazolam, 5–15 mg/h continuous IV infusion
Neuromuscular blockade	Vecuronium, 6–8 mg/h IV
Management of autonomic dysfunction	Labetalol, 0.25–1.0 mg/min continuous IV infusion
	or
	Magnesium sulfate, 70 mg/kg IV loading, then 1–4 g/h continuous infusion to maintain blood level of 2.5–4 mmo/L
	Morphine sulfate, 0.5–1.0 mg/kg per h
	Clonidine, 300 µg every 8 h per NG tube

sion. Animal bites contracted outside the United States in an undeveloped country should be considered at high risk for rabies transmission.

Rabid wildlife species include skunks, bats, raccoons, cows, dogs, foxes, and cats. Rodents (squirrels, chipmunks, rats, mice, etc.) and lagomorphs (rabbits, hares, etc.) have never been implicated as carriers, and bites by these animals are not at risk for transmission. Most rabid animals are agitated and labile, may indiscriminately attack anything that moves and may wander aimlessly. Feeble bark, drooling, stupor, and convulsions mark more advanced disease preceding death of the animal.

Clinical Features

As human rabies has decreased in the United States, the proportion of rabies patients without animal-bite exposure has increased. In 60% of the cases in the 1980s, a source of infection was not identified. In such untreated rabid bites, the risk of contracting rabies ranges from 5% to 80%. Rabid hand and foot bites carry a 15% to 20% mortality; rabid head and neck bites carry a 50% mortality.

Incubation periods average 35 to 64 days; periods as short as 12 days or as long as 700 days have been reported and are dependent on the size of the viral inoculum, host immunity, and bite location.

The initial symptoms of human rabies are nonspecific: fever, malaise, headache, anorexia, nausea, sore throat, cough, and pain or paresthesias at the bite site (80%) may last for 1 to 4 days. Subsequently CNS involvement becomes apparent, with restlessness and agitation, altered mental status, painful bulbar and peripheral muscular spasms, opisthotonos, and bulbar or focal motor paresis. Alternatively, in 20% an ascending, symmetric, flaccid and areflexic paralysis, comparable to the Landry–Guillain–Barré syndrome may be seen. Hypersensitivity to sensory stimuli and hydrophobia may occur at this stage, the latter resulting from the sight, sound, swallowing, or even mention of water. Progressively, lucid and confused intervals may become interspersed, cholinergic nervous abnormalities may manifest (hyperpyrexia, mydriasis, and increased lacrimation and salivation), and brainstem dysfunction (dysphagia, optic neuritis, and facial palsies) with hyperreflexia and extensor plantar responses may occur, mimicking many toxidromes and botulism. Common complications include adult respiratory distress syndrome, diabetes insipidus, SIADH, hypovolemia, electrolyte abnormalities, pneumonia and cardiogenic shock with hypotension and arrhythmia from rabies myocarditis. Coma, convulsions, and apnea are the final manifestations of rabid death.

Death universally occurs in 4 to 7 days in untreated patients, which may be prolonged to 25 days if supportive care is instituted. There are three reported cases of neurologically intact survivors of rabies, who received rabies vaccine before onset of symptoms and intensive supportive care. In these patients, supportive care maintained vital functions while the patient's stimulated immune response eradicated the infection. Such recoveries, however, are exceedingly rare.

Diagnosis and Differential

The diagnosis of rabies in animals and humans is made by postmortem analysis of brain tissue. Analysis for Negri bodies is highly specific, but carries a 5% false-negative rate. Fluorescent antibody testing (FAT) has become the procedure of choice due to low cost, speed, and reliability when performed in a competent laboratory. More recently, enzyme-linked immunosorbent assay techniques have been employed, with results comparable to those with FAT and tissue culture. Serum antibody titers in unimmunized patients become positive between days 6 and 19, and a fourfold increase in these patients in antibody titers is considered diagnostic. CSF titers for rabies antibodies become positive between days 8 and 169 with titers of 1:100 or higher being diagnostic. Elevated CSF protein and a mononuclear pleocytosis are also seen. In vaccinated patients, CSF analysis for rabies antibodies suggests the diagnosis, as immunizations alone rarely produce detectable antibodies in the CSF.

The differential diagnosis includes viral or other infectious encephalitis, polio, tetanus, viral process, meningitis, brain abscess, septic cavernous sinus thrombosis, cholinergic poisoning, and the Landry–Guillain–Barré syndrome. The diagnosis is especially difficult without history of exposure but should be considered in patients with a picture of progressive and unexplained encephalitis.

Emergency Department Care

The treatment of rabies exposure consists of assessment of risk of rabies, public health and animal control notification and, if warranted, the administration of specific immunobiological products to protect against rabies. These measures are usually performed in the ED together but may at times require time between modalities, although never at the risk of patient infection. Since no fetal abnormalities have been reported, and because of the possibilities of rabies infection without passive and active protection, pregnant patients should receive the same treatment as nonpregnant individuals. A unified approach to such management is outlined in Figure 85-1 and the treatment is summarized below.

1. Local wound care—Debridement of devitalized tissue, if any, is important in reducing the viral inoculum. Wounds of special concern should not be sutured as this promotes rabies virus replication.
2. Prophylactic antibiotics—May be indicated for other reasons but have no effect on the replication of rabies virus.
3. Tetanus prophylaxis—Tetanus should always be considered and primary or reimmunization prophylaxis should be administered.

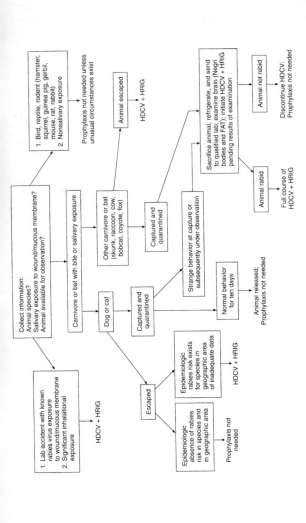

FIG. 85-1. Clinical guidelines for administration of rabies postexposure prophylaxis. FAT, fluorescent antibody test; HDCV, human diploid cell vaccine. HRIG, human rabies immune globulin. (Adapted from Mann JM. Rabies risk: Systematic evaluation and management of animal bites. *Comp Ther* 7:53, 1981. Used by permission.)

4. Human Rabies Immune Globulin (HRIG)—Administered once at the onset of therapy. The dose is 20 IU/kg, with half of the dose (based on volume constraints) infiltrated locally at the exposure site and the remainder administered intramuscularly. Each vial of HRIG contains 2 ml (300 IU) for passive immunization.
5. Human Diploid Cell Vaccine—For active immunization, it produces excellent IgG and IgM antibody responses by day 7 after initial administration. Administered in 5 1-ml doses on day 0, 3, 7, 14, and 28. The World Health Organization recommends a sixth dose on day 90, but this is not universally accepted.
6. Quarantine of animals inflicting wounds—Ordinarily withheld for domestic dogs and cats with normal behavior, and quarantined for 10 days, which is sufficient for the disease to manifest if the animal is infected. If no signs become apparent, the animal can be considered nonrabid. The principal indication for the initiation of prophylaxis is a bite wound by an uncaptured dog or cat in an endemic area, or a bite wound by an uncaptured bat or appropriate species of carnivore.
7. Notify state and local health department and animal control agencies—State or local officials should be consulted regarding the possibility of rabies in local dog or cat populations before decisions on initiating postexposure rabies prophylaxis are made. Both animal bites and rabies are reportable entities in all states. Animal bites should be reported to the local animal control unit or police departments so that appropriate animals can be captured and quarantined for observation in a timely fashion.

If Standard Treatment Fails

Rabies antibody titers are not recommended following the fifth dose on day 28 for healthy individuals but are recommended for an incomplete immunization course or immunocompromised patients (particularly those on corticosteroids). Both RIG and HDCV should be administered in the deltoid muscle rather than in the gluteal area due to vaccine failures at the latter site.

Adverse reactions following the use of HRIG are limited to local pain and low-grade fever, which are transient and can be treated with salicylates or NSAIDs. HDCV can precipitate similar local reactions and may manifest mild headache, nausea, dizziness, and myalgias; booster recipients have experienced an immune complex-like reaction. Rabies prophylaxis should not be stopped because of mild reactions, but serious neuroparalysis or anaphylaxis during treatment poses a therapeutic dilemma. Postexposure assessment of the clinical risk of rabies must be weighed against the risks of treatment with continuation of therapy, switching to an alternative vaccine, pretreatment with antihistamine for hypersensitive patients, or discontinuation of treatment. Both the CDC and state or county health departments can provide assistance in the management of complications.

Recent reviews suggest that initial presentations of active rabies in humans is so nonspecific that it is almost always missed, resulting in significant exposure of ED staff to infectious secretions. Universal precautions should always be utilized in patients with unexplained encephalopathy. Management of exposure to such patients is beyond the scope of this chapter and reader is referred for guidance to federal and state health officials.

For further reading in *Emergency Medicine, A Comprehensive Study Guide*, see Chapter 123, Tetanus, by Donna L. Carden; and Chapter 124, Rabies, by Louis S. Binder.

With increased international travel to tropical locales, more Americans are contracting malaria. A diagnosis of malaria must be considered in any person returning from the tropics with an unexplained febrile illness.

Etiology

Four species of the protozoa *Plasmodium* infect humans: *P. vivax, P. ovale, P. malariae,* and *P. falciparum.* The organism is transmitted by the bite of a female anopheline mosquito, found in tropical and subtropical regions. Plasmodial sporozoites travel to the liver where asexual reproduction occurs (exoerythorocytic stage). After several weeks, the liver cell ruptures, releasing daughter merozoites into the blood where they rapidly invade erythrocytes (erythrocytic stage). In *P. vivax* and *P. ovale* infections, some intrahepatic forms are not released and stay dormant for months. These forms can later activate, causing relapse. The clinical manifestations of malaria first appear in the erythrocytic stage. Merozoites mature in erythrocytes in various forms, including early ring forms, trophozoites, and schizonts (masses of new merozoites). Eventually the erythrocyte lyses, and new merozoites invade more red cells, continuing the infection. These cycles tend to occur at regular intervals, giving rise to the classic periodicity of symptoms. After several cycles, some merozoites become sexual forms, or gametocytes. Upon ingestion by another feeding mosquito, these forms undergo sexual reproduction, ready for reintroduction into a human host.

Malaria may also be transmitted by blood transfusion or passed transplacentally from mother to fetus.

Malaria transmission occurs in large areas of Central and South America, the Caribbean, sub-Saharan Africa, the Indian subcontinent, Southeast Asia, the Middle East, and Oceania. More than half of all U.S. cases of malaria, including most cases caused by *P. falciparum,* arise from travel to sub-Saharan Africa. Resistance of *P. falciparum* to chloroquine continues to spread, and strains exist that resist other agents as well. The CDC has a 24-h hotline (404-332-4555), which can provide the most recent information on resistance patterns. Although malaria is largely preventable through mosquito protection measures and chemoprophylaxis, malaria can be contracted or can recur.

Clinical Features

The incubation period ranges from one to several weeks. Partial chemoprophylaxis or incomplete immunity can markedly prolong the incubation period to months or even years. The hallmark of malaria is the recurring febrile paroxysm, which corresponds to hemolysis of infected erythrocytes. With *P. falciparum*, hemolysis can be very high, since red cells of all ages are affected. Infected red cells lose flexibility and are removed in the microcirculation with resultant obstruction and tissue anoxia.

Patients develop a prodrome of malaise, myalgias, headache, and low-grade fever and chills. The early manifestations are nonspecific and may resemble viral illness, influenza, or hepatitis. Illness progresses to high fever, severe chills, orthostatic dizziness, and extreme weakness. The malarial paroxysm—rigor and fever followed by profuse diaphoresis and exhaustion—occurs at regular intervals that correspond to the length of the asexual erythrocytic cycle. The paroxysms may not be present in *P. falciparum* malaria.

The findings on physical exam are also nonspecific. Most patients look acutely ill, with high fever, tachycardia, tachypnea. Splenomegaly is common. In falciparum infections, hepatomegaly, edema, and icterus occur often. Laboratory features include normocytic normochromic anemia, hemolysis, and thrombocytopenia. The WBC is normal or low.

Complications of malaria can occur rapidly, particularly with *P. falciparum*. All forms cause hemolysis and splenomegaly and predispose to splenic rupture. An immune mediated glomerulonephritis occurs most often in *P. malariae* infections. With its high degree of parasitemia, *P. falciparum* infections are especially virulent and can be fatal. Cerebral malaria, characterized by somnolence, coma, delirium, and seizures, has a mortality rate over 20%. Other life-threatening complications associated with *P. falciparum* include noncardiogenic pulmonary edema and metabolic abnormalities, including lactic acidosis and profound hypoglycemia. Blackwater fever is a severe renal complication seen almost exclusively in *P. falciparum* infections, associated with massive intravascular hemolysis, jaundice, hemoglobinuria, and acute renal failure.

Diagnosis

The definitive diagnosis is established by visualization of the parasite on Giemsa-stained thin and thick smears. In early infection, especially *P. falciparum* in which parasitized red cells are often sequestered from the bloodstream, parasitemia may be undetectable initially. Parasitemia also fluctuates over time and is highest during chills and as the fever is on the rise. Not being able to detect parasitemia is not an indication to withhold therapy. If parasitemia is not seen in the thin smear, a thick smear which concentrates the parasites may improve the yield, but interpretation requires expertise, as artifacts are common. If parasites are not visualized, repeated smears should be taken at least twice daily for 3 days to fully exclude malaria.

Once malaria is diagnosed, the two major issues that the smear answers are the degree of parasitemia, which correlates with prognosis, and whether *P. falciparum* is present. Most patients with *P. falciparum* should be hospitalized, as should any patient with more than 3% parasitemia. Clues to *P. falciparum* infection include small ring forms with double chromatin knobs within the red cell, multiple rings in individual red cells, a paucity of trophozoites and schizonts on smear, the pathognomonic crescent or banana-shaped gametocyte, and parasitemia exceeding 4%.

Emergency Department Care

If *P. falciparum* can be excluded, most patients can be treated as outpatients with close followup, including repeated blood smears. Patients with significant hemolysis or with underlying diseases that can be aggravated by high fevers or hemolysis are best hospitalized, as are infants and pregnant women.

The drug of choice for treatment of infection due to *P. vivax*, *P. ovale*, and *P. malariae* is chloroquine. Table 86-1 summarizes recommended treatment regimens. With treatment, the parasite load should decrease significantly over the first 24 to 48 h. No asexual forms of the parasite should persist 3 to 4 days after treatment is completed. Gametocytes, the sexual form, may persist for several weeks after treatment and do not represent treatment failure. Chloroquine has no effect on the exoerythrocytic parasites, which remain dormant in the liver in infection due to *P. vivax* and *P. ovale*. Unless further treatment with primaquine is given, relapse will occur. Primaquine should be avoided in patients with G6PD deficiency because it can cause hemolysis. Despite treatment with both chloroquine and primaquine, persistence of infection or relapse may still occur.

P. falciparum infections are best managed in the hospital. Unless certain that the patient could not be chloroquine-resistant based on geographic exposure, it is best to assume that the infection is resistant and initiate treatment with a combination of quinine and pyrimethamine–sulfadoxine or doxycycline. Mefloquine is also an effective therapy for chloroquine resistant *P. falciparum* (and the asexual erythrocytic phase of other plasmodial species). Halofantrine, a new agent, is especially useful for self-treatment of presumptive malaria acquired in Southeast Asia if multiple drug resistance is suspected.

Patients presenting with complications of *P. falciparum*, or with high parasitemia but unable to tolerate oral medication, should receive intravenous treatment. Exchange transfusions have been life-saving in some patients with parasitemia over 10%. Quinidine is probably the intravenous drug of choice. Parenteral quinine is only available from the CDC. Both drugs are associated with severe hypoglycemia and are contraindicated in patients with cardiac disease. Because cinchona alkaloids are myocardial depressants, cardiac monitoring is recommended during administration. Terminal treatment with primaquine is not necessary in *P. falciparum* because of lack of dormant forms in the liver.

For further reading in *Emergency Medicine, A Comprehensive Study Guide*, see Chapter 125, Malaria, by Jeffrey D. Band.

TABLE 86-1. Treatment Regimens for Malaria

Clinical Setting	Drug	Dosage Guidelines	
		Adults	Children
Uncomplicated infection with *P. vivax, P. ovale, P. malariae,* and chloroquine-sensitive *P. falciparum*	Chloroquine phosphate	1-g load (600-mg base), then 500 mg (300-mg base) in 6 h, then 500 mg (300-mg base) per day for 2 days (total dose 2.5 g)	10 mg/kg base to maximum of 600 mg load, then 5 mg/kg base in 6 h and 6 mg/kg base per day for 2 days
	plus		
	Primaquine-phosphate[a]	26.3 mg load (15-mg base) per day for 14 days upon completion of chloroquine therapy	0.3 mg/kg base for 14 days upon completion of chloroquine therapy
Uncomplicated infection with chloroquine-resistant *P. falciparum*	Quinine sulfate	650 mg PO tid for 5–7 days	8.3 mg/kg PO tid for 5–7 days[b]
	plus		
	Pyrimethamine-sulfadozine (Fansidar)[c]	3 tablets (75 mg/1500 mg) PO × 1 dose	plus Over 2 months old: >50 kg 3 tabs 30–50 1 tab 15–29 1 tab 10–14 ½ tab 4–9 ¼ tab
	plus		
	Doxycycline	100 mg PO bid for 10 days	Contraindicated in children <8 y of age
	or		
	Mefloquine	1250 mg PO × 1	1 tablet/10 kg PO × I[d]
	plus		
	Doxycycline	See above	See above
	or		
	Halofantrine[f]	500 mg 6 h apart for 3 doses (repeat again in 1 wk)	8 mg/kg salt orally, given q 6 h for 3 doses (repeat again in 1 wk)

Complicated infection with chloroquine-resistant *P. falciparum*	Quinidine gluconate	10 mg/kg load over 2 h then 0.02 mg/kg per min continuous infusion until patient stabilizes and is able to tolerate PO therapy	Same as adults[g]
	plus		
	Doxycycline	100 mg IV q 12 h until tolerating PO therapy	Contraindicated in children <8 y of age

[a]Terminal treatment of *P. vivax* and *P. ovale* only.
[b]If unable to administer with doxycycline due to patient's age, extend treatment to full 10 days.
[c]Optional; of unlikely value if acquisition in area with Fansidar resistance.
[d]Not formally approved yet by FDA in this setting.
[e]Optional; many experts feel comfortable with mefloquine alone.
[f]Although FDA approved, halofantrine is not yet commercially available in the United States. (Contact SmithKline Beecham at 1-800-366-8900.) Becoming drug of choice for self-treatment of presumptiver malaria in Thai–Cambodian and Myanmar borders *if* access to medical care is not available. In these areas, may need to extend treatment to 3 days instead of 1 day.
[g]Consult an expert in pediatric infectious disease immediately for guidance.

In the United States, parasitic disease is increasingly common due to immigration from developing countries, increased travel abroad, and increased infection in immunosuppressed persons, especially those with HIV. This chapter reviews selected helminths and protozoa.

History and Clinical Features

In considering parasitic diseases, ask about travel to or immigration from high-risk areas. Parasites flourish in warm, moist climates with poor sanitation and nutrition. Children are more often infected than adults because of their poor hygiene, oral behavior, and inability to ward off arthropod vectors. Parasitic disease should be considered in any patient with fever, abdominal pain, diarrhea, skin rash, ulcers, or eosinophilia. Symptoms may be protean, as listed in Table 87-1, making diagnosis more difficult because there may be a latent period of months to years between exposure and symptoms. Certain specific areas of the world may implicate particular parasites. Hmong tribesmen from Southeast Asia often harbor the lung fluke *Paragonimus*, whereas vistors to Leningrad or the Rockies may return with *Giardia*. The presence of historical risk factors can also provide clues (Table 87-2).

Diagnosis

Multiple symptoms are associated with parasitic infections. Diarrhea is a particularly common symptom; testing the stool for ova and parasites is the best way to detect intestinal parasites. Ideally, three specimens should be collected on different days, with the stool free of substances such as barium, bismuth, and mineral oil. Antimicrobial agents should be stopped at least 1 wk prior to collection. Fresh specimens are best, and specimens over 1 h old should be preserved with formalin or polyvinyl alcohol. Obviously, these conditions are often quite difficult to achieve in the ED. Other specialized tests include acid-fast stain of stool specimens, useful for detection of *Cryptosporidia, Isospora*, and *Cyclospora*. For pinworms, the most useful test is a cellophane tape swab of the perianal area. Occasionally, *Giardia, Cryptosporidia*, and the larvae of *Strongyloides* may be detected by examining a duodenal aspirate or by having the patient swallow a string with a gelatin capsule (Entero-test).

HELMINTHS

Helminths are multicellular worms. A useful characteristic is that helminths, unlike protozoa, usually induce eosinophilia, an important clue to infection.

TABLE 87-1. Common Symptoms of Parasitic Disease

Symptom	Possible Cause
Urticaria	*Ascaris, Strongyloides, Dracunculus, Trichinella, Fasciola*
Diarrhea	Hookworm, *Strongyloides, Trichuris, Trichinella, Schistosoma, Fasciola, Fasciolopsis, Taenia, Hymenolepis, Entamoeba, Giardia, Dientamoeba, Palantidium, Leishmania donovani*
Abdominal pain	*Ascaris,* hookworm, *Trichuris, Schistosoma, Entamoeba, Clonorchis, Fasciola, Taenia, Hymenolepis, Diphyllobothrium, Giardia*
Pruritis	*Enterobius, Trichuris,* filariae (*Onchocerca volvulus*), *Dientamoeba, Leishmania*
Nausea and vomiting	*Ascaris, Trichuris, Trichinella, Taenia, Entamoeba, Giardia, Leishmania*
Skin ulcers	*Dracunculus,* hookworm (*Ancylostoma duodenale*), *L. donovani, Trypanosoma*
Splenomegaly	*Babesia, Toxoplasma, Plasmodium* species
Intestinal obstruction	*Ascaris, Strongyloides,* fluke (*Fasciolopsis buski*), *Taenia, Diphyllobothrium*
Eosinophilia	*Strongyloides,* hookworm, *Trichuris, Dracunculus, Fasciola, Toxocara, Ascaris, Trichinella,* filariae (*W. bancrofti, B. malayi*) *Hymenolepis, Schistosoma,* fluke (*P. westermani, C. sinensis, Fasciolopsis leuski*), *Taenia*
Fever	*Ascaris, Toxocara,* hookworm, *Trichuris, Trichinella,* filariae (*W. bancrofti*), *Schistosoma,* fluke (*C. sinensis*), *Fasciola, Entamoeba, Giardia, Trypanosoma, L. donovai, Babesia, Plasmodium* species
Hepatomegaly	*trypanosoma, L. donovani, Toxocara, Schistosoma,* fluke (*C. sinensis, O. viverrini, Fasciola*), tapeworm (*Echinococcus*), *Plasmodium* species

Nematodes (Roundworms)

Nematodes are cylindrical, elongated white worms. Humans are infected by egg ingestion (Ascaris, Enterobius), skin penetration (Necator), and insect bite (filiariae). The intestinal nematodes include hookworm, roundworm, and whipworm, in which a soil phase is needed for fecally passed eggs to develop. Thus, these infections usually occur in areas of poor sanitation. (Pinworm eggs are infectious when passed so person-to-person spread can occur.) The tissue nematodes include filiarae, arthropod-borne worms, which induce lymphatic, ocular, and skin disease but are much less common in the United States and will not be further discussed here.

TABLE 87-2. Risk Factors for Parasitic Disease

Blood transfusion—*Plasmodium* species, *Trypanosoma, Babesia, Toxoplasma*
Intravenous drug use—*Plasmodium* species
Homosexuality—*Entamoeba* (often seen after colonic irrigation therapy), *Giardia, Cryptosporidium*
Immunocompromised host—*Toxoplasma, Pneumocystis, Strongyloides, Cryptosporidium, Microsporidium, Isospora,* and *Cyclospora*
Institutionalization—*H. nana, Entamoeba histolytica, Giardia*
Day care centers—*Giardia, Cryptosporidium*
Livestock workers—*Cryptosporidium*
Pica—*Toxocara* (visceral larva migrans), hookworm (*Necator Americanus*)
Consumption of raw food
Sushi, sashimi, gefilte fish—*Diphyllobothrium, Anisakis*
Pork—*Taenia solium, Trichinella, Sarcocystis*
Beef—*Taenia saginata, Toxoplasma, Sarcocystis*

Ascaris (Roundworm)

After ingestion of *Ascaris* eggs, the larvae migrate through the lungs; they are then swallowed and mature into worms in the small intestine. During the lung phase, patients may develop pulmonary infiltrates (Loffler's syndrome), with fever, cough, dyspnea, and hemoptysis. Adult worms in the intestines are often asymptomatic, despite their large size (10–35 cm), but they may produce intestinal obstruction in heavy infections, especially in children. Worm migration into the biliary tract can also cause biliary obstruction and pancreatitis. Treatment is with **mebendazole** (100 mg po bid × 3 days), **albendazole** (400 mg po single dose), or **pyrantel pamoate** (11 mg/kg single dose, up to 1.0 gm). Surgery may be needed for intestinal obstruction.

Enterobius (Pinworm)

Adult pinworms inhabit the intestines after humans ingest their eggs. The gravid female travels to the anus at night where it causes intense itching. Pinworm most often affects children. The diagnosis is confirmed with cellophane tape swab of the anus. Eosinophilia is usually absent, unlike *Ascaris* and *Necator*. Treatment is with **pyrantel pamoate** (11 mg/kg single dose, up to 1.0 gm), **mebendazole** (100 mg/ po bid × 3 days), or **albendazole** (400 mg po single dose, repeated in 2 wks). All close household contacts of the patient should be treated.

Strongyloides (Threadworm)

Because this worm enters the body through the skin, allergic manifestations occur, including itching and rash. Migration through the lungs can cause cough, dyspnea, and pneumonia. The intestinal phase produces diarrhea and abdominal pain. A unique feature of this worm is its ability to reproduce in the host without reinfection. This means that strongyloides may persist for decades. In immunosuppressed persons, the reproductive cycle may be magnified, leading to hyperinfection, which is often fatal. Diagnosis is made by finding larvae in the stool or duodenal contents. Treatment is with **thiabendazole** (22 mg/kg up to 1.5 gm po bid × 2 days) or **ivermectin** (200 mcg/kg/day × 2 days).

Necator americanus (Hookworm)

Hookworm is more common in the South and is associated with use of human fertilizer and lack of shoes and latrines. Infection is percutaneous and may induce rash. There may be pulmonary and gastrointestinal symptoms related to worm migration. This worm also ingests blood and infection may lead to iron-deficiency anemia. Diagnosis is by stool testing for eggs. Treatment is with **mebendazole** (100 mg po bid × 3 days), **pyrantel pamoate** (11 mg/kg single dose, up to 1.0 gm), or **albendazole** (400 mg po single dose).

Trichuris trichiura (Whipworm)

Trichuris is most common in the rural South, most often in children who play in the soil. If symptoms occur, they are usually gastrointestinal. *Trichuris* can result in rectal prolapse or colitis in children. Diagnosis is made by stool testing. **Mebendazole** (100 mg po bid × 3 days) and **albendazole** (400 mg po single dose) are the drugs of choice.

Trichinella spiralis

Trichinosis is common in Mexico and the United States and comes from eating infected pork. In the early enteric stage, GI symptoms predominate. Later, larvae travel to muscle where encystment starts 3 wks after infection. Symptoms include periorbital edema, splinter and subconjunctival hemorrhages, myalgia, urticaria, headache, weakness, and fever. Although encystment occurs only in striated muscle, inflammation occurs in the heart, lungs, and nervous system also, with myocarditis, bronchopneumonia, and CNS disturbances. Laboratory clues include eosinophilia and elevation of muscle enzymes. The triad of periorbital edema, myalgias, and eosinophilia strongly suggests trichinosis. The diagnosis can be confirmed serologically. Biopsy of involved muscle may be helpful after the fourth week. Stool specimens are only helpful early. Mebendazole (100 mg po bid × 3 days) is indicated for the intestinal phase but may not be effective after encystment. Steroids are indicated for serious CNS disease and myocarditis but not routinely. Most cases are mild, self-limited, and resolve without specific therapy.

Trematodes (Flukes)

These are leaflike symmetrical flatworms that live in intermediate hosts like snails, crabs, and fish in the tropics. *Clonorchis*, the liver fluke, is endemic in the Far East and causes biliary disease. *Paragonimus*, the lung fluke, produces hemoptysis and lung disease. The most common fluke-borne disease is schistosomiasis. Schistosomes penetrate the skin, inducing dermatitis. Acute disease (Katayama fever) includes fever, cough, hepatosplenomegaly, urticaria, and eosinophilia. Chronic disease occurs from egg deposition in the bladder, intestines, and liver, with resultant scarring. In *S. hematobium*, dysuria, hematuria, and infection occur. With the other schistosomes, there is cirrhosis and portal hypertension. The diagnosis is made by finding eggs in urine or stool or by rectal biopsy. **Praziquantel** (75 mg/kg/day divided tid × 1 day) is the treatment of choice.

Cestodes (Flatworms)

Commonly referred to as tapeworms, these worms grow by segmentation, producing new proglottids, which can be detected in stool specimens. The most common tapeworm in the U.S. is the dwarf tapeworm, *Hymenolepsis nana*, which often occurs in children and in institutions. Other tapeworms seen in the U.S. include:

Taenia

Taenia solium (pork tapeworm) occurs occasionally in the U.S. in immigrants from Central America or the Middle East. *Taenia saginita* (beef tapeworm) is more common, seen in persons who eat raw beef. Adult worms live in the small intestine. Infections may be asymptomatic or cause gastrointestinal distress, weight loss, and weakness. Eggs or proglottids may be identified in the stool, or eggs may be detected by perianal tape application. **Praziquantel** (25 mg/kg, single dose) is the treatment of choice. *T. solium* can also cause another, more serious disease, cystocercosis, in which eggs encyst in multiple organs. When the cysts degenerate, a host reaction occurs, including inflammation, necrosis, and calcification. The most serious forms involve the eye, heart, and brain. X-rays show curvilinear calcifications in soft tissues (like puffed rice), and CT also demonstrates the cysts. The drugs of choice are **albendazole** (7.5 mg/kg po tid × 8 days) and **praziquantel** (20 mg/kg po tid × 14 days).

Diphyllobothrium

This fish tapeworm occurs where raw fish (sushi, sashami, gefilte fish) are eaten. The worm competes with the host for vitamin B12, so patients may present with vitamin B12 deficiency. Treatment is the same as for *taenia*.

PROTOZOA

Amebiasis

Amebiasis, caused by *E. histolytica*, is associated with poor sanitation. Transmission is by fecal–oral contamination. Outbreaks have been reported at institutions and in homosexuals. Amebae inhabit the cecum and ascending colon, where they cause inflammation and ulcers. An ameboma can rarely develop in the liver and mimic abscess. Half of all infected patients are asymptomatic. Symptoms include nausea, vomiting, diarrhea, fever, and abdominal pain. As with other protozoan infections, there is no eosinophilia. The diagnosis is made by stool testing. Serologic tests are helpful, especially for extraintestinal disease. Treatment is with **metronizadole** (35–50 mg/kg/day divided tid up to 750 mg tid × 10 days) or **tinazadole** (50 mg/kg/day divided bid up to 1 gm bid × 3 days).

Giardia

This protozoan is the most common intestinal parasite in the US. It inhabits the proximal small intestine. Cysts are ingested in fecally contaminated water and food. Water-borne outbreaks are increasingly common because cysts resist chlorination. Outbreaks by person-to-person spread have also occurred in day-care centers and institutions. Many infected persons are asymptomatic. Acute symptoms include watery diarrhea, abdominal cramps, nausea, fever, burping, and flatus, and stools are greasy and malodorous. Chronic diarrhea with weight loss and malabsorption may also occur. Diagnosis is by stool testing. Occasionally, duodenal aspiration, string testing, or small bowel biopsy may be needed. Treatment is with **metronidazole** (15 mg/kg/day divided tid up to 250 mg tid × 5 days).

Trypanosoma

American trypanosomiasis (Chagas disease) is transmitted by the reduvid (kissing) bug, although it can also be transmitted by transfusion. A nodular swelling appears at the site of bite. The acute phase lasts several months and includes fever, headache, conjunctivitis, rash and, in severe cases, myocarditis or meningoencephalitis. Chronic infection leads to cardiac disease with heart failure and rhythm disturbances, as well as gastrointestinal disease with megacolon and megaesophagus. During the acute phase, blood smear and serology may be helpful. In the chronic phase, serology or biopsy of the liver, spleen, or marrow can be diagnostic. **Nifurtimox** (8–10 mg/kg/day po divided qid × 120 days) is the drug of choice.

Babesia

Babesia microti is transmitted by ixodes ticks, the same vector as Lyme disease, and occasionally by blood transfusion. In the U.S., babesiosis occurs most commonly in the Northeast. Patients present with fevers, splenomegaly, hemolysis, and jaundice. Infection can be fatal in splenectomized patients. Diagnosis is made by blood smear, but may be mistaken for malaria. Also in the differential is Lyme disease and Rocky Mountain spotted fever. Treatment is with **clindamycin** (600 mg po tid × 7 days) and **quinine** (650 mg po tid × 7 days).

Cryptosporidium

Previously regarded as a disease of immunosuppressed persons, *Cryptosporidium* is now recognized as an important cause of diarrhea worldwide. Water-borne transmission is well-documented. *Cryptosporidium* can also affect cows; runoff from dairies may contaminate reservoirs. *Cryptosporidium* alters small intestinal villi. The diarrhea is profuse and watery, usually without blood or fecal leukocytes. There may be abdominal cramping, nausea, vomiting, and fever. In normal hosts, the illness lasts several days to wks, but immunocompromised patients, particularly with AIDS, have protracted diarrhea, with dehydration, malabsorption, and weight loss. Diagnosis is made by stool testing with an acid-fast stain. Treatment is **Paromomycin** 500–750 mg qid in adults. Infection is self-limited in normal hosts.

Protozoan Infections in the Immunocompromised Host

Respiratory Tract

Pneumonia in the immmunocompromised host is often due to *Pneumocystis carinii*. Patients present with fever, dyspnea, and dry cough. Blood gases show hypoxia or widened A-a gradient. The LDH is often elevated. Early, the chest x-ray may be normal. Later, the chest x-ray classically shows symmetrical interstitial infiltrates in the mid- and lower lung zones. *P. carinii* occurs in premature or debilitated infants, AIDS patients, organ transplant patients, and patients on immunosuppressive agents. Diagnosis is usually made by sputum exam, lung lavage, or biopsy. Treatment is with **trimethoprim/sulfamethoxazole** (DS tablet po qd × 21 days) or **pentamidine** (300 mg by aerosol, every 4 wks). If respiratory compromise is present ($PO_2 < 70$ mmHg or elevated A-a gradient), steroids are also beneficial in addition to trimethoprim/sulfamethoxazole (20 mg/kg/day divided q8h IV) or pentamidine (4 mg/kg/day for 21 days).

Gastrointestinal Tract

Most patients with AIDS develop diarrhea, which is often protracted and life-threatening at some time in their disease. Among the protozoal causes are *Cryptosporidium* and closely related pathogens *Isospora*, *Microsporidia*, and *Cyclospora*. *Isospora belli* can be detected with acid-fast stain of the stool; treatment is **trimethoprim/sulfamethoxazole** (DS tablet po qid × 10 days, then bid × 21 days). *Microsporidium* also presents with diarrhea, but hepatitis, peritonitis, and keratitis have also been described. Diagnosis by stool exam is difficult due to the small spore size, so intestinal biopsy is sometimes required. There is no standard treatment; octreotide, metronidazole, and albendazole may be tried.

Central Nervous System

Toxoplasma is an intracellular parasite of mammals, which can be devastating in immunocompromised patients. Infection occurs from oocyst ingestion in undercooked meats, placental transfer, following organ transplant, or transfusion. Cats are a common source of infection for humans. During acute infection, transient lymphadenopathy and splenomegaly can occur but is often asymptomatic. Reactivation can result in encephalitis, chorioretinitis, myocarditis, and pneumonia. Symptoms of cerebral toxoplasmosis include headache, seizures, confusion, lethargy, and focal deficits. An ELISA test for *Toxoplasma* antibodies is available but is less reliable in AIDS patients due to low titers. CT typically reveals lesions with ring enhancement following contrast. MRI is even more sensitive. The treatment of choice is **pyrimethamine** (200 mg po loading dose, then 50–75 mg qd × 3–6 wks) plus **sulfadiazine** (4–8 gms po qd × 3–6 wks).

Gregory S. Hall

In the United States, ticks are responsible for more vector-borne diseases than any other arthropod agent. Ticks can transmit infections caused by bacteria, viruses, rickettsia, and parasites, and indeed the incidence of such diseases has been increasing in the U.S. Be suspicious about any patient in an endemic area with symptoms suggestive of one of these illnesses, as the patient may not give a history of recent tick bite. Lyme disease and Rocky Mountain spotted fever are the most commonly reported tick-borne infections in humans in the U.S. Additional diseases encountered include tularemia, Ehrlichiosis, relapsing fever, Colorado tick fever, and tick paralysis.

LYME DISEASE

Lyme disease, the most frequently transmitted vector-borne infection in the U.S., is caused by the spirochete bacteria, *Borrelia burgdorferi.* Small mammals (rodents and rabbits), as well as deer, serve as host reservoirs in the wild, and although the majority of cases have been reported in New England, the mid-Atlantic, and south Atlantic regions, cases have been reported in almost all of the mainland states. Most infections occur in the late spring and early summer and less than one third of patients can recall a tick bite.

Clinical Features

Lyme disease is an infection affecting multiple organ systems and can generally be divided into 3 stages, although not all patients may have all stages and stages may overlap. Also there may be remissions between any stage. Stage I is identified by a skin lesion, *erythema chronicum migrans* (ECM), an annular, erythematous lesion with central clearing which develops at the site of the tick bite. ECM generally appears 7 to 10 days after the bite. ECM is found in 60% to 70% of patients and may be accompanied by (in decreasing order of frequency) generalized malaise and fatigue, headache, fever and chills, stiff neck, arthralgias, and constitutional symptoms. If untreated, ECM and other symptoms usually abate spontaneously in about 4 wks.

Stage II represents disseminated infection and usually occurs within days to a few wks after primary infection. Stage II symptoms include multiple secondary annular skin lesions, fever, adenopathy, splenomegaly, and constitutional symptoms. About 10% of untreated stage II patients develop neurologic symptoms, including headache, meningoencephalitis, and unilateral or bilateral facial nerve palsy. Some patients may develop first-, second-, or third-degree AV node block. Stage II consists of chronic persistent infection with findings of chronic arthritis, chronic central nervous system disease, or chronic dermatitis. Arthritis typically presents with brief but recurrent episodes of migratory oligoarthritis with remissions that often last longer than the exacerbations. The most common joints affected in order of frequency are the knee (which may have swelling), shoulder, TMJ, ankle, wrist, hip, and small joints of the hands and feet.

Diagnosis and Differential

Because sensitive and specific diagnostic tests for Lyme disease are not available, the diagnosis must be based on clinical findings in a patient exposed to ticks in an endemic area. The best diagnosis remains culture isolation of *B. burgdorferi* from ECM lesions, but this requires special media, has a low sensitivity, and is not widely available.

Emergency Department Care

Early Lyme disease seems to respond well to antimicrobial therapy, especially if begun early. A variety of agents may be effective in early disease, but therapy for late-stage Lyme disease remains controversial, as does prophylaxis for patients in an endemic area with a known tick bite but no symptoms.

1. *Erythema chronicum migrans* may be treated with **doxycycline** (100 mg po bid), **amoxicillin** (500 mg po tid), or **cefuroxime** (500 mg po bid). Pediatric cases should be treated with **amoxicillin** (25–50 mg/kg body wt per day in 3 divided doses).
2. Bell's palsy, mild arthritis, or mild cardiac manifestations may be similarly managed as with ECM, using oral doxycycline or amoxicillin (amoxicillin is preferred for children).
3. Oral regimens are generally prescribed for 10 to 30 days.
4. Serious CNS disease (meningitis, encephalitis, encephalopathy, or neuropathy), serious cardiac manifestations, or serious arthritis are probably best managed with hospital admission for supportive care and a 14 to 21 day course of IV ceftriaxone or penicillin G.
5. Timely consultation with an infectious disease specialist is highly desirable for any patient who presents to the ED with suspected Lyme disease.

If Standard Treatment Fails

Reconsider the diagnosis, provide aggressive supportive care, consider parenteral antimicrobials if the patient has failed to respond to oral therapy, and consider immediate consultation with an infectious-disease expert.

ROCKY MOUNTAIN SPOTTED FEVER

Rocky Mountain spotted fever (RMSF), the most common rickettsial disease in the U.S., is caused by *Rickettsia rickettsii*, a small, obligate intracellular coccobacillus. In recent years the highest number of cases have been reported in a band running from North and South Carolina horizontally to Oklahoma and Kansas, however, more than 40 states reported cases in 1993. An overwhelming majority of cases occur between April 1 and September 30, and the highest incidence of cases occur in children aged 5 to 9 y.

Clinical Features

RMSF is a disease affecting multiple organ systems with most patients developing moderate to severe illness unless treated early. The usual incubation period is 4 to 10 days, and the onset may be abrupt or insidious. Initial symptoms are nonspecific and include fever, malaise, severe headache, myalgias, nausea, vomiting, anorexia, abdominal pain, and photophobia.

Rash, the hallmark of RMSF, typically appears between the 3rd and 5th days of illness. Early on the rash is maculopapular, but as it evolves it becomes more defined and petechial. It typically begins on the extremities, often at the wrists and ankles, and often involves the palms and soles. It then spreads centripetally to the trunk, usually sparing the face. The rash may be absent in 5% to 15% of cases with so-called spotless fever, more often seen in African–Americans, the elderly, and severe fatal cases. GI symptoms are often prominent, and since they may precede the onset of rash they may lead to a misdiagnosis of gastroenteritis or even acute abdomen. Pneumonitis is a common and potentially fatal feature of RMSF and presents with cough, dyspnea, pulmonary edema, and systemic hypoxia. The CNS is another potentially critical target of RMSF, with serious neurologic involvement occurring in 23% to 38% of cases. Symptoms include confusion, stupor, ataxia, coma, and seizures. Renal and cardiac dysfunction are other important clinical manifestations.

Diagnosis and Differential

The ED physician must maintain a high index of suspicion for RMSF in the appropriate clinical setting since a definitive rash may be an absent or late finding, the early symptoms are nonspecific and misleading, and the patients are frequently unable to remember a tick bite. Early definitive diagnosis of RMSF requires demonstration of rickettsiae in biopsy samples of the rash using fluorescent antibody techniques (sensitivity 70%, specificity 100%). Serologic tests may help confirm RMSF, but the clinical diagnosis must be based on symptoms, findings, and epidemiological factors as serology will not become reliably positive for 6 to 10 days after onset of the clinical symptoms. Some laboratory findings may be useful in suggesting diagnosis of RMSF, but these are usually not found until the second week of the illness. Most patients will have a normal leukocyte count but a left shift may be seen in about 70%.

Anemia is found in 30% and mild thrombocytopenia has been seen in 30% to 50%. Severe thrombocytopenia (<20,000 platelets/uL) has been reported in 10%; hyponatremia is noted in about 20% of patients; a low serum albumin may also be found; and The CSF often has an elevated protein or pleocytosis. The differential includes viral illnesses (measles, rubella, hepatitis, mononucleosis, enteroviral exanthem), gastroenteritis, acute abdomen, streptococcal pharyngitis, disseminated gonorrhea, meningitis (meningococcal), secondary syphilis, pneumonia, leptospirosis, typhoid fever, and encephalitis.

Emergency Department Care

Early therapy with appropriate antimicrobials dramatically reduces mortality associated with RMSF.

1. Appropriate coverage for adults includes **doxycycline** (100 mg po bid), **tetracycline** (500 mg po qid), or **chloramphenicol** (50–75 mg/kg body wt. per day IV in 4 divided doses).
2. Appropriate therapy for children (<45 kg or 100 lbs) includes doxycycline (4.4 mg/kg po in 2 divided doses on day 1, followed by 2.2 mg/kg per day po in a single dose). Alternatives include tetracycline (30–40 mg/kg per day po in 4 divided doses [for children >8 y old]) and **chloramphenicol** (100 mg/kg body wt. per day [up to total of 3 grams] IV in 4 divided doses, (which may be later switched to oral therapy). Doxycycline has been used for short courses in children with insignificant staining of the teeth, but these cosmetic risks must be balanced against the potentially serious adverse effects of chloramphenicol. It is probably best to discuss these risks with the parents and the child's primary care provider at the onset of therapy to decide about which therapy to use. Chloramphenicol has also been advocated for use in pregnant patients.
3. Antimicrobial therapy is generally administered for 5 to 7 days, continuing until the patient is afebrile and has shown clinical progress for 2 days.
4. Parenteral agents should be used in any patient with nausea, vomiting, or significant systemic disease. Patients with all but the most minor of symptoms of RMSF should probably be admitted for continued observation and antimicrobial therapy. Seriously ill patients require aggressive supportive care and detailed attention to fluid and electrolyte imbalances. Those discharged should have prompt and close followup care to ensure their clinical improvement.

If Standard Treatment Fails

Reconsider the diagnosis of RMSF, carefully review the patient's fluid and electrolyte state and renal function, and consider immediate consultation with an infectious-disease expert. Patients initially managed as outpatients who deteriorate or fail to improve rapidly with oral antimicrobial agents should be admitted for parenteral therapy.

TULAREMIA

Tularemia (rabbit skinners disease) is caused by *Francisella tularensis*, a small gram-negative coccobacillus. In addition to tick bites, it may be transmitted by the bite of the deerfly. Natural reservoirs of this disease include many small animals, particularly rabbits, hares, muskrats, beavers, some domestic animals, and hard ticks. Although widespread throughout the U.S., tularemia seems to have its highest incidence in Arkansas, Missouri, and Oklahoma. Cases occur all year, but they may be more common in adults in early winter and in children in the summer. Methods of transmission can include arthropod bites, animal bites, inoculation of skin, conjunctivae, or oral mucosa by blood or tissue from infected animals or insects, or by handling or ingestion of inadequately cooked rabbit or hare meat. It may also be acquired by drinking contaminated water or by inhalation of contaminated soil, grain, or hay.

Clinical Features

Tularemia has an average incubation period of 3 to 5 days and begins suddenly with fevers, chills, headache, anorexia, malaise, and fatigue. Additional symptoms include myalgias, cough, vomiting, pharyngitis, abdominal pain, and diarrhea. Fever usually persists for several days, stops for a brief period, and then recurs. Several clinical syndromes of tularemia may be seen with features that vary somewhat depending on the mode of transmission. *Ulceroglandular fever* follows tick bites and animal contact and is characterized by enlarged tender lymphadenopathy. A papule develops at the site of inoculation, becomes necrotic, and leaves a tender ulcer with a raised border. *Glandular tularemia* consists of tender regional lymphadenopathy without a local skin lesion. *Oculoglandular tularemia* presents with photophobia, lacrimation, eyelid edema, and painful conjunctivitis. Preauricular, submandibular, and cervical adenopathy may also be present. *Pharyngeal tularemia* is acquired from contaminated food or water and presents with exudative pharyngitis or tonsillitis. *Typhoidal tularemia* can occur with any mode of transmission. Multiorgan symptoms may be seen, including fever, headache, chills, myalgias, pharyngitis, nausea and vomiting, diarrhea, abdominal pain, and cough. Hepatomegaly or splenomegaly may be present. Secondary pneumonitis can occur in up to 45%. *Tularemia pneumonia* can occur with inhalation of the organism; symptoms are fever, non- or minimally productive cough, substernal chest tightness, and pleuritic chest pain. Physical findings may be nonspecific or may include rales, consolidation, or pleural rub.

Diagnosis and Differential

The key to the diagnosis of tularemia in any of its clinical forms is obtaining a thorough history of potential exposure. Serologic studies (ELISA is preferred) to determine acute and convalescent titers are useful for confirmation. *F. tularensis* may also be cultured on special media from blood, lymph nodes, wounds, sputum, and pleural fluid. The multiple clinical variations of tularemia can be confusing and lead to misdiagnosis. The differential of the glandular and ulceroglandular forms includes pyogenic bacterial infection, cat-scratch disease, rat-bite fever, syphilis, tuberculosis, atypical mycobacterial infection, sporotrichosis, toxoplasmosis, anthrax, and plague. The differential for tularemic pneumonia includes viruses, *Mycoplasma, Legionella*, plague, anthrax, Q fever, and psittacosis. The *typhoidal* form is challenging to diagnose and has a differential including *salmonella* infection, brucellosis, Q fever, disseminated mycobacterial or fungal disease, rickettsial infection, malaria, and endocarditis.

Emergency Department Care

The drug of choice for the treatment of tularemia is **streptomycin** (7.5–10 mg/kg body wt IM q12h for 7–14 days). The pediatric dose is 30 to 40 mg/kg IM in 2 divided doses. Gentamicin is an alternative; tetracycline and chloramphenicol have been used for oral therapy, but relapse rates are high. Patients generally should be admitted for close supportive care and adequate antimicrobial therapy.

If Standard Treatment Fails

Reconsider the diagnosis of tularemia. Consider consultation with an infectious-diseases expert.

EHRLICHIOSIS

Ehrlichiosis is caused by *Ehrlichia chaffeensis*, a small gram-negative, pleomorphic coccobacillus member of the *Rickettsia* family, which infects circulating leukocytes. Most cases have occurred in the south central and south Atlantic regions of the U.S., especially in Oklahoma, Missouri, and Georgia. About 75% of cases occur between May and July. Men are more commonly infected and the incidence increases with age.

Clinical Features

Just over two thirds of patients can give a history of tick bites in the preceding 3 wks. The incubation period ranges from 1 to 21 days with a median of 7 days. Patients usually present with a nonspecific febrile illness. The most common symptoms are high fever and headache, but malaise, nausea, vomiting, rigors, myalgias, and anorexia are also frequent. A maculopapular or petechial rash develops in about 35% of cases, rarely involving the palms or soles. Unusual but severe potential complications include renal failure, disseminated intravascular coagulation, cardiomegaly, seizures, and death.

Diagnosis and Differential

The diagnosis of Ehrlichiosis depends primarily on its clinical features, but serology may provide confirmation. Laboratory findings are most prominent at 5 to 7 days and include leukopenia, absolute lymphopenia, thrombocytopenia, elevated serum hepatic enzymes and, rarely, CSF pleocytosis. The differential includes, most importantly, other rickettsial diseases and meningitis.

Emergency Department Care

The drug of choice is tetracycline or its analogues, but chloramphenicol may be used as an alternative. Doses and duration of therapy should be similar to the treatment of RMSF. Most patients will probably require admission, since bacterial meningitis will often have to be excluded.

If Standard Treatment Fails

Reconsider the diagnosis of Ehrlichiosis and consider consultation with an infectious disease expert.

COLORADO TICK FEVER

Colorado tick fever, an acute viral illness, is caused by an RNA virus of the genus coltivirus. It has been reported from the mountainous western regions of the U.S. Most infections occur between late May and early July.

Clinical Features

Colorado tick fever begins suddenly approximately 3 to 6 days after a tick bite, with fever, chills, severe headache, photophobia, and myalgias. Symptoms usually last for 5 to 8 days and spontaneously resolve. Fifty% of patients experience a secondary phase with similar symptoms, beginning about 3 days after the primary phase ends. This secondary phase lasts about 2 to 4 days, and it may be accompanied by a transient petechial or macular rash.

Diagnosis and Differential

The diagnosis may be confirmed by serologic studies or by isolation of the virus from blood or CSF inoculated into suckling mice. Lab abnormalities include leukocytosis and thrombocytopenia. The differential includes meningitis and rickettsial infections such as Rocky Mountain spotted fever.

Emergency Department Care

No specific therapy exists, and supportive care alone will usually suffice. Recovery is spontaneous and usually takes about 3 wks.

If Standard Treatment Fails

Reconsider the diagnosis and particularly consider the other potential causes of acute meningitis. Consider consultation with an infectious-disease expert.

TICK PARALYSIS

Tick paralysis, a relatively uncommon tick-borne disease, is important to recognize because it is easily curable and potentially fatal if unrecognized. It is most likely caused by a neurotoxic venom secreted from the female tick salivary glands, which produces a conduction block at the peripheral motor end plate. The incidence is highest in spring to late summer and it seems to occur more commonly in children, girls more than boys.

Clinical Features

Symptoms begin within 4 to 7 days after attachment by the female tick. Initial findings include irritability, restlessness, and hand or foot paresthesias. Within 1 to 2 days these symptoms are followed by a symmetric, ascending flaccid paralysis, accompanied by a loss of deep tendon reflexes. Poor coordination and ataxia may indicate cerebellar involvement. In severe, untreated cases, bulbar and respiratory paralysis may ensue, resulting in death.

Diagnosis and Differential

Diagnosis consists of recognition of clinical features coupled with discovery of an attached tick. The patient must be carefully searched for a tick with particular attention paid to the scalp. The differential includes other causes of ascending paralysis, most notably Guillain-Barré disease.

Emergency Department Care

The key to therapy is discovery of the causative tick and its prompt removal. Most patients begin showing signs of spontaneous recovery within h after tick removal, and complete recovery is expected within 48 to 72 h. Aggressive supportive care, including most notably ventilatory support, is indicated for patients who have developed respiratory compromise prior to tick removal.

If Standard Treatment Fails

If the patient fails to improve within a few h after tick removal or, if after a thorough but unsuccessful search has been made for a tick, reconsider the diagnosis. Consider the possibility of Guillain–Barré syndrome and other causes of flaccid paralysis.

For further reading in *Emergency Medicine, A Comprehensive Study Guide*, see Chapter 127, Tick-Borne Diseases, by David J. Weber and Susan Isbey.

Management of the transplant patient in the ED can be divided into two general areas—disorders specific to the transplanted organ, and disorders common to all transplant patients due to their immunosuppressed state. Compromised response to infection and other side-effects of immunosuppressive medication are common to all transplant recipients. Disorders specific to the transplanted organ are manifestations of acute rejection, surgical complications specific to the procedure performed, and altered physiology (most important in cardiac transplantation). Also, the management of routine injuries or illness may be complicated by the patient's immunosuppressed state or medication. Before prescribing any new drug for a transplant recipient, discuss your treatment plan with a representative from the transplant team.

POST-TRANSPLANT INFECTIOUS COMPLICATIONS

Infections after transplantation are a common and feared complication. Predisposing factors include ongoing immunosuppression in all patients and the presence of diabetes mellitus, advanced age, obesity, and other host factors in some. Table 89-1 displays the broad array of potential infections and the time after transplant they are most apt to occur.

The most common life-threatening infection in recipients of solid organs, especially in bone-marrow graft recipients, is cytomegalovirus (CMV). This infection may manifest with daily fever and malaise in its mildest form. Progressively more serious disease manifestations include leukopenia, hepatopathy (elevated transaminase enzymes), enteropathy (epigastric pain and diarrhea), and pneumonitis. Mortality associated with CMV pneumonitis exceeds 50%. CMV infection occurs most commonly 4 to 12 wks after transplant surgery. A patient presenting with a febrile illness at that time should have as part of their assessment a complete blood count, chest x-ray, and measurement of liver function. During active CMV infection, immunosuppression is maintained at the minimum possible level, and if liver, gut, or pulmonary involvement is documented, intravenous ganciclovir therapy, often in conjunction with immune globulin, is prescribed.

The initial presentation of a potentially life-threatening infectious illness may be quite subtle in transplant recipients. The transplant recipient receiving glucocorticoids may not mount an impressive febrile response. A nonproductive cough with little or no findings on physical examination may be the only clue to emerging *P. carinii* pneumonia or CMV pneumonia. The threshold for obtaining chest x-rays for these patients should be low. Central nervous system (CNS) infections are

TABLE 89-1. Infectious Complications of Whole-Organ Transplantation

First Mo Post-Transplant

Bacterial
 Wound infection
 Pneumonia
 Urinary tract infection
 Line-related sepsis
Viral
 Herpes simplex
Fungal
 Candidal pharyngitis, esophagitis, cystitis

Second to Sixth Mo Post-Transplant

Bacterial
 Pneumonia: pneumococcal and other community acquired pneumonitis
 Urinary tract infection
 Nocardial infection
 Listeriosis
Viral
 Cytomegalovirus, EBV, HSV, varicella zoster
 Adenovirus
 Hepatitis A, B, C
Fungal
 Aspergillosis
 Candidal pharyngitis, esophagitis, cystitis
Other opportunistic infection
 Pneumocystis carinii pneumonia, tuberculosis, toxoplasma

Beyond Sixth Mo Post-Transplant

Bacterial
 Pneumonia: pneumococcal and other community-acquired pneumonitis
 Urinary tract infection
 Listeriosis
Viral
 Cytomegalovirus chorioretinitis
 Varicella zoster
 Hepatitis C, B
Fungal
 Cryptococcal
Other opportunistic infection
 Pneumocystis carinii pneumonia

more common in transplant recipients than in other patients. Common etiologies include *Listeria monocytogenes* and cryptococci. Complaints of recurrent headaches, therefore, with or without fever, should be investigated vigorously, first with a structural study to exclude a mass lesion (CNS lymphomas occur with increased frequency too), then with a lumbar puncture. Finally, a significant subset of renal transplant recipients have undergone intentional splenectomy to improve allograft survival. Although this procedure is no longer routinely practiced, these patients, as in other postsplenectomy patients, are at particularly high risk for overwhelming sepsis caused by encapsulated bacteria such as pneumococci or meningococci.

Management of Infection

1. Alternatives for therapy are listed below, however, drug choice, dose, and ultimate management should be accomplished in consultation with the transplant team. For skin and superficial wounds, probable offending organisms are gram-positive cocci, especially *Staphylococcus aureus*, and treatment should be with a penicillinase-resistant penicillin (e.g., nafcillin or oxacillin) or a first-generation cephalosporin (e.g., cefazolin), unless there is a suspicion for methicillin-resistant organisms or sensitivity to ß-lactams, in which case vancomycin should be used.

2. Nosocomial pneumonia is likely due to gram-negative organisms such as *E. coli*, *Enterobacter*, or *Pseudomonas* and should be treated with a broad-spectrum antibiotic (e.g., cefoxitin, cefotetan, cefotaxime, ceftriaxone, ceftazidime). Community-acquired pneumonia should be treated as such, with the proviso that opportunistic infection may also be present.

3. Intra-abdominal infection may be due to enterococci, gram-negative bacilli, or anaerobes. Triple coverage may be necessary empirically, with ampicillin or vancomycin plus an aminoglycoside to treat enterococci; a broad-spectrum penicillin or second- or third-generation cephalosporin to treat gram-negative organisms; and piperacillin, cefoxitin, cefotetan, clindamycin, or metronidazole to treat anaerobes. Penicillins with ß-lactamase inhibitors (e.g., sulbactam and clavulanic acid) have broad coverage against gram-positive cocci, gram-negative bacilli, and anaerobes.

4. Meningitis is frequently due to *L. monocytogenes*, and patients with suspected meningitis should be treated with a third-generation cephalosporin and ampicillin.

5. The mainstay of fungal treatment has been amphotericin B.

6. Viral therapy depends on the disease syndrome and the offending agent. CMV disease is treated with ganciclovir, which is only available intravenously. Mean duration of treatment is 16 days, with a dose of 5 mg/kg IV bid, adjusting the dose for renal insufficiency. Varicella and HSV are typically treated with acyclovir, which has renal excretion; the dose must be adjusted for renal insufficiency. Epstein–Barr virus (EBV) is typically treated with a reduction in the immunosuppression regimen.

7. Treatment of choice for *P. carinii* pneumonia is cotrimoxazole, with pentamidine reserved as an alternative therapy if cotrimoxazole is

not tolerated. Toxoplasmosis is treated with pyrimethamine/sulfadia-
zine or clindamycin.

Complications of Immunosuppressive Agents

Therapeutic immunosuppression is accompanied by a number of side-
effects and complications (Table 89-2). Combined toxicities can produce
or worsen pre-existing renal insufficiency, hypertension, and hyperglycemia. Elevated cyclosporine levels cause renal arteriolar constriction,
reducing glomerular blood flow and stimulating the renin–angiotensin
system, and elevated blood pressure. Glucocorticoids promote renal salt
and water retention, which further aggravate hypertension. A headache
syndrome often indistinguishable from migraine is common in transplant
recipients and usually develops within the first 2 mo of immunosuppression. An important differential must include infectious causes and malignancy when headache first presents and usually requires a head CT scan
with subsequent biochemical analysis of cerebrospinal fluid.

ORGAN SPECIFIC REJECTION SYNDROMES AND COMPLICATIONS

Cardiac Transplantation

Transplantation results in a denervated heart that does not respond to
tachycardia in response to stress or exercise, but does respond to circulat-

TABLE 89-2. Drug Side-Effects

Cyclosporine
　Nephrotoxicity—worsened by aminoglycosides, H_2-blockers, NSAIDs,
　trimethoprim/sulfamethoxazole, amphotericin B
　Neurotoxicity—tremors, seizures, headaches
　Hyperkalemia
　Hyperuricemia
　Hypertension
　Anorexia
　Increased bilirubin
　Cholestasis
　Gastric dysmotility
Prednisone
　Cushing syndrome
　Osteoporosis
　Adrenal suppression
　Hypertension
　Hyperglycemia
　Peptic ulcer disease
　Myopathy
　Poor wound healing
Imuran
　Leukopenia
　Thrombocytopenia
　Cholestatic jaundice
　Alopecia

ing catecholamines and increased preload. Patients may complain of fatigue or shortness of breath with the onset of exercise, which resolves with continued exertion as an appropriate tachycardia develops.

The donor heart is implanted with its sinus node intact to preserve normal atrioventricular conduction. The technique of cardiac transplantation also results in the preservation of the recipient's sinus node at the superior cavoatrial junction. The atrial suture line renders the two sinus nodes electrically isolated from each other. Thus, ECGs will frequently have two distinct P waves. The sinus node of the donor heart is easily identified by its constant 1:1 relationship to the QRS complex, whereas the native P wave marches through the donor heart rhythm independently.

Clinical Features of Rejection and Acute Illness after Cardiac Transplantation

Because the heart is denervated, myocardial ischemia does not present with angina. Instead, recipients present with heart failure secondary to silent myocardial infarctions or with sudden death. Transplant recipients who present with new-onset shortness of breath, chest fullness, or symptoms of CHF should be evaluated, in routine fashion with ECG and serial cardiac enzymes, for the presence of myocardial ischemia or infarction.

Although most episodes of acute rejection are asymptomatic, symptoms can occur. The most common presenting symptoms are arrhythmias and generalized fatigue. The development of either atrial or ventricular arrhythmias in a cardiac transplant recipient must be assumed due to acute rejection until proven otherwise.

Emergency Department Care

1. Consultation—Differentiating rejection from other acute illness in the transplant patient can be difficult. Treatment for rejection without biopsy confirmation is contraindicated except when the patient is hemodynamically unstable.
2. Rejection—Management of acute rejection is 1 gram of methylprednisolone IV, after consultation with the transplant center. The patient may need further cytotoxic therapy, but this should be guided by a representative from the transplant center.
3. Arrhythmias—If patients are hemodynamically compromised by arrhythmias, empiric therapy for rejection with methylprednisolone (Solu-Medrol), 1 g IV, may be given after consultation with the transplant center. Atrial arrhythmias may respond to treatment with digoxin or calcium channel blockers. Ventricular arrhythmias may respond to lidocaine or other class I-C agents. Frequently arrhythmias will be controlled only with antirejection therapy. Atropine has no

effect on the denervated heart; isoproterenol is the drug of choice for bradyarrhythmias in these patients.

4. Hypotension—Low-output syndrome or hypotension should be treated with inotropic agents such as dopamine or dobutamine when specific treatment for rejection is instituted.

5. Hospitalization—Transplant patients suspected of having rejection or acute illness should be hospitalized, preferably at the transplant center, if stable for transfer.

LUNG TRANSPLANTATION

Clinical Features of Rejection and Acute Illness after Lung Transplantation

Clinically, the patient may have cough, chest tightness, fatigue, and fever ($>0.5°C$ above baseline). Acute rejection may be manifest with frightening rapidity, causing a severe decline in patient status in only a day. Isolated fever may be the only finding; on the other hand, spirometry may show a 15% drop in FEV_1, and examination may reveal rales and adventitious sounds. Chest x-ray may demonstrate bilateral interstitial infiltrates, septal lines, and effusions. The chest x-ray may be normal, however, when rejection occurs late in the course. The longer period of time a patient is from transplant, the less classic a chest x-ray may appear for acute rejection. Infection, such as interstitial pneumonia, may present with a clinical picture similar to acute rejection. Diagnostically, bronchoscopy with transbronchial biopsy is usually needed not only to confirm rejection but to exclude infection.

Two late complications of lung transplant are obliterative bronchiolitis and post-transplant lymphoproliferative disease (PTLD). Obliterative bronchiolitis presents with episodes of recurrent bronchitis, small airway obliteration, wheezing and, eventually, respiratory failure. PTLD is associated with Epstein-Barr virus and presents with painful lymphadenopathy and otitis media (due to tonsillar involvement), or may present with malaise, fever, and myalgia.

Evaluation of the lung-transplant patient should include chest x-ray, ABG, CBC, serum electrolytes, creatinine, magnesium and, in some cases, a cyclosporine level.

Emergency Department Management

1. Consultation—Communicate directly with the transplant center (often a nurse coordinator). The coordinator should have the patient's current medication doses, recent infection history, and a knowledge of complications for which the patient may be at risk.

2. Rejection—If clinically indicated (i.e., infection is excluded), large doses of glucocorticoids are given (1 g IV Solu-Medrol on day 1, followed by 500 mg Solu-Medrol IV qd for 2 days). Treatment

should result in improved symptoms and clinical parameters in 1 to 2 days. Failure to respond to glucocorticoids suggests an alternative diagnosis. Patients who have a history of seizures associated with the administration of high-dose glucocorticoids will also need concurrent benzodiazepines to prevent further seizure episodes.

3. Late complications—Obliterative bronchiolitis is treated with increased immunosuppression, whereas PTLD is treated with reduced immunosuppression. These decisions should be made by physicians from the transplant center.

RENAL TRANSPLANT

Clinical Features of Rejection and Acute Illness after Renal Transplantation

Diagnosis and treatment of acute rejection is most critical. Without timely recognition and intervention, allograft function may deteriorate irreversibly in a few days.

The renal transplant recipient, when symptomatic from acute rejection, will complain of vague tenderness over the allograft (in the left or right iliac fossa, a heterotopic location in contrast to the orthotopic location of liver or heart transplants). The patient may also describe decreased urine output, rapid weight gain (from fluid retention), low-grade fever, and generalized malaise. Physical may disclose worsening hypertension, allograft tenderness, and peripheral edema. *The absence of these symptoms and signs, however, does not exclude the possibility of acute rejection.* With improved methods of maintenance immunosuppression, the only clue may be an asymptomatic decline in renal function, as assessed by a rising serum creatinine level. Therefore, even small asymptomatic changes in serum creatinine cannot be dismissed as unimportant and must be investigated. Even a change in creatinine from 1.0 mg/dL to 1.2 or 1.3 mg/dL may be important. When such changes in creatinine are reproducible, a careful workup consists of complete urinalysis, renal ultrasonography, and a trough level of cyclosporine, in addition to a careful history and examination. It is critical to interpret changes in renal function in the context of prior data (e.g., trends of recent serum creatinine levels, recent history of rejection, or other causes of allograft dysfunction). Evaluation should consider the multiple etiologies of decreased renal function in the renal transplant recipient. The two most common causes, apart from acute rejection causing an increase in creatinine, are volume contraction and cyclosporine-induced nephrotoxicity.

Emergency Department Management

1. Consultation—Communicate directly with the transplant center (often a nurse coordinator). The coordinator should have the patient's

current medication doses, recent infection history, and a knowledge of complications for which the patient may be at risk.
2. Rejection—Treatment of allograft rejection is high dose glucocorticoids, typically methylprednisolone (250–500 mg intravenously for 3 to 4 days).

LIVER TRANSPLANT

Clinical Features of Rejection and Diagnosis of Acute Illness

Though frequently subtle in presentation, a syndrome of acute rejection includes fever, liver tenderness, lymphocytosis, eosinophilia, liver enzyme elevation, and a change in bile color or production. In the perioperative period, the differential diagnosis must include infection, acute biliary obstruction, or vascular insufficiency. Diagnosis can be made with certainty only by hepatic ultrasound and biopsy, which usually requires referral back to the transplant center for management and followup.

Two possible surgical complications in liver transplant patients are biliary obstruction or leakage and hepatic artery thrombosis. Biliary obstruction follows three typical presentations. The most common is intermittent episodes of fever and fluctuating liver function tests. The second is a gradual worsening of liver-function tests without symptoms. Finally, obstruction may present as acute bacterial cholangitis with fever, chills, abdominal pain, jaundice, and bacteremia. Presentation can be difficult to distinguish clinically from rejection, hepatic artery thrombosis, CMV infection, or a recurrence of a pre-existing disease, especially hepatitis.

If a biliary complication is suspected, all patients should have a CBC with platelet count and differential; serum chemistries, including liver-function tests and amylase and lipase levels; cultures of blood, urine, bile, and ascites, if present; chest x-ray; and abdominal ultrasound. Ultrasound rules out the presence of fluid collections, screens for the presence of thrombosis of the hepatic artery or portal vein, and identifies any dilatation of the biliary tree.

Biliary leakage is associated with a 50% mortality. It occurs most frequently in the third or fourth postoperative wk. The high mortality may be related to a high incidence of concomitant hepatic-artery thrombosis, infection of leaked bile, or difficult bile repair where the tissue is inflamed. Patients most often present with peritoneal signs and fever, but these signs may be masked by concomitant use of steroids and immunosuppressive agents. Presentation is signaled by elevated PT and transaminase levels and little or no bile production, but this complication may also present as acute graft failure, liver abscess, unexplained sepsis, or a biliary tract problem (leak, obstruction, abscess, or breakdown of the anastomosis).

Emergency Department Management

1. Consultation—Communicate directly with the transplant center (often a nurse coordinator). The coordinator should have the patient's current medication doses, recent infection history, and a knowledge of complications for which the patient may be at risk.
2. Rejection—Acute rejection is managed with high-dose glucocorticoid bolus, followed by a rapid taper over 5 to 7 days.
3. Surgical complications are best managed at the transplant center. Biliary obstruction is managed with balloon dilatation, and all patients should receive broad spectrum antibiotics against gram-negative and -positive enteric organisms. Biliary leakage is treated with reoperation, and hepatic artery thrombosis is treated with retransplantation.

For further reading in *Emergency Medicine, A Comprehensive Study Guide*, see Chapter 63, Cardiac Transplantation, by Michael R. Mill; Chapter 73, Lung Transplants, by L.J. Paradowski and M.K. Robbins; Chapter 89, Liver Failure and Transplantation, by Steven Kronick and Rawden Evans; and Chapter 93, The Renal Transplant Patient, by Leslie Rocher and Warren Kupin.

90 | General Management of the Poisoned Patient

Dexter L. Morris

It is estimated that over four million poisonings occur in the U.S. annually. Whereas most of these are not fatal, the ED physician will see a substantial number of serious poisonings, mostly self-inflicted. An organized approach to the poisoned patient is essential.

Clinical Features

Poisoned patients often present with clinical features associated with a specific toxin (toxic syndromes). Examples of toxic syndromes include anticholinergic syndrome, cholinergic syndrome, and sympathomimetic syndrome, all of which will be discussed in subsequent chapters. Table 90-1 lists basic elements of the common toxic syndromes. Identification of a particular syndrome can direct the ED physician to specific treatment. Whether or not a syndrome is identified, the physician must address the three organ systems most likely to cause immediate morbidity or mortality.

The respiratory system is usually not affected directly by the toxin but an altered level of consciousness may compromise ventilation. Decreased respiratory effort or apnea is common and the loss of gag reflex may compromise the airway as well. Direct effects on the respiratory system are less common and can be seen in aspiration of some hydrocarbons, bronchospasm from specific toxins and, rarely, pulmonary edema or Adult Respiratory Distress Syndrome.

Cardiovascular complications of poisoning are mainly rhythm disturbances. Tachyarrhythmias are common but are not usually associated with serious perfusion problems unless caused by agents that prolong the QT interval. These agents (quinidine, amiodarone, and sotalol) can produce torsades de pointes. Older individuals may also have difficulty with tachycardia secondary to underlying cardiovascular disease. Bradyarrhythmias are uncommon and often associated with hypoxia or acidosis. Hypotension secondary to decreased vascular tone is common and associated with toxins that decrease central sympathetic outflow (benzodiazepines) or direct vasodilation (calcium channel blockers). Hypertension is also seen and may be accompanied by cerebrovascular hemorrhage in severe cases.

Altered level of consciousness is a common complication of poisonings and may range from mild drowsiness or agitation to coma and death. Seizures also can occur as a direct effect of the toxin or from underlying perfusion or metabolic problems.

Other organ systems can be affected, depending on the individual nature of the toxin. These are discussed in the chapters on individual

501

TABLE 90-1. Toxic Syndromes (Multiple-Cause Symptom Complexes)

Syndrome	Causes			Manifestations
Narcotic	Alphaprodine	Ethylmorphine	Normeperidine	CNS depression
	Anileridine	Ethohepatazine	(meperidine metabolite)	Pinpoint pupils
	Codeine	Fentanyl	Opium	Slowed respirations
	Cyclazocine	Heroin	Oxycodone	Hypotension
	Dextromethorphan	Hydromorphone	Oxymorphone	Response to naloxone
	Dextromoramide	Levorphanol	Pentazocine	Pupils may be dilated and excitement
	Diacetylmorphine	Meperidine	Phenazocine	may predominate
	Dihydrocodeine	Methadone	Phenazine	Normeperidine: tremor, CNS excitation,
	Dihydrocodeinone	Metopon	Piminodine	seizures
	Dipaone	Morphine	Propoxyphene	
	Diphenoxylate (Lomoul)		Racemorphan	
Sympathomimetic	Aminophylline	Ephedrine	Methylphenidate	CNS excitation
	Amphetamines	Epinephrine	(Ritalin)	Seizures
	Caffeine	Fenfluramine	Pemoline	Hypertension
	Catha edulus (Khat)	Levaterenol	Phencyclidine	Hypotension with caffeine
	Cocaethylene	Metaraminol	Phenmetrazine	Tachycardia
	Cocaine	Methamphetamine	Phentermine	
	Dopamine	Methcathinone		
Withdrawal	Alcohol	Ethchlorvynol	Methyprylon	Diarrhea, mydriasis, piloerection,
	Barbiturates	Glutethimide	Opioids	hypertension, tachycardia, insomnia,
	Benzodiazepines	Meprobamate	Paraldehyde	lacrimation, muscle cramps,
	Chloral hydrate	Methaqualone		restlessness, yawning, hallucinosis
	Cocaine			Depression with cocaine

Adapted from Done AK. *Poisoning—A Systematic Approach for the Emergency Department Physician.* Presented Aug. 6–9, 1979, at Snowmass Village, CO. Symposium sponsored by Rocky Mountain Poison Center. Used by permission.

toxins. A general plan for the initial treatment of all poisonings is described below.

Diagnosis and Differential

Diagnosis of poisoning is based on history and clinical presentation. Recognition of toxic syndromes are often useful in putting together a clinical picture. When there is a question of ingestion, having the actual container, remnant pills, or liquids is very important. Having family, friends, or emergency personnel retrieve these items is essential. A thorough physical exam is necessary and can lead to diagnosis. Laboratory studies may be useful but often serve only to confirm the diagnosis. Drug screens may be useful in unknown ingestions but rarely alter management. Acetaminophen and aspirin are common coingestions in suicide attempts, so consideration should be given to testing for these drugs. Other tests that may be useful include EKG, ABG, complete blood count, electrolytes, and glucose.

Emergency Department Care and Disposition

Management of the poisoned patient in the ED involves airway management, supportive care (assuring adequate breathing and circulation), decontamination, and definitive care (antidotes and elimination of toxin).

As in any ED patient, care starts with the ABCs. Particular attention should be paid to gag reflex and quality of the respirations. Consideration should be given to early intubation, particularly as most patients will need gastric lavage. Respiratory status should be continuously monitored.

Hypotension should be treated with fluids, and only rarely are vasopressors required. Ventricular arrhythmias should be managed aggressively with standard agents unless treatment for a particular toxin specifies alternative treatment. Bradycardia can be treated with atropine but may require pacing.

Once the ABCs have been addressed, patients with altered mental status should receive oxygen, a fingerstick glucose test, naloxone (2 mg IV), and thiamine (100 mg IV), and have IV access secured. The routine use of a benzodiazepine antagonist, flumazenil, is not recommended. Appropriate laboratory studies can then be obtained. Unconscious patients should have a Foley catheter placed.

Gastric lavage is the preferred method of gastric decontamination. Ipecac is no longer recommended. A large-bore (36-40 Fr for adults), orogastric tube with connections for infusion and drainage should be used. The patient should be placed in a left lateral decubitus position with the head lower than the feet. Infusion of 250 ml aliquots of tap water until the return is clear, followed by an infusion of 1 gm/kg of activated charcoal and removal of the tube is an effective protocol. A cathartic (sorbitol) may be added to the charcoal although the utility of this has not been clearly demonstrated. When large-bore orogastric lavage is not possible or indicated, charcoal can be administered through an NG tube or can be mixed with juice or soda and sipped by the patient. Whole-bowel irrigation is also a treatment option and may be particularly useful for packages of toxic drugs (body packers) or slow-release tablets such as iron. Non-absorbable polyethylene glycol at a rate of 1 to 2 liters an h (500 mL/h for pediatric patients) is administered by mouth or NG tube.

Surface decontamination should be done as soon as feasible for absorbed toxins such as pesticides. Care should be taken to avoid exposing other individuals.

Either simultaneously or once decontamination is underway, definitive treatment should be instituted. A list of antidotes to specific substances is listed in Table 90-2. In addition to these antidotes, specific treatments may exist for increasing the elimination of a toxin or for preventing complications such as alkalization for tricyclic-antidepressant overdose or hemodialysis for other toxins. Calling the regional poison control center is an excellent option for suggestions about definitive treatment and other aspects of patient care.

Other problems needing immediate treatment include seizures and agitation. Seizures should be treated with benzodiazepines initially, followed by phenobarbital for longer acting control or prophylaxis (phenytoin is less useful for the poisoned patient). Agitated patients should be physically restrained as necessary. Also, sedation with short-acting benzodiazepines or haloperidol can be used. Finally, patients who are actively suicidal need to be kept in the ED until an appropriate psychiatric evaluation has been completed.

Disposition of patients depends on the nature of the exposure and underlying conditions. Consideration should be given to delayed effects and absorption of toxins. Psychiatric consultation should be obtained for all intentional overdoses. Poisonings in children over 5 years old should be considered suspicious and warrant social-work consult or law-enforcement involvement of law enforcement. Patients and families should be given instructions on prevention of poisonings.

If Standard Treatment Fails

Consider the presence of other toxins or underlying conditions (myocardial infarction, trauma). These may cloud the clinical picture. Also consider delayed absorption of the toxin or incomplete decontamination.

For further reading in *Emergency Medicine: A Comprehensive Study Guide*, 4th edition, see Chapter 129, General Management of the Poisoned Patient, by Michael V. Vance.

TABLE 90-2. Emergency Antidotes

Poison	Antidote	Adult Dosage*	Comments
Acetaminophen	N-Acetylcysteine	Initial dose: 140 mg/kg	Most effective within 16 h
Arsenic	See Mercury		
Atropine	Physostigmine	Initial dose: 0.5–2 mg IV	Can produce convulsions, bradycardia
Carbon monoxide	Oxygen	Inhale contents of crushed pearl for 30 s; breath oxygen for 30 s	Methemoglobin-cyanide complex
Cyanide	Amyl nitrite;	10 mL of 3% solution over 3 min IV in adults	
	then Sodium nitrite	0.33 mL (10 mg 3% sol)/kg initially in children	Causes hypotension. Dosage assumes normal level hemoglobin
	Sodium thiosulfate	25% solut on—50 mL IV over 10 min in adults; 1.65 mL/kg in children	Forms harmless sodium thiocyanate
Ethylene glycol	See methyl alcohol		
Gold	See mercury		
Iron	Deferoxamine	Initial dose: 10–15 mg/kg per hour IV	Deferoxamine merylate—forms excretable ferrioxamine complex
Lead	Calcium disodium edetate or	1 ampoule/250 mL D5W over 1 h	5-mL ampoule IV 20% solution. Dilute to less than 3% solution. Calcium displaced by lead
	Dimercaptosuccinic acid	250 mg PO	
Mercury (arsenic, gold)	BAL (British anti-Lewisite)	5 mg/kg IM as soon as possible	Each mL BAL in oil has dimercaprol, 100 mg, in 210 mg (21%) benzyl benzoate and 680 mg peanut oil. Forms stab e nontoxic excretable cyclic compound
	Dimercaptosuccinic acid (DMSA; succimer)	250 mg PO	Oral, water soluble preparation of BAL

(Table continues)

505

TABLE 90-2. Continued

Poison	Antidote	Adult Dosage*	Comments
Methyl alcohol (ethylene glycol)	Ethyl alcohol in conjunction with dialysis	1 mL/kg of 100% ethanol initially in glucose solution; maintain blood level of 100 mg/100 mL	Competes for alcohol dehydrogenase; prevents formation of toxic metabolites
Nitrites	Methylene blue	0.2 mL/kg of 1% solution IV over 5 min	Exchange transfusion may be needed for severe methemoglobinemia
Opiates	Naloxone	0.4–0.8 mg IV in adults; up to 8–22 mg 0.01 mg/kg IV in children	Higher doses may be required for certain high-affinity substances such as propoxyphene (Darvon) and diphenoxylate (Lomoil)
Organophosphates	Atropine	Initial dose: 2–5 mg IV in adults; 0.05 mg/kg IV in children	Physiologic: blocks acetylcholine at muscarinic receptor sites). Up to 5 mg IV every 15 min (or more) may be necessary in the critical adult patient
	Pralidoxime (2-PAM chloride)(Protopam)	Initial dose: 1 g IV in adults; 25–30 mg/kg IV in children	Specific: breaks alkyl phosphate-cholinesterase bond, regenerating acetylcholinesterase activity

*Dosages listed may require modification according to specific clinical conditions.
Adapted from the American College of Emergency Physicians poster on poisoning, Dallas, TX, 1980.

91 | Anticholinergic Toxicity

C. Crawford Mechem

Anticholinergic toxicity is commonly seen in the ED. Causative agents include tricyclic antidepressants, phenothiazines, antihistamines, antiparkinson drugs, and some plants, including Jimsonweed (Table 91-1).

Clinical Features

Clinical features include mydriasis, hypo- or hypertension, absent bowel sounds, tachycardia, flushed skin, urinary retention, hyperthermia, dry skin and mucous membranes, cardiogenic pulmonary edema, seizures, and mental status changes.

Diagnosis and Differential

The diagnosis must be based on clinical presentation. Routine laboratory studies are normal. The most common electrocardiographic abnormality is sinus tachycardia. Comprehensive toxicologic screens are of little value.

The differential diagnosis includes delirium tremens, acute psychiatric disorders, and sympathomimetic toxicity.

Emergency Department Care and Disposition

Supportive therapy is the mainstay of treatment. Symptomatic patients should be placed on a cardiac monitor and vascular access obtained.

1. Gastric emptying may be effective even after several h.
2. Activated charcoal with a cathartic may be useful to decrease drug absorption.
3. Hyperthermia and hypertension are controlled by conventional methods.
4. Seizures can be treated with benzodiazepines and barbiturates.
5. Arrhythmias are treated with standard antiarrhythmics. Class Ia agents should be avoided.
6. Agitation is treated with benzodiazepines. Phenothiazines should be avoided.
7. The use of physostigmine is controversial. Indications include seizures or hemodynamically unstable arrhythmias unresponsive to conventional therapy, uncontrollable agitation, coma with respiratory depression, malignant hypertension, or refractory hypotension. The initial dose is 0.5 to 2.0 mg IV over 5 min. Patients should be observed for cholinergic symptoms. Contraindications include cardiovascular disease, bronchospasm, and intestinal or bladder obstruction.

Patients with mild symptoms of anticholinergic toxicity can be discharged after 6 h of observation if their symptoms are improving.

TABLE 91-1. Anticholinergic Substances

Antihistamines
  Ethanolamines
    Dimenhydrinate (Dramamine)
    Diphenhydramine (Benadryl)
  Ethylenediamines
    Tripelennamine
      (Pyribenzamine)
  Alkylamines
    Chlorpheniramine (Teldrin)
  Piperazines
    Astemizole (Hismanal)
    Terfenadine (Seldane)
    Loratadine (Claritin)
    Cyclizine (Marezine)
    Meclizine (Antivert)
  Phenothiazines
    Promethazine (Phenergan)
Antiparkinsonian drugs
  Benztropine mesylate (Cogentin)
  Biperiden (Akineton)
  Ethopropazine (Parsidol)
  Trihexyphenidyl (Artane)
  Procyclidine (Kemadrin)
Antipsychotics
  Phenothiazines
    Chlorpromazine (Thorazine)
    Thioridazine (Mellaril)
    Perphenazine (Trilafon)
  Nonphenothiazines
    Molindone (Moban)
    Loxapine (Loxitane)
Antispasmodics
  Clidinium bromide (Quarzan,
    Librax)
  Dicyclomine (Bentyl)
  Methantheline bromide
    (Banthine)
  Propantheline bromide (Pro-
    Banthine)
  Tridihexethyl chloride (Pathilon)
Plants
  Deadly nightshade
  Mandrake
  Jimsonweed
Belladonna alkaloids, synthetic
  congeners
  Atropine (Hyoscyamine)
  Belladonna alkaloid mixtures
  Glycopyrrolate (Robinul)

Homatropine (Dia-Quel,
  Malcotran)
Methscopolamine bromide
  (Pamine)
Scopolamine hydrobromide
  (Hyoscine)
Antidepressants
  Amitryptiline hydrochloride
    (Elavil, Amitril, Endep)
  Desipramine hydrochloride
    (Norpramin, Pertofrane)
  Doxepin hydrochloride
    (Sinequan, Adapin)
  Imipramine hydrochloride
    (Tofranil, Pramine)
  Nortriptyline hydrochloride
    (Aventyl, Pamelor)
  Protriptyline hydrochloride
    (Vivactil)
  Trimipramine (Surmontil)
  Maprotiline hydrochloride
    (Ludiomil)
  Zimelidine hydrochloride
  Fluoxetine (Prozac)
  Amoxapine (Asendin)
Ophthalmic products
  Atropine and scopolamine
    solutions
  Cyclopentolate hydrochloride
    (Cyclogyl)
  Tropicamide (Mydriacyl)
OTC medications (including
  antihistamines and belladonna
  alkaloids)
  Analgesics—Excedrin PM,
    Percogesic
  Cold remedies—Actifed,
    Allerest, Coricidin, Dristan,
    Flavihist, Romex, Sine-Off
  Hypnotics—Compoz, Sleep-Eze,
    Sominex
  Menstrual products—Pamprin,
    Premesyn PMS
Skeletal muscle relaxants
  Orphenadrine citrate (Norflex)
  Cyclobenzaprine hydrochloride
    (Flexeril)
Mushrooms
  Amanita muscaria
  Amanita pantherina

Adapted from LR Goldfrank, et al, 1990.

Patients receiving physostigmine usually require admission for at least 24 h.

For further reading in *Emergency Medicine: A Comprehensive Study Guide,* 4th edition, see Chapter 157, Anticholinergic Toxicity, by Leslie R. Wolf.

Keith L. Mausner

TRICYCLIC ANTIDEPRESSANTS

Tricyclic antidepressants (TCAs) are widely prescribed drugs with a low therapeutic-to-toxic ratio. The mortality rate for intentional overdose is between 2% to 5%, and TCAs cause more intentional overdose deaths than any other group of medications.

Clinical Features

Ingestions of greater than 2 to 4 mg/kg may be toxic, and fatalities in adults are commonly associated with ingestions of greater than 1 gram. Coingestants are involved in approximately 50% of TCA overdoses.

Anticholinergic signs (dry mucus membranes and axillae, mydriasis, sinus tachycardia, diminished bowel sounds, urinary retention) are common in TCA toxicity, but are not uniformly present. Mild-to-moderate TCA toxicity may be associated with drowsiness, confusion, slurred speech, ataxia, anticholinergic signs, myoclonus, or hyper-reflexia. Serious toxicity is almost always seen within 6 h of ingestion, and is associated with coma, hypotension, respiratory depression, cardiac disturbances, and seizures. Seizures are usually generalized, single, and brief. Complications of severe toxicity include aspiration pneumonia, anoxic encephalopathy, and rhabdomyolysis.

Common EKG abnormalities include prolongation of the PR, QRS, and QT intervals, PVCs, and supraventricular or ventricular dysrhythmias. Conduction blocks, right-axis deviation, and nonspecific ST and T wave changes also are seen. There is much variability in EKG findings with TCA toxicity. Only 70% of symptomatic patients have sinus tachycardia. Widening of the QRS interval > 100 ms is seen in 20% to 50% of patients with TCA toxicity. A significant percentage of normal individuals, however, have a QRS interval > 100 ms. Widening of the QRS interval in the context of other signs and symptoms of TCA toxicity indicates a patient at high risk for serious complications.

Diagnosis and Differential

A qualitative toxicology screen may be confirmative of TCA ingestion. Not all TCAs are detected by all screening test batteries, however. It is crucial to be familiar with your hospital lab's limitations. Quantitative TCA levels are not useful in assessing acute overdoses.

Differential diagnosis includes three main classes of drugs. First, there are those that produce seizures, wide QRS sinus rhythm, and anticholinergic symptoms. These include carbamazepine, phenothiazines, antihistamines, quinidine, procainamide, and disopyramide. Secondly, drugs that produce seizures and wide QRS, complex rhythm but are not anticholinergic include propranolol, class IC antiarrhythmics, cocaine, local anesthetics, lithium, and propoxyphene. Thirdly, sympathomimetics can produce narrow-complex tachycardia, hypertension, and seizures, but are not anticholinergic.

Emergency Department Care and Disposition

All patients with decreased level of consciousness require immediate attention to airway, breathing, and circulation. Oxygen, peripheral IV access, and cardiac monitoring should be instituted. Quickly assess glucose with a bedside test and oxygenation with pulse-oximetry. Administer thiamine, and consider the use of naloxone. Flumazenil may precipitate seizures and is contraindicated in TCA overdose. Always consider the possibility of occult head or neck trauma.

Gastric lavage is recommended in the first 1 to 2 h after an overdose, or if the patient has diminished bowel sounds. Following gastric lavage, administer activated charcoal (1 gram/kg). Asymptomatic patients with a reliable history of minimal ingestion can be administered activated charcoal alone. Repeat doses of activated charcoal may enhance elimination, but caution is advised with decreased GI motility. The role of cathartics (e.g., sorbitol or magnesium citrate) is controversial, although they are commonly given with the first dose of activated charcoal.

Sodium bicarbonate therapy is indicated in the setting of QRS prolongation, ventricular dysrhythmias, or hypotension refractory to isotonic fluid resuscitation. It is administered in boluses of 1 to 2 mEq/kg IV until clinical improvement is noted, or until an arterial pH of 7.5 to 7.55 is achieved. Alkalinization beyond 7.55 can be deleterious. A continuous infusion of sodium bicarbonate is administered as 2 ampules (50 mEq/50 mL each) in 1 liter of D_5W or 0.5 NS at 2 cc/kg/hr. Infusion rate is adjusted according to pH, serum sodium, and response to treatment. Hypokalemia may result from sodium bicarbonate therapy and serum potassium should be monitored.

Alkalinization also can be achieved in the intubated patient through hyperventilation. Sodium bicarbonate appears to be more effective, however, possibly because sodium infusion has beneficial effects independent of alkalinization.

Agitation may occur secondary to central anticholinergic receptor stimulation. It is usually effectively treated with reassurance, decreased environmental stimuli, and benzodiazepines. Physostigmine has been used in severely agitated patients when other measures have failed, but its use has been associated with potentially life-threatening adverse cardiovascular, pulmonary, and CNS effects.

Seizures usually occur in the first 3 h after ingestion. Single and brief seizures do not require anticonvulsant therapy, unless they are associated with amoxapine or maprotiline. These agents may produce status epilepticus unless immediate treatment is initiated. Focal seizures are not typical of TCA toxicity and require neurologic evaluation.

Benzodiazepines (lorazepam, diazepam) are the first drugs of choice in the treatment of TCA-induced seizures. Barbiturates (e.g., phenobarbital) are second-line therapy. Phenobarbital is administered IV in a dose of 10 to 15 mg/kg. This dose can be repeated as necessary and as long as the patient maintains an adequate blood pressure. Patients not responding to this therapy may require paralysis, EEG monitoring, and further anticonvulsant therapy (see Chap. 131, Seizures and Status Epilepticus in Adults). Phenytoin, physostigmine, and bicarbonate are ineffective against TCA-induced seizures.

Hypotension is initially treated with isotonic crystalloid boluses of 10 cc/kg at a time. Care must be taken not to precipitate pulmonary edema. Sodium bicarbonate therapy is the next line of treatment, regardless of QRS duration. Norepinephrine, the most effective vasopressor in TCA toxicity, is third-line treatment. Dopamine is less effective and may occasionally lower systolic blood pressure because of vasodilation from its beta-adrenergic effects. Patients not responsive to the above treatment require pulmonary-artery-catheter monitoring to optimize therapy.

Asymptomatic patients with sinus tachycardia, isolated QT prolongation, or first-degree AV block do not require treatment. Patients with conduction blocks greater than first degree, which can rapidly progress to complete heart block, as well as patients with QRS duration > 100 ms, should receive sodium bicarbonate therapy.

Ventricular dysrhythmias are initially treated with sodium bicarbonate. Lidocaine and bretylium are second-and third-line therapies. Torsades de points is treated with 2 grams of magnesium sulfate IV over 15 to 20 min. Overdrive pacing and isoproterenol infusion may also be effective. Synchronized cardioversion is indicated for unstable rhythms. Class IA and IC antiarrhythmics, as well as beta blockers, calcium-channel blockers, and phenytoin are contraindicated.

Patients who have a normal physical examination and are completely asymptomatic 6 h after ingestion do not require admission for toxicologic reasons. They should receive appropriate psychiatric evaluation. All symptomatic patients should be admitted to a monitored bed. An NG tube or Foley catheter may be necessary in patients with ileus or urinary retention. Patients with moderate to severe toxicity require ICU admission.

Laboratory evaluation should include an acetaminophen level to rule out coingestion of this common drug. Consider obtaining electrolytes, creatinine, glucose, CPK, and an ABG on patients who are admitted. Chest x-ray is indicated in patients who have been intubated, or if aspiration pneumonia is suspected.

If Standard Treatment Fails

TCA-induced cardiovascular collapse is potentially reversible. In the appropriate circumstance, a trial of cardiopulmonary bypass, overdrive pacing, or aortic balloon pump support may be indicated.

NEWER ANTIDEPRESSANTS AND SEROTONIN SYNDROME

The toxicology and pharmacology of the newer antidepressants is distinct from that of TCA and MAOIs. In general, they have lower toxicity and fewer adverse effects and drug interactions.

Clinical Features, Diagnosis, and Differential

The newer antidepressants are not detected on routine toxicology screening tests. Symptoms and signs of toxicity are in general nonspecific, and diagnosis depends on history and clinical suspicion. These agents are not significantly cardiotoxic and are not associated with anticholinergic side-effects.

Trazodone

Clinical Features

Adverse effects include sedation, orthostatic hypotension, dizziness, dry mouth, nausea, and peripheral edema. Trazodone is the most common cause of drug-induced priapism, affecting as many as 1 in 1000 patients on routine therapy.

Serious toxicity in adults is usually seen with ingestions of greater than 2 g and commonly presents as CNS depression, ataxia, dizziness, nausea, vomiting, dry mouth, and nonspecific abdominal pain. Important drug interactions occur with alcohol, CNS depressants, and beta blockers. Seizures, coma, respiratory depression, and overdose fatalities are usually seen in mixed drug ingestions.

Trazodone has low cardiotoxicity but can be arrhythmogenic in patients with underlying conduction abnormalities or ischemic heart disease. Reported arrhythmias include sinus arrest, sinus bradycardia, A-V blocks, complete heart block, atrial fibrillation, PVCs, ventricular tachycardia, and torsades de pointes. Orthostatic hypotension is frequently seen. Sinus tachycardia occurs in approximately 25% of overdoses.

Emergency Department Care and Disposition

An intravenous line and cardiac monitoring should be instituted. Isolated ingestions of less than 1000 mg have a low risk of toxicity, and administration of 1 gram per kg of activated charcoal is adequate. Consider gastric lavage in ingestions of 1 to 2 g if the patient presents less than 2 h after overdose. Gastric lavage and activated charcoal are recommended in overdoses of more than 2 g. Most patients require only monitoring and supportive care. Asymptomatic patients after 6 h of observation may be discharged with appropriate psychiatric evaluation. ICU admission is indicated for patients with neurologic or cardiac symptoms after 6 h of observation. Telemetry admission is adequate for asymptomatic patients with risk factors for complications such as cardiovascular disease or coingestants that may have delayed or prolonged effects.

Bupropion

Clinical Features

At the maximum daily recommended dose of 450 mg, bupropion is associated with a 0.4% incidence of seizures and at doses of > 450 mg, a 4% incidence. The most common adverse effects are dry mouth, nausea, headache, constipation, tremor, anxiety, confusion, blurred vision, and increased motor activity. Adverse drug interactions may occur with levodopa, lithium, SSRIs, MAOIs, and phenothiazines.

Bupropion has a low toxic-to-therapeutic ratio. Toxicity may be seen with ingestions of > 5 mg/kg. The most common findings are lethargy, tremor, generalized seizures, confusion, and vomiting. Sinus tachycardia may occur, but no significant arrhythmias or conduction abnormalities have been reported. Hypotension and coma have only been seen in mixed drug overdoses. Mild hypokalemia has been reported.

Emergency Department Care and Disposition

Intravenous access and cardiac monitoring should be instituted. Gastric lavage is recommended if the patient presents 1 to 2 h after overdose. All patients should receive 1 g/kg of activated charcoal. Ipecac is contraindicated because of risk of seizures.

Seizures usually occur 1 to 4 hours after ingestion but may be delayed up to 8. They are typically generalized, single, and brief and may occur in otherwise asymptomatic patients. Self-limited seizures do not require treatment. Repetitive seizures, or those lasting more than 5 min, respond best to benzodiazepines, with phenobarbital as a second-line drug. Dilantin is not usually effective. (For further guidance on seizure management, see chap. 131.)

Patients should be observed for at least 8 h. Asymptomatic patients can be discharged with appropriate psychiatric evaluation. Symptomatic patients, including those with sinus tachycardia, should be admitted to a monitored or ICU bed.

Selective Serotonin Reuptake Inhibitors (SSRIs)

Clinical Features

Three SSRIs are currently available in the US—fluoxetine (Prozac), sertraline (Zoloft), and paroxetine (Paxil). Fluoxetine is the most frequently prescribed antidepressant in the US.

Serotonin syndrome is the most serious adverse effect seen in both routine therapy and overdose. Nausea, vomiting, diarrhea, and constipation are common. Other adverse effects include headache, sedation, insomnia, dizziness, weakness, tremor, and nervousness. Sexual dysfunction is common. Extrapyramidal symptoms (EPS) including akathisia, dystonic reactions, and parkinsonian symptoms also may occur. Less common adverse reactions include dry mouth, increased sweating, visual blurring, hyponatremia, and hypoglycemia. Seizures occur in 0.2% of patients taking fluoxetine.

Fluoxetine may elevate the levels of carbamazepine, valproic acid, clozapine, haloperidol, perphenazine, diazepam, lithium, and tricyclic antidepressants. There is an increased risk of serotonin syndrome when SSRIs are combined with serotonergic drugs, especially MAOIs. The SSRIs have a high toxic to therapeutic ratio. Virtually all overdose experience is with fluoxetine, but all SSRIs appear to be similar in overdose. Significant toxicity in adults is expected with ingestions > 1500 mg fluoxetine. Deaths have occurred with fluoxetine overdose but have usually been associated with mixed-drug overdose.

The most serious reactions in overdose are generalized seizures and serotonin syndrome. EKG is usually normal, except for sinus tachycardia. Laboratory studies are usually normal, except for rare cases of hyponatremia associated with chronic therapy.

Emergency Department Care and Disposition

Institute intravenous access and cardiac monitoring on all patients. Activated charcoal administration, 1 g/kg, is adequate for isolated fluoxetine ingestions of less than 1000 mg. Gastric lavage followed by activated charcoal are recommended for ingestions greater than 1000 mg and for mixed drug overdoses. Comparable doses for sertraline and paroxetine have not yet been established.

Most SSRI overdose patients require only monitoring and supportive care. Patients at high risk for complications include those with a seizure history, symptoms of serotonin syndrome, and mixed-drug ingestions. Patients who are tachycardic, lethargic, or otherwise symptomatic should be admitted to a monitored or ICU bed. Asymptomatic patients may be discharged with appropriate psychiatric evaluation after a 6-h observation period.

Venflaxine

Clinical Features

Venflaxine is the newest antidepressant in the U.S. Adverse effects and toxicity appear to be similar to the SSRIs. Coma has occurred in ingestions of > 750 mg; generalized seizures have been seen; no fatalities have been reported.

Emergency Department Care and Disposition

At the present time, the same management guidelines used for SSRI overdose are recommended.

TABLE 92-1. Symptoms of Serotonin Syndrome

Cognitive–behavioral
  Agitation, anxiety
  Drowsiness, coma
  Confusion, delirium
  Euphoria, hypomania
  Headache, insomnia
  Seizures
Autonomic nervous system
  Nausea, salivation
  Sinus tachycardia, ventricular tachycardia
  Diaphoresis, diarrhea, abdominal cramps
  Hyperthermia, hypertension, mydriasis
  Cutaneous piloerection, flushed skin
Neuromuscular
  Ankle clonus, hyperreflexia
  Restlessness, rigidity
  Shivering, teeth chattering, tremor
  Dysarthria, ataxia, incoordination (clumsiness)
  Head twitching, hyperactivity
  Muscle joint pain; muscle twitching, myoclonic jerks
  Myoclonus, jaw quivering
  Nystagmus, paresthesias
  Babinski (bilateral) sign

Serotonin Syndrome

Clinical Features

Serotonin syndrome is characterized by autonomic nervous system dysfunction, and alterations in behavior, cognitive ability, and neuromuscular activity. Table 92-1 summarizes the major clinical findings. Rhabdomyolysis may occur secondary to severe muscle rigidity and hyperthermia. The symptoms of serotonin syndrome are nonspecific and can be attributed to other disorders. There are no pathognomonic diagnostic tests.

Serotonin syndrome can be precipitated by agents that increase CNS serotonin activity. MAOIs and SSRIs are the most commonly implicated agents. Other associated drugs, especially when used in combination, include meperidine, dextromethorphan, venlaxine, clomipramine, lithium, amphetamines, cocaine, bromocriptine, levodopa, and buspirone.

Emergency Department Care and Disposition

Discontinue all serotonergic agents and institute cardiac monitoring and supportive care. Benzodiazepines are nonspecific serotonin antagonists and may decrease patient discomfort. (See chap. 136, for guidelines on muscle rigidity and hyperthermia management.) Admission is indicated until all symptoms have resolved, and most patients improve significantly within 24 h.

MONOAMINE OXIDASE INHIBITORS (MAOIs)

The psychiatric and neurologic indications for MAOIs have expanded, and their use is increasing. MAOIs are associated with numerous side effects, dietary and drug interactions, and severe toxicity in overdose.

Clinical Features

Phenelzine (Nardil), tranylcypromine (Parnate), and isocarboxazid (Marplan) are the only MAOI antidepressants currently available in the U.S. Sergyline (Eldepryl) is a MAOI used as an adjunct in treatment of Parkinson's disease. Pargyline, an antihypertensive, furazolidone, an antimicrobial, and procarbazine, an antineoplastic, also have MAOI activity.

MAOI toxicity is usually precipitated by overdose, drug interaction, or dietary interaction. Tyramine is a biogenic amine metabolized by monoamine oxidase. It is in numerous foods, especially unfresh meat or fish, sauerkraut, aged meats and cheeses, alcohol (especially Chianti wine and vermouth), pickled fish, yeast extracts, and broad beans.

A tyramine reaction typically occurs 30 to 90 min after ingestion of tyramine-containing food. Symptoms and signs include severe head-ache, diaphoresis, mydriasis, neck stiffness, neuromuscular excitation, and hypertension. Symptoms usually resolve in 6 to 12 h. Fatalities are usually due to intracranial hemorrhage or myocardial infarction.

MAOIs may have severe interactions with numerous medications, which are only partially listed in this text, due to space constraints (see Table 92-2). Currently available MAOIs in the U.S. irreversibly bind monoamine oxidase. Before administration of any contraindicated drugs, a two-wk wash-out period is necessary to allow enzyme activity to recover. Table 92-3 lists drugs considered safe to coadminister with MAOIs.

MAOIs increase the amount of norepinephrine in presynaptic nerve terminals. The indirect acting sympathomimetics displace norepineph-rine from presynaptic nerve terminals. A dangerously augmented sym-pathetic discharge can therefore occur when these classes of drugs are combined. Direct acting sympathomimetics, such as norepinephrine, are metabolized outside of the neuron by a different enzyme and are therefore not contraindicated.

MAOIs in combination with beta blockers, phenothiazines, theophyl-line, caffeine, and ketamine may precipitate cardiovascular complica-tions. MAOIs may potentiate the action of oral hypoglycemics. Seroto-nin syndrome may be precipitated when MAOIs are administered with numerous drugs.

MAOIs have a low toxic-to-therapeutic ratio. Spontaneous hyperten-sive episodes are occasionally seen with therapeutic doses, and over-doses of 2 to 3 mg/kg may be lethal. In overdose there is a characteristic

TABLE 92-2. Drugs Contraindicated with MAOIs*

Indirect sympathomimetics
  Amphetamines
  Bretylium
  Cocaine
  Cylert
  Dopamine
  Ephedrine
  Flenfluramine
  Guanethidine
  Metaraminol
  Methyldopa
  Methylphenidate
  Phencyclidine
  Phenylephrine
  Phenylpropanolamine
  Pseudoephedrine
  Reserpine
  Tyramine
Miscellaneous drugs
  Anticholinergics
  Beta blockers
  Caffeine
  Codeine
  Dextromethorphan
  Disulfiram
  Ketamine
  Levodopa
  Meperidine
  Oral hypoglycemic agents
  Phenothiazines
  Serotonin reuptake inhibitors
  Theophylline
  Tricyclic antidepressants
  Tryptophan

* See Table 131-1, *Emergency Medicine: A Comprehensive Study Guide,* 4th ed., for additional list of drugs that cause serotonin syndrome.

delay of symptom onset of 6 to 12 h, but as long as 29 h has been reported.

Initial symptoms include headache, agitation, restlessness, nausea, palpitations, and tremor. Early signs include sinus tachycardia, hyperreflexia, fasciculations, mydriasis, hyperventilation, nystagmus, and cutaneous flushing. Findings in moderate toxicity include opisthotonos, muscle rigidity, diaphoresis, chest pain, hypertension, diarrhea, hallucinations, combativeness, confusion, and marked hyperthermia. In severe toxicity there may be progression to bradycardia, hypotension, hypoxia, seizures, and coma. Hypotension is an ominous finding and is usually resistant to treatment.

TABLE 92-3. Drugs Considered Safe with MAOIs

Direct sympathomimetics
  Albuterol
  Clonidine
  Dobutamine
  Epinephrine
  Isoproterenol
  Methoxamine
  Norepinephrine
  Salbutamol
  Terbutaline
Miscellaneous drugs
  Acetaminophen
  Antibiotics
  Aspirin
  Barbiturates
  Benzodiazepines
  Butyrophenones
  Calcium channel blockers
  Corticosteroids
  Lidocaine
  Metoclopromide
  Morphine
  Nitroglycerin
  Nonsteroidal anti-inflammatory drugs
  Ondansetron
  Procainamide
  Sumatriptan

Diagnosis and Differential

MAOIs are not detected on most drug screens, and their toxicity is not associated with any specific laboratory abnormalities or EKG findings. Laboratory tests are useful to detect complications such as hypoxia, rhabdomyolysis, renal failure, hyperkalemia, acidosis, hemolysis, and DIC. The most common EKG abnormality is sinus tachycardia, and T-wave abnormalities are not uncommon.

All drugs and medical conditions that produce hyperadrenergic states are in the differential diagnosis of MAOI toxicity. These include cocaine, PCP, amphetamines, phenylpropanolamine, methylphenidate, theophylline, strychnine, nicotine, and anticholinergics. Withdrawal from alcohol, sedative hypnotics, beta blockers, and clonidine may produce a similar picture. Also, consider neuroleptic malignant syndrome, serotonin syndrome, and malignant hyperthermia. Medical conditions in the differential diagnosis include hypoglycemia, hyperthyroidism, pheochromocytoma, heat stroke, meningitis, encephalitis, sepsis, tetanus, and rabies.

Emergency Department Care and Disposition

Institute an intravenous line and cardiac monitoring. If less than 4 h since ingestion, gastric lavage followed by 1 g/kg of activated charcoal are recommended. Activated charcoal alone is adequate if more than 4 h have elapsed since ingestion. Ipecac is contraindicated. Repeat charcoal dosing, hemodialysis, hemoperfusion, and peritoneal dialysis have no current role.

In cases of severe hypertension, an arterial line is recommended. The drug of choice is nitroprusside, started at an initial rate of 1 mcg/kg/min and titrated to response. Phentolamine is an alternative, and is dosed 2.5 to 5 mg IV every 10 to 15 min, until BP is controlled. Phentolamine may also be given as continuous infusion. Nitroglycerin is indicated for treatment of angina.

Hypotensive patients have a poor prognosis. Initial treatment is with isotonic fluid boluses of 10 to 20 ml/kg. Norepinephrine is the vasopressor of choice for resistant hypotension.

Sinus tachycardia rarely requires treatment unless it produces ischemia. Bradycardia may be treated with atropine, isoproterenol, dobutamine, or pacing. Lidocaine, procainamide, and phenytoin are the most effective antiarrhythmics. Bretylium is contraindicated. Beta blockers may precipitate severe hypertension because of unopposed vasoconstriction.

Seizures are initially treated with benzodiazepines, and then barbiturates. Phenytoin is generally ineffective.

Hyperthermia treatment includes cooling blankets, mist spray, and fans. Benzodiazepines may reduce muscle hyperactivity. Dantrolene (2.5 to 10 mg/kg IV divided q 6 h) may be effective in resistant cases of muscle rigidity.

All intentional MAOI overdoses, accidental overdoses greater than 2 ml/kg, or any patients with symptoms of toxicity, should be admitted to the ICU. Asymptomatic accidental ingestions should be admitted to a monitored bed due to the possibility of delayed onset of toxicity. Patients with tyramine reactions should be observed a minimum of 6 h, and those with persistent symptoms should be admitted.

If Standard Treatment Fails

Seizures unresponsive to treatment may require neuromuscular paralysis combined with general anesthesia to prevent neurologic sequelae, metabolic acidosis, hyperthermia, and rhabdomyolysis. Resistant hyperthermia also may require neuromuscular paralysis. A nondepolarizing paralytic, such as vecuronium, should be used.

NEUROLEPTICS

Neuroleptics are primarily used in the treatment of psychotic disorders. They are also used in the treatment of nausea, headaches, and various involuntary motor disorders, such as hiccoughs and Tourette's syndrome.

Clinical Features

Adverse reactions to neuroleptics are related to their antidopaminergic, anticholinergic, and antiadrenergic actions. Table 92-4 summarizes the major classes of neuroleptics and their potency in relation to dopaminergic, muscarinic (anticholinergic), and adrenergic antagonism. Dopamine antagonism may result in a variety of movement disorders, including dystonias, akathisia, drug-induced parkinsonism, tardive dyskinesia, and NMS. Table 92-5 summarizes the major clinical features of these disorders and their treatment.

Neuroleptic overdose causes CNS depression. Coingestion of other CNS depressants increases the risk of coma and respiratory depression. Hypothermia or, less commonly, hyperthermia may occur secondary to hypothalamic dysfunction. Pinpoint pupils may be seen in phenothiazine ingestion. The motor disorders described above may be seen. Seizures also may occur.

Anticholinergic signs and symptoms may be present. Hypotension and reflex tachycardia are common secondary to alpha-adrenergic blockade. Ventricular arrhythmias, including torsades de pointes (especially with the piperidine phenothiazines), supraventricular tachycardia, and AV dissociation, may occur.

Emergency Department Care and Disposition

Assess airway and ventilation. Institute an intravenous line and cardiac monitoring. Check serum glucose level and consider naloxone administration in patients with altered level of consciousness.

Administer activated charcoal (1 g/kg) to all patients. Gastric lavage should be considered on a case-by-case basis. Patients presenting early (1–2 h) after overdose, those with delayed gastric emptying from anticholinergic effects, and those with the finding of radiopaque pills in the stomach, may benefit from lavage (phenothiazine pills may be radiopaque). Multidose charcoal (0.5 g/kg q 4 h) may enhance elimination by removing the drug from the enterohepatic circulation. Hemodialysis and forced diuresis are not helpful.

After initial stabilization, a qualitative urine drug screen may confirm the presence of a neuroleptic. Blood levels are not useful in management of overdose. A 12-lead EKG should be obtained on all patients. Electrolytes and renal-function tests also may be useful.

The drugs of choice for ventricular arrhythmias are class IB antiarrhythmics (e.g., lidocaine) and bicarbonate therapy, which is summarized in the section on tricyclic antidepressants. Class IA antiarrhythmics (disopyramide, quinidine, and procainamide) are contraindicated. Torsades de pointes is treated with magnesium, isoproterenol, or overdrive pacing. Seizures are treated initially with benzodiazepines. Phenobarbital and phenytoin are second- and third-line drugs.

After a 4 h observation period, asymptomatic patients except those ingesting a piperidine phenothiazine, may be discharged from the ED

TABLE 92-4. The Five Neuroleptic Classes

Class	Dose Range, mg/day	Dopaminergic Antagonism	Muscarinic Antagonism	Adrenergic Antagonism
Butyrohenone				
Haloperidol	1–100	High	Low	Moderate
Droperidol	1.25–10	High	Low	Moderate
Dibenzoxazepines				
Loxapine	10–300	Low	Low	Low
Dihydroindolone				
Molindone	15–225	Low	Low	Low
Phenothiazines				
Aliphatics				
Chlorpromazine	25–2000	Low	High	High
Promethazine	50–150	Low	High	Moderate
Piperidines				
Mesoridazine	75–400	Low	High	High
Thioridazine	50–800	Low	High	Moderate
Piperazines				
Prochlorperazine	15–150	Moderate	Moderate	Low
Fluphenazine	1–25	High	Moderate	Moderate
Thioxanthenes				
Thiothixene	6–60	High	Low	Moderate

522

TABLE 92-5. Adverse Reactions to Neuroleptics

Type of Disorder	Presentation	Incidence, %	Treatment
Dystonic reaction Torticollis, facial grimacing, opisthotonos oculogyric crisis, laryngeal spasm	Early	12 >males	Diphenhydramine, 50 mg or benztropine, 2 mg IM/IV
Akathisia Restlessness, jittery feeling, insomnia	Early	20 >females	Lower dose or change to less potent drug; benztropine, amantadine, or propranolol
Parkinsonism Resting tremor, rigidity, masked facies	Early	13 >females	Lower dose or change to less potent drug; benztropine or amantidine
Tardive dyskinesia Lip smaking, tongue protrusion, grimacing, chewing motion	Late	30 >tfemales	No proven treatment
NMS Hyperthermia, rigidity, altered mental status, autonomic instability	Variable	<3 >males	ABC, muscle relaxation, cooling, rehydration

523

with appropriate psychiatric evaluation. All patients who are symptomatic or have a vital-sign abnormality after 4 h of observation should be admitted to an ICU or monitored bed. All patients who ingest a piperidine phenothiazine should be admitted and monitored, even if asymptomatic, because of the risk of delayed dysrhythmias.

LITHIUM

Lithium is a widely prescribed psychotropic used in the treatment of bipolar and affective disorders. It has a low therapeutic index, with a mortality rate as high as 10% to 20% in serious overdoses.

Clinical Features

Lithium has numerous potential side-effects, listed in Table 92-6; the major signs and symptoms of acute lithium toxicity are summarized

TABLE 92-6. Potential Side-Effects of Lithium Therapy

Initial side effects
  Polydipsia
  Polyuria
  Dry mouth
  Nausea
  Fine tremor of hands
Chronic effects
  Ophthalmologic
    Tearing
    Blurring of vision
    Scotomatas
    Exophthalmos
    Papilledema (pseudotumor cerebri)
  Renal
    Lowered urine osmolarity
    Naphrogenic diabetes insipidus
    Nephrotic syndrome
    Structural damage ($+/-$)
  Endocrine
    Nontoxic goiter
    Hyperparathyroidism
  Teratogenesis (lithium crosses placenta and is excreted in breast milk)
    Ebstein anomaly or other heart defects
    Neonatal diabetes insipidus
  Dermatologic
    Acne
    Localized edema
    Cutaneous ulcers
  Hematologic
    Neutrophilia
    Aplastic anemia (rare)

TABLE 92-7. Signs and Symptoms of Acute Lithium Toxicity

CNS/Neuromuscular
 Tremor
 Neuromuscular irritability:
  muscle twitching, hyperreflexia, clonus, fasciculations
 Ataxia
 Transient neurologic asymmetries
 Lethargy
 Dysarthria
 Confusion
 Stupor
 Convulsions
 Coma
Gastrointestinal
 Nausea and vomiting
 Diarrhea
Cardiovascular:
 ST-T-wave changes
 Sinus bradycardia
 Conduction defects
 Ventricular arrhythmias
 Hypertension (rare)

in Table 92-7. At therapeutic doses, side-effects or toxicity may be precipitated if lithium renal clearance is diminished. Lithium clearance is decreased in the setting of impaired kidney function and water or sodium depletion. Diabetes mellitus, hypertension, renal failure, advanced age, and a low sodium diet all increase the risk of lithium toxicity. Diuretics and NSAIDs may precipitate toxicity.

Lithium blood levels greater than 2.0 mEq/l are considered toxic. Patients on chronic therapy have intracellular stores of lithium not reflected in the blood level. They may demonstrate toxicity at lower blood levels than patients not previously taking lithium. Peak blood levels usually occur 8 to 12 h after ingestion.

Emergency Department Care and Disposition

Intravenous line and cardiac monitoring should be instituted. Gastric lavage is recommended in all patients. In overdose of sustained release preparations, repeat lavage in 2 to 4 h as well as whole-bowel irrigation, may be effective. Activated charcoal does not bind lithium, but a dose of 1 g/kg is recommended because of the risk of a multiple drug ingestion. Close monitoring of electrolytes, renal function, and volume status is essential. Intravenous normal saline increases sodium ion concentration and may promote lithium excretion. The development of lithium toxicity may be delayed. All patients with significant ingestions or with symptoms of toxicity should be admitted to a monitored or ICU bed.

If Standard Treatment Fails

Hemodialysis effectively removes lithium ions from the serum. Repeated dialysis is often necessary as lithium reaccumulates in serum from tissue stores. Indications for hemodialysis are:

1. Severe toxicity or progression of symptoms
2. Renal failure or decreasing urine output
3. Lack of expected drop in lithium level of 20% in 6 h
4. Lithium level > 4.0 mEq/l

For further reading in *Emergency Medicine: A Comprehensive Study Guide*, 4th ed., see Chapter 130, Tricyclic Antidepressants, by Kirk C. Mills; Chapter 131, Newer Antidepressants and Serotonin Syndrome, by Kirk C. Mills; Chapter 132, Monoamine Oxidase Inhibitors, by Kirk C. Mills; Chapter 133, Neuroleptics, by William P. Kerns II; and Chapter 134, Lithium, by P. J. Ryan.

93 | Sedative-Hypnotics

C. Crawford Mechem

Sedative–hypnotics include barbiturates, benzodiazepines, and nonbenzodiazepine agents such as buspirone, zolpidem, and meprobamate. They are used in the induction of anesthesia and in the management of seizure disorders, alcohol withdrawal, anxiety, insomnia, and elevated intracranial pressure. Their ingestion can result in serious morbidity or mortality, alone or in combination with other agents.

BARBITURATES

Clinical Features

Mild to moderate barbiturate intoxication is characterized by lethargy, emotional lability, impaired thinking, slurred speech, incoordination, and nystagmus. Severe toxicity generally follows ingestion of 10 times the hypnotic dose and presents with central nervous system (CNS) depression ranging from lethargy to coma and a flat EEG. Respiratory depression, vasodilatation, hypotension, shock, hypothermia, muscle flaccidity, depressed deep tendon reflexes, slowed gastrointestinal motility, and skin bullae may also be seen.

Emergency Department Care and Disposition

The key to recovery is the management of multiple depressed organ systems until the patient metabolizes and clears the drug.

1. Airway management in patients with severe overdose frequently involves intubation. Serial arterial blood gases and chest radiographs should be obtained.
2. Gastric lavage is used for gastric emptying, after ensuring a protected airway. Ipecac is contraindicated because of the potential for barbiturate-associated CNS depression.
3. Activated charcoal is administered after the completion of adequate lavage. In phenobarbital overdoses, the use of multiple doses of charcoal, 30 gm every 6 h by nasogastric tube for 6 doses, decreases the elimination half-life.
4. An intravenous fluid challenge with crystalloid solutions is the first treatment for hypotension. Low doses of may be required if the pressure does not respond to fluid resuscitation.
5. Forced diuresis and alkalinization of the urine using sodium bicarbonate, (1–2 mEq/kg IV every 4 to 6 h) to maintain urine pH at 7.5 or higher significantly increases the phenobarbital excretion rate. This is not effective for intermediate- or short-acting barbiturates. The patient should be observed for evidence of fluid overload.
6. Hemodialysis and charcoal hemoperfusion are more effective than forced diuresis and alkalinization in removing phenobarbital. Be-

cause of potential complications, they should be reserved for the most critical overdoses or in patients with underlying hepatic or renal insufficiency.

BENZODIAZEPINES

Clinical Features

The predominant manifestations of benzodiazepine toxicity are neurologic and include drowsiness, dizziness, slurred speech, confusion, ataxia, and impairment of intellectual function. Coma is atypical and should prompt a search for coingestants or a nontoxin-related medical problem. Respiratory depression and hypotension may be seen, generally after parenteral administration and most commonly, in the elderly. Paradoxical reactions, including excitement, anxiety, aggression, hostile behavior, rage, and delirium may be seen. Other effects include headache, nausea, vomiting, chest pain, joint pain, diarrhea, and incontinence. Extrapyramidal reactions, as well as allergic, hematologic, and hepatotoxic reactions are seen uncommonly. In general, benzodiazepines have no long-term organ system toxicity.

Benzodiazepine withdrawal may be seen on abrupt discontinuation following prolonged use in high doses. Symptoms include anxiety, irritability, insomnia, nausea, vomiting, anorexia, tremor, and sweating. More serious manifestations, including confusion, psychosis, and seizures, have been reported.

Emergency Department Care and Disposition

As with all victims of overdoses, initial management involves stabilizing the patient's airway, breathing, and circulatory status.

1. Administration of thiamine and naloxone should be considered in all patients with altered mental status, and the serum blood glucose should be determined.
2. Gastric emptying is performed by lavage. Ipecac is contraindicated because of the risk of benzodiazepine-mediated CNS depression.
3. Activated charcoal should be administered routinely.
4. Flumazenil is a selective antagonist of the central effects of benzodiazepines. Its use in benzodiazepine toxicity may obviate the need for intubation. In the ED it is useful mainly in reversing the effects of benzodiazepines administered for diagnostic and therapeutic procedures. The initial dose is 0.2 mg IV, followed by a second dose of 0.3 mg, and a third dose of 0.5 mg, as needed. Its plasma elimination half-life is approximately 1 h. As a consequence, recurrent benzodiazepine toxicity may result once its effects have worn off. Generalized seizures have occurred in patients given flumazenil after coingestion of benzodiazepines and seizure-inducing agents, particularly cyclic antidepressants. Seizures have also occurred after

administration of flumazenil to patients physically dependent on benzodiazepines or who are taking them for control of a seizure disorder. Flumazenil also is contraindicated with elevated intracranial pressure, such as following severe head trauma.

5. Withdrawal symptoms may be treated by administration of a benzodiazepine and subsequent tapering.

NONBENZODIAZEPINE SEDATIVE–HYPNOTICS

Ethchlorvynol (Placidyl; street named pickles, jelly beans, Mr. Green Jeans)

Clinical Features

Although now widely replaced by safer sedative-hypnotic agents, intentional overdose of ethchlorvynol is still seen occasionally. Clinical manifestations of toxicity vary according to the method and chronicity of abuse. The chronically-dependent patient complains of neurologic disabilities, such as facial numbness, incoordination, tremors, confusion, slurred speech, muscle weakness, diplopia, or visual disturbances resulting from macular degeneration or chiasmal optic neuritis. With acute IV injection, noncardiogenic pulmonary edema is commonly seen. Acute oral overdose produces a mint-like taste in the mouth, dyspnea, a dry cough, nystagmus, and profound CNS depression, including coma and a flat EEG. Hemodynamic instability with bradycardia and hypotension may be seen. Other findings following oral overdose include hypothermia, pulmonary edema, bullae, sudden painless bilateral blindness, hemolysis, cholestatic jaundice, and pancytopenia. Ethchlorvynol coingested with ethanol or other CNS depressants can produce respiratory arrest.

Meprobamate (Miltown, Equanil)

Clinical Features

Although widely replaced by safer benzodiazepines, meprobamate is still seen in cases of intentional overdose and chronic long-term abuse among the elderly. Clinical manifestations include CNS depression leading to coma, as well as hypotension, tachycardia, bradycardia, pulmonary edema, and bullous skin lesions. Myoclonus and seizures are seen rarely.

Glutethimide (Doriden; street names sets, hits, loads, packs, three's and eight's, four doors)

Clinical Features

Clinical manifestations include CNS and myocardial depression. A unique feature of glutethimide is its ability to cause anticholinergic toxicity. Profound, cyclical coma lasting up to 100 h may be seen as a result of enterohepatic circulation of active metabolites and the anticholinergic effect of the parent compound on gut motility. Other anticholinergic manifestations include dry mucous membranes, mydriasis, tachycardia, hypertension, ileus, urinary retention, hyperpyrexia, delirium, agitation, and seizures. Hypotension, pulmonary edema, and bullous skin lesions have also been reported.

Methaqualone (Quaalude, Parest, Mequin, Sopor; Mandrax-a combination with diphenhydramine; street names quads, ludes, sopers, mandies, soapers, the love drug, wallbanger)

Clinical Features

Mild intoxication is characterized by slurred speech, slow and uncoordinated movements, and nystagmus. Higher doses lead to CNS depression, as well as a paradoxical increase in muscle tone with hyperreflexia, myoclonus, and seizures. Painful hyperacusis is a helpful, discriminating feature. Pulmonary edema is frequently seen in large overdoses. Methaqualone induces thrombocytopenia and hypoprothrombinemia, which may lead to conjunctival, retinal, gastrointestinal, and bullous skin hemorrhages.

Chloral Hydrate (Noctec; street name Mickey Finn when combined with ethanol)

Clinical Features

Mild toxicity presents with sedation and incoordination. A pear-like odor may be noted on the patient's breath. Other findings include GI bleeding, hepatitis, and skin lesions such as purpura and bullae. Severe cardiovascular complications account for the majority of deaths from this drug and include depressed myocardial contractility, a prolonged refractory period, and increased sensitivity of myocardial cells to catecholamines. Refractory dysrhythmias and death may follow.

Buspirone (BuSpar)

Clinical Features

Buspirone is less sedating than diazepam and interacts less with other sedatives such as ethanol. The most common manifestations of toxicity are drowsiness and dysphoria. Hypotension, bradycardia, paresthesias, seizures, GI upset, hepatotoxicity, dystonic reactions, and priapism have also been reported.

Zolpidem (ambien, stilnox, bikalm, niotal)

The primary effects of toxicity are CNS and respiratory depression. Effects are dose-related and exacerbated by the coingestion of other

CNS depressants such as ethanol. Psychotic reactions have been reported at therapeutic doses. Other manifestations of toxicity are dizziness, amnesia, and vomiting.

Diagnosis and Differential

The diagnosis of ethchlorvynol overdose may be aided by the detection of a pungent vinyl or sweet odor on the patient's breath. Blood ethchlorvynol levels correlate with symptoms but may not be readily available. This is also the case with meprobamate and 4–HG, the active metabolite of glutethimide. In methaqualone overdoses, plasma levels do not correlate well with clinical findings. Because chloral hydrate is radiopaque, abdominal x-rays may confirm ingestion and guide intestinal decontamination. Chloral hydrate and zolpidem levels are not useful in guiding management.

Emergency Department Care and Disposition

Most oral overdoses of the non-benzodiazepine sedative–hypnotics involve multiple agents. Careful search for other treatable ingestions, such as acetaminophen or salicylates, is therefore mandatory. In addition, all of these agents with the possible exception of buspirone cause physical dependence with chronic use. Development of a life-threatening withdrawal state following treatment of acute toxicity therefore must be anticipated. Meticulous supportive care is the mainstay of treatment. Several general principles apply.

1. The patient's airway must be secured before attempts at decontamination.
2. Intravenous crystalloid solutions are used initially to manage hypotension. Vasopressors are indicated early on because many of these agents cause pulmonary edema.
3. The IV administration of glucose, naloxone, and thiamine should be considered in all patients with altered mental status.
4. Decontamination is performed by gastric lavage, followed by administration of activated charcoal (1 g/kg) and sorbitol (1 g/kg) or other cathartic. Repeat doses of charcoal may be useful in comatose patients or in cases of glutethimide toxicity. Multiple-dose charcoal or whole-bowel irrigation is contraindicated in patients with ileus.
5. Hemoperfusion is more effective than hemodialysis in enhancing elimination.
6. In cases of ethchlorvynol overdose, ibuprofen may reduce lung injury from noncardiogenic pulmonary edema.
7. Because meprobamate tends to form concretions in the GI tract, whole-bowel irrigation using 2 L/h polyethylene glycol (40 mL/kg per h in children) until the rectal effluent is clear should be considered.

8. In glutethimide overdoses, hyperthermia, agitation, and seizures should be treated aggressively to prevent rhabdomyolysis and neurologic injury. Physostigmine to reverse anticholinergic toxicity is not recommended.

9. Hypertonicity and seizures due to methaqualone toxicity can be treated with benzodiazepines. Severe muscle contractions may necessitate use of neuromuscular paralytic agents. Platelets, vitamin K, and fresh frozen plasma are administered to control hemorrhage.

10. Ventricular dysrhythmias due to chloral hydrate may respond to lidocaine, phenytoin, propranolol, or overdrive pacing. If vasopressors are required for pressure support, pure alpha-acting agents such as norepinephrine should be used. Agents with beta-agonist properties should be avoided because they can exacerbate dysrhythmias.

11. Flumazenil (0.2 mg IV over 30 s) has been effective in reversing the CNS and respiratory actions of zolpidem. If adequate consciousness is not obtained within 30 s, a second dose of 0.3 mg may be administered over 30 s. Additional doses of 0.5 mg may be administered at 1–min intervals up to a maximum dose of 3 mg. Contraindications include known or suspected coingestion of cyclic antidepressants, known seizure disorder, or chronic benzodiazepine dependence.

For further reading in *Emergency Medicine: A Comprehensive Study Guide*, 4th edition, see Chapter 135, Barbiturates, by P.J. Ryan; Chapter 136, Benzodiazepines, by George M. Boss; and Chapter 137, Nonbenzodiazepine Sedative–Hypnotics, by Suzanne R. White.

Michael P. Kefer

In discussing the toxicity of common alcohols, an understanding of the osmolal gap is important. The presence of an osmolal gap suggests the presence of a low molecular weight substance such as ethanol, isopropanol, methanol, or ethylene glycol.

The Osmolal gap = Osm measured − Osm calculated (normal Osm gap < 10 mOsm/L)

Osm measured is determined in the lab by freezing point depression
Osm calculated = 2(Na) + BUN/2.8 + glucose/18

ETHANOL

The costs of ethanol to society are well known. Although acute ethanol intoxication may cause death directly from respiratory depression, morbidity and mortality are usually related to accidental injury from impaired cognitive function caused by ethanol. Ethanol intoxication predisposes patients to trauma and complicates the medical evaluation of the injured patient. Intoxicated patients are more likely to undergo major diagnostic procedures and studies due to inability of the physician to get a reliable history and physical. On average, non-drinkers eliminate ethanol from the bloodstream at a rate of 15–20 mg/dL/hr, chronic drinkers at 25–35 mg/dL/hr.

Ethanol Intoxication

Clinical Features

Signs and symptoms of ethanol intoxication include slurred speech, disinhibited behavior, CNS depression, and altered coordination and motor control. Manifestations of serious head injury may be identical to or clouded by ethanol intoxication. Ethanol use is associated with abuse of other elicit drugs.

Emergency Department Care and Disposition

The mainstay of treatment is observation of the patient until clinically sober. Perform a careful physical exam to evaluate for complicating injury or illness. Exclude hypoglycemia by measuring fingerstick glucose. Administer thiamine.

A CT scan of the head is indicated in any intoxicated patient who has a history of significant head injury and a Glasgow Coma Scale < 15, deterioration of mental status while under observation, or no improvement in mental status after 3 h of observation. Discharge once intoxication has resolved to the extent that the patient does not pose a threat to self or others. Those who drive themselves should have ethanol levels approaching zero.

Ethanol Withdrawal

Clinical Features

Signs and symptoms include tremor, anxiety, autonomic hyperactivity, sinus tachycardia or atrial fibrillation, seizures, and hallucinations, usually peaking in intensity 48 h after the last drink.

Emergency Department Care and Disposition

Volume repletion and sedation are the mainstays of treatment. Magnesium is administered because hypomagnesemia associated with tremor and possibly with seizures.

Sedate the patient with phenobarbital (260 mg IV over 15 min, followed by 130 mg q 30–45 minutes prn). Alternatively, lorazepam (2–4 mg IV followed by 2 mg q 30–45 min prn) may be used. Administer 1 l D_5NS with 100 mg thiamine and 2 to 4 grams of $MgSO_4$ over 1 to 2 h

Patients with alcohol withdrawal and complicating medical problems should be admitted, as should patients who require high doses of sedatives. Patients in mild withdrawal who respond well to ED treatment may be discharged. Those treated with phenobarbital require no outpatient prescription as the drug has a long half-life, 24 to 96 h. Patients treated with benzodiazepines may be prescribed a tapering dose if it is not thought they will immediately resume drinking.

ISOPROPANOL

Isopropanol is commonly found in rubbing alcohol, solvents, skin and hair products, paint thinners, and antifreeze. Its CNS-depressant effects are twice as potent and twice as long-lasting as ethanol. Acetone is the principle metabolite.

Clinical Features

Clinically, isopropanol intoxication manifests similar to ethanol intoxication except the duration is longer and the CNS depressant effects are more profound. The smell of rubbing alcohol may be noted on the patient's breath. Severe poisoning is marked by early onset coma, respiratory depression, and hypotension. Hemorrhagic gastritis is a characteristic finding, causing nausea, vomiting, and abdominal pain; upper GI bleeding may be severe. Other less common complications include hepatic dysfunction, acute tubular necrosis, and rhabdomyolysis.

Laboratory investigation reveals ketonemia and ketonuria, from accumulation of acetone, without hyperglycemia or glycosuria. Mild acidosis may be present from acetone metabolism to acetate and formate. Ketonemia and an osmolal gap, with or without a minimal metabolic acidosis, is a unique characteristic.

Diagnosis and Differential

Diagnosis is based on clinical presentation and laboratory findings of ketonemia and ketonuria and an osmolal gap with or without a minimal metabolic acidosis. Diagnosis is confirmed by an elevated isopropanol level. Isopropanol intoxication is distinguished from that of other common alcohols by the significant osmolal gap without a significant anion gap metabolic acidosis and a negative ethanol level.

Emergency Department Care and Disposition

General supportive measures are indicated. As with any patient who presents with altered mental status, administration of glucose, thiamine, and naloxone should be considered. Laboratory evaluation includes serum electrolytes, BUN, creatinine, glucose, acetone, ABGs and hepatic aminotransferases. An isopropanol level is used mainly to confirm the diagnosis; it does not usually influence management.

Charcoal does not bind alcohols, so it is useful only if there is coingestion of an adsorbable substance.

Hypotension usually responds to IV fluids. Severe hemorrhagic gastritis may require transfusion.

Hemodialysis is indicated for refractory hypotension or when the predicted peak level of isopropanol is > 400 mg/dL. Hemodialysis removes both isopropanol and acetone.

Patients with prolonged CNS depression require admission. Those who are asymptomatic after 6 to 8 h of observation can be discharged or referred for psychiatric evaluation if indicated.

METHANOL AND ETHYLENE GLYCOL

Methanol (wood alcohol) is commonly found as a solvent in paint products, windshield washing fluids, and antifreeze. Ethylene glycol is commonly used as a coolant and preservative and is found in polishes and detergents. Toxicity from these alcohols is due to formation of their toxic metabolites which results in a high anion gap metabolic acidosis (Na -[Cl- + HCO_3] $> 12 \pm 4$ mEq/L). Prognosis is related to the severity of the acidosis.

Clinical Features of Methanol

Methanol metabolism results in formation of formaldehyde and formic acid. Symptoms may not appear for 12 to 18 h after ingestion because these toxic metabolites must accumulate. Time to symptom onset may be longer if ethanol is consumed, as ethanol inhibits methanol metabolism.

Symptoms include CNS depression, visual disturbances (classically the patient complains of looking at a snowstorm), abdominal pain, nausea, and vomiting. The GI symptoms may be due to mucosal irritation or pancreatitis. On exam, CNS signs can vary from lethargy to coma.

Fundoscopic exam may show retinal edema or hyperemia of the optic disk.

Laboratory investigation reveals a high anion gap metabolic acidosis with a high osmolal gap.

Clinical Features of Ethylene Glycol

Ethylene glycol poisoning often exhibits three distinct clinical phases after ingestion due to the toxic metabolites glycolate, glyoxalate, and oxalate. First, within 12 h, CNS effects predominate. The patient appears intoxicated without the odor of ethanol on the breath. Second, 12 to 24 h after ingestion, cardiopulmonary effects predominate. Elevated heart and respiratory rate and blood pressure are common. CHF, respiratory distress syndrome, and circulatory collapse are also noted. Third, 24 to 72 h after ingestion, renal effects predominate. Flank pain with CVA tenderness is noted. Acute tubular necrosis with acute renal failure occurs if appropriate treatment is not received.

Hypocalcemia may result from precipitation of calcium oxalate into tissues and may be severe enough to cause tetany and typical EKG changes. Calcium oxalate crystals are noted on urinalysis. Elevated CPK may be seen, and leukocytosis is common.

Diagnosis and Differential

The diagnosis of toxicity is based on the clinical presentation and laboratory findings of a high anion gap metabolic acidosis and a high osmolal gap. The diagnosis may be confirmed by elevated levels of methanol or ethylene glycol.

The differential diagnosis includes other causes of an anion gap metabolic acidosis, recalled by the acronym MUDPILES (see Table 118-1). Ethylene glycol poisoning differs from methanol poisoning in that visual disturbances and fundoscopic abnormalities are absent in ethylene glycol poisoning, and calcium oxalate crystals in the urine are present.

Emergency Department Care and Disposition

Treatment is based on preventing formation of the toxic metabolites and removing them from the body. General supportive measures are indicated including the administration of glucose, thiamine, and naloxone in the patient with altered mental status.

Charcoal does not bind the alcohols and is useful only if there is coingestion of an adsorbable substance. Bicarbonate is administered to correct acidosis; large amounts may be required.

Ethanol should be administered as soon as the diagnosis is suspected. Ethanol competitively inhibits metabolism of methanol and ethylene glycol by alcohol dehydrogenase. Because ethanol has a 10 to 20 times greater affinity for alcohol dehydrogenase than methanol and 100 times that of ethylene glycol, formation of toxic metabolites is inhibited. Indications for ethanol treatment are: (1) suspected methanol or ethylene glycol poisoning; (2) the presence of an anion gap metabolic acidosis with an osmolal gap; (3) a methanol or ethylene glycol level > 20 mg/dL; and (4) any patient requiring hemodialysis (see below). Administer ethanol (0.6 gm/kg IV) as a loading dose, followed by a maintenance dose of 0.11 gm/kg/h in the average drinker, 0.15 gm/kg/h in the heavy drinker. The maintenance infusion is adjusted accordingly to keep the blood ethanol level at 100 to 150 mg/dL.

If necessary, oral therapy with commercial alcoholic beverages can be initiated. The amount of ethanol contained in these is calculated by: grams ethanol = ml beverage x 0.9 x (proof/200).

Ethanol administration is continued until the methanol or ethylene glycol level is zero and the acidosis has resolved. Hypoglycemia may be induced, especially in children.

Dialysis eliminates both methanol and ethylene glycol and their toxic metabolites. Indications for dialysis are: (1) signs or symptoms of significant toxicity; (2) methanol or ethylene glycol level > 20–25 mg/dL; (3) presence of a metabolic acidosis; and (4) signs of nephrotoxicity in ethylene glycol poisoning. Peritoneal dialysis is considered only when hemodialysis is not available.

Ethanol is dialyzable, therefore, during dialysis, the maintenance rate of ethanol will need to be increased (doubled initially) and readjusted accordingly to maintain a blood alcohol level of 100 to 150 mg/dL. Dialysis and ethanol are continued until methanol and ethylene glycol levels are zero and acidosis has resolved.

Vitamin therapy is thought to play an important role in treatment as well. In methanol poisoning, folate is a cofactor for the conversion of formic acid to carbon dioxide, therefore, administer folate (50 mg IV q 4 h). In ethylene glycol poisoning, pyridoxine and thiamine are cofactors for the conversion of toxic metabolites to nontoxic compounds. Both thiamine and pyridoxine (100 mg IV or IM q day), are administered to drive the metabolism of ethylene glycol to nontoxic metabolites.

Basic laboratory investigation includes a CBC, serum electrolytes, BUN, creatinine, ABGs, urinalysis, calcium, and magnesium and levels of ethanol, isopropanol, methanol, and ethylene glycol.

Any patient with serious signs or symptoms of toxicity should be admitted to the ICU at a facility with hemodialysis capabilities. Asymptomatic individuals should be admitted for observation because of possible delayed onset of toxic symptoms.

For further reading in *Emergency Medicine: A Comprehensive Study Guide*, 4th edition, see Chapter 138, Alcohols, by William A. Burke and Wilma V. Henderson.

95 | Drugs of Abuse

Judith Linden

Commonly abused psychoactive drugs include narcotics, cocaine, amphetamine-like drugs, and hallucinogens. While patients who ingest a single drug often present with typical signs or symptoms, multiple drug ingestions may confound the clinical picture. Drug preparations are often adulterated with substances (such as quinine, lactose, procaine, mannitol and talc). Many other complications (such as infections) are the result of drug abuse. Withdrawal syndromes may be present with certain classes of drugs (opiates, amphetamines).

Clinical Features and Emergency Department Care and Disposition

The clinical features and management vary, and are presented by class of drug.

Narcotics. The most commonly abused narcotic is heroin. Other narcotic preparations include methadone, meperidine (Demerol), morphine, codeine, hydromorphone (Dilaudid), and oxycodone (Percocet, Percodan). Hypoventilation and pinpoint pupils are characteristic of opiate intoxication. Other signs of narcotic abuse may be present, including injection sites (needle track marks). Heroin users may attempt to treat overdoses by injecting milk, or packing the axilla with icepacks. Opiate overdose is treated with **naloxone** (Narcan) 2 mg (0.01 mg/kg. in children), which can be given IV, IM, or endotracheally. A smaller test-dose of Narcan (0.5–1 mg) may be given to avoid precipitating violent withdrawal symptoms. The half-life of Narcan is 1 hour, and it has a 2 to 3 hour duration of action. Naloxone IV drip (2 mg/500 cc of D5W (0.004 mg/mL) may be administered at 0.4 mg/hr if a long acting opiate (methadone) has been ingested.

Common complications of chronic narcotic abuse are often infectious sequelae. Cellulitis and abscesses, caused by skin flora (staph, strep), pseudomonas, gram negative and anaerobic organisms may form at injection sites. Hand infections may require surgical drainage. Mycotic aneurysms may form in the groin or neck; these sites should be carefully inspected and palpated for bruits before incision and drainage is attempted. Necrotizing fasciitis should be suspected if the limb is dusky, or the patient appears septic, tachycardic and febrile. Rapid surgical debridement and IV antibiotics are crucial. Endocarditis, which may present with septic emboli to brain, lung, skin, kidneys, or liver, should be suspected in an IV drug user with a fever. Brain abscess or meningitis present with fever and mental status changes. Fever, focal back pain, and leukocytosis suggests an epidural abscess, and mandates prompt MRI or CT scan with contrast. Septic arthritis and osteomyelitis has a predilection for the axial skeleton, spine, and sterno-clavicular joints. Blood-borne infectious diseases such as HIV and hepatitis are common in IV drug users who share needles.

Non-cardiogenic pulmonary edema may be the initial presentation of an opiate overdose. The etiology is unknown (but may be related to an allergic reaction, the toxic effects of heroin, or hypoxia). Treatment consists of respiratory support and naloxone. Symptoms resolve within 1 to 2 days. Lasix and digoxin are not helpful.

Narcotic withdrawal presents with flu-like symptoms (chills, myalgias and arthralgias, rhinorrhea, lacrimation, abdominal pain and confusion). Withdrawal is not life-threatening, and is treated with Methadone (later tapered) or **Clonidine** (0.1–0.2 mg po). Clonidine ameliorates, but does not eliminate symptoms of withdrawal by blocking two adrenergic sites. Side effects include hypotension, dizziness, and dry mouth.

Cocaine Cocaine may be insufflated, smoked, or injected intravenously. The peak effect occurs within 30 minutes, and lasts 1 to 3 hours when insufflated. Inhalation and intravenous administration produce peak effect of 30 seconds to 2 minutes, and duration of 15 to 30 minutes. The major metabolite of cocaine, benzoylecgonine, may be detected in the urine for 24 to 72 hours by the usual assays.

Cocaine intoxication presents with signs of adrenergic stimulation. Tachycardia, tachypnea, hypertension, diaphoresis, mydriasis, and occasionally hyperthermia are often present. Paranoia, mania, agitation, or coma may be present. Symptoms during acute intoxication often include chest pain, palpitations, shortness of breath, headache, seizure, or focal neurologic deficits.

Complications of acute cocaine intoxication include myocardial ischemia and infarction, arrhythmias, stroke (hemorrhagic or bland) secondary to vasoconstriction or vasculitis, spinal cord infarction, pneumomediastinum, pulmonary edema (adrenergic mediated), and rhabdomyolysis.

Treatment of acute cocaine intoxication includes **benzodiazepines** for sedation (Ativan 1 to 2 mg IV, or diazepam 2.5 to 5 mg IV), and cooling if hyperthermic. Hypertension not controlled with sedation should be treated with **nipride** (0.5–10 mcg/kg/min IV) or **phentolamine** (5 mg IV). Beta-blockers (including labetalol) are not recommended since beta-blockade leaves unopposed alpha stimulation, increasing vasoconstriction. Symptoms of chest pain mandate ECG, as myocardial infarction may occur secondary to coronary vasoconstriction (especially if there is coexisting coronary artery disease). Chest pain should be treated with benzodiazepines, oxygen, and sublingual nitroglycerin, if pain is unrelieved. Pneumothorax and pneumomediastinum should be ruled out with chest radiograph if chest pain is pleuritic. Seizures are treated with benzodiazepines and dilantin. CT scan of the head should be performed, as intracranial pathology may be present.

Body packers and body stuffers may present to the ED. Body stuffers ingest well-wrapped packages with a large amount of drugs for smuggling. Body stuffers may ingest poorly wrapped packets of cocaine containing smaller amounts of drug to hide evidence. Body stuffers are treated with **activated charcoal** (1 gm/kg) and observation with symptomatic treatment. Body packers often ingest a larger dose of drug and are treated with charcoal, **whole bowel irrigation (PEG, or Go-LYTELY)**, and are hospitalized until the packets are passed. If the patient begins exhibiting signs of toxicity, surgical intervention for removal of drug packets is recommended. Endoscopic removal is *not* recommended, as the remaining packets may break open, releasing toxic amounts of drug.

Amphetamines Amphetamines include illicit drugs and over-the-counter drugs which have similar action, including phenylpropanolamine, l-methamphetamine (Vicks nasal inhaler), ephedrine, and pseudoephedrine. Acute intoxication presents with hyperautonomic sympathetic signs and symptoms, such as mydriasis, tachycardia, hypertension, hyperthermia, restlessness, anorexia, insomnia, repetitive or stereotyped behavior, and occasionally paranoid psychosis. Seizures may occur. Peak plasma levels occur 1 to 2 hours after oral ingestion.

Treatment includes a quiet room, dim lighting, and benzodiazepines for sedation. Hypertension that does not respond to sedation is treated with phentolamine or nipride. Psychosis that does not respond to sedation may be treated with **Haldol** (5–10 mg IM or IV). Hyperthermia is treated with sedation, cooling, and occasionally Dantrolene (1 mg/kg that may be repeated for a maximum dose of 10 mg/kg) for malignant hyperthermia. Seizures not responding to benzodiazepines are treated with dilantin and phenobarbital, as needed. While urinary acidification will theoretically increase drug excretion, this is not recommended, as renal failure may be precipitated if myoglobinuria is present. Urinary alkalinization is recommended for myoglobinuria.

Amphetamine withdrawal may present with depression, increased appetite, abdominal cramps, diarrhea, nausea, and headache.

Hallucinogens Hallucinogens have the effect of creating a sensory experience which does not exist outside of the mind. The hallucinations may be visual, auditory, or tactile. This class includes a wide variety of drugs, including LSD, PCP, mescaline, mushrooms, anticholinergics, and certain amphetamines.

Clinical features and complications of intoxication are listed in Table 95-1. Other causes of hallucinations such as hypoglycemia, drug and alcohol withdrawal, and infection should be considered. Treatment is primarily supportive with quiet surroundings and benzodiazepines as needed for agitation. Haldol (5–10 mg IV every 10 to 15 minutes) or droperidol (2.5 to 5 mg IV every 10 to 15 minutes) may be administered

TABLE 95-1. Clinical Features of Hallucinogens*

Drug	Clinical features	Complications
PCP	Mild: nystagmus, ataxia, emotional lability, violent behavior Moderate: muscular rigidity, hypertension, tachycardia Severe: coma, hyperpyrexia	Muscle rigidity seizures, coma, rhabdomyolysis, hyperthermia, flashbacks
LSD	paranoia, anxiety, psychosis	Flashbacks
Peyote (Mescaline)	nausea, vomiting, abdominal pain, diaphoresis, headache, anxiety, paranoia	rare
Hallucinogenic Amphetamines	excitement, agitation, hallucinations, confusion, anorexia	Muscle rigidity, seizures, coma, IC hemorrhage, hyperthermia, rhabdomyolysis, vasculitis
Anti-cholinergics	agitation, tachycardia, urinary retention, ileus, mydriasis	SVT, hypertension, seizures, hyperthermia
Marijuana	Euphoria, relaxation, impaired motor performance, paranoia, panic, conjunctival injection	Rare
Nutmeg	Nausea, vomiting, mydriasis, abdominal pain, hallucinations, delirium, stupor	Rare

* Hallucinations may be present with all.

for extreme agitation. Multiple dose activated charcoal every 6 hours is recommended for PCP intoxication.

Hallucinogen ingestions should be admitted if hyperthermia, cardiovascular instability, seizures, rhabdomyolysis, or metabolic abnormalities are present. Asymptomatic patients may be discharged after a short observation period since there is no delayed toxicity. Mild to moderate ingestion may be managed in the ED with an observation period of 4 to 8 hours. Psychiatric evaluation should be considered when the patient is medically cleared and able to think more clearly. Substance abuse counseling should be offered.

For further reading in *Emergency Medicine: A Comprehensive Study Guide,* 4th edition, see Chapter 139, Narcotics, by James A. Smith and George L. Sternbacher; Chapter 140, Cocaine, by Jeanmarie Perrone and Robert S. Hoffman; Chapter 141, Amphetamine and Amphetaminelike Drugs, by George Braitburg and Donald B. Kunkel; and Chapter 142, Hallucinogens, by James E. Cisek.

Salicylates, acetaminophen, and NSAIDs are analgesics found in a wide variety of prescription and nonprescription pain-relief, cough, and cold preparations. Acute overdoses of NSAIDs in otherwise healthy adults are rarely fatal and usually require only supportive care. Acetaminophen and salicylate poisonings, on the other hand, are potentially life-threatening and require rapid identification and treatment.

SALICYLATES

Clinical Features

Acute ingestion is frequently accompanied by gastroenteritis from direct irritation to the GI tract, with persistent vomiting and upper GI bleeding. Neurologic manifestations include tinnitus, confusion, lethargy, convulsions, coma, and brain death. Cerebral edema is a common cause of death. Cardiac toxicity is due to impaired ATP production, acidosis, electrolyte abnormalities and, rarely, hyperthermia and presents with CHF and potentially life-threatening dysrhythmias. The most serious pulmonary manifestation of toxicity is pulmonary edema, usually noncardiogenic, and is seen more commonly in adults than children. Salicylates directly stimulate respiratory centers in the brainstem. In very high doses, however, respiratory depression may be seen.

Chronic salicylate poisoning is the result of excessive ingestion over a period of 12 h or longer. Patients are usually brought in by family because of changes in mentation, including disorientation, lethargy, or hallucinations. Noncardiogenic pulmonary edema is common. Patients usually do not have significant gastroenteritis, although dehydration can be severe.

Diagnosis and Differential

Laboratory abnormalities in acute salicylate poisoning include a mixed respiratory alkalosis and metabolic acidosis. Elevated serum ketoacids may be seen. Serum glucose may be normal, elevated, or low, with hypoglycemia more common in children. Patients with chronic salicylate toxicity frequently have an elevated prothrombin time. Elevation of liver function tests may also be seen.

Determination of the serum salicylate level is an important part of patient management. The Done nomogram can be used to assist in predicting the degree of toxicity associated with a given serum level (Fig. 96-1). Because of salicylate pharmacokinetics, a serum level should not be plotted on the nomogram unless it was drawn at least 6 h after ingestion. The Done nomogram should also not be used in acute ingestions when salicylate has been taken within the last 24 h, in acute

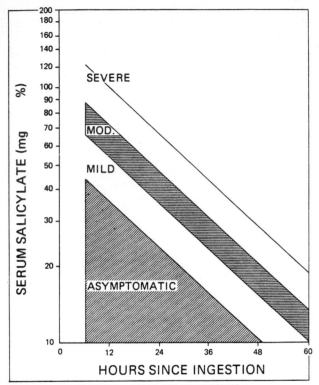

DONE NOMOGRAM FOR SALICYLATE POISONING

FIG. 96-1.   The Done nomogram can be used to assist in determining the likelihood of toxicity. It can only be used after a single, acute ingestion of aspirin in which no salicylate has been taken previously in the last 24 h. Nontoxic levels drawn before 6 h cannot be used to determine degree of toxicity. This monogram cannot be used in chronic salicylate poisoning or after the ingestion of enteric-coated aspirin. (From Done AK: Salicylate intoxication: Significance of salicylate in blood in cases of acute ingestion. *Pediatrics* 26:800, 1960. Used by permission)

overdoses when salicylate was ingested over several h, after ingestion of enteric-coated aspirin tablets, or in chronic salicylate poisoning. A patient suffering from chronic salicylate toxicity can have a therapeutic serum salicylate level. In these patients it is therefore important to treat the patient and not the serum salicylate level.

The differential diagnosis of salicylate poisoning includes theophylline toxicity, caffeine overdose, acute iron poisoning, Reyes syndrome, diabetic ketoacidosis, sepsis, and meningitis.

Emergency Department Care and Disposition

After addressing the patient's airway, breathing, and circulatory status, blood should be sent for determination of electrolytes, glucose, BUN, creatinine, salicylate level, prothrombin time, hemoglobin, and hematocrit. An arterial blood gas should be drawn to determine the acid-base status. Bedside determination of serum glucose is indicated in all patients with CNS depression or seizures.

1. Decontamination is accomplished with oral administration of **activated charcoal** (1 gm/kg body weight).
2. Intravenous fluid challenges with saline or colloid should be given to all patients with evidence of dehydration. After adequate hydration, intravenous solutions should include adequate amounts of sodium and potassium to replenish depleted body stores. Children should never receive plain 5% dextrose in water as an intravenous fluid.
3. **Alkalinization** of the serum and urine enhances salicylate binding to protein as well as urinary excretion. This can be accomplished by giving intravenous boluses of sodium bicarbonate (1 mEq/kg) until arterial pH is at least 7.5. A continuous infusion is then started at 2 to 3 times maintenance rate using 1 L D5W to which is added 50 to 100 mmol sodium bicarbonate and 40 mmol potassium chloride. Potassium is required, in addition to bicarbonate, to produce an alkaline urine. Serum electrolytes, urine pH, and arterial blood gases should be monitored every 2 to 4 h. Serum salicylate levels should be followed until a consistent downward trend is noted. Furosemide can be given for evidence of fluid overload or to enhance urine output.
4. Carbonic anhydrase inhibitors (e.g., acetazolamide) are contraindicated in salicylate poisoning. Whereas they alkalinize urine, they also alkalinize CSF, trapping salicylate in the CNS.
5. **Hemodialysis** is indicated in the patient who is deteriorating despite supportive care and alkaline diuresis, in deteriorating patients in whom an alkaline urine cannot be successfully produced, in patients with renal failure, in the encephalopathic or comatose patient, or in one with significant cardiac toxicity, and in the patient with noncardiogenic pulmonary edema in whom the salicylate levels are not rapidly falling. Peritoneal dialysis is much less effective and

should only be used if hemodialysis is unavailable. If peritoneal dialysis is used, the dialysate should contain 5% albumin to enhance salicylate binding to protein.
6. Parenteral vitamin K can be given for a prolonged prothrombin time.
7. Antacids may be required for the treatment of upper GI bleeding.
8. Standard antiarrhythmic drugs are used to treat ventricular dysrhythmias. Dysrhythmias will usually resolve with correction of acid-base abnormalities.

If the serum salicylate level drawn 6 h after ingestion falls in the asymptomatic portion of the Done nomogram, the patient has minimal or no symptoms, and if a repeat serum determination shows the levels to be dropping, the patient can be discharged. Patients whose levels fall in the mild range can be discharged if they have minimal symptoms, if nausea and vomiting have resolved, if salicylate levels are falling, and if adequate followup can be assured. All other patients should be admitted. Because of the potential for delayed absorption and toxicity, anyone who has taken more than 150 mg/kg of enteric-coated aspirin should also be admitted.

ACETAMINOPHEN

Clinical Features

The clinical course of patients who become poisoned by a single overdose of acetaminophen (APAP) can be divided into four stages. Stage I is characterized by nausea and vomiting. During stage II, signs, symptoms, and laboratory evidence of hepatic toxicity become apparent. Gastrointestinal symptoms may improve, followed by the development of right upper quadrant abdominal pain with liver enlargement and tenderness. Oliguria may be noted, either due to dehydration or APAP-mediated nephrotoxicity. In Stage III, nausea and vomiting may reappear or worsen and liver function abnormalities peak. Stage IV is characterized by either recovery or progressive deterioration with death from fulminant hepatic failure.

Since APAP does not cause direct cardiovascular or respiratory abnormalities and only causes CNS depression in the setting of massive overdose, the ingestion of other substances should be suspected if these findings are observed.

Diagnosis and Differential

Laboratory abnormalities in APAP poisoning include elevation of ALT (SGPT) and AST (SGOT) to over 10,000 IU/ml, more than 100 times the normal level. Lesser elevations of alkaline phosphatase and glutathione-S-transferase (GST) are often seen. The serum bilirubin may increase, particularly the indirect fraction, and the prothrombin time (PT) may become prolonged. Elevation of serum BUN and creatinine along with proteinuria, glucosuria, hematuria, pyuria, and granular casts on urinalysis are consistent with renal toxicity. Hypoglycemia and elevated serum ammonia levels may be seen in deteriorating patients.

Serum APAP level measuring 4 to 24 h after a single large overdose is the best predictor of hepatotoxicity. The Rumack–Matthew nomogram depicts this relationship (Fig. 96-2), with 150 mg/mL being the potentially toxic 4-h level. An APAP level falling above the lower line of the nomogram, in the possible or probable toxicity areas, warrants antidotal therapy. If a serum APAP concentration is not readily available, patients should be considered at risk for hepatotoxicity if they have ingested more than 140 mg/kg or 7.5 gm.

The differential diagnosis of APAP poisoning includes viral hepatitis, alcoholic hepatitis, hepatobiliary disease, and other drug- or toxin-induced hepatitides. Acute APAP poisoning can often be distinguished from other causes of hepatitis by the presence of very high aminotransferase levels, its acute onset, and its rapid progression.

Emergency Department Care and Disposition

Children who ingest less than 140 mg/kg of APAP, and adults who ingest less than 7.5 gm may be managed at home if the history is certain. No treatment is necessary if less than 100 mg/kg has been ingested. For those ingesting between 100 and 140 mg/kg, ipecac-induced vomiting or activated charcoal (AC) is recommended if fewer than 4 h have passed since the time of ingestion. Telephone followup over the next 24 h is mandatory. All other patients, including those who may have taken an intentional overdose, should be evaluated in the ED, with initial stabilization of airway, breathing, and circulatory status. Laboratory evaluation should include measurement of serum amylase, electrolytes, ALT, AST, bilirubin, PT, creatinine, BUN, and urinalysis. Arterial blood gas analysis may be beneficial in patients with a recent massive overdose who are clinically ill. In those with vague or unreliable histories or with intentional ingestions, toxicology screening tests are advisable.

1. **Activated charcoal** (AC) is the preferred method of decontamination and should be given within 4 h of overdose, if possible. The value of cathartics in the treatment of APAP overdose is uncertain. The combined use of gastric lavage and AC may be optimal for the decontamination of patients with mixed ingestions.
2. Hepatic or renal failure should be treated by standard, supportive measures.
3. Vitamin K is effective for patients with a prolonged PT.
4. **N-acetylcysteine** (NAC, Mucomyst) is antidotal and virtually 100% effective in preventing fatalities when given within 8 to 10 h of overdose to patients whose APAP levels are predictive of toxicity. NAC is given orally in a loading dose of 140 mg/kg followed by

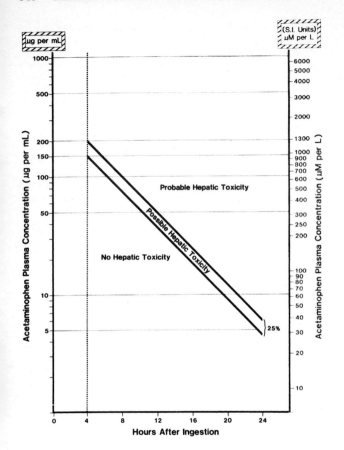

**RUMACK – MATTHEW NOMOGRAM
FOR ACETAMINOPHEN POISONING**

FIG. 96-2.   Semilogarithmic plot of plasma acetaminophen levels versus time. Adapted from Rumack BH, Matthew H: Acetaminophen poisoning and toxicity. *Pediatrics* 55:873.

17 doses of 70 mg/kg every 4 h. Since it is foul-smelling (rotten eggs), NAC should be diluted to a 5% solution with soft drink or fruit juice. Nausea and vomiting are frequent side-effects. The dose should be repeated if vomiting occurs within 1 h of administration. Metoclopramide (Reglan, 0.1 mg/kg IV) or ondansetron (Zofran, 0.15 mg/kg IV over 15 min), can be used to prevent or treat vomiting. Although activated charcoal absorbs NAC, this effect is unlikely to be clinically important. If multiple doses of activated charcoal are given for treatment of coingestant poisoning, however, alternating doses of charcoal and NAC at 2–h intervals is recommended. Intravenous NAC has been successfully used in Europe and Canada with a dosage schedule identical to the oral protocol but stopping after 12 doses. Because this route is not recommended by its manufacturer, it should only be used in potentially life-threatening situations where oral NAC is not tolerated and only after informed consent is obtained.

Candidates for NAC therapy require admission. A floor bed is acceptable provided that the patient is otherwise clinically stable and has not coingested a potentially life-threatening substance. Patients with intentional overdoses should have psychiatric evaluation prior to discharge.

NONSTEROIDAL ANTI-INFLAMMATORY AGENTS (NSAIDs)

Clinical Features

Therapeutic doses of nonsteroidal anti-inflammatory agents (NSAIDs) can cause GI intolerance, nephrotoxicity, tinnitus, peripheral edema, platelet dysfunction, anaphylactic shock, and premature closure of the ductus arteriosus in the fetus. Overdose can result in nausea, vomiting, epigastric abdominal pain, and GI hemorrhage, especially in elderly patients. Renal vasoconstriction leading to nephrotoxicity and acute renal failure may also be seen. Patients with congestive heart failure, cirrhosis, or volume contraction secondary to diuretic use are most susceptible. Acute interstitial nephritis with papillary necrosis can result from chronic NSAID use. These patients often present with hematuria and flank pain, with or without rash or fever. NSAID use or abuse can also lead to a variety of cutaneous manifestations, including generalized exanthems and pruritus, Stevens–Johnson syndrome, toxic epidermal necrolysis, bullous eruptions, photosensitivity, urticaria, and pustular psoriasis. Common neurologic symptoms in acute overdose include drowsiness, dizziness, and lethargy. Seizures and coma have also been reported.

Diagnosis and Differential

Severe metabolic acidosis and hyperkalemia may result from NSAID overdose. Abnormal renal function tests will be present in the setting of NSAID-induced nephrotoxicity. Prolonged bleeding times and thrombocytopenia have been reported. A transient rise in liver enzymes may result through a hypersensitivity response. Blood levels of the specific NSAIDs should not be routinely ordered because they do not correlate with outcome.

The most common symptoms of NSAID poisoning are consistent with many other diseases and poisonings. The mild metabolic acidosis frequently seen should prompt consideration of a recent seizure, in addition to poisoning with methanol, isoniazid, ethylene glycol, salicylates, and iron.

Emergency Department Care and Disposition

Initial stabilization should follow the airway, breathing, and circulation protocol. Altered mental status should be treated with standard measures. Patients with evidence of severe toxicity, including hypovolemia and hyperkalemia, should have continuous cardiac monitoring.

1. Hypovolemia should be treated with boluses of normal saline or Ringer's lactate.
2. Symptomatic bradycardia should respond to atropine.
3. Severe metabolic acidosis is treated with bicarbonate.
4. Hypotension unresponsive to fluids can be treated with norepinephrine.
5. Decontamination with gastric lavage and **activated charcoal** or charcoal alone should be initiated in patients presenting after acute ingestions. Syrup of ipecac is contraindicated, as NSAIDs may predispose to seizures.
6. Hemodialysis may be required in NSAID-induced renal failure.
7. NSAID-induced seizures are treated with benzodiazepines.
8. Antacids or H_2 blockers can be employed in patients with GI distress or bleeding.

Any patient who develops symptoms after a NSAID ingestion needs evaluation and observation for at least 24 h. All asymptomatic patients ingesting potentially toxic doses (several times the therapeutic dose of mefenamic acid or phenylbutazone, 5 times the therapeutic dose of other agents in pediatric ingestions, or 10 times the therapeutic dose of other agents in adult ingestions) should be observed in the ED for at least 4 to 6 h. Asymptomatic patients with possible ingestions of other substances should be worked up on an individual basis.

For further reading in *Emergency Medicine: A Comprehensive Study Guide,* 4th edition, see Chapters 143, Salicylates, by Steven C. Curry; Chapter 144, Acetaminophen, by Christopher H. Linden; and Chapter 145, Nonsteroidal Anti-Inflammatory Agents, by Gregory Almond and Richard F. Clark.

Xanthines

Greg Mears

Theophylline and caffeine are the two most common xanthines that produce major toxicity. The cardiovascular, neurologic, metabolic, and GI systems can be affected.

Clinical Features

Even at therapeutic levels (10–20 μg/ml), theophylline can cause significant side-effects. Cardiac effects include sinus tachycardia, premature atrial contractions, atrial fibrillation, and atrial flutter. Premature ventricular contractions and ventricular tachycardia may occur with elevated levels (40–60 μg/ml) and are more common in older patients. Hypotension can occur. Neurologic symptoms include agitation, headache, irritability, sleeplessness, tremors, and muscular twitching. Seizures have been reported, especially in patients with a history of seizure disorder. Toxicity may produce hallucinations and psychosis. Metabolic changes associated with acute toxicity include elevated levels of catecholamines, glucose, fatty acids, insulin, and WBC counts. Hypokalemia may occur. Gastrointestinal effects most commonly include nausea and vomiting, which can occur with therapeutic levels, and GI bleeding.

Caffeine produces many of the same effects of theophylline. Premature ventricular contractions and paroxysmal atrial tachycardia can occur. Neurologic effects include seizures, agitation, and coma. GI effects include abdominal pain, nausea, and vomiting. Metabolic effects include rhabdomyolysis, hyperglycemia, leukocytosis, and metabolic acidosis.

Diagnosis and Differential

In pediatric cases a thorough history may reveal access to over-the-counter caffeine products. Serum theophylline levels of 10 to 20 μg/ml are considered therapeutic but may still produce toxic effects. Levels above 30 μg/ml are much more likely to produce significant toxicity. Cimetidine, erythromycin, congestive heart failure, and chronic obstructive lung disease will increase the half-life of theophylline. Caffeine doses of 1 gm in adults or 80 mg/kg in children may produce toxicity.

Emergency Department Care and Disposition

The treatment of xanthine toxicity consists of initial stabilization, gastric decontamination and elimination, treatment of life-threatening toxic effects, and in severe cases hemoperfusion or dialysis. Patients should be placed on a cardiac monitor and noninvasive BP device with intravenous access established.

1. Gastric emptying should be initiated with gastric lavage. The use of ipecac may complicate other therapy and can be dangerous if mental status deteriorates.
2. **Activated charcoal** in doses of 50 to 100 gms in adults combined with a cathartic such as sorbitol should be given as soon as gastric emptying is achieved. The charcoal should be repeated every 2 to 4 h since theophylline undergoes hepatobiliary enteric circulation.
3. **Ranitidine** (50 mg IV) is useful to control nausea and vomiting associated with toxicity.
4. Intravenous diazepam, phenobarbitol, and phenytoin may be helpful in controlling seizure activity.
5. Hypotension typically will respond to IV crystalloids. In patients who are unresponsive to fluid resuscitation or who have life-threatening cardiac arrythmias, ß-blocking agents such as labetalol, esmolol, or propranolol may be given cautiously. Verapamil, diltiazem, lidocaine, phenytoin, and digoxin have been shown to be effective as well. Adenosine should be used with caution due to the potential to induce bronchospasm. Hemoperfusion or hemodialysis are effective in increasing clearance rate of xanthines. It should considered in any patient with a life-threatening toxicity that does not respond to standard therapy. These patients usually have serum levels greater than 30 µg/ml.

For further reading in *Emergency Medicine: A Comprehensive Study Guide*, 4th edition, see Chapter 146, Xanthines, by Charles L. Emerman.

Keith L. Mausner

DIGITALIS GLYCOSIDES

Digitalis glycosides have an extremely low toxic-to-therapeutic ratio. They are widely prescribed for the treatment of supraventricular tachydysrhythmias and congestive heart failure, and naturally occurring cardiac glycosides are found in plants such as foxglove, oleander, and lily of the valley.

Clinical Features

Acute digitalis toxicity occurs in the setting of accidental or intentional overdose. Chronic digitalis toxicity occurs most commonly in elderly patients on digoxin therapy and diuretics. Underlying conditions that predispose to digitalis toxicity include renal insufficiency, hepatic dysfunction, hypothyroidism, and chronic obstructive pulmonary disease. Hypokalemia, hypomagnesemia, and hypercalcemia, as well as quinidine and calcium channel blockers, may precipitate or worsen digitalis toxicity. Table 98-1 summarizes the clinical features of acute and chronic digitalis toxicity. Patients also may complain of visual disturbances, including seeing yellow halos around objects.

TABLE 98-1. Clinical Presentation of Digitalis Toxicity

Acute toxicity
  Clinical history—Intentional or accidental ingestion
    GI effects—Nausea and vomiting
    CNS effects—Headache, dizziness, confusion, coma
    Cardiac effects—Predominantly supraventricular tachydysrythmias with AV block
  Bradydysrythmias
    Electrolyte abnormalities—Hyperkalemia
    Digoxin level—Marked elevation
Chronic toxicity
  Clinical history—Typically an elderly cardiac patients taking diuretics. May have renal insufficiency
    GI effects—Nausea, vomiting, diarrhea, abdominal pain
    CNS effect—Fatigue, weakness, confusion, delirium, coma
    Cardiac effects—Ventricular dysrhythmias are common; almost any ventricular or supraventricular dysrhythmia can occur
    Electrolyte abnormalities—Hypokalemia or normal serum potassium, hypomagnesemia
    Digoxin level—Minimally elevated or therapeutic range

Almost any cardiac dysrhythmia may be seen in digitalis toxicity. The most common dysrhythmia is frequent PVCs. Supraventricular tachycardia with AV block is highly suggestive of digitalis toxicity, and AV block and junctional escape rhythms also are seen. Although bidirectional ventricular tachycardia, which has a right bundle branch block morphology, is highly specific for digitalis toxicity, it is rarely seen.

Diagnosis and Differential

Therapeutic digoxin levels are 0.5 to 2.0 ng/mL. Digoxin levels do not necessarily correlate with toxicity. Chronic toxicity may occur in the setting of a low digoxin level. In acute ingestion, a patient with a high level may be asymptomatic if the digoxin has not distributed into the tissue compartment. The serum digoxin level is most reliable 6 h after ingestion when distribution to tissues is complete. The standard digoxin assay may detect naturally occurring plant digitalis glycosides, but the extent of cross reactivity is unknown, and no relationship has been established between their level and toxicity.

In acute overdose, serum potassium level may be the best marker of the severity of toxicity; poisoning of the Na/K − ATPase pump may lead to significant hyperkalemia. Hypokalemia or normal potassium is more common in chronic toxicity.

Ingestions that may present similarly to digitalis toxicity by producing bradydysrhythmias include calcium channel blockers, beta blockers, procainamide, quinidine, clonidine, and organophosphate insecticides.

Emergency Department Care and Disposition

Institute an intravenous line and cardiac monitoring. Assess airway, breathing, and circulation. Gastric lavage is indicated in massive ingestions, or in patients presenting 1 to 2 h after overdose. Be cautious in the setting of cardiac toxicity, since vagal stimulation from lavage may worsen bradydysrhythmias. Administer 1 g/kg of activated charcoal to all patients. Ipecac is contraindicated because of the risk of obtundation. Forced diuresis, hemodialysis, and hemoperfusion do not effectively eliminate digitalis glycosides.

Initial treatments for bradydysrhythmias are atropine and cardiac pacing. Phenytoin may be the antiarrhythmic of choice for digitalis-related ventricular arrhythmias. Lidocaine and bretylium may also be effective. Class IA antiarrhythmics (e.g., quinidine and procainamide) may worsen digitalis-induced cardiac toxicity and are contraindicated. Electrical cardioversion may result in intractable ventricular fibrillation; use only as a last resort, with low energies (10 to 25 J).

Assess for and rapidly correct hypoxia, hypoglycemia, volume depletion, and electrolyte abnormalities. Hyperkalemia mandates rapid treatment: intravenous dextrose, insulin, sodium bicarbonate, and enteral potassium binding resin. Calcium administration for hyperkalemia may worsen digitalis toxicity and is contraindicated.

Digoxin-specific antibodies or Fab fragments (Digibind, Burroughs-Wellcome), are highly effective at reversing severe toxicity and have been effective in digitoxin and oleander poisoning. Indications for Fab fragment therapy are ventricular dysrhythmias, bradydysrhythmias with hemodynamic compromise unresponsive to standard therapy, and serum potassium greater than 5.5 mEq/L.

There have been few reported adverse effects from Fab fragment therapy. No cases of anaphylaxis or serum sickness have been reported, but mild hypersensitivity reactions have occurred. Fab fragment therapy may result in an increase in the ventricular response rate of underlying atrial fibrillation, and cardiogenic shock has been reported in patients dependent on digitalis for inotropic support. Hypokalemia also may occur as digitalis toxicity is reversed.

Fab fragment dose is based on the total body digoxin load. If the ingested dose is unknown, 5 to 10 vials are recommended as the initial dose. Fab fragments are administered IV through a 0.22 micron filter over 30 min. In cardiac arrest, administer as a bolus.

One vial of Fab fragments (40 mg) binds 0.6 mg of digoxin. The dose of Fab fragments may also be calculated:

$$\text{Digoxin total body load} = \text{amount ingested (mg)} \times 0.80 \text{ (the bioavailability of digoxin)}$$

$$\text{Total body load also} = \frac{(\text{serum digoxin level in ng/mL}) \times (5.6 \text{ L/kg}) \times (\text{patient weight in kg})}{1000}$$

$$\text{Number of vials required} = \frac{\text{total body load}}{0.6}$$

A simple formula is:

$$\text{Number of vials required} = \frac{(\text{serum digoxin level}) \times (\text{patient weight in kg})}{100}$$

Asymptomatic patients with acute ingestions should be observed at least 12 h in the ED or admitted to a monitored bed, since onset of toxicity may be delayed for many h. Patients with signs or symptoms of toxicity should be admitted to an ICU.

BETA BLOCKERS

Beta blockers are widely prescribed medications with significant cardiovascular toxicity in overdose.

Clinical Features

Standard release preparations are rapidly absorbed, with onset of symptoms between 20 min and 2 h after overdose. Long-acting preparations may have delayed-onset toxicity.

EKG changes with toxicity include bradycardia, AV block, widened QRS, peaked T waves and ST changes. Hypotension results from bradycardia and negative inotropic effects. Tachycardia has been reported in practolol, pindolol, and sotalol overdose.

Delirium, coma, and seizures may occur. Bronchospasm, CHF, and pulmonary edema may be precipitated. Beta blockers also may precipitate, interfere with recovery from, and mask warning symptoms of acute hypoglycemia and hypovolemia secondary to trauma.

Emergency Department Care and Disposition

Institute an intravenous line and cardiac monitoring. In any patient with altered mental status, assess airway, breathing, and circulation; perform a rapid glucose assay, and consider naloxone and thiamine administration.

Gastric lavage should be considered in patients presenting soon after ingestion. Administer **activated charcoal**, 1 g/kg in all patients. In symptomatic patients, pretreatment with atropine prior to gastric lavage may prevent vagal effects, which may worsen bradycardia.

Specific agents to counter the effects of beta-blockade include atropine, dopamine, norepinephrine, epinephrine, and dobutamine. Isoproterenol may worsen hypotension by causing vasodilation. Optimal doses of the vasopressors in overdose may be higher than the usual recommended clinical doses.

Glucagon may be the drug of choice in beta blocker overdose. It enhances myocardial contractility, rate, and conduction. Administer glucagon as a 3 to 10 mg bolus over 1 min, followed by an infusion of 2 to 5 mg/h. Titrate infusion to clinical response; no upper dose limit has been established.

Seizures are treated in a standard fashion, with benzodiazepines, phenytoin, or phenobarbital, as needed. Hypoglycemia is treated with a glucose infusion and, if resistant, may respond to glucagon. Treat bronchospasm with a beta-2-agonist therapy.

Laboratory evaluation in beta-blocker overdose should include an EKG, glucose, BUN, creatinine, and electrolytes. Toxicology screens for beta blockers are usually not rapidly available and therefore do not play an important role in diagnosis or management.

Patients with significant ingestions should be admitted to an ICU until symptoms and signs of toxicity have resolved. Asymptomatic patients with ingestions of sustained-release preparations should be admitted to a monitored bed.

If Standard Treatment Fails

Hemodialysis or charcoal hemoperfusion may enhance elimination of some of the beta blockers. In the setting of pharmacologically-resistant hypotension, administer isotonic fluid boluses with caution to avoid precipitating CHF. Swan–Ganz and arterial pressure monitoring will help optimize therapy. A pacemaker is indicated for resistant bradycardia. In severe cases, balloon pump or cardiopulmonary bypass may be effective. Successful resuscitation has been reported even after prolonged CPR.

CALCIUM CHANNEL BLOCKERS

Calcium channel blockers are the leading cause of overdose death from cardiovascular drugs in the U.S. The three most commonly prescribed agents are verapamil, diltiazem, and nifedipine.

Clinical Features

The potential toxic effects of these drugs include AV nodal conduction defects (i.e., third-degree block), decreased sinus node discharge, impaired cardiac contractility, and marked vasodilation with hypotension. Verapamil and diltiazem frequently cause bradycardia and conduction delays. Nifedipine and many of the newer agents are potent vasodilators and have less effect on conduction. Nifedipine overdose typically produces reflex tachycardia secondary to hypotension.

Symptoms of toxicity include lethargy, nausea, vomiting, respiratory depression, and coma. Hypoperfusion can cause lactic acidosis. Hyperglycemia is common with verapamil overdose.

Emergency Department Care and Disposition

Institute an IV line and cardiac monitoring. Consider gastric lavage in patients presenting soon after overdose. Administer 1 g/kg of **activated charcoal** to all patients. Whole-bowel irrigation may be effective in overdose of sustained release preparations.

Calcium chloride or **calcium gluconate** may be effective against conduction defects and hypotension. A 1-g (10 mL) vial of 10% calcium chloride contains 272 mg of calcium, and a 1-g (10 mL) vial of calcium gluconate contains 93 mg of calcium. Administer 10 mL of calcium chloride or 30 mL of calcium gluconate IV over 15 min. The chloride component of calcium chloride may worsen an underlying metabolic acidosis. Therefore, calcium gluconate is preferable in patients with acidosis. The optimum dose of calcium has not been established. Three or four repeat doses may be administered if necessary. If multiple doses are administered, monitor serum calcium to avoid hypercalcemia.

Bradycardia and conduction defects also may respond to atropine, isoproterenol, or cardiac pacing. Treat hypotension with IV fluids and pressors. Dopamine and norepinephrine have been effective, although higher doses than usual may be required.

Verapamil-induced hypoglycemia usually does not require treatment and resolves within 24 h. Marked hyperglycemia may require insulin therapy.

All symptomatic patients should be admitted to a monitored bed or ICU. All overdoses of sustained-release preparations should be admitted and monitored. Overdose of sustained-release verapamil has resulted in significant toxicity more than 15 h after ingestion.

If Standard Treatment Fails

Glucagon infusion has been effective in severe toxicity in isolated case reports (see section on beta-blockers for dosage). Aminopyridine may be an effective antidote but is not yet available in the U.S. Hemodialysis and charcoal hemoperfusion are probably not beneficial.

CLONIDINE

Clonidine is a commonly prescribed antihypertensive, is an adjunct in the treatment of opiate, nicotine, and alcohol withdrawal, and is used in the treatment of various neurologic and psychiatric disorders.

Clinical Features

The minimum toxic dose of clonidine is not known. Pediatric patients are particularly susceptible, with significant toxicity reported in a 24 mo old infant who ingested 0.1 mg. Symptoms of toxicity usually occur within 2 h of ingestion and resolve within 72 h.

Common manifestations of clonidine toxicity include lethargy, coma, respiratory depression, apnea, hyporeflexia, hypotonia, and hypothermia. Miosis is the most common pupillary finding, but mydriasis has been reported. Seizures occur only rarely. Cardiovascular effects include hypotension, sinus bradycardia, and AV block. Transient hypertension followed by hypotension may be seen in large ingestions.

Diagnosis and Differential

Most toxicology screening tests do not detect clonidine but may detect coingestants or other agents responsible for the clinical picture. Several drugs and pesticides may produce similar toxidrome.

The triad of coma, miosis, and respiratory depression is most commonly associated with narcotics overdose, but phenobarbital and chloral-hydrate ingestion must be considered as well. Beta-blockers may cause bradycardia, hypotension, and coma. Phenothiazine ingestion may produce miosis, coma, and hypotension. Pesticide toxicity may include miosis, coma, and bradycardia.

Emergency Department Care and Disposition

Institute an intravenous line, as well as cardiac and respiratory monitoring. In all obtunded patients evaluate serum glucose and consider dextrose, naloxone, and thiamine administration.

Gastric lavage is recommended in patients presenting 1 h or less after ingestion. Administer 1 g/kg of **activated charcoal** to all patients. Ipecac is contraindicated because of the potential for the patient to become rapidly obtunded. Forced diuresis, urinary pH manipulation, dialysis, and hemoperfusion are not clinically useful.

All patients with clonidine ingestions should be monitored for at least 4 h. Patients without signs or symptoms of toxicity may then be discharged with appropriate psychiatric evaluation. All patients with symptoms or vital-sign abnormalities should be admitted to a monitored bed or ICU.

Supportive care is the most important aspect of treatment. Children are especially vulnerable to apnea, and may require intubation. Hypothermia generally resolves with passive rewarming. Symptomatic bradycardia usually responds to standard doses of atropine. Hypertension, which is transient and followed by hypotension, should only be treated if there is evidence of end-organ damage. Nitroprusside is the agent of choice, since it is short-acting. Hypotension should be treated initially with Trendelenburg position and boluses of normal saline, followed by dopamine if necessary. Seizures are rare, so it is important to rule out other etiologies such as hypoglycemia or hypoxia. Prolonged seizures are treated with benzodiazepines and phenytoin.

Naloxone may reverse some of the CNS and cardiovascular toxicity of clonidine. In addition, naloxone is the antidote of choice in narcotics overdose, and it is difficult to distinguish clonidine and narcotic toxicity. The recommended initial dose of naloxone is 2 to 4 mg IV in adults and 0.01 mg IV in children.

Tolazoline is a nonselective alpha-adrenergic blocker that was investigated as a possible antidote to clonidine and found not to be consistently effective. The only reported death in a clonidine overdose occurred after a patient was administered tolazoline. Tolazoline has been associated with seizures, hypotension, GI hemorrhage, and death in other settings and is not recommended as an antidote.

Abrupt discontinuation of chronic clonidine therapy may result in a withdrawal syndrome, which may present as early as 12 h after the last dose and last for 5 to 7 days. Clonidine withdrawal may be prevented by tapering the drug over 3 to 5 days. Acute overdose is not associated with withdrawal.

Manifestations of clonidine withdrawal include anxiety, diaphoresis, headache, nausea, abdominal pain, tachycardia, and hypertension. Ventricular arrhythmias, hypertensive encephalopathy, and death have been reported in severe cases. The treatment of choice is restarting clonidine. Nitroprusside may be indicated for severe hypertension. Beta-blockers may worsen hypertension because of unopposed alpha-adrenergic vasoconstriction.

For further reading in *Emergency Medicine: A Comprehensive Study Guide,* 4th edition, see Chapter 147, Digitalis Glycosides, by Mark A. Kirk; Chapter 148, Beta Blockers, by Peter Viccellio and Mark Henry; Chapter 149, Calcium Channel Blockers, by Louis J. Ling; and Chapter 150, Clonidine, by E. Martin Caravati.

Greg Mears

Clinical Features

Phenytoin toxicity is dependent on route of administration, duration of exposure, and dosage used. The most important association with toxicity is with intravenous administration. Following IV administration, cardiovascular (bradycardia, hypotension, asystole) toxicity may develop. This is more common in the elderly and in those with previous heart disease but may occur in young, healthy patients as well. Tissue necrosis and sloughing, following extravasation at the intravenous access, site can occur.

Oral preparation toxicity is typically dose related and predictable at higher plasma concentrations. Vestibular, ocular, and cerebellar signs appear early. These include nystagmus, dysdiadokinesia, and ataxia. As plasma levels increase, central nervous system (CNS) depression and other cognitive effects such as confusion, dizziness, loss of concentration and memory may occur. Very high levels may produce seizures. Clinically, the presentation for an acute oral overdose consists of nystagmus, nausea and vomiting, ataxia, and CNS depression. Death from oral ingestion of phenytoin is extremely rare.

Hypersensitivity reactions to phenytoin usually occurs in the first few months of therapy. This syndrome includes fever, rashes, blood dyscrasias and, rarely, hepatitis.

Diagnosis and Differential

Therapeutic phenytoin levels are between 10 and 20 μg/mL (40 to 80 μmol/L) with a free phenytoin level of 1 to 2 μg/mL. The therapeutic range is relatively narrow, and individual variation in toxicity is a function of baseline neurologic status, individual response to the drug, and the free-drug fraction. Patients with underlying brain disease are predisposed to toxicity and may become toxic at much lower levels than others. Many drugs have an effect on the serum level of phenytoin (Table 99-1).

Altered mental status may occur at levels below 20 μg/mL (Table 99–2). Nystagmus usually presents with phenytoin levels of 20 μg/mL but can occur at lower or higher levels. Ataxia usually begins at about 30 μg/mL, and lethargy at 40 μg/mL. Patients who have phenytoin-induced seizures will have levels greater than 30 μg/mL. Toxicity is noted with free phenytoin levels of 2.0 μg/mL and are severe above 5.0 μg/mL.

CNS toxicity typically begins with nystagmus. Vertical, bidirectional, or alternating nystagmus may occur with severe intoxication. Decreased level of consciousness is routine, with initial sedation, lethargy, ataxic gait, and dysarthria progressing to confusion, coma, and even apnea in

TABLE 99-1. Phenytoin-Drug Interactions

Phenytoin *increases* serum level of
  Acetaminophen
  Oral anticoagulants
  Primidone

Phenytoin *decreases* serum level of:

Amiodarone	Disopyramide
Carbamazepine	Mexiletine
Levodopa	Doxycycline
Methadone	Furosemide
Contraceptives	Quinidine
Glucocorticoids	Theophylline
Cyclosporine	Valproic acid

Phenytoin levels are *increased* by:

Amiodarone	Fluconazole
Oral anticoagulants	Phenylbutazone*
Chloramphenicol	Sulfonamide*
Isoniazid	Valproic acid*
Cimetidine	High-dose salicylate*
Disulfiram	Tolbutamide*
Trimethoprim	

Phenytoin levels are *decreased* by:

Antineoplastic drugs	Theophylline
Diazoxide	Phenobarbital
Folic acid	Diazepam
Rifampin	Ethanol
Sucralfate	Calcium

*These drugs displace phenytoin from its protein-binding sites, thus increasing the free phenytoin fraction, although the total phenytoin level may decrease.

TABLE 99-2. Correlation of Plasma Phenytoin Level and Side Effects

Plasma level, μm/mL	Side-Effects
< 10	Usually none
10–20	Occasional mild nystagmus
20–30	Nystagmus
30–40	Ataxia, slurred speech, nausea and vomiting
40–50	Lethargy, confusion,
> 50	coma, seizures

large overdoses. Acute dystonias and movement disorders, including opisthotonos and chroeoathetosis, may occur. Depressed or hyperactive deep tendon reflexes, clonus, and extensor toe responses may be noted. Psychosis, toxic delirium, visual and auditory hallucinations, euphoria, irritability, agitation, and combativeness have all been reported with toxicity.

Significant cardiovascular toxicity after oral phenytoin overdose in an otherwise healthy patient has never been reported and, if observed,

TABLE 99-3. Toxicity of Phenytoin
<hr>

Intravenous
  Loading dose is 18 mg/kg
  Mix total dose in 75–100 mL of normal saline
  Administer through a milipore filter using an infusion pump
  Rate of administration should not exceed 30 mg/min (less in patients with cardiovascular disease)
  Monitor the blood pressure and cardiac rhythm continually during the infusion
  In the event of complications, immediately stop the infusion and administer isotonic crystalloid and other treatment as indicated
Oral
  Loading dose is 20 mg/kg
  Phenytoin tablets or suspension may be used
  Patient must be conscious with an intact gag reflex and not actively seizing or vomiting
  Administer the total amount in one dose
  Check phenytoin level 6–8 h after administration
<hr>

should mandate a rapid assessment of other causes. Hypotension with decreased peripheral vascular resistance, bradycardia, conduction delays progressing to complete AV nodal block, ventricular tachycardia, primary ventricular fibrillation, and asystole have been reported after IV phenytoin administration. ECG changes include increased PR interval, widened QRS interval, and altered S-T and T-wave segments. Bradycardia, hypotension and syncope in healthy individuals has been reported after small IV doses. Most of the complications are attributed to rapid intravenous administration of the propylene glycol diluent fraction and are avoidable with cautious administration (Table 99-3).

It is important to note the toxic effect of phenytoin on tissue secondary to IV extravasation. Tissue necrosis requiring skin grafting, compartment syndrome, gangrene, amputation, and death have been reported. The propylene glycol diluent, strong alkalinity of the intravenous solution, and crystallization of the drug contribute to this toxicity.

Hypersensitivity reactions usually occur within 1 to 6 wks of beginning phenytoin therapy. Reactions can include fever, systemic lupus erythematosus, erythema multiforme, toxic epidermal necrolysis, Stevens–Johnson syndrome, hepatitis, rhabdomyolysis, acute interstitial pneumonitis, lymphadenopathy, leukopenia, disseminated intravascular coagulation, and renal failure. It is important to obtain a history of previous hypersensitivity reactions before administering phenytoin.

Other side-effects of phenytoin include gingival hyperplasia, hirsutism, hypocalcemia, osteomalacia, megaloblastic anemia, lymphoma, and hemorrhagic disease of the newborn responsive to vitamin K. Gingival hyperplasia is common and is a marker for noncompliance. Hyperglycemia can occur and complicate diabetic therapy. Phenytoin is teratogenic and should never be initiated in a pregnant patient without consultation and followup by a neurologist and obstetrician.

Intoxication with almost any CNS-active or sedative–hypnotic drug may mimic early phenytoin toxicity. These drugs include ethanol, carbamazepine, benzodiazepines, barbiturates, and lithium. Hyperglycemia, Wernicke's encephalopathy, and posterior fossa hemorrhage or tumor can mimic toxicity as well. Seizures can occur with toxic phenytoin levels, but other sources and epileptogenic drug overdoses should be considered.

Emergency Department Care and Disposition

The treatment of phenytoin toxicity consists of initial stabilization, activated charcoal, and observation. Serial phenytoin levels should be obtained to determine if the level has peaked. Patients should be placed on a cardiac monitor, noninvasive BP device, pulse-oximetry monitor, and an IV line.

1. Administer sufficient oxygen to maintain a pulse-oximetry reading of 95% O_2 saturation. Respiratory acidosis should be avoided.
2. Crystalloid IV fluids should be given initially for hypotension. Intravenous infusion of phenytoin should be discontinued.
3. **Activated charcoal** (50 g) mixed with a cathartic should be administered every 4 h for the first 24 h due to poor GI absorption of phenytoin.
4. Seizures may be treated with a benzodiazepine or phenobarbital.
5. Bradyarrhythmias associated with intravenous phenytoin may require atropine.

Patients with serious complications (seizures, coma, altered mental status, and ataxia) following oral ingestion should be admitted. The absorption of phenytoin is long and erratic, which requires more than a single serum level to determine if the danger of toxic effects has passed. Patients with symptomatic chronic intoxication should be admitted for observation unless signs are minimal, adequate care can be obtained at home, and they are 8 to 12 h from their last therapeutic dose. Phenytoin should be stopped in all cases until levels have been evaluated in 2 to 3 days.

For further reading in *Emergency Medicine: A Comprehensive Study Guide*, 4th edition, see Chapter 151, Phenytoin Toxicity, by Harold H. Osborn.

100 | Iron

O. John Ma

Iron toxicity from intentional or accidental ingestion is a common poisoning. Prompt and aggressive management of these patients is essential to prevent morbidity and mortality. When determining the amount of iron ingested, elemental iron must be used in calculations. Ferrous sulfate, ferrous fumarate, and ferrous gluconate contain about 20%, 33%, and 12% elemental iron, respectively.

Clinical Features

Based on clinical findings, iron poisoning can be divided into four stages. It is imperative to note that patients can die in any stage.

The first stage develops within the first few hours after the ingestion. The direct corrosive effects of iron on the GI tract produce abdominal pain, vomiting, and diarrhea. Hematemesis is not unusual. Stage 1 toxicity may result in lethargy, shock, and a metabolic acidosis secondary to hypovolemia and tissue hypoperfusion.

During the second stage, which may continue for up to 12 h following ingestion, the patient's GI symptoms may resolve, thereby giving a false sense of security despite toxic amounts of iron being absorbed into the body.

The third stage may appear either early in poisonings or develop h after the second stage. Shock and a metabolic acidosis can be due to persistent hypovolemia, anemia from GI hemorrhage, hepatic dysfunction, heart failure, and renal failure.

The fourth stage develops days to wks after recovery from iron poisoning. It is characterized by gastric outlet or small-bowel obstruction secondary to GI tract scarring from the initial corrosive effects of the iron.

Diagnosis and Differential

The diagnosis of iron poisoning is based on the clinical picture and the history provided by the patient, significant others, or prehospital care providers. Obviously, a symptomatic patient requires evaluation and possible treatment regardless of history. Opinions vary as to what constitutes a toxic dose of iron. Some patients become symptomatic after ingestion of only 20 mg/kg of elemental iron. Serious poisoning often can be seen after ingestion of greater than 40 mg/kg.

For symptomatic patients, laboratory work should be done for serum electrolytes, blood urea nitrogen, serum glucose, coagulation studies, CBC, serum iron level, and total iron binding capacity (TIBC). It is crucial to note that the determination of a single serum iron level does not reflect what iron levels have been previously, in which direction they are going, or the degree of iron toxicity in the tissues.

A plain radiograph of the kidneys, ureters, and bladder (KUB) may reveal iron in the GI tract; however, 50% of children who develop serum iron levels in excess of 300 μg/dL have a negative KUB film.

Emergency Department Care and Disposition

Patients who have remained asymptomatic for 6 h after ingestion of iron and who have a completely normal physical exam do not need medical treatment for iron toxicity.

Patients who present with minimal symptoms after ingestion do well with supportive care. If the patient remains nontoxic after several h observation, and a repeat serum iron level 3 to 5 h after ingestion is well below 350 μg/dL, the patient can be medically cleared of acute iron poisoning. The repeat serum iron level during the ED course helps to ensure that the iron level is not rising.

For patients who present after a significant ingestion of iron (about 20 mg/kg or greater), they should:

1. Receive supplemental oxygen, be placed on a cardiac monitor, and have two large-bore IVs established.
2. Undergo gastric lavage. Activated charcoal does not bind unchelated iron salts.
3. Receive **intravenous fluids** to help correct hypovolemia and tissue hypoperfusion.

Deferoxamine mesylate is a chelating agent that can remove iron from tissues and can remove free iron from plasma. Deferoxamine combines with iron to form water-soluble ferrioxamine, which is excreted in the urine. The preferred route of administration is as an intravenous infusion at a rate of 15 mg/kg per h.

Indications for deferoxamine therapy (after adequate hydration) include:

1. Any moderately or severely symptomatic patient (e.g., one with hypotension, severe gastroenteritis, lethargy), even if iron levels are below the TIBC, have not yet returned, or are not available. One should never wait for the results of a serum iron level or TIBC to decide whether to give deferoxamine to a significantly symptomatic patient.
2. Any patient whose serum iron level is greater than the TIBC.
3. Any patient with a serum iron level greater than 350 to 400 μg/dL.

Deferoxamine therapy should be continued until the patient demonstrates no signs of systemic iron toxicity and serum iron levels are normal. Hypotension due to vasodilation is occasionally seen with deferoxamine therapy. This is usually not a problem if infusion rates are kept below 45 mg/kg per h.

If Standard Treatment Fails

Dialysis and charcoal hemoperfusion can remove ferrioxamine. Dialysis should be initiated in the face of acute renal failure during acute iron poisoning. Deferoxamine infusion should be continued; however, the elimination half-life is prolonged markedly with renal failure so the deferoxamine infusion rate should be decreased appropriately.

For further reading in *Emergency Medicine: A Comprehensive Study Guide*, 4th edition, see Chapter 152, Iron, by Steven C. Curry.

Hydrocarbons

Judith Linden

Hydrocarbons are a diverse group of organic compounds composed of carbon and hydrogen atoms. This group includes fuels, lighter fluids, paints, paint removers, glues, lubricants, spot removers, degreasers, and pesticides. Exposure may be unintentional (occupational exposure to fumes) or intentional (glue sniffers, 'huffing' or 'bagging' TCE, or toluene) in an attempt to get high or achieve a spiritual experience. Exposure can produce life-threatening toxicity.

Clinical Features

Toxicity depends on the route of exposure (ingestion, inhalation or dermal exposure), physical characteristics (volatility, viscosity, surface tension), chemical characteristics (aliphatic, aromatic, hydrogenated; see Table 101-1), and the presence of toxic additives (lead, pesticides). Pulmonary and cardiac toxicity are the most common. Toxicity is discussed below according to organ system.

TABLE 101-1. Chemical Toxicity

Chemical Composition	Example	Commercial Use	Toxicity
Aliphatic (open chain)	Short chain Methane Butane		Pulmonary
			Negligible GI absorption
	Intermediate chain Gasoline Kerosene Mineral seal oil	Motor fuel Stove fuel Furniture polish	Gas/kerosene hemolysis
	Long chain Tar		N-Hexane, butyl ketone polyneuropathy
Aromatic (benezene ring)	Benzene Toluene Xylene	Gasoline Airplane glue Cleaning agent, degreaser	Arrhythmias
			Benzene-aplastic anemia, CML
Halogenated (substituted halogen group)	Carbon-tetrachloride Chloroform TCE, TCA	Refrigerant, propellant Solvent Spot remover, degreaser, Typewriter correction fluid	Arrhythmias
			Hepatic toxicity Acute Renal Failure TCE-Hemolysis

Pulmonary Aspiration of low viscosity liquids, or inhalation of gases may cause a chemical pneumonitis, the most frequent complication of aliphatic hydrocarbon exposure. Pulmonary edema, alveolar membrane injury, and alterations in surfactant result in hypoxemia. Pneumatocele, pneumothorax, and pneumomediastinum also are associated with aliphatic hydrocarbon exposure. Symptoms are usually present within 30 minutes, including cough, dyspnea, choking and gasping. Physical exam may reveal tachypnea, tachycardia, cyanosis, grunting, wheezing, and decreased breath sounds. Radiographic changes may lag behind clinical signs and symptoms, but are usually present within 4 to 6 hours.

Neurologic CNS toxicity occurs most frequently with the inhalation of highly volatile petroleum distillates and solvents. These hydrocarbons have an affinity for lipids, and thus are able to cross the blood-brain barrier. Symptoms include CNS depression, ataxia, slurred speech, obtundation, and lethargy progressing to coma. CNS excitation consists of euphoria and giddiness, and often progresses to tremor, agitation, seizures, hallucinations, and psychosis. Chronic sequela include cerebellar ataxia, emotional lability, and cognitive and psychomotor impairment. Peripheral nervous system toxicity may be delayed for months to years after exposure, and presents as a peripheral polyneuropathy (foot and wrist drop), which is most common with 6–carbon aliphatic hydrocarbons (n-hexane and n-butyl ketone).

Toxicity also may affect the cardiac, hepatic, GI, renal, and hematologic systems (Table 101-2). Cardiac toxicity (most common with halogenated and aromatic hydrocarbons) may present with life-threatening arrhythmias, resulting from increased myocardial sensitivity catecholamines. The sudden release of endogenous catecholamines may be the etiology of sudden death in glue sniffers. Hepatocellular injury is most common with the halogenated hydrocarbons (carbon tetrachloride and chloroform), and is caused by metabolites formed by the cytochrome P-450 enzyme system. Elevated transaminases occur within 24 hours, with jaundice in 48 to 96 hours. Drugs which induce the P-450 system, such as phenobarbital and alcohol, should be avoided. Cirrhosis has been associated with chronic exposure. Carbon monoxide toxicity may result from methylene chloride exposure, with CO levels increasing after removal from the source of exposure, as methylene chloride is metabolized to CO.

Emergency Department Care and Disposition

Small unintentional ingestions of hydrocarbons that are asymptomatic may not need hospital evaluation. Patients who are symptomatic or have been exposed to a large amount of hydrocarbons should be evaluated in the ED. Mental obtundation is treated with glucose, naloxone, and thiamine (for reversible causes). Hypotension is treated with aggressive fluid resuscitation, with avoidance of catecholamines (dopamine, epi-

TABLE 101-2. Toxicity Side-Effects

Organ System	Toxicity (Side Effects)	Organic Compound
Cardiac	Arrhythmias, sudden death	Halogenated, aromatic hydrocarbons
Pulmonary	Chemical pneumonitis, pneumothorax, pneumatoceles	Aliphatic hydrocarbons
CNS	Euphoria, giddiness, tremor, agitation, seizures, obtundation	Halogenated, aromatic HC
	Peripheral neuropathy	Aliphatic (N-hexane, N-butyl ketone)
Gastrointestinal	Nausea and vomiting Oral mucosal burning	
Dermal	Erythema, vesicles, scarlatiniform rash, exfoliative dermatitis	
Hepatic	Hepatocellular injury, elevated transaminases Chronic cirrhosis	Halogenated hydrocarbons (carbon tetrachloride and chloroform)
Renal	Renal tubular acidosis (hypokalemia, anion-gap acidosis) Proteinuria, renal insufficiency	Toluene
Hematologic	Hemolysis	Kerosene, TCE
	AML, CML, aplastic anemia	Chronic benzene exposure

nephrine), which can precipitate life-threatening arrhythmias. GI decontamination should be performed for hydrocarbons which are absorbed from the GI tract, or with toxic additives (CHAMP - Camphor, Halogenated HC, Aromatic HC, Metals and Pesticides), and wood distillate (turpentine, pine oil) ingestions. Aliphatic hydrocarbons are poorly absorbed from the GI tract and have an increased risk of toxicity when aspirated during attempted decontamination, and thus should not be treated with decontamination measures. A small nasogastric tube may be used for liquid ingestions who present immediately after ingestion. Activated charcoal and cathartics are of no benefit. Useful laboratory tests in include arterial blood gas, chest x-ray, and EKG, baseline BUN, creatinine and hematocrit. An abdominal x-ray may be helpful if radiopaque substances (such as chlorinated hydrocarbons) have been ingested. Beta-blockers are used to treat tachyarrhythmias. Hyperbaric oxygen therapy may be helpful in methylene chloride ingestions with high carbon monoxide levels or mental status changes.

Hospital admission is recommended for halogenated and aromatic hydrocarbon ingestions causing delayed toxicity, and for aliphatic ingestions with respiratory symptoms. Aliphatic ingestions who are asymptomatic may be released after an observation period of 4 to 6 hours. All patients who express suicidal ideation should be evaluated by psychiatry.

For further reading in *Emergency Medicine: A Comprehensive Study Guide,* 4th edition, see Chapter 153, Hydrocarbons, by Paul M. Wax.

Strong acids and bases are found in many household and industrial items. Common acids include sulfuric acid and hydrochloric acid. Household items containing acids include toilet bowl cleaners and drain openers. Common alkali include lye (Drano, Liquid Plumber), sodium hydroxide, and ammonium hydroxide. Household bleach (5% sodium hypochlorite) is relatively dilute and weak. Clinitest tablets (used in urine ketone tests) are a solid alkaline compound found in the home. Button batteries contain alkali and mercury.

Clinical Features

Significant acid and alkali ingestions present acutely with orofacial burns, drooling, vomiting, and odynophagia (suggesting esophageal and gastric involvement), dyspnea, hoarseness, and stridor (suggesting laryngeal or epiglottic involvement). Acids are extremely irritating and foul-tasting, and, therefore, usually present with small ingestions and vomiting. Alkali are relatively tasteless and odorless and present with increased tissue exposure. Hypotension and shock may result from third spacing, vomiting, or hematemesis. Abdominal pain and peritonitis suggests gastric or esophageal perforation.

Acids cause coagulation necrosis and immediate eschar formation, thus limiting the depth of penetration and esophageal injury. The acid then pools in the antrum of the stomach, causing pylorospasm and extensive damage to the antrum. Immediate presentations include hematemesis, melena, acidemia, hemolysis and, occasionally, gastric perforation with peritonitis. Late complications include gastric-outlet obstruction (presenting with early satiety and weight loss)

Alkaline exposures cause liquefaction necrosis with potential for extensive deep-tissue injury and full-thickness esophageal burns. Household bleach is relatively weak and may cause emesis and superficial mucosal erythema, but rarely causes significant injury when ingested in small amounts. Patients often present with odynophagia, and may have a soapy film over the oropharynx. The absence of visible oral lesions does not, however, rule out more extensive esophageal injury (10%–30% of patients with significant esophageal injury have no identifiable oropharyngeal burns). Chest pain suggests esophageal perforation with mediastinitis. Immediate injury is followed by tissue sloughing in 2 to 3 days and collagen deposition with granulation tissue formation in 5 to 14 days (contributing to increased risk of perforation). Delayed stricture formation occurs after 21 days. Significant alkali-injured patients have a risk of esophageal cancer 1000 times the general population.

Emergency Department Care and Disposition

Out-of-hospital treatment includes dermal and oropharyngeal decontamination, with irrigation of external surfaces. Oral dilution with milk or water remains controversial. Animal studies suggest decreased tissue damage, but the risk of vomiting and aspiration increases. *Ipecac is absolutely contraindicated.*

ED treatment includes **early orotracheal intubation** with paralysis and direct visualization if signs of laryngeal edema or airway compromise are present. Cricothyrotomy may be necessary if extensive edema prevents orotracheal intubation. Two large-bore intravenous catheters should be placed and crystalloid infused if volume depletion or shock is present. Product information and the local poison center should be consulted early. If chest pain or peritonitis are present, immediate surgical consultation is indicated. Helpful laboratory tests include ABG (to detect acidemia in acid ingestions), CBC, type and crossmatch, and an upright chest x-ray (looking for aspiration, pneumomediastinum, free air under the diaphragm). NG tube placement is controversial. Most authorities recommend placement in acid ingestions, and placement under direct visualization in alkali ingestions. Sodium bicarbonate should be administered if pH is less than 7.1 to 7.2.

Significant acid and alkali ingestions should be admitted for observation. **Early endoscopy** within 12 to 24 h is recommended in alkali ingestions to identify the extent of esophageal injury. The endoscope should be advanced until third-degree or circumferential second-degree burns are visualized. Early esophagectomy with colonic interposition may be considered if severe second- and third-degree burns are present. Treatment of second-degree burns with steroids (40 mg methyl prednisolone every 8 h for 2 to 3 wks, then tapered) is controversial and may increase the risk of infection. Antibiotics are given if steroids are started or fever is present but are otherwise with held (penicillin, VK 12 million units in divided doses over 24 h, or ampicillin, 8 to 12 g in divided doses over 24 h). Delayed complications include stricture formation in 3 wks to 1 y and increased risk of esophageal cancer. Stricture is treated with dilatation or esophagectomy with colonic interposition in severe cases.

Clinitest tablets represent a unique ingestion, since they consist of alkali in solid form (sodium hydroxide, sodium bicarbonate, copper sulfate, and citric acid), thus may have prolonged contact with tissues, causing extensive full-thickness burns. Dilution with milk or water is recommended in patients who can maintain an airway. Button batteries, which are ingested by toddlers are another unique ingestion. They contain alkaline corrosive material and mercury. An x-ray will identify the location of the battery. Batteries in the esophagus should be removed endoscopically. Batteries that have passed beyond the gastroesophageal junction are followed closely as an outpatient. Cathartics decrease transit time. If signs of obstruction or perforation occur, immediate surgical removal is indicated. Stool samples are followed for elimination.

For further reading in *Emergency Medicine: A Comprehensive Study Guide,* 4th edition, see Chapter 154, Caustic Ingestions, by Monica Parraga and Diane Sauter.

Charles J. Havel, Jr.

Widespread use of both organophosphates and carbamates as insecticides is likely responsible for the frequency with which they cause toxicity. Mass poisoning with organophosphates may also be associated with the use of various nerve agents in chemical warfare. Both classes of compounds can cause illness through oral, dermal, conjunctival, gastrointestinal, or respiratory contact. Acute exposure generally results in symptoms within 12 to 24 h; however, some more lipid-soluble compounds may exhibit delayed onset, but prolonged duration of effects and chronic low-grade exposure may produce a nonspecific and long-lasting symptom complex.

Clinical Features

The symptoms and signs of cholinergic excess derived from the inhibition of cholinesterase by organophosphates and carbamates can be divided into muscarinic, nicotinic, and CNS effects (Table 103-1). Muscarinic overstimulation results in the sludge syndrome (Salivation, Lacrimation, Urination, Defecation, Gastrointestinal, Emesis). Pronounced nicotinic activity may override the bradycardia characteristic of muscarinic activity, causing tachycardia and hypertension. It should be noted that CNS effects often predominate in pediatric patients, who may show little in the way of muscarinic or nicotinic signs.

Diagnosis and Differential

The diagnosis of organophosphate or carbamate poisoning is generally made on clinical grounds. The typical presentation is that of altered mental status or coma, diaphoresis, miosis, muscle fasiculations, bradycardia, and varying degrees of respiratory distress. Patients may have the odor of garlic or petroleum products about them. Definitive laboratory testing involves an assay of both serum and RBC cholinesterase activity that should be obtained regardless, bu these results seldom become available for decisionmaking in the ED. Further limitations of the test are that individuals vary widely in their baseline levels, and significant poisoning may occur with normal levels. Other routine laboratory testing is nondiagnostic but may reveal hyperglycemia, hypokalemia, leukocytosis, hyperamylasemia, glycosuria, or proteinuria. In severe cases, a chest X-ray may show signs of pulmonary edema. Electrocardiographic findings are variable and include tachydysrrhythmias, ventricular blocks, bradydysrrhythmias, or asystole.

The cholinergic toxidrome associated with organophosphate and carbamate toxicity is generally distinctive and thus the differential is narrow. Muscarinic signs can also be seen with exposure to pilocarpine,

TABLE 103-1. Classification of the Symptoms and Signs of Acute Organophosphate or Carbamate Poisoning According to Receptor Site and Type

Muscarinic	Nicotinic	Central*
Miosis**	Muscle fasiculations**	Unconsciousness
Blurred vision	Striated muscle	Confusion
Nausea, vomiting	Paralysis	Toxic psychosis
Diarrhea	Muscle weakness	Seizures
Salivation	Hypertension	Fatigue
Lacrimation	Tachycardia	Respiratory depression
Bradycardia	Pallor	Dysarthria
Crampy	Mydriasis (rare)	Ataxia
Abdominal cramping		Anxiety
Diaphoresis		
Wheezing		
Urinary incontinence		
Fecal incontinence		

*Most specific findings.
**Less prominent with carbamate exposure.

mushrooms (specifically *Amanita muscaria*), betel nut, and carbachol. Nicotinic effects can be seen with tobacco toxicity and black widow spider envenomation.

Emergency Department Care and Disposition

Asymptomatic patients with a history of exposure require observation only, generally for 6 to 8 h. Symptomatic patients require aggressive attention to airway protection and ventilation with supplemental oxygen to maintain saturation to > 95%. Tracheal intubation and mechanical ventilation with high oxygen concentrations may be necessary in severe poisoning. Continuous cardiac and pulse oximetry monitoring, noninvasive BP monitoring, and intravenous access are essential.

1. The mainstay of treatment is atropinization with intravenous administration of **atropine** sulfate. Adult dosing should approximate 2 mg IV every 5 to 15 min. The pediatric dose is 0.05 mg/kg every 15 min, as needed. An atropine drip titrated to effect can be useful for maintenance of atropinization. The most useful clinical endpoint for assessing adequacy of atropinization is the drying of secretions.
2. For dermal exposure, **decontamination of the skin** is important to prevent ongoing exposure. Clothing should be removed and the skin should be washed thoroughly with soap and water. Gastrointestinal decontamination for ingestions should, at the minimum, involve administration of activated charcoal. For large ingestions, gastric lavage may be useful (ipecac for emesis should be avoided), as well as multiple doses of activated charcoal.

3. **Pralidoxime** (2–PAM chloride) is indicated for additional treatment, primarily for known organophosphate or mixed organophosphate/carbamate poisoning. Its role in treating pure carbamate exposure is controversial and it is not suggested for asymptomatic patients. Pralidoxime dosing for adults is 1 g IV, and for pediatric patients 20 to 50 mg/kg, either given over 15 to 30 min. Subsequent doses can be given 1 to 2 h after, then every 10 to 12 h, as needed; alternatively, a continuous infusion (0.5 gm/h for adults, 10–20 mg/kg/h for children) may be used after administration of the first bolus dose.

If Standard Treatment Fails

If the diagnosis is firmly established, persistence of symptoms generally is due to inadequate dosing of atropine, as significant amounts (up to 10–12 mg/h in adults) may be required for serious poisoning. Seizures can be treated conventionally with lorazepam or diazepam. Ventricular dysrrhythmias refractory to lidocaine, bretylium, or cardioversion may respond to overdrive pacing or intravenous isoproterenol.

Long-term sequelae of organophosphate and carbamate poisoning may be observed. A so-called intermediate syndrome can result after recovery from the acute cholinergic phase, consisting of a motor polyneuropathy, with generalized hyporeflexia and muscle weakness. Respiratory muscle involvement may cause mechanical ventilation to be required for an extended period. Other patients may manifest long-term neuropsychiatric abnormalities for which there is no specific treatment.

For further reading in *Emergency Medicine: A Comprehensive Study Guide*, 4th edition, see Chapter 155, Organophosphate and Carbamate Poisoning, by James Roberts and John Tafuri.

Charles J. Havel, Jr.

CARBON MONOXIDE

Carbon monoxide (CO) is a colorless, odorless, nonirritating gas that displaces oxygen from hemoglobin, resulting in tissue hypoxia. Sources of exposure to carbon monoxide include the incomplete combustion of organic fuels, tobacco smoke, the metabolism of methylene chloride (contained in the vapors of paint removers), and the low-grade physiological endogenous production of CO.

Clinical Features

The initial clinical picture, though nonspecific, corresponds well to the severity of poisoning and to carboxyhemoglobin levels (Table 104-1). Patients will often present with vague symptoms that may suggest a variety of conditions that may be misleading (Table 104-2). Fetuses and neonates are particularly susceptible to the toxic effects of CO due to the process of fetal hemoglobin and an oxygen dissociation curve that is already shifted to the left. Children are frequently affected and make up almost 40% of patients treated with hyperbaric-oxygen therapy.

TABLE 104-1. Symptoms and Signs at Various Carboxyhemoglobin Concentrations

COHb Level (%)	Symptoms and Signs
0	Usually none
10	Frontal headache
20	Throbbing headache, dyspnea with exertion
30	Impaired judgment, nausea, dizziness, visual disturbances, fatigue
40	Confusion, syncope
50	Coma, seizures
60	Hypotension, respiratory failure
70	Death

Diagnosis and Differential

The primary key to the diagnosis is maintaining a high degree of clinical suspicion. Victims of house fires with appropriate symptoms and signs must be evaluated specifically for CO poisoning. Particularly in colder months, patients with headache, nausea, weakness, fatigue, difficulty in concentrating, dizziness, chest pain, abdominal pain, and the like must also be considered as possible victims.

The most useful laboratory test is the determination of the blood carboxyhemoglobin level. Adjunctive testing may include other toxicologic assays and assessment of acid-base status. For patients with cardiac symptoms, EKG and cardiac enzyme determinations are indicated.

577

TABLE 104-2. Reported Complications of Carbon Monoxide Poisoning

System Involved	Complication
Neuropsychiatric	Coma, seizures, agitation, leukoencephalopathy, cerebral edema, behavioral disorders, decreased cognitive ability, Tourette-like syndrome, mutism, fecal and urinary incontinence, parietal lobe dysfunction, ataxia, muscular rigidity, parkinsonism, peripheral neuropathy, psychosis, memory impairment, gait disturbance, abnormal EEG, personality changes
Cardiovascular	Angina, tachycardia, ST-segment changes, hypotension, arrhythmias, myocardial infarction, heart block
Pulmonary	Pulmonary edema and hemorrhage, unilateral diaphragmatic paralysis
Ophthamologic	Flame-shaped retinal hemorrhages, decreased light sensitivity, decreased visual acuity, cortical blindness, retrobulbar neuritis, papilledema, pancentral scotomata
Vestibular and auditory	Central hearing loss, tinnitus, vertigo, nystagmus
Gastrointestinal	Vomiting, diarrhea, hepatic necrosis, hematochezia, melena
Dermatologic	Bullae, alopecia, sweat gland necrosis, cherry-red skin color, edema, cyanosis, pallor, erythematous patches
Hematologic	Disseminated intravascular coagulation, thrombotic thrombocytopenic purpura, leukocytosis
Musculoskeletal	Rhabdomyolysis, myonecrosis, compartment syndrome
Renal	Acute renal failure secondary to myoglobinuria, proteinuria
Metabolic	Lactic acidosis, nonpancreatic hyperamylasemia, diabetes insipidus, hyperglycemia, hypocalcemia
Fetal	Death, cerebral atrophy, microcephalus, low birth weight, psychomotor retardation, seizures, spasticity

Chest radiographs are generally obtained for fire victims, and other pulmonary function testing may be helpful as well. In patients with focal neurologic signs, CT or MRI may identify specific lesions or generalized cerebral edema. Psychometric testing can detect subtle deficits in patients and assess for indications for hyperbaric oxygen therapy.

Emergency Department Care and Disposition

Table 104-3 delineates appropriate treatment guidelines for CO poisoning. Initially, patients must be removed from the source of exposure,

TABLE 104-3. Treatment Guidelines Based on Severity of CO Poisoning

Mild Poisoning

Criteria— COHb levels < 30%

No symptoms or signs of impaired cardiovascular or neurologic function

May complain of headache, nausea, or vomiting

Treatment—Admission of patients with COHb levels > 25%

Symptomatic medication

100% oxygen by non-rebreathing mask until COHb remains < 5%

Patients with underlying heart disease should be admitted and cardiac function appropriately monitored regardless of COHb level

Moderate Poisoning

Criteria— COHb levels from 30–40%

No signs or symptoms of impaired cardiovascular or neurologic function

Treatment—Admission

Cardiovascular status should be followed closely even in the absence of clear cardiac effects, especially in those patients with underlying heart disease

Determination of acid-base status (will be corrected by high-flow oxygen) 100% oxygen by nonrebreathing mask until COHb remains <5%

Severe Poisoning

Criteria— COHb levels > 40%

or

Cardiovascular or neurologic impairment at any COHb level

Treatment—Admission

Cardiovascular function monitoring

Acid-base status monitoring

100% oxygen by non-rebreathing mask

Transport to a hyperbaric oxygen facility immediately if available, or if no improvement in cardiovascular or neurologic function is seen within 4 h

placed on **100% oxygen** (administered with a tight-fitting mask with a reservoir) and have cardiac monitoring instituted. Intravenous access and noninvasive blood pressure monitoring are also required for management. Indications for initiating **hyperbaric oxygen therapy** include severe CO poisoning, pregnancy, extremes of age, neurologic deficits, cardiovascular abnormalities, and metabolic acidosis. It is valuable not only for treatment of acute toxicity but also to prevent delayed neuropsychiatric sequelae.

If Standard Treatment Fails

Concomitant poisoning must be considered; for fire victims, this includes the possibility of cyanide exposure. Neurologic symptoms from

CO exposure can be caused by cerebral edema that may require administration of mannitol or tracheal intubation and hyperventilation. Severe metabolic acidosis (pH < 7.20) with cardiovascular compromise may be judiciously treated with intravenous sodium bicarbonate.

CYANIDE

Cyanide is a naturally occurring and potent cellular toxin. Acute poisoning results from accidental occupational exposures, accidental or suicidal nonoccupational exposure to substances converted to cyanide (e.g., burning wool, silk, polyurethane, vinyl), ingestion of plants or foods containing naturally occurring cyanogenic glycosides, or iatrogenic toxicity due to prolonged nitroprusside therapy.

Clinical Features

The hallmark of cyanide poisoning is apparent hypoxia without cyanosis. Metabolic acidosis is prominent with high lactate levels due to failed oxygen utilization. Awake patients complain of breathlessness and anxiety. In more severe cases, loss of consciousness (often with seizures) and tachydysrhythmias are apparent, proceeding on to bradycardia with apnea, then to asystolic cardiac arrest. Other clues to cyanide toxicity are bright red retinal blood vessels, oral burns from ingestions, the smell of bitter almonds on the patient's breath, and high peripheral venous oxygen saturations. Absorption of cyanide gas is immediate and ingestion of cyanide salts may cause symptoms within min. At the other end of the spectrum, however, ingestion of cyanogenic compounds may not cause ill effects for h.

Diagnosis and Differential

The diagnosis of cyanide toxicity should always be entertained in the poisoned patient with profound metabolic acidosis. Further support for the diagnosis is any finding consistent with decreased oxygen utilization. Laboratory testing has a limited role in diagnosing cyanide poisoning. Whole blood levels should be obtained, but results will not generally be available for decisionmaking. Arterial blood gas assays can identify acid-base disturbances and the presence of an oxygen saturation gap, whereas serum lactate levels may provide additional, though nonspecific, supporting evidence. The differential diagnosis includes other cellular toxins, such as carbon monoxide, hydrogen sulfide, and simple asphyxiants. In the setting of an ingestion, other possibilities are methanol, ethylene glycol, iron, and salicylates. Severe isoniazid or cocaine poisoning may also mimic the effects of cyanide, causing severe metabolic acidosis and seizures.

Emergency Department Care and Disposition

All patients should have frequent BP and continuous cardiac monitoring, administration of **100% oxygen,** and IV access. Those with altered

TABLE 104-4. Treatment of Cyanide Poisoning

Children

Amyl nitrite inhaler—crack and inhale 30 s / min*
Administration of IV sodium nitrite and sodium thiosulfate

Hb, g/100 ml	3% NaNO2, ml/kg	25% Na2S2O3
7	0.19	0.95
8	0.22	1.10
9	0.25	1.25
10	0.27	1.35
11	0.30	1.50
12	0.33	1.65
13	0.36	1.80
14	0.39	1.95

May repeat once at half dose
Monitor methemoglobin to keep level less than 30%

Adults

Amyl nitrite; crack and inhale 30 s / min*
Sodium nitrite—10 mL IV (10 mL ampule of 3% solution = 300 mg)
Sodium thiosulfate—50 mL IV (50 mL ampule of 25% solution = 12.5 g)
May repeat once at half dose

* Administration of amyl nitrite is only necessary if venous access has not been obtained

mental status must be considered for IV glucose, thiamine, and naloxone administration. Gastric lavage and administration of activated charcoal are standard for ingestions; dermal contacts require skin decontamination and inhalational exposures require removal from the source. Specific treatment with the **nitrite–thiosulfate antidote** in the Lilly Cyanide Antidote Kit must be considered (Table 104-4). Asymptomatic patients or those with minimal symptoms should be observed and treated only if deterioration in their condition is noted, while severely toxic patients with a clear history of exposure demand full and immediate treatment. Due to the potential side-effects of hypotension and induction of methemoglobinemia, hypotensive acidotic patients without clear cyanide toxicity or with smoke inhalation are best served by administration of IV sodium thiosulfate only.

If Standard Treatment Fails

Consideration of concomitant poisoning ought to be considered in cases when further deterioration occurs despite specific antidote administration. Other less standard treatments for cyanide toxicity include hydroxycobalamin (vitamin B_{12a}), dicobalt edetate (Kelocyanor), and 4-dimethylaminophenol (DMAP).

For further reading in *Emergency Medicine: A Comprehensive Study Guide*, 4th edition, see Chapter 171, Carbon Monoxide Poisoning, by Earl J. Reisdorf and John G. Wiegenstein; and Chapter 156, Cyanide, by Kathleen Delaney.

LEAD

Lead is the most common cause of chronic heavy metal poisoning. Children between 1 and 5 y old and the economically disadvantaged are at greatest risk. Sources of lead include lead-based paint, solder, ceramic lead glaze in pottery, moonshine and certain industries (smelting, battery reclamation, radiator repair). Poisoning is usually chronic.

Clinical Features

Lead poisoning mainly affects the nervous and hematopoietic system. CNS symptoms can include such vague complaints as headache, irritability, depression, fatigue, and memory and sleep disturbances. Encephalopathy (particularly in children), however, can also occur, with confusion, obtundation, seizures, and coma. Cerebellar and cranial nerve function is usually normal. Peripheral effects can include motor weakness (rarer in children), with wrist drop, depressed DTRs, and paresthesias. Sensory function is unaffected. Hematopoietic effects can include hypoproliferative or hemolytic anemias. Other clinical features include abdominal pain, vomiting, decreased libido, and fertility problems.

Diagnosis and Differential

Lead poisoning should be suspected in patients, particularly children and the economically disadvantaged who present with the symptoms cited above. A history of potential exposure is useful. The differential diagnosis for lead poisoning is large, making routine screening less useful for this relatively rare condition. Lead poisoning is diagnosed by blood lead levels (normal range being below 10 ug/dL). Adults can tolerate somewhat higher levels.

Emergency Department Care and Disposition

Treatment recommendations depend on the blood lead level, symptomatology, age, and the nature of the exposure. Several new agents are becoming available and the physician should consult a toxicologist or Poison Control Center prior to starting treatment. **Chelation therapy** is usually started in asymptomatic children when the levels are >45 ug/dL and is considered when levels are between 20 and 45 ug/dL. Symptomatic children and adults are always treated. Asymptomatic adults may be watched, depending upon the level and the exposure. General guidelines for chelation are given below.

Children without encephalopathy or vomiting—2,3–dimercaptosuccinic acid (DMSA), 10 mg/kg every 8 h for 5 days, followed by the same dose every 12 h for 14 days.

Children with encephalopathy or vomiting and all adults—Dimercaprol (BAL), 75 mg/m2 IM initially, followed 4 h later by CaNa2–EDTA, 1500 mg/m2 per 24 h in a continuous IV infusion. BAL is continued every 4 h. It must be give prior to CaNa2–EDTA to prevent exacerbation of CNS toxicity. (For adults without CNS toxicity some recommend CaNa2–EDTA alone. DMSA, currently approved only for children in the U.S., is used for asymptomatic adults in Europe.)

Other measures should include whole-bowel irrigation with polyethylene glycol electrolyte solution if lead is detected radiographically in the bowels (100–500 mL/h for children, 1000–2000 mL/h for adults till clear.) Of greatest importance is finding and removing the source of lead. Other individuals exposed to the same source should be tested.

Children with symptoms or with lead levels > 70 ug/dL and adults with CNS symptoms should be admitted to the hospital. Admission should also be considered for patients for whom returning to the usual environment would pose a risk.

ARSENIC

Arsenic is the most common cause of acute heavy-metal poisoning and a major cause of chronic heavy-metal poisoning. Arsenic is found in insecticides, rodenticides, herbicides, and antiparasitical medicines, as well as in several industrial processes.

Clinical Features

Arsenic poisoning can present with a wide variety of clinical pictures, depending on whether the ingestion was acute or chronic and the amount and form of arsenic. Acute poisoning manifests with severe nausea, vomiting, and choleralike diarrhea, which can last several days to wks. Patients may complain of a metallic taste. There may be prolonged QT, and ventricular tachycardia may result. Severe poisonings may have encephalopathy, seizures, coma, pulmonary edema, acute renal failure and rhabdomyolysis. Patients with chronic toxicity present with peripheral neuropathy (stocking–glove sensory progressing to motor), skin rash, malaise, and weakness. Hyperpigmentation and hyperkeratosis of the palms and soles can be seen as well as white transverse lines (Mee lines) in the nails. Chronic encephalopathy and Korsakoff–like symptoms can also be present.

Diagnosis and Differential

Arsenic poisoning is difficult to diagnose because of its rarity and nonspecific symptoms. Hypotension preceded by gastroenteritis of unknown etiology should warrant consideration of arsenic poisoning. Patients with unexplained peripheral neuropathy, typical skin manifestations, or recurrent bouts of unexplained gastroenteritis may warrant testing for arsenic. Definitive diagnosis of acute poisoning is made with 24–h urine levels of arsenic. Hair and nail analysis can be done for chronic poisoning. Other laboratory findings suggestive of arsenic poisoning include relative eosinophilia, basophilic stippling, a prolonged QT, and metallic flecks seen on abdominal radiographs.

Emergency Department Care and Disposition

Hypotension and arrhythmias are the most acute problems encountered in arsenic poisoning. Hypotension is usually due to volume depletion and should be treated with aggressive crystalloid replacement, invasive hemodynamic monitoring, and pressor therapy (dopamine). Overhydration should be avoided. Ventricular tachycardia and fibrillation should be treated by standard methods, except drugs that prolong the QT (procainamide, etc.) should be avoided. Potassium, calcium, and magnesium levels should be monitored. Seizures can be treated with standard therapy, and gastric lavage followed by 1g/kg activated charcoal should be initiated. Although charcoal does not absorb arsenic well, it may absorb the carriers. Whole-bowel irrigation should also be considered.

Chelation therapy should be instituted immediately in all cases of known or suspected acute poisonings. The most effective therapy depends on the nature of the ingestion, and a Poison Control Center should be consulted. BAL has been the standard therapy, with doses of 3 to 5 mg/kg IM every 4 h for 2 days to start. Other agents in use include DMSA and D-penicillamine. Hemodialysis is minimally effective.

Patients should be hospitalized if they have acute or life-threatening poisonings, chronic poisonings requiring BAL therapy, and if suicidal or homicidal intent is suspected. Intentional poisonings are reportable to police by law in many states.

If Standard Treatment Fails

If hypotension persists, consider invasive monitoring. Also consider concomitant illnesses such as myocardial infarction or ingestion of other substances.

MERCURY

Clinical Features

Mercury poisoning is rare and its manifestations vary considerably depending upon the form. Short-chained alkyl compounds and methyl-/ethylmercury have the most effect on the CNS, followed by elemental mercury. Erethism, (anxiety, depression, irritability, mania, memory loss) is a common finding, along with various types of tremor. Paresthesias, ataxia, spasticity, rigidity, and visual or hearing problems can also be found. Little GI toxicity is noted. Mercury salts have little effect on the

CNS but can cause severe corrosive gastritis followed by cardiovascular collapse and acute renal failure. Several forms of mercury can cause acrodynia in children. Swallowing mercury from a glass thermometer does not produce poisoning.

Diagnosis and Differential

Diagnosis of mercury poisoning is by history and clinical suspicion. A blood level > 1.5 ug/dL suggests toxicity. Because of the wide variety of symptoms, the differential diagnosis is large and many other diseases must be considered unless there is overwhelming evidence of mercury ingestion.

Emergency Department Care and Disposition

Treatment consists mainly of general supportive therapy. Acute poisoning with mercury salts should be treated with aggressive GI decontamination, including instillation of milk or egg whites to bind the mercury, lavage, and activated charcoal. A Poison Control Center should be contacted for information on chelation therapy and other treatments. Patients should be hospitalized if mercury salt ingestion is suspected, mercury vapor inhaled, or BAL therapy initiated.

For further reading in *Emergency Medicine: A Comprehensive Study Guide*, 4th edition, see Chapter 158, Heavy Metals, by Marsha D. Ford.

Kent N. Hall

Frostbite and hypothermia constitute a spectrum of illness. Frostbite and its related entities (chilblains, trench foot) are localized skin damage caused by cold injury, with or without associated factors. Hypothermia is defined as a core temperature less than 35°C (95°F).

Clinical Features

Clinical entities in the spectrum of focal cold related injuries include chilblains, trench foot, and frostbite. Chilblains is a painful, inflamed skin lesion caused by chronic, intermittent exposure to damp, nonfreezing ambient temperatures. Manifestations are edema, erythema, cyanosis, plaques, nodules, ulcerations, vesicles, and/or bullae that develop up to 12 hours after acute exposure. Patients often complain of burning paresthesias and pruritus. Blue nodules may develop upon rewarming and may last for several days.

Trench foot results from cooling of soft tissues, and is accelerated by wet conditions. Tingling and numbness develop in the affected area. Initially the area appears pale and mottled, and is anesthetic, pulseless, and immobile. A hyperemic phase occurs hours after rewarming, and is associated with a severe burning sensation and return of sensation in the proximal area. Edema and bullae develop in the area over the next 2–3 days. Anesthesia of the area may be permanent. Long-term hyperhidrosis and cold sensitivity are common.

Frostbite can occur on any skin surface, but is usually limited to the exposed skin. The spectrum of injuries seen in frostbite is seen in Table 106-1. Frostnip is a less severe form of frostbite, associated with discomfort that resolves with rewarming and no tissue loss.

Hypothermia is caused by the factors listed in Table 106-2. In mild hypothermia (defined as a body temperature between 32° and 35°C (90° to 95°F)), heart rate and blood pressure rise, and shivering occurs. When body temperature falls below 32°C, shivering ceases and the heart rate and blood pressure begin to fall. Below 32°C (86°F) the patient is prone to ventricular dysrhythmias, the incidence increasing as body temperature falls. The classic ECG finding of hypothermia is the Osborn (J) wave, a slow positive deflection at the end of the QRS complex.

Pulmonary effects of hypothermia include initial tachypnea, followed by progressive decrease in respiratory rate and tidal volume. Bronchorrhea, and loss of the cough and gag reflex also occur. Hypothermia causes a depression of the central nervous system, initially manifested by incoordination followed by confusion, lethargy and coma. Renal effects include a cold diuresis which can cause a significant volume loss, exacerbated by a plasma shift to the extravascular space. This can

TABLE 106-1. Classification of Cold Injury According to Severity

Thickness	Symptoms
Superficial	

First degree—partial skin freezing
  Erythema, edema, hyperemia
  No blisters or necrosis
  Occasional skin desquamation
(5–10 d later)
	Transient stinging and burning
	Throbbing and aching possible
	May have hyperhidrosis

Second degree—full-thickness injury Erythema, substantial edema, vesicles with clear fluid Blisters that desquamate and form blackened eschar	Numbness; vasomotor disturbances in severe cases
Deep	

Third degree—full-thickness skin
and subcutaneous freezing
  Violaceous/hemorrhagic blisters
  Skin necrosis
  Blue-gray discoloration
	Initially no sensation
	Tissue feels like block of wood
	Later, shooting pains, burning,
	throbbing, aching

Fourth degree—full-thickness skin, subcutaneous tissue, muscle, tendon, and bone freezing Little edema Initially mottled, deep red, or cyanotic Eventually dry, black, mummified	Possible joint discomfort

result in hemoconcentration, intravascular thrombosis, and disseminated intravascular coagulation.

Emergency Department Care and Disposition

Management of the patient with chilblains and trench foot is supportive. Affected skin should be rewarmed, bandaged and elevated. Nifedipine (20 mg tid), topical corticosteroids, and oral prednisone have been

TABLE 106-2. Causes of Hypothermia: Clinical Settings

Accidental (environmental)
Metabolic
Hypothalamic and CNS dysfunction
Drug-induced
Sepsis
Dermal disease
Acute incapacitating illness

shown to be helpful in ameliorating the symptoms of chilblains. Affected areas are more prone to reinjury.

Rapid rewarming is the most important aspect of **frostbite** therapy. Placement of the involved extremity in gently recirculating water at a temperature of 40° to 42°C (104° to 108°F) for 30 minutes results in complete thawing. Severe pain is associated with this therapy, and parenteral narcotics should be administered and titrated to effect. Current recommendations are to debride all clear blisters, but to leave hemorrhagic blisters intact. All blisters should be treated with topical aloe vera q6h. Prophylactic use of penicillin G at a dose of 500,000 units q6h for 48–72 h has been beneficial in some published protocols. Early surgical intervention is not indicated, and, in fact, may result in greater tissue loss. However, early escharotomy for circumferential lesions may be limb-saving. All patients with more than isolated and superficial frostbite lesions should be admitted to the hospital. Transfer to a tertiary care burn center should be considered for severe cases.

Management of the patient with hypothermia includes both supportive measures and specific rewarming techniques. Supportive measures include attention to the ABCs of resuscitation. If indicated for oxygenation, ventilation, or pulmonary toilet, gentle endotracheal intubation rarely results in complications. **Oxygen and intravenous fluids should be warmed.** The patient's core body temperature should be monitored using an electronic or glass thermometer capable of recording in the severe hypothermic ($<32°C$) range. Most rhythm disturbances in the severely hypothermic patient are not immediately life-threatening. Ventricular fibrillation, when present, is usually refractory to therapy until the patient's core temperature is above 30°C (86°F). Current American Heart Association guidelines recommend countershock three times if ventricular fibrillation occurs. If these are unsuccessful, CPR is begun and rapid rewarming instituted.

Rewarming techniques include passive external, active external, and active core. Passive rewarming uses the patient's endogenous heat production for rewarming and is the most physiologic. When intrinsic thermoregulatory mechanisms are not intact, metabolic heat production does not occur, and passive rewarming will not work.

Active external rewarming provides exogenous heat to the body, and includes the use of warm water immersion, heating blankets, heated objects, and/or radiant heat. Core temperature after-drop occurs when this technique is used, due to peripheral vasodilation and shunting of cold blood to the central circulation. The importance of this phenomenon is unknown. Washout of lactic acid from the periphery into the central circulation may increase demands on the circulatory system with no reserve, further increasing tissue hypoxia and acidosis.

Active core rewarming allows the heart to be preferentially warmed, decreasing myocardial irritability and returning cardiac function. Active core rewarming techniques include inhalation rewarming, heated IV fluids, GI, bladder, peritoneal, pleural and mediastinal lavage, and extra-corporeal rewarming. Inhalation rewarming (using warmed, humidified oxygen by mask or endotracheal tube) and use of warmed intravenous fluids provide for only a small amount of heat transfer, but should be used on every moderately or severely hypothermic patient. Lavage of the GI tract and bladder is simple, and large volumes of warmed fluid may be used rapidly.

Peritoneal and pleural lavage have been shown to be effective in animal studies and human cases, and can be instituted quickly in the ED with readily available material. In the case of peritoneal lavage, potassium free saline is warmed in a microwave oven to 42°C and instilled in the peritoneal cavity through a peritoneal dialysis or diagnostic peritoneal lavage catheter. Similar fluid can be instilled into the left chest through a thoracostomy tube placed in the 2nd left intercostal space at the midclavicular line. An effluent tube placed in the 5th or 6th intercostal space at the midaxillary line allows the fluid to drain.

Rewarming through an extracorporeal circuit is the method of choice in the severely hypothermic patient in cardiac arrest. This requires placement of bypass catheters, usually in the femoral vessels. Rapid rewarming rates, circulatory support, and oxygenation are achieved with this technique. Unfortunately, specialized equipment and personnel are required.

A general approach to rewarming takes into account the degree of hypothermia and the patient's cardiovascular status. If endogenous heat production mechanisms are functional, gradual rewarming without active modalities is usually sufficient. When the patient has severe hypothermia, but has a stable cardiac rhythm, active external rewarming in conjunction with inhalational and heated IV fluids may be attempted, although some authorities recommend active core rewarming in this setting. In the presence of cardiovascular insufficiency, rapid rewarming is required and active core techniques should be used.

For further reading in *Emergency Medicine: A Comprehensive Study Guide*, 4th edition, see Chapter 159, Frostbite and Other Localized Cold-Related Injuries, by Mark Rabold; and Chapter 160, Hypothermia, by Howard Bessen.

HEATSTROKE

Heatstroke (HS) is a true emergency, as failure to lower body temperature promptly can lead to significant end-organ damage. The very young and the very old are at greatest risk, particularly those without home air-conditioning. Amateur athletes, military recruits, and people who work in hot environments are also at risk. Drugs associated with HS include cocaine, amphetamines, and tricyclic antidepressants.

Clinical Features

Patients with HS present with hyperpyrexia (core temperature >40.5° C), CNS dysfunction, and anhidrosis. Although anhidrosis is common, sweating may still occur in the early stages of HS. Typically patients present with an elevated core temperature, lack of sweating, confusion, and a history of heat exposure. Neurologic abnormalities can vary, though, ranging from confusion and ataxia to posturing, hemiplegia, status epilepticus, and coma.

Diagnosis and Differential

Heatstroke is a diagnosis of exclusion. A core temperature of >40.5° C and an abnormal neurologic exam are necessary for the diagnosis. Anhidrosis and a history of environmental heat exposure should make the clinician strongly suspect HS. There are a large number of conditions, however, including infection, alcohol withdrawal, toxic ingestions (cocaine, PCP, amphetamine, salicylate, and anticholinergics), and neuroleptic malignant syndrome (NMS), which also produce fever and neurologic abnormalities. These conditions need to be considered before assuming a diagnosis of HS.

Emergency Department Care and Disposition

The overall goal of ED management is cooling, but initial attention must be to the airway, breathing, and circulation. Continuous pulse oximetry, cardiac monitoring, IV access, and a Foley catheter are needed. Serial monitoring of core temperature is crucial. The following treatments are indicated.

1. High-flow supplemental oxygen.
2. IV fluids–NS or LR at 250 mL/h, with close monitoring. Vigorous fluid resuscitation should not be initiated automatically. These patients are prone to CHF and cerebral edema, and volume expansion may worsen their condition.
3. **Cooling**—This is the most important treatment and should be initiated immediately. Evaporative cooling, in conjunction with other

methods, is the treatment of choice. The patient should be completely undressed and moistened or sprayed with tepid water. Fans directed across the patient accomplish the cooling. Wet sheets on top of the patient should not be used. Adjunct methods included ice packs in the groin or axilla, gastric lavage with cold water if the airway is protected (intubated or wide awake), and Foley irrigation with cool water. Other methods of cooling include peritoneal lavage (very effective) and immersion cooling (technically difficult). Shivering during cooling can be treated with benzodiazepines and, secondarily, with phenothiazines. Cardiac electrodes can be applied to the patients if adhesion is problematic. Cooling efforts should be discontinued when the core temperature reaches 40°C. Antipyretics are not useful in HS.

4. Laboratory studies—Including complete blood count, electrolytes, BUN, creatinine, calcium, magnesium, coagulation profile, ABG, urinalysis, and urinary myoglobin should be obtained. A toxicology screen, blood cultures, CT scan of the head, and lumbar puncture may also be indicated.

5. Admission—Patients with HS should be admitted to nonmonitored, monitored, or ICU bed, depending upon clinical status. Rarely, a young patient with HS and rapidly clearing mental status may be discharged with appropriate followup after prolonged observation in the ED. Complications of HS include heart failure, pulmonary edema, cardiovascular collapse, mild hepatic injury, acute tubular necrosis, rhabdomyolysis, and a wide variety of hematologic disorders. These should be treated according to standard therapies.

If Standard Treatment Fails

When core temperature fails to drop, make sure the cooling methods are appropriate (patient undressed, fan, etc.) Consider an alternative diagnosis, such as toxins (body packing cocaine or unsuspected anticholinergics), or other syndromes such as NMS or brain lesions.

MINOR HEAT ILLNESSES

Although HS is the most serious heat-related illness, patients will present to the ED more frequently with one of the minor heat illnesses. These rarely require hospitalization.

Heat exhaustion This condition is characterized by vague symptoms, including dizziness, malaise, myalgias, headache, fatigue, nausea, vomiting, and lightheadedness. Clinically, patients present with syncope, orthostatic hypotension, tachycardia, tachypnea, and diaphoresis. Core temperature can range from normal to 40°C. Importantly, neurologic exam, including mental status, is normal. They may present immediately after the heat exposure or up to 48 h later. Laboratory studies are necessary only to exclude other diagnosis and may show hemoconcentration, as well as minor electrolyte abnormalities. Treatment includes volume and electrolyte replacement and rest. Rapid administration of 1 to 2 l of IV fluid is usually effective, although oral fluids can be used in minor cases. Patients can be safely discharged with instructions for heat avoidance and fluid replacement. It is important to remember that if the patient has altered mental status, they have the more serious diagnosis of heat stroke.

Heat cramps These are painful, involuntary contractions of the calf, thigh, or shoulder muscles, which often occur in unconditioned or nonacclimated individuals. They are self-limiting and cause no permanent damage. Treatment is fluid and electrolytes. Although this can be accomplished orally, patients usually respond more rapidly to an IV infusion of NS. Rest, fluid replenishment, and heat avoidance should be prescribed on discharge.

Heat syncope This type of syncope is a variant of postural hypotension resulting from peripheral vasodilatation, decreased vasomotor tone, and minor volume depletion. It occurs usually early in the stages of heat exposure. Treatment consists of removal of the patient from the source of heat and oral or IV fluids. Examination of the patient for injuries from the fall and consideration of other types of syncope, particularly in older patients, should be undertaken. Patients do not need to be admitted unless another etiology of the syncope is suspected.

Prickly heat (heat rash) This is a pruritic, maculopapular, erythematous rash found on clothed areas of the body. It is an acute inflammation of the sweat glands caused by blockage of the pores. Itching is the main reason for presentation and can be treated with antihistamines. Prevention involves the use of clean, light, loose-fitting clothing and avoidance of sweating. The use of powder is of no benefit. Occasionally, the sweat ducts become secondarily infected with bacteria. Chlorhexidine cream or lotion is an acceptable treatment. If heat rash progresses, white papules will be present and the rash will not be pruritic. This requires oral dicloxacillin or erythromycin and desquamation of the skin with 1% salicylic acid 3 times a day.

Heat edema This is a mild swelling and tightening of the hands and feet that occurs in the first few day of heat exposure. It is more common in the elderly and in patients moving from a cold to a hot environment. It usually resolves spontaneously in a few days but can last as long as 6 wks. No treatment is necessary. Other potential causes for edema should be considered.

For further reading in *Emergency Medicine: A Comprehensive Study Guide*, 4th edition, see Chapter 161, Heat Emergencies, by James S. Walker and Michael V. Vance.

HYMENOPTERA (WASPS, BEES, AND ANTS)

Wasps, bees, and ants that sting are members of the order Hymenoptera. Both local and generalized reactions may occur in response to an encounter.

Clinical Features

Local reactions consist of edema contiguous with the sting site. Although it may involve neighboring joints, local reactions cause no systemic symptoms. Severe local reactions increase the likelihood of serious systemic reactions if the patient is exposed again in the future.

Toxic reactions are a nonantigenic response to multiple stings. They have many of the same features seen in true systemic (allergic) reactions, but there is greater frequency of GI disturbance, and bronchospasm and urticaria do not occur.

Systemic or anaphylactic reactions are true allergic reactions that range from mild to fatal. In general, the shorter the interval between the sting and the onset of symptoms, the more severe the reaction. Initial symptoms usually are itching eyes, urticaria, and cough. As the reaction progresses, patients may experience respiratory failure and cardiovascular collapse.

Delayed reactions may appear 10 to 14 days after a sting. Symptoms of delayed reactions resemble serum sickness and include fever, malaise, headache, urticaria, lymphadenopathy, and polyarthritis.

Emergency Department Care and Disposition

The treatment for all Hymenoptera encounters is the same. First, any bee stinger remaining in the patient should be removed immediately. Scraping is the preferred technique since squeezing may force more venom from the stinger sac into the wound. The wound should be cleansed, and ice packs may reduce swelling. Erythema and swelling seen in local reactions may be difficult to distinguish from cellulitis. As a general rule, infection is present in a minority of cases. For minor local reactions, oral antihistamines and analgesics may be the only treatment needed.

More severe reactions, such as chest constriction, nausea, presyncope, or a change in mental status, require treatment with **1:1000 epinephrine** subcutaneously (0.3 mL–0.5 mL adult dose, 0.01 mL/kg for a child, 0.3 mL maximum). Some patients may require a second epinephrine injection in 10 to 15 min. Parenteral **antihistamines** (e.g., diphenhydramine) and **steroids** (e.g., methylprednisolone) should be rapidly administered. Bronchospasm is treated with inhaled beta-agonists and, possibly, an infusion of aminophylline over 20 to 30 min. Hypotension should be treated aggressively with a crystalloid infusion, although dopamine and other vasopressors may be required. Patients with minor symptoms who respond well to conservative measures may be discharged after monitoring for several h. Severe reactions require admission. All patients with Hymenoptera reactions should be referred to allergists for further evaluation and possible immunotherapy.

SPIDER BITES

Brown Recluse Spider (*Loxosceles reclusa*)

Clinical Features

The *L. reclusa* bite causes a mild, erythematous lesion that may become firm and heal over several days to wks. Occasionally a severe reaction, with immediate pain, blister formation, and bluish discoloration, may occur. Lesions often become necrotic over the next 3 to 4 days and form eschars from 1 to 30 cm in diameter. *Loxoscelism* is a systemic reaction that may occur 1 to 2 days after envenomation. Symptoms include fever, chills, vomiting, arthralgias, myalgias, petechiae, and hemolysis; severe cases progress to seizures, renal failure, disseminated intravascular coagulation, and death. The diagnosis of *L. reclusa* envenomation is sometimes made solely on clinical grounds, since the spider may not be found. All patients with suspected *L. reclusa* envenomation should have the following tests: CBC, BUN, creatinine, electrolytes, coagulation profile, and urinalysis for hemoglobinuria.

Emergency Department Care and Disposition

Treatment of the brown recluse spider bite includes the usual supportive measures. Currently, there is no commercially available antivenom. Tetanus prophylaxis, analgesics, and antibiotics may be offered when appropriate. Surgery is reserved for lesions greater than 2 cm and is deferred for 2 to 3 wks following the bite. An intravenous dose of methylprednisolone, followed by a 5-day course of oral prednisone, should be given. **Dapsone,** 50 to 200 mg per day, may prevent ongoing local necrosis. Patients with systemic reactions must be hospitalized and monitored for consideration of red-cell transfusion and hemodialysis.

Black Widow Spider Bites

Clinical Features

Black-widow bites are initially painful, and within 1 h, the patient may experience erythema, swelling, and diffuse muscle cramps. Large muscle groups are involved, and painful cramping of the abdominal-wall musculature can mimic peritonitis. Severe pain may wax and wane for up to 3 days, but muscle weakness and spasm can persist for wks to months. Serious complications include hypertension, respiratory failure, shock, and coma.

Emergency Department Care and Disposition

Initial therapy includes local wound treatment and supportive care. **Analgesics** and **benzodiazepines** will relieve pain and cramping, and some patients may benefit from intravenous calcium gluconate. An **antivenin** derived from horse serum is very effective for severe envenomation. If the patient tolerates placement of a standard cutaneous test dose, the usual intravenous dose is 1 to 2 vials over 30 min. Major complications, including anaphylaxis, have occurred with this therapy.

Tarantula

The typical tarantula bite causes local pain and swelling without any systemic reaction. Local wound care is the only treatment. The South American tarantula, also known as the *banana spider*, may cause a systemic reaction; an antitoxin is available for this bite.

FLEA, LICE, AND SCABIES BITES

Flea Bites

Flea bites are frequently found in zigzag lines, especially on the legs and waist. They are intensely pruritic lesions with hemorrhagic puncta, surrounding erythema, and urticaria. Discomfort is relieved with starch baths (1 kg starch in a tub of water), calamine lotion, and oral antihistamines. Severe irritation may require topical steroid creams. Patients may develop impetigo and other local infections from scratching. Fingernails should be cut short, and infections should be treated in the standard manner.

Lice

Body lice concentrate on the waist, shoulders, axillae, and neck. Their bites produce red spots that progress to papules and wheals. They are so intensely pruritic that linear scratch marks are suggestive of infestation. The white ova of head lice are adherent to the hair shaft, and can therefore be distinguished from dandruff. Pubic lice are spread by sexual contact and also cause intense pruritus with small white eggs (nits) visible on the hair shafts. Reactions to lice saliva and feces may cause fever, malaise, and lymphadenopathy. Treatment of any lice infestation consists of a thorough application of pyrethrin with piperonyl butoxide (RID Lice Killing Shampoo), with mandatory reapplication in 10 days. A fine toothed comb will aid in removal of dead lice and nits. Clothing, bedding, and personal articles must be sterilized to prevent reinfestation.

Scabies

Scabies bites are concentrated in the web spaces between fingers and toes. Other common areas include the penis, children's faces and scalps, and the female nipple. Transmission is typically by direct contact. The distinctive feature of scabies infestation is intense pruritus with *burrows*. These white, thread-like channels form zigzag patterns with small gray spots at the closed ends, where the parasites rest. A burrow can be traced with a hand lens, and the female mite is easily scraped out with a blade edge. Associated vesicles, papules, crusts, and eczematization may obscure the diagnosis. Adult treatment of scabies infestation consists of a thorough application of permethrin (Elimite) from the neck down; infants may require additional application to the scalp, temple, and forehead. The patient should first bathe in warm soapy water, apply the medication, then bathe again in 12 h. Reapplication is only necessary if mites are found 2 wks following treatment.

Kissing Bug Bites

Cone-nose or kissing bugs feed on blood at night, commonly on the exposed surface of a sleeping victim. Proper identification is difficult if the insect is not recovered. The initial bite is painless, and the victim may be unaware of the attack. Bites are often multiple and result in wheals, or hemorrhagic papules and bullae. Anaphylaxis may occur in the sensitized individual. Treatment consists of local wound care and analgesics. Allergic reactions must be treated as previously outlined for Hymenoptera envenomation. Hypersensitive individuals should be referred to an allergist for immunotherapy.

Puss Caterpillar Stings

The puss caterpillar has stinging spines on its body that provoke immediate, intense, and rhythmic pain. Local edema and pruritus with vesicles, red blotches, and papules may follow. Infrequently, fever, muscle cramps, anxiety, and shock-like symptoms may occur. Lymphadenopathy with local desquamation may develop in a few days. Treatment consists of immediate spine removal with cellophane tape. Intravenous calcium gluconate, 10 mL of a 10% solution, is effective in relieving pain. Mild cases may respond to an antihistamine such as tripelennamine (PBZ; 25–50 mg every 4 to 6 h in adults; 5 mg/kg/day in divided doses for children).

Blister Beetle Stings

Blister beetles produce local irritation and blistering within hours of contact and provoke intense GI disturbances if ingested. Treatment consists of an occlusive dressing to protect the bullae from trauma.

Large bullae should be drained and covered with a topical antibiotic ointment.

SNAKE BITES

Pit Viper

There are approximately 8000 venomous snake bites each year in the United States, but only about ten deaths result. In fact, 25% of bites are dry strikes, with no effect from the venom. Except for imported species, the only venomous North American snakes are the pit vipers (e.g., rattlesnakes, copperheads, water moccasins, and massasaugas) and coral snakes. Pit vipers are identified by their two retractable fangs and by the heat-sensitive depressions (pits) located bilaterally between each eye and nostril.

Clinical Features

The clinical effects of envenomation depend on the size and species of snake, the age and size of the victim, the time elapsed since the bite, and the characteristics of the bite itself. The degree of poisoning following an encounter is therefore variable; bites that seem innocuous at first may rapidly become severe. The hallmark of pit-viper envenomation is fang marks with local pain and swelling. Degree of swelling, systemic involvement, and coagulopathy determines the severity of the strike. Envenomation is graded on a continuum. Minimal envenomation describes cases with local swelling, no systemic signs, and no laboratory abnormalities. Moderate envenomation causes increased swelling that spreads from the site, together with systemic signs, such as nausea, paresthesia, hypotension, and tachycardia. Coagulation parameters may be abnormal, but there is no significant bleeding. Severe envenomation causes extensive swelling, potentially life-threatening systemic signs (hypotension, altered mental status, respiratory distress), and markedly abnormal coagulation parameters that may result in hemorrhage. In general, all patients who have been envenomated will have swelling within 30 min, although some may take several hours. The diagnosis is based on the clinical findings and corroborating laboratory data, including anemia, thrombocytopenia, elevated prothrombin time (PT), elevated partial thromboplastin time (PTT), and decreased fibrinogen levels.

Emergency Department Care and Disposition

All patients bitten by a pit viper must be evaluated at a medical facility. Consultation with a specialist familiar with snake bite is recommended for all but the simplest cases (one state's resource is the Arizona Poison Control Center at [520] 626–6016). The patient should minimize physical activity, remain calm, and immobilize any bitten extremity in a neutral position below the level of the heart. Establish intravenous access, resuscitate the patient aggressively per ACLS protocols, and obtain specimens for a CBC, PT, PTT, urinalysis, and blood typing. Local wound care and tetanus immunization should be given, but prophylactic antibiotics and steroids have no proven benefit. Limb circumference at several sites above and below the wound should be checked every 30 min, and the border of advancing edema should also be marked. Any patient with progression of local swelling, systemic effects, or coagulopathy should immediately receive equine-derived **antivenin (Crotalidae) polyvalent.** An intradermal skin test (0.03 mL of 1:10 diluted antivenin) must be placed before the patient is treated; a 10 mm wheal within 30 min is considered positive. A positive skin test warrants a risk–benefit analysis before any antivenin is administered; these cases should be discussed with a toxicologist at once. The starting dose of antivenin is 10 vials IV; severe cases require 20 vials. The antivenin package insert will guide in administration, and the physician must be prepared to treat severe allergic and anaphylactic reactions. The endpoint of antivenin therapy is the arrest of progression of the coagulopathy and symptoms. Laboratory determinations are repeated every 4 h or after each course of antivenin, whichever is more frequent. Additional 10-vial doses of antivenin are warranted if the patient's condition worsens.

Compartment syndromes may occur secondary to envenomation. If suspected, determine the compartment pressure. Pressures over 30 mm Hg require limb elevation and mannitol (1–2 g/kg IV over 30 min) if no contraindications exist. Repeated dosing of antivenin is the most effective therapy for elevated compartment pressures; give an additional 10 to 15 vials over 60 min and reassess the pressure. Persistently elevated pressure may require consultation for emergent fasciotomy.

All patients with a pit-viper bite must be observed for at least 8 h. Patients with severe bites and those receiving antivenin must be in the ICU. Patients with mild envenomation who have completed antivenin therapy may be admitted to the general ward. Patients with no evidence of envenomation after 8 h may be discharged. All patients who receive antivenin should also be counseled about serum sickness, since this occurs in nearly all patients in 7 to 14 days following therapy.

Coral Snakes

Coral snakes are brightly colored, with a pattern of black, red, and yellow bands. All true coral snakes have their yellow bands directly touching the red bands; nonpoisonous impostors have an intervening black band. Only the bite of the eastern coral snake (*Micrurus fulvius fulvius*) requires significant treatment; the bite of the Sonoran (Arizona) coral snake is mild and only needs local care. Eastern coral-snake venom is neurotoxic, causing tremor, salivation, respiratory paralysis, seizures, and bulbar palsies (dysarthria, diplopia, dysphagia). Patients with possible envenomation must be admitted to the hospital for 24 to 48 h of observation. Toxic effects of coral-snake venom may be preventable, but they are not easily reversed. Therefore, all patients who have potential envenomation should receive 3 vials of **antivenin (Micrurus Fulvius).** Additional doses are required if symptoms appear and these patients must be admitted to an ICU.

GILA MONSTER BITE

Gila monster bites result in pain and swelling. Systemic toxicity is rare but may cause diaphoresis, paresthesia, weakness, and hypertension. The bite may be tenacious, and the reptile should be removed as soon as possible. If the reptile is still attached, it may loosen its bite when placed on a solid surface that no longer suspends it in mid-air. Other techniques include submersion of the animal, use of a cast spreader, and local application of an irritating flame. Once removed, standard wound care should be performed, including a search for implanted teeth. No further treatment is required.

SCORPION STING

Of all scorpion species, only the bark scorpion (*Centruroides exilicauda*) produces effects other than local pain. Scorpion stings produce immediate burning and stinging although no local injury is visible. Systemic effects are infrequent and mainly occur at extremes of patient age. Findings may include tachycardia, excessive secretions, roving eye movements, opisthotonos, and fasciculations. The diagnosis may be elusive if the scorpion is not seen, although roving eye movements are pathognomonic. Treatment is supportive, including local wound care. Patients with pain in the absence of other toxic symptoms may be briefly observed before they are discharged home with analgesics. Muscle spasm and fasciculation often responds to benzodiazepines. (Severe cases should receive antivenin produced by Arizona State University; this is an unlicensed product available only in Arizona.)

For further reading in *Emergency Medicine: A Comprehensive Study Guide,* 4th edition, see Chapter 162, Insect and Spider Bites, by Richard F. Salluzzo; and Chapter 163, Reptile Bites and Scorpion Bites, by Richard C. Dart and Hernan F. Gomez.

Trauma and Envenomations from Marine Fauna

Keith L. Mausner

Exposure to hazardous marine fauna primarily occurs in tropical areas, but may occur as far north as 50°N latitude. Exposure also may occur in home aquariums.

Clinical Features

Shark attacks are rare, and death is usually due to hemorrhagic shock or drowning. Other marine animals reported in attacks include great barracudas, moray eels, giant groupers, sea lions, seals, crocodiles, alligators, needle fish, wahoos, piranhas, and triggerfish. Injuries include abrasions, puncture wounds, lacerations, and crush injuries.

Coral cuts are the most common underwater injury. Coral poisoning is a painful local reaction with raised welts and pruritus, which may progress to cellulitis with ulceration.

Ocean water contains many potential bacterial pathogens, including *Aeromonas hydrophilia, Bacteroides fragilis, Chromobacterium violaceum, Clostridium perfringens, Erysipelothrix rhusopathiae, Escherichia coli, Mycobacterium marinum, Pseudomonas aeruginosa, Salmonella enteriditis, Staphylococcus aureus, Streptococcus* species, and *Vibrio* species. *Vibrio vulnificus* and *parahemolyticus* may cause a severe cellulitis, myositis, or necrotizing fasciitis. *Vibrio vulnificus* is also associated with sepsis in chronically ill patients, especially those with liver disease; it has 60% mortality.

Numerous invertebrate and vertebrate marine species are venomous. The most important invertebrates are in five phyla: *Cnidaria, Porifera, Echinodermata, Annelida,* and *Mollusca. Cnidaria* includes fire corals, Portuguese men-of-war, jellyfish, sea nettles, and anemones. Most of these organisms have tentacles with nematocysts that release venom upon contact. Most reactions are localized, with pain, erythema, and other cutaneous manifestations. The anemones, jellyfish, and men-of-war may produce severe systemic signs and symptoms that occur in minutes to hours. Envenomation by the Indo-Pacific box jellyfish has a 15% to 20% mortality rate.

Porifera consists of sponges that produce allergic dermatitis. Venomous inhabitants of the sponges may also produce local reactions. Spicules of silica or calcium carbonate that become embedded in the skin may also produce dermatitis. In severe reactions, erythema multiforme with systemic manifestations may occur.

Echinodermata include starfish, sea urchins, and sea cucumbers. Sea urchins have spines that produce immediate pain, then erythema, muscle aches, and local swelling. Severe envenomations may cause nausea, vomiting, paresthesias, paralysis, abdominal pain, syncope, respiratory distress, and hypotension. Starfish envenomation produces a painful local reaction. Possible systemic manifestations include nausea, vomiting, paresthesias, and paralysis. Sea cucumbers produce mild contact dermatitis, but eye exposure may produce a severe reaction.

Annelida include bristleworms, which leave bristles embedded in the skin, causing pain and erythema. *Mollusca* include cone shells and octopuses. Mild cone-shell envenomations are similar to hymenoptera stings. Severe reactions produce muscle paralysis and respiratory failure. Octopus bites may produce paresthesias, paralysis, and respiratory arrest.

The most common vertebrate envenomations involve stingrays. The stinging spine may become embedded and produce a puncture or laceration, causing a severe, painful local reaction. Potential systemic manifestations include weakness, nausea, vomiting, diarrhea, syncope, seizures, paralysis, hypotension, and arrhythmias. The scorpionfish (including the lionfish and stonefish) also have venomous spines, and the toxin may produce paralysis of skeletal or cardiac muscle. Other spined venomous fish include the catfish, weeverfish, surgeonfish, horned sharks, toadfish, ratfish, rabbitfish, stargazers, and leatherbacks.

Sea-snake venom contains a neurotoxin that causes paralysis and a myotoxin. Muscle aches, ophthalmoplegia, ascending paralysis, and respiratory failure may be seen. Myoglobinuria and elevated SGOT are common.

Emergency Department Care and Disposition

Attend to airway, breathing, circulation, hemorrhage control, treatment of life-threatening injuries, volume resuscitation, and correction of hypothermia. Lacerations and bites require copious irrigation, exploration for foreign matter, and debridement, if necessary, in the operating room. Soft-tissue x-rays may help to locate foreign bodies. Most wounds should undergo delayed primary closure. Tetanus prophylaxis is indicated if the patient is not immunized.

Prophylactic antibiotics are not recommended for minor lacerations or abrasions in healthy patients. In immunocompromised patients, prophylaxis with trimethoprim-sulfamethoxazole, tetracycline, cefuroxime, or ciprofloxacin is recommended. In grossly contaminated or extensive wounds, prophylaxis with an initial parenteral dose of trimethoprim-sulfamethoxazole, a third-generation cephalosporin, aminoglycoside, or chloramphenicol, is recommended. Infected wounds may have retained foreign bodies. Culture infected wounds for aerobes and anaerobes; always alert the lab, since special media may be needed. Institute **empiric antibiotic coverage.** Always cover for *Staphylococcus* and *Streptococcus* species. In ocean-related infections also cover for *Vibrio* species with a third-generation cephalosporin, trimethoprim-sulfamethoxazole, tetracycline, or ciprofloxacin. Fresh-water infections require an aminoglycoside or imipenem to cover for *Aeromonas* species. Imipenem–cilastin also may be indicated for sepsis or severe infections.

Cnidaria envenomations are treated symptomatically and with local measures to deactivate and remove nematocysts. Rinse the affected area with saline (avoid fresh water, which may cause further envenomation). **Acetic acid** (vinegar, 5%) or **isopropyl alcohol** (40 to 70%) inactivate the venom. Apply the solution for 30 min or until the patient is pain free. After the nematocyst is deactivated, remove it by applying shaving cream or talcum powder and shaving the area with a razor or blade. Patients with systemic manifestations should be observed for at least 8 h. There is an antivenin for box jellyfish envenomations. Sponge-induced dermatitis is treated with gentle drying of the skin and removal of spicules with adhesive tape. Acetic acid or isopropyl alcohol solution also may be helpful. Topical steroids are helpful only after acetic acid treatment.

Echinodermata envenomations are treated by immersion in hot water (45° C), as tolerated, for 30 to 90 min, or until there is pain relief. Promptly remove embedded spines. In *Annelida* envenomations, remove bristles with tape or forceps. Acetic acid or isopropyl alcohol may be helpful in sea cucumber and *Annelida* envenomations. *Mollusca* envenomations are treated with supportive and wound care.

With stingray, scorpionfish, and other vertebrate envenomations, immerse the affected area in hot water and remove spines. Subsequent thorough exploration and debridement is necessary. Observe the patient for 4 h to rule out systemic toxicity. With sea-snake bites keep the injured area immobilized and dependent. Incision and suction are not recommended. Supportive care, including ventilatory support, may be necessary. If no symptoms develop after 8 h, envenomation did not occur. Sea-snake antivenin is beneficial up to 36 h after envenomation. Also, the neurotoxin is dialyzable.

For further reading in *Emergency Medicine: A Comprehensive Study Guide*, 4th edition, see Chapter 164, Trauma and Envenomations from Marine Fauna, by Daniel G. Guenin and Paul S. Auerbach.

High altitude syndromes are primarily due to hypoxia; the risk of occurrence is influenced by the rapidity and height of ascent.

Clinical Features

Acute mountain sickness (AMS) is usually seen in unacclimated people making a rapid ascent to over 2000 m (6600 ft) above sea level. The earliest symptoms are lightheadedness and mild breathlessness. Symptoms similar to a hangover may develop within 6 h after arrival at altitude but may be delayed as long as 1 day. These include bifrontal headache, anorexia, nausea, weakness, and fatigue. Worsening headache, vomiting, oliguria, dyspnea, and weakness indicate progression of AMS. There are few specific physical findings. Postural hypotension and peripheral and facial edema may occur. Localized rales are noted in 20% of cases.

High-altitude cerebral edema (HACE) is an extreme progression of AMS. It presents with altered mental status, ataxia, stupor, and progression to coma. Focal neurologic findings such as 3rd- and 6th-cranial nerve palsies may be present.

High altitude neurologic syndromes distinct from HACE include high altitude syncope, cerebrovascular spasm (migraine equivalent), cerebral vascular thrombosis, transient ischemic attack, and cerebral hemorrhage. These syndromes typically have more focal findings than HACE. Previously asymptomatic brain tumors may be unmasked by ascent to high altitude. Underlying epilepsy may be worsened by hyperventilation, which is part of the normal acclimatization response.

High altitude pulmonary edema (HAPE) is the most lethal of the high altitude syndromes. Risk factors include heavy exertion, rapid ascent, cold exposure, excessive salt intake, use of sleeping medications, and previous history of HAPE. Table 110-1 summarizes the classification, symptoms, and findings in the different stages of HAPE. Low-grade fever (38.5° C) is common and may make it difficult to distinguish HAPE from pneumonia.

High altitude may adversely affect COPD, heart disease, sickle cell disease, and pregnancy. COPD patients may require supplemental O_2, or an increase in their usual O_2 flow rate. Patients with atherosclerotic heart disease do surprisingly well at high altitude, but there may be a risk of earlier onset of angina and worsening of CHF. Ascent to 1500 to 2000 m may cause a vaso-occlusive crises in individuals with SC disease or sickle thalassemia. Individuals with sickle cell trait usually do well at altitude, but splenic infarction has been reported during heavy exercise. Pregnant long-term high altitude residents have an increased risk of hypertension, low-birth-weight infants, and neonatal jaundice.

TABLE 110-1. Severity Classification of HAPE

Grade	Symptoms	Signs	Chest film
1 Mild	Dyspnea on exertion, dry cough fatigue while moving uphill	Heart rate (HR) (rest) < 90–100, respiratory rate (RR) (rest) < 20, dusky nailbeds, localized rales, if any	Minor exudate involving less than ¼ of one lung field
2 Moderate	Dyspnea, weakness, fatigue on level walking, raspy cough, headache, anorexia	HR 90–100, RR 16–30, cyanotic nailbeds, rales present, ataxia may be present	Some infiltrate involving 50% of one lung or smaller area of both lungs
3 Severe	Dyspnea at rest, productive cough, orthopnea, extreme weakness stupor, coma, blood-tinged sputum	Bilateral rales, HR > 110, RR > 30, Facial and nailbed cyanosis, ataxia	Bilateral infiltrates > 50% each lung

Hultgren HN: High altitude pulmonary edema, in Staub NC (ed): *Lung Water and Solute Exchange.* New York, Marcel Dekker, 1978, pp. 437–469.

607

No increase in pregnancy complications, however, has been reported in pregnant visitors who engage in reasonable activities at high altitude.

Diagnosis and Differential

The differential diagnosis of the high altitude syndromes includes hypothermia, carbon monoxide poisoning, pulmonary or CNS infections, dehydration, and exhaustion. HACE may be difficult to distinguish in the field from the other high altitude neurologic syndromes. HAPE must be distinguished from pulmonary embolus, cardiogenic pulmonary edema, and pneumonia. A key to diagnosis is the clinical response to treatment.

Care and Disposition (in the Field and Emergency Department)

Mild AMS usually improves or resolves in 12 to 36 h if further ascent is delayed and acclimatization is allowed. A decrease in altitude of 500 to 1000 m may provide prompt relief of symptoms. **Oxygen** relieves symptoms, and nocturnal low-flow O_2 (0.5 to 1 L/min) is helpful. Patients with mild AMS should not ascend to a higher sleeping elevation. **Descent** is indicated if symptoms persist or worsen. Immediate descent and treatment is indicated if there is a change in the level of consciousness, ataxia, or pulmonary edema.

Acetazolamide causes a bicarbonate diuresis, leading to a mild metabolic acidosis. This stimulates ventilation and pharmacologically produces an acclimatization response. It is effective in prophylaxis and treatment. Specific indications for acetazolamide are: (1) prior history of altitude illness; (2) abrupt ascent to over 3000 m (10,000 ft); (3) treatment of AMS; (4) symptomatic periodic breathing during sleep at altitude. The adult dose is 250 mg twice a day or a 500-mg extended-release tablet per day. Treatment is for 3 to 4 days as prophylaxis or until symptoms resolve.

Dexamethasone (4 mg po, IM, or IV q 6 h) is effective in moderate to severe AMS. Tapering of the dose over several days may be necessary to prevent rebound. Aspirin or acetaminophen may improve headache. Prochlorperazine (5 to 10 mg IM or IV) may help with nausea and vomiting. Diuretics may be useful for treating fluid retention.

HACE mandates immediate descent or evacuation. Administer oxygen. Start dexamethasone (8 mg po, IM, or IV, then 4 mg q 6 h). **Furosemide** (40 to 80 mg) may help reduce brain edema. **Mannitol** (1 g/kg IV) has not been used extensively but should be considered in severe cases not responding to treatment. Intubation and hyperventilation also are necessary in severe cases. Carefully monitor ABGs to prevent excessive lowering of pCO_2 (below 25 to 30 mmHg), which may cause cerebral ischemia.

HAPE should also be treated with immediate descent. Oxygen may be lifesaving if descent is delayed. The patient should be kept warm, and exertion should be minimized. Drugs are second-line treatment after descent and oxygen. Nifedipine (10 mg po q 4 to 6 h), as well as morphine, and furosemide, may be effective. These patients are usually volume depleted, and care should be taken not to precipitate drug-induced hypotension.

Hospitalization is indicated for cases of HAPE that do not respond immediately to descent. Severe cases may require **intubation** and **PEEP**. Pulmonary artery catheterization may be necessary to exclude cardiogenic pulmonary edema in patients with heart disease.

If Standard Treatment Fails

An expiratory positive airway pressure (EPAP) mask may be useful in the field and, without supplemental O_2 can increase oxygen saturation by 10% to 20%. Portable fabric inflatable hyperbaric chambers have shown promise in the field when immediate descent or evacuation is not possible.

For further reading in *Emergency Medicine: A Comprehensive Study Guide,* 4th edition, see Chapter 165, High Altitude Medical Problems, by Peter H. Hackett and Mark Rabold.

Keith L. Mausner

Dysbarism is most commonly encountered in scuba divers and refers to complications associated with changes in environmental ambient pressure and with breathing compressed gases.

Clinical Features

Barotrauma is the most common diving-related affliction and is caused by the direct mechanical effects of pressure. Middle-ear squeeze, or barotitis media, is the most commonly encountered form of barotrauma and occurs secondary to eustachian tube dysfunction. The diver complains of ear fullness or pain. If the dive is not aborted or pressure is not equalized, the eardrum may rupture, and the diver may have a sensation of escaping air bubbles from the ear, with nausea and vertigo. On physical exam there may be blood around the ear and mouth, mild conductive hearing loss, and TM hemorrhage or perforation. External ear squeeze is less common and occurs when the external canal is occluded by cerumen, debris, or ear plugs. Sinus squeeze most commonly affects the frontal and maxillary sinuses. Squeeze may also affect the conjunctiva, sclera, and periorbital areas if a diver does not exhale into his mask and equalize pressure during descent.

The most rare ear affliction is inner ear barotrauma, which usually occurs after an overly forceful valsalva maneuver or with very rapid ascent. This may lead to inner-ear damage including hemorrhage, fistula formation, or rupture of Reissner's membrane. Inner-ear barotrauma may present with tinnitus, vertigo, and deafness, as well as a feeling of ear fullness, nausea, and vomiting. Hearing loss is sensorineural as opposed to conductive.

Barotrauma during ascent is due to expansion of gas in body cavities. Although rare, reverse squeeze may affect the ear or sinuses during ascent. Alternobaric vertigo (ABV) can occur during ascent due to unbalanced vestibular stimulation from unequal middle-ear pressures. Tooth squeeze may be noted during ascent from air-filled dental cavities.

Pulmonary overpressurization syndrome (POPS) may occur during ascent, resulting in mediastinal and subcutaneous emphysema. After the dive these patients may have gradual onset of increasing hoarseness, neck fullness, substernal chest pain, dyspnea, and dysphagia. Syncope and pneumothorax also may be seen.

Air embolism is the most severe form of pulmonary barotrauma. Gas bubbles may enter the systemic circulation through ruptured pulmonary veins and occlude distal circulation. This typically presents immediately on surfacing in a diver who ascends too rapidly. Cardiac arrest and arrhythmias may occur. The neurologic picture may be consistent with acute stroke affecting multiple areas of cerebral circulation. Multiplegias, sensory disturbances, confusion, vertigo, seizures, or aphasia may be seen.

Decompression sickness (DCS) is not a form of barotrauma. It is due to gas bubble formation as inert gas comes out of solution in blood and tissues, if ascent is too rapid, without adequate time for decompression. In conventional compressed-air diving, nitrogen is the culprit. DCS is a multiorgan system disorder, due to the direct effects of nitrogen bubbles on circulation and cells, as well as to secondary inflammatory responses and activation of clotting mechanisms. Severe, aching joint pain is a common symptom. A multitude of neurologic complications can occur, and common findings are bladder dysfunction and lower extremity paraplegia, paraparesis, and paresthesias. Chest pain, cough, dyspnea, pulmonary edema, and shock also may occur. Risk factors for DCS include advanced age, obesity, dehydration, recent alcohol intake, cold water diving, vigorous underwater exercise, and multiple repetitive dives.

Diagnosis and Differential

The time of symptoms onset in relation to the dive and descent and ascent may assist in diagnosis. During descent, the most common maladies are the squeeze syndromes. Breathing-gas problems, such as carbon monoxide poisoning or hypoxia, are also more likely to present early, during descent. During the ascent phase, barotrauma or ABV are most likely to occur. DCS, if severe, may become symptomatic during ascent.

Onset of severe symptoms within 10 min of surfacing is an air embolism until proven otherwise. Onset of symptoms after 10 min is DCS until proven otherwise. Most cases of DCS become symptomatic 1 to 6 h after surfacing, but there may be a delay of up to 48 h. Mild POPS and other forms of barotrauma may also present in the immediate hours after a dive.

Emergency Department Care and Disposition

Stabilize all patients in relation to airway, breathing, and circulation, and attend to immediately life-threatening injuries. Administer high-flow oxygen. Evaluate and treat for hypothermia. If air embolism is suspected, place the patient in a supine position. The Trendelenburg and left lateral decubitus positions are no longer recommended because of concerns about interfering with breathing and aggravating cerebral edema.

Patients with suspected DCS or air embolism should receive **recompression-chamber therapy** as quickly as possible. Patients should be transported in an aircraft that flies at an altitude of less than 1000 ft or that can be pressurized to 1 atmosphere. Most DCS patients are volume depleted; administer fluids if not otherwise contraindicated.

Patients with middle ear and other squeeze syndromes should stop diving until symptoms resolve. Decongestants and antihistamines may be useful for eustachian tube dysfunction. Antibiotics are indicated if the eardrum is ruptured, and diving is contraindicated until the eardrum has healed. Treatment of sinus squeeze is similar to middle-ear squeeze. Antibiotics are usually indicated with frontal-sinus squeeze. External-ear squeeze is best treated by keeping the canal dry and administering antibiotics if there is evidence of infection or eardrum rupture. Inner-ear barotrauma mandates ENT consultation since surgical repair may be indicated. These patients should avoid straining and be at bed rest with the head elevated. Administer analgesia and other symptomatic treatment as needed.

POPS may require needle thoracostomy and chest tube if pneumothorax occurs. POPS usually resolves with rest and supplemental oxygen, and rarely requires recompression therapy.

If Standard Treatment Fails

For assistance in treating dive-related conditions, and for the location of the nearest recompression unit, call the National Diving Alert Network at Duke University, 24 h a day, at (919) 684–8111.

For further reading in *Emergency Medicine: A Comprehensive Study Guide*, 4th edition, see Chapter 166, Dysbarism, by Kenneth W. Kizer.

112 | Near Drowning
Stephen W. Meldon

Drowning often affects young, healthy individuals. Although prevention is the most important way to reduce associated morbidity and mortality, once near drowning has occurred the patient's prognosis is dependent on early rescue and resuscitation.

Clinical Features

Respiratory failure and hypoxic neurologic injury dominate the clinical course. Initial hypoxemia results from alveolar flooding and impairment of gas exchange or laryngospasm and glottal closure. Aspiration of water leads to surfactant loss, atelectasis, ventilation perfusion mismatch and alveolar capillary membrane damage. Noncardiogenic pulmonary edema results. Metabolic acidosis from poor perfusion and hypoxemia is common. Respiratory insufficiency may be shown by dyspnea, tachypnea, or use of accessory muscles of respiration. Physical exam may reveal wheezing, rales, or rhonchi. Neurologic status may range from full alertness to coma. Hypothermia is common and may occasionally be severe, with core temperatures less than 30°C.

Diagnosis and Differential

The diagnosis of near drowning is usually known because of the history or evidence of submersion. Evidence of other injuries should be sought, especially cervical spine injuries associated with diving accidents. Essential diagnostic tests include chest x-rays (CXR) and arterial blood gas (ABG) analysis. CXR may show generalized pulmonary edema, perihilar infiltrates, and other patterns, or be normal. Since the CXR may not correlate with the arterial PO_2, an ABG to assess oxygen saturation and metabolic acidosis is important. Complete blood counts, electrolytes, and renal function should be measured, although abnormalities are seldom significant. Regarding the differential diagnosis, occasionally an acute cardiovascular (e.g., arrhythmia, myocardial infarction) or neurologic (e.g., hypoglycemia, seizure) event may precipitate submersion and near drowning.

Emergency Department Care and Disposition

ED care should emphasize initial resuscitation, treatment of respiratory failure, and evaluation of associated injuries.

1. Airway, ventilation, and oxygenation should be assessed. Stabilization/evaluation of the patient's cervical spine may be indicated.
2. All patients should receive supplemental oxygen. An IV, cardiac monitoring, and continuous pulse oximetry should be established. An ABG and CXR should be obtained.

3. **Intubation** and mechanical ventilation should be instituted for patients with continuing hypoxemia (PaO_2 less than 60 mmHg in adults or 80 mmHg in children) despite high-flow oxygen (40% to 50%). Positive end-expiratory pressure (PEEP) is generally required and neuromuscular paralysis may be needed in some patients.
4. An NG tube and Foley catheter should be placed, and core body temperature should be measured.
5. Standard therapy for bronchospasm, seizures, arrhythmias, and hypothermia should be instituted as needed. Prophylactic antibiotics and steroids are not indicated.

Since survival and neurologic outcome may be unpredictable, all patients requiring CPR should have advanced life support and resuscitation initiated. Patients with severe hypoxia, the need for mechanical ventilation, and severe neurologic deficits require ICU admission. Patients with mild to moderate hypoxemia corrected by supplemental oxygen should be admitted and monitored closely. Those with minimal or no symptoms and normal CXR and ABG should be observed in the ED for several hours and then discharged if stable.

If Standard Treatment Fails

In some patients mechanical ventilation can be avoided, and oxygenation increased by continuous positive airway pressure (CPAP). Candidates for mask CPAP ventilation must be alert and unlikely to vomit. Also standard resuscitation treatments are often ineffective in the setting of severe hypothermia. These patients should be rewarmed to 30° to 32.5°C before resuscitation efforts are abandoned.

For further reading in *Emergency Medicine: A Comprehensive Study Guide*, 4th edition, see Chapter 167, Near Drowning, by Bruce E. Haynes.

Thermal and Chemical Burns

Stephen W. Meldon

THERMAL BURNS

Approximately 2 million patients present to the ED with burn injuries each year, and about 5% of these patients require admission. Burns are the second leading cause of accidental death, with higher death rates seen in patients less than 4 and greater than 65 years of age.

Clinical Features

Burns are defined by their size and depth. Burn size is quantified as a percentage of total body surface area (TBSA). The most common method of approximating the percentage of TBSA burned is the *rule of nines* (Fig. 113-1). Smaller burns can be estimated by using the area at the back of the patient's hand as approximately 1% of the TBSA.

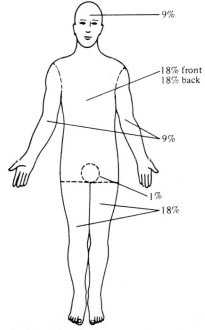

FIG. 113-1. Rule of nines.

A more precise estimation, especially in infants and children, is to use a Lund–Browder burn diagram (Fig. 113-2). Burn depth is described as first, second, or third-degree. First-degree burns are painful and red,

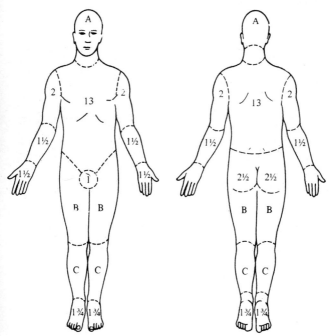

Relative Percentages of Areas Affected by Growth (Age in Years)

	0	1	5	10	15	Adult
A: half of head	$9\frac{1}{2}$	$8\frac{1}{2}$	$6\frac{1}{2}$	$5\frac{1}{2}$	$4\frac{1}{2}$	$3\frac{1}{2}$
B: half of thigh	$2\frac{3}{4}$	$3\frac{1}{4}$	4	$4\frac{1}{4}$	$4\frac{1}{2}$	$4\frac{3}{4}$
C: half of leg	$2\frac{1}{2}$	$2\frac{1}{2}$	$2\frac{3}{4}$	3	$3\frac{1}{4}$	$3\frac{1}{2}$

Second degree _____ and

Third degree _____ =

Total percent burned ____

FIG. 113-2.   Classic Lund and Browder chart.

with no blister formation. Healing occurs in 7 days. Second-degree, or partial-thickness burns, are very painful and have blister formation, under which the skin is red and moist. They heal in 2–3 wks and may scar. Third-degree, or full-thickness burns, result in full epidermal and dermal layer injury. The skin is charred, pale, leathery, and painless. These burns require skin grafting to heal. Burns may also be associated with smoke inhalation injuries. Signs of pulmonary injury, which can have a delayed presentation for 12 to 24 h, include cough, wheeze, and respiratory distress. Thermal injury to the upper airway can occur and result in hoarseness, stridor, and significant upper airway edema. Carbon monoxide (CO) poisoning should be suspected in all patients with smoke inhalation. Clinical signs include headache, vomiting, confusion, lethargy, and coma.

Diagnosis and Differential

Burns can also be diagnosed as major, moderate, or minor. Examples of major burns include third-degree burns greater than 10% TBSA or partial-thickness burns greater than 20% or 25% TBSA. Burns involving the face, hands, feet, or perineum are also major. Minor burns involve less than 10% or 15% TBSA, or third-degree burns less than 2% TBSA. Moderate burns are those not meeting criteria for either major or minor burns. The diagnosis of smoke inhalation is suggested by the history of a fire in an enclosed space. Physical signs include soot in the mouth or nose, carbonaceous sputum, and respiratory symptoms. Chest x-ray may be normal initially. Bronchoscopy may be helpful in determine the extent of injury. Carboxyhemoglobin levels should be obtained if CO poisoning is suspected.

Emergency Department Care and Disposition

Attention to the ABCs, appropriate fluid resuscitation, and accurate burn assessment are critical.

1. Administer 100% oxygen. **Intubate** for signs of airway compromise. Obtain an ABG and a carboxyhemoglobin level and a CXR.
2. Establish IV lines. **Initial fluid resuscitation** is 2 to 4 mL/kg per %TBSA per 24 h. Half the calculated amount is given in the first 8 h since burn and the remainder over the next 16 h. Lactated Ringer's solution is appropriate. A Foley catheter and NG tube should be placed. Monitor resuscitation by assessment of the patient's urinary output (0.5 to 1.0 mL/kg per h) and other signs of perfusion.
3. Assess burn and look for evidence of other trauma. Cover burns with moist saline dressing. IV narcotic analgesia and a tetanus booster should be administered.
4. Patients who require admission (Table 113-1) should generally be transferred to a hospital with a burn unit.

TABLE 113-1. Admission Criteria
_____

1. Patients between 10 and 50 years old with partial-thickness burns > 15% TBSA, or full-thickness burns > 5% TBSA.
2. Patients less than 10 or greater than 50 years old with partial-thickness burns > 10% TBSA, or full-thickness burns > 3% TBSA.
3. Patients with burns to face, hands, feet, or perineum, or burns across major joints or circumferential limb burns.
4. Electrical burns.
5. Chemical burns.
6. Burns with inhalation injury.
7. Burns in patients with underlying medical problems.
8. Burns associated with other trauma.
_____

5. Outpatient management of minor burns is appropriate. Burns should be cleansed and covered with a topical antibiotic (e.g., bacitracin) and sterile dressing. Dressings should be changed daily. Oral analgesics (e.g., ibuprofen) should be prescribed. Initial followup should be in 24 h.

If Standard Treatment Fails

Circumferential burns of limbs or chest may require escharotomy to relieve compromise of distal circulation or mechanical restriction of ventilation. Minor burns can be managed with commercial occlusive dressings such as Biobane, if daily dressing changes aren't feasible.

CHEMICAL BURNS

Chemical burns can occur in a variety of settings, including the home, industry, and school or research laboratories. More than 25,000 products are capable of producing chemical burns.

Clinical Features

Clinical features of chemical burns depend on the agent, concentration, and duration of exposure. Acids generally result in coagulation necrosis of the involved area. Superficial to full-thickness burns may result. An exception is hydrofluoric acid (HF), which rapidly penetrates intact skin causing severe pain and progressive, deep-tissue damage. The involved skin may develop a blue-gray appearance with surrounding erythema. Signs and symptoms may not develop, however, until 12 to 24 h after exposure. Oxalic acid may result in hypocalcemia and renal impairment. Alkalis generally cause liquefaction necrosis and deeper tissue destruction. Soft, gelatinous brownish eschars often result. Wounds that initially appeared superficial may progress to full-thickness burns. Pepper mace exposure causes mucous membrane, ocular, and upper airway irritation; bronchospasm may occur. Lastly, systemic toxicity may result from chemical burns. Hypocalcemia, acidosis, hypotension, and renal and hepatic necrosis can occur, depending on the agents involved.

Diagnosis and Differential

Diagnosis is usually made by a history of exposure to a chemical agent. Acids with a pH less than 2 and alkalis with a pH greater than 12 are considered strong corrosives. Careful questioning regarding possible exposures (especially in the home setting) and agents involved is important. Chemical burns should be considered in all cases of pain and irritation to the skin. This is especially true with HF acid burns, where skin findings may be minimal.

Emergency Department Care and Disposition

The first priority is to stop the burning processes. Hydrotherapy is the cornerstone of initial treatment for chemical burns. Dry chemical particles should be brushed away before irrigation. Treatment ideally should begin at the scene of the accident.

1. Remove offending chemical, including contaminated garments.
2. Copious irrigation is indicated for alkalis, acids, and pepper-mace exposure.
3. Exceptions to irrigation include: elemental metals (sodium, lithium, magnesium), which should be covered with mineral oil, or extinguished with a class-D fire extinguisher; and phenol which should be decontaminated with PEG300, glycerol, or isopropyl alcohol.
4. HF acid burns often require additional treatment. **Calcium gluconate** can be used topically if mixed with DMS0. Subcutaneous and intra-dermal injections of a 5% to 10% solution into the affected skin is recommended. A maximum dose of 0.5 mL of 10% calcium gluconate per square cm of burned skin is recommended.
5. Cardiac monitoring and evaluation of electrolytes, renal functions, and calcium levels is indicated in significant HF, chromic, and oxalic acid burns.
6. After initial specific measures, treat as a thermal burn, with IV fluid replacement, analgesics, and tetanus prophylaxis.

If Standard Treatment Fails

HF acid burns may require an intra-arterial infusion of calcium gluconate. Ten mL of 10% solution should be diluted with 40 mL of 5% dextrose and infused over 2 to 4 h.

For further reading in *Emergency Medicine: A Comprehensive Study Guide*, 4th edition, see Chapter 168, Thermal Burns, by Lawrence R. Schwartz; and Chapter 169, Chemical Burns, by Marcus L. Martin and Fred P. Harchelroad, Jr.

ELECTRICAL INJURIES

Electrical injuries present with a wide spectrum of damage, ranging from simple skin burns to multisystem injury and sudden death. It is important to suspect occult damage to tissue and organs in the path of the current. As expected, most electrical injuries occur in children under 6, adolescent males, and workers exposed to electrical hazards.

Clinical Features

Electricity causes tissue damage by the direct effects of the current upon the cells and by thermal damage from the heat generated by the resistance of the tissues. Electrical energy is greatest at the contact point, thus the skin often has the greatest observable damage. The exit wound site is often larger than the entrance site. As the current flows through the body, nerves, blood vessels, and muscles sustain the greatest damage. This may result in coagulation necrosis, neuronal death, and damage to blood vessels (thrombosis and disruption of the intima or media). As a result of these types of injury, the overall picture resembles a crush injury more than a burn injury. Since the size of the skin lesions does not correlate with the amount of underlying damage, a careful search for underlying injury is necessary.

Cardiopulmonary arrest, the primary cause of immediate death from electrical injury, may result from several mechanisms, including direct electrical disruption of the heart, coronary artery spasm, and primary respiratory arrest from central or local (chest-wall muscle or diaphragmatic tetany) causes. Asystole or ventricular fibrillation are often the initial presenting rhythm. Survivors of the initial injury can manifest the full spectrum of cardiac arrhythmias. Although the majority of serious dysrhythmias occur immediately following the event, a few have been noted up to 12 h postinjury. Actual myocardial damage is rare except with extensive body-surface involvement or transthoracic current flow.

Neurologic findings of electrical injuries include temporary loss of consciousness, confusion, coma, seizures, headache, tinnitus, stroke, and spinal cord injurylike presentations. Peripheral nerve injury is common, often involving the median nerve.

Cutaneous burns are almost always present with a charred central area, a white-to-gray middle zone with an outer region of severe erythema. Entry wounds are usually small and found in the upper extremities; exit wounds are often larger.

Vascular problems may include pulseless extremities, decreased peripheral perfusion, compartment syndrome, and venous thrombosis.

Delayed rupture of injured vessels also may occur. A unique electrical injury is the oral and perioral burns that occur in children who suck on a live wire. Temperatures of > 2000°C can be produced, and a burn or oval ulcer at the corner of the mouth with surrounding edema is present. Systemic damage is rare but must be ruled out. These children are at risk for scarring, deformation of lips and mouth, impaired jaw growth, and abnormal speech. Delayed presentation (7–14 days) of hemorrhage from the labial artery may arise.

Other types of injury may include trauma from being thrown by the electrical current, falling from a height after the injury, or stress of the tetanic contractures. Fractures occur in about 10% of patients with electrical shock.

Diagnosis and Differential

Diagnosis of electrical injury is usually based on history. The type of current (high-tension wires produce the greatest injury) and surrounding circumstances, such as falls and intoxication, should be noted. In unclear cases, characteristic skin lesions or oral lesions in children may be helpful. A thorough physical exam to search for occult injuries to muscle, nerves, and blood vessels must be undertaken. Bones should be examined for fractures or dislocation even in the absence of a history of trauma. The absence of findings on initial exam does not rule out serious underlying damage.

Laboratory studies should include a complete blood count, electrolytes, calcium, BUN, creatinine, coagulation studies, ABG, myoglobin, creatinine kinase, and CK–MB (CK–MB may be elevated without cardiac damage due to extensive muscle injury). Urinalysis should include a screen for myoglobin. Liver functions and amylase are indicated for suspected abdominal injury. Type and crossmatching for packed RBCs is indicated for those suffering severe injuries. An EKG should be performed along with radiographic studies of sites with suspected injuries. Cranial CT scanning is indicated for those presenting with severe head injury, coma, or unresolving altered mental status.

Emergency Department Care and Disposition

Treatment of electrical shock begins with stabilization of the airway, breathing, and circulation. **Cervical-spine immobilization** should be instituted in cases of unwitnessed events or when there is a potential for cervical-spine injury. Patients should have continuous cardiac monitoring, pulse oximetry, noninvasive BP monitoring, and at least one large-bore intravenous line. Treatment should include:

1. High-flow oxygen by face mask.
2. Ventricular fibrillation, asystole, or ventricular tachycardia should be treated by **standard ACLS protocols.** Other arrhythmias are usually transient and do not need immediate therapy.

3. IV crystalloid fluid should be given with an initial bolus of 10 to 20 mL/kg. Fluid requirements are generally higher than that of thermal burn patients. Urine output should be maintained at 1.0 mL/kg/h. A Foley catheter for urine-output measurement is helpful in severely injured patients.

4. If evidence of myoglobinuria is present, **urinary alkalinization** should be accomplished by administering approximately 50 mEq of sodium bicarbonate per l of IV fluids. Blood pH should be maintained at 7.45 and urinary output at 1.5 to 2 mL/kg/h. Mannitol should be avoided in patients with thermal burns.

5. Tetanus prophylaxis should be given.

6. Antibiotics are not necessary initially unless large open wounds are present.

7. Seizures can be treated with standard therapy.

8. Fractures and dislocations should be reduced and splinted as appropriate.

It is appropriate to consult a general surgeon if there is any evidence of systemic or deep-tissue injury. These patients may require formal wound exploration, debridement, or fasciotomy and long-term care. Children with oral injuries should be evaluated by a plastic surgeon or otolaryngologist.

Patients with severe electrical injuries should be admitted to a regional burn or trauma center. Admission to a monitored setting is also indicated for all patients with high-tension (>1000 V) current exposure, regardless of injuries, and patients with low-tension (< 1000 V) current exposure who have evidence of complications. Disposition of patients with brief exposures to low-intensity current is controversial, but it appears that asymptomatic patients who have a normal EKG, normal urinalysis, and no evidence of significant electrothermal burns, may be discharged after 6 to 8 h of observation. Patients with an unclear history of exposure or degree of injury should be admitted. Children with isolated oral injuries can usually be discharged.

LIGHTNING INJURIES

There are about 1500 lightning injuries reported each year in the U.S., with about 25% of them being fatal. Unlike the electrical injuries discussed above, extensive tissue damage and renal failure are rare.

Clinical Features

Lightning injuries can vary in severity depending on the circumstances of the strike. Minor injuries produce a stunned patient. These people will appear well. Their vital signs will be normal, or they will exhibit a mild tachycardia or hypertension. They may have signs of confusion, amnesia, and short-term memory difficulties. Other symptoms include headache, muscle pain, paresthesias, and temporary visual or auditory problems. Most patients with minor lightning injuries have a gradual improvement and little long-term sequelae.

More serious lightning injuries can cause a large variety of cardiopulmonary problems. These include direct muscle damage, coronary artery spasm, atrial and ventricular dysrhythmias, global cardiac dysfunction, pericardial effusion, and pulmonary edema. Neurologic injuries are frequent as well and may have immediate or delayed onset. Loss of consciousness, occurring in 70% of patients, is the most common neurologic event. It is usually brief and accompanied by confusion and amnesia for the event. The causes of coma include brain injury from the lightning itself, cerebral anoxia prior to resuscitation, and cerebral edema, infarction, ischemia, or hemorrhage. Keraunoparalysis (transient flaccid paralysis of the lower extremities), with sensory and vasomotor changes of the lower extremities, can occur but usually resolves in 24 h.

Other problems that occur commonly with lightning exposure include otologic and ophthalmologic injuries. Over 50% of victims sustain bilateral or unilateral tympanic membrane rupture. Cataracts often occur within several days of the injury, but they may develop up to 2 y after the incident. Vision loss, diplopia, corneal lesions, uveitis, iritis, retinal detachment, and optic-nerve injury may occur. Dilated, unresponsive pupils may be the result of ocular autonomic disturbances. Cutaneous injuries, which arc generally superficial, are related to the specific area struck or the ignition of clothing. Fernlike erythematous streaks (keraunographic skin marking) are pathognomonic for lightning injury. Victims may also suffer from a variety of blunt trauma related to the force generated by the strike or from falls.

Diagnosis and Differential

The diagnosis of lightning injuries is based on history. A lightning injury should be considered in a patient found unconscious or in cardiopulmonary arrest who was outdoors during appropriate weather conditions. Ruptured tympanic membranes or characteristic skin markings should alert the physician to potential lightning injuries. A careful physical exam should be performed to asses neurologic status, otologic and ophthalmologic injuries, and blunt trauma. Diagnostic tests should include an ECG in all patients and a complete blood count, urinalysis, and CK levels with MB fraction in most patients. Tests for those with more severe injuries should include an ABG, electrolytes, calcium, magnesium, BUN, creatinine, coagulation studies, and myoglobin levels. Consideration should be given to performing cranial CT scanning, chest radiograph, and cervical spine films.

Emergency Department Care and Disposition

Unlike other trauma, priority should be given to people who appear clinically dead when there are multiple victims. Aggressive resuscitation measures are indicated, as survival has been reported after prolonged respiratory arrest. **Cervical-spine immobilization** should be placed in cases of unwitnessed events or when there is potential cervical-spine injury. Patients should have continuous cardiac monitoring, pulse oximetry, noninvasive BP monitoring, and at least one large-bore IV line. Treatment, particularly in moderate to severe cases, should include:

1. High-flow oxygen by face mask.
2. Ventricular fibrillation, asystole, or ventricular tachycardia should be treated by standard **ACLS protocols**.
3. Fluid resuscitation is usually unnecessary.
4. Tetanus prophylaxis should be given.
5. Seizures can be treated with standard therapy.
6. Fractures and dislocations should be reduced and splinted as appropriate.

Extensive debridement of wounds is usually not necessary. Patients with severe or moderate lightning injuries should be admitted to a critical care unit with appropriate consultation. Most patients with minor lightning injuries should be admitted for close monitoring of cardiac and neurologic status.

For further reading in *Emergency Medicine: A Comprehensive Study Guide*, 4th edition, see Chapter 170, Electrical and Lightning Injuries, by Phil Fontanarosa.

Radiation Injuries

Keith L. Mausner

The use of potentially dangerous radioactive isotopes in industry and medicine is widespread, and there are numerous nuclear power plants around the country. Emergency physicians should have a basic understanding of radiation injuries and their treatment.

Clinical Features

Ionizing radiation can cause significant damage to living tissue. X-rays, gamma rays, and alpha and beta particles are common types of ionizing radiation. Radiation exposure is measured in terms of the rad (radiation absorbed dose), which equals 100 ergs of energy in 1 g of material. The rem (roentgen equivalent man) equals the dose in rads, multiplied by a factor that accounts for biologic destructiveness. Rad and rem for x-rays, gamma rays and beta particles, for example, are equivalent. However, 1 rad of alpha particles may be 20 times more destructive and represent an exposure of 20 rem.

The lethal dose of whole-body ionizing radiation to 50% of those exposed is 400 rem. Exposure to 600 rem is nearly 100% lethal. In addition to dose, the period of time over which exposure occurs is critical. A 100-rem exposure over 1 y is much less harmful than over 1 sec.

Table 115-1 summarizes the clinical features of increasing doses of acute whole-body ionizing radiation. The timing of the onset of symptoms and signs of radiation illness correlates with the dose absorbed. Early onset of symptoms indicates a greater dose and poorer prognosis. Onset of nausea and vomiting within 2 h indicates a 400-rem or greater dose; onset of these symptoms more than 2 h after exposure indicates less than a 200-rem exposure; and absence of these symptoms after 6 h points to less than a 50-rem exposure. Skin exposure of greater than 300 rem causes erythema in hours, which progresses over days. Nausea, vomiting, and general malaise generally subside over hours to days, followed by a latent period of 1 or more wks, after which serious GI, hematopoietic, and infectious complications occur.

Lymphocyte counts 48 h after exposure are prognostic. A lymphocyte count of greater than 1200/µL at 48 h is associated with a good prognosis. A fair prognosis is associated with a count of 300 to 1200/µL, and counts below 300/µL have a poor prognosis.

Emergency Department Care and Disposition

The first priority in all radiation accident victims is to address airway, breathing, circulation, and life-threatening injuries. After stabilization, evaluate the patient with a GM counter for **surface contamination**

625

TABLE 115-1. Dose-Effect Relations Following Acute Whole Body Irradiation (X- or γ-Ray)

Whole body dose, rad	Clinical and laboratory findings
5–25	Asymptomatic. Conventional blood studies are normal. Chromosome aberrations detectable.
50–75	Asymptomatic. Minor depressions of white cells and platelets detectable in a few persons, especially if baseline values established.
75–125	Minimal acute doses that produce prodromal symptoms (anorexia, nausea, vomiting, fatigue) in about 10–20% of persons within 2 days. Mild depressions of white cells and platelets in some persons.
125–200	Symptomatic course with transient disability and clear hematologic changes in a majority of exposed persons. Lymphocyte depression of about 50% within 48 h.
240–340	Serious, disabling illness in most persons, with about 50% mortality if untreated. Lymphocyte depression of about ≥75% within 48 h.
500 +	Accelerated version of acute radiation syndrome with GI complications within 2 wks, bleeding, and death in most exposed persons.
5000 +	Fulminating course with cardiovascular, GI, and CNS complications resulting in death within 24–72 h.

From Mettler FD: Emergency management of radiation accidents. *JACEP* 7:302, 1978. Used by permission.

and, by history, determine whether radioactive matter was inhaled or ingested. External and internal decontamination, fluid replacement, and supportive care are the emergency treatments most likely to assure long-term survival. Patients exposed to nonparticulate ionizing radiation such as x-rays and gamma rays are not radioactive and do not require decontamination.

Cover open wounds to avoid contaminating them while disrobing and washing the patient. The patient should be carefully washed with soap and water, and contaminated water should be collected in secure containers. The goal is to avoid the incorporation of radioactive materials into wounds and to prevent them from being inhaled or ingested.

Decorporation is the removal of radioactive material from the body, primarily the GI tract. Transuranic elements and heavy metals, which may be encountered in nuclear fuel processing plants and military nuclear weapons facilities, may be chelated with diethylenetriaminepentaacetic acid (DTPA).

Potassium iodide prevents the uptake of radioactive iodine by the thyroid if given within hours of exposure. It is recommended in exposures of greater than 10 to 30 rem of radioactive iodine. The dose is 130 mg po q day for 14 days for ages 13 and older. Pregnant women and children ages 3 to 12 should receive 65 mg a day and younger children 32.5 mg a day.

Primary wound closure is acceptable only if adequate decontamination is achieved. Extensive debridement, delayed closure and, on rare occasions, amputation of severely contaminated extremities may be required. Radiation burns, like electrical burns, may have minimal findings on initial presentation. Excision and full-thickness skin grafting may be necessary, especially with beta-particle burns.

Radiation accident victims may also be exposed to hazardous chemicals such as beryllium, lead, or plastic fumes from nuclear weapons facilities. These materials have potentially severe respiratory, CNS, and multiorgan system toxicity.

Patients with exposures of less than 125 rem have a good prognosis. Patients with exposures of less than 200 rem generally recover and require only supportive and symptomatic treatment. Patients with exposures greater than 200 rem should be placed in reverse isolation and require extensive supportive care, aggressive treatment of bacterial, fungal, and viral infections and, occasionally, bone-marrow transplantation.

All facilities that may receive radiation-accident victims should have a disaster and decontamination plan, and appropriate protective gear and dosimeters. It is recommended that providers of care should not be exposed acutely to more than 5 rem, except to save a life. Exposure to individuals can be minimized by rotating care among several providers. Anyone caring for patients contaminated with radioactive iodine should take prophylactic potassium iodide.

If Standard Treatment Fails

The Radiation Emergency Assistance Center/Training Site (REAC/TS), Oak Ridge, Tennessee, may be contacted 24 h a day at (615) 576-1004. Radiation Management Consultants (RMC) may also be of assistance, and can be reached at (215) 537-0672.

For further reading in *Emergency Medicine: A Comprehensive Study Guide*, 4th edition, see Chapter 173, Radiation Injuries, by H. Arnold Muller.

Plants and mushrooms have evolved a diverse array of metabolites that are harmful to humans. Chemicals applied to cultivated plants may also cause toxicity. Mushroom ingestion can lead to morbidity and even mortality among amateur foragers and recreational drug users, with *Amanita* species responsible for most fatalities.

Clinical Features

The signs and symptoms of plant toxicity are highly variable and depend on which part of the plant is ingested or contacted. In most cases patients are asymptomatic or have mild GI symptoms. Nausea, vomiting, hematemesis, abdominal pain, and diarrhea, at times bloody, may follow ingestion of *Actaea* (baneberry), aloe, *Conium* (poison hemlock), *Convallaria* (Lily of the valley), Daphne, *Euphorbia* (poinsettia), rhododendron, *Ricinus*, *Solanum* (nightshades), and *Taxus* (yews). Resultant electrolyte abnormalities can be fatal.

Direct irritation and chemical burns to the oropharynx have been reported after ingestion of *Actaea*, *Abrus* (rosary pea), *Capsicum* (ornamental peppers), Daphne, *Dieffenbachia*, and rhododendron. *Capsicum*, *Laportea*, and *Urtica* can also cause a contact dermatitis.

Cardiovascular symptoms, including hypotension, dysrhythmias, and conduction defects, have been reported after ingestion of *Convallaria*, *Taxus*, rhododendron, and oleander and may be life-threatening.

Hallucinations may follow ingestion of *Datura* (jimson weed) seeds or smoking its leaves and are attributable to the plant's anticholinergic properties. Hallucinations have also been associated with *Actaea* ingestion. Seizures may be seen after ingestion of *Conium* and *Actaea*.

Poisonous mushrooms can be divided into 8 groups based on their clinical toxicity. Amatoxin poisoning presents with nausea, vomiting, diarrhea, and abdominal pain 6 to 48 h after ingestion. Dehydration, hypotension, tachycardia, and oliguria may result. One to three days after ingestion, the patient may develop manifestations of hepatic failure, intestinal necrosis, and renal failure.

Gyromitrin poisoning presents with nausea, vomiting, diarrhea, abdominal cramps, severe headache, and altered mental status 6 to 24 h after ingestion. Hepatitis progressing to hepatic failure may ensue. Another complication is methemoglobinemia.

Orellanine and orelline poisoning is characterized by the development of gastrointestinal symptoms 1 to 3 days after ingestion. Patients may subsequently develop renal toxicity, with back pain, polyuria or oliguria, and flank tenderness.

Ingestion of ethanol after consuming coprine-containing mushrooms results in a disulfiramlike reaction, with gastrointestinal distress, diaphoresis, dyspnea, flushed skin, hypotension, chest tightness, palpitations, arrhythmias, and weakness.

Mushrooms containing ibotenic acid and muscimol are generally consumed for their mind-altering effects. Toxicity develops within 2 h and includes vomiting, severe headache, lethargy, ataxia, euphoria, delirium, visual hallucinations, and psychosis. Muscle fasciculations and cholinergic and anticholinergic manifestations may be seen.

Muscarine poisoning begins within 15 min to 2 h of ingestion. Evidence of cholinergic hyperactivity is seen, with gastrointestinal symptoms, miosis, increased secretions, urinary frequency, skin flushing, bradycardia, hypotension, seizures, and wheezing.

Psilocybin- and psilocin-containing mushrooms are also consumed for their mind-altering effects. Symptoms begin with 60 min and include ataxia, confusion, headache, visual hallucinations, aggressive or suicidal behavior, paresthesias, and weakness. Physical signs include hyperreflexia, pulse and BP abnormalities, and miosis.

Miscellaneous unidentified toxins cause gastroenteritis lasting 4 to 48 h. Less common complaints include bloody diarrhea, chills, diaphoresis, dyspnea, headache, myalgias, lightheadedness, carpopedal spasm, paresthesias, and weakness.

Diagnosis and Differential

Because the signs and symptoms of plant and mushroom poisoning may be nonspecific and easily attributed to gastroenteritis, patients at risk should be routinely asked about plant consumption. Important historical information includes the type and quantity of plant consumed. In the case of mushroom poisoning, determining the time between consumption and onset of symptoms is especially useful. An interval less than 6 h suggests ibotenic acid/muscimol, muscarine, psilocin/psilocybin, or miscellaneous unidentified toxins; greater than 6 h suggests amatoxin, gyromitrin, or orellanine/orelline. An association between mushroom ingestion and ethanol consumption suggests coprine toxicity.

Physical exam should include assessment of the patient's hydration status and evaluation for evidence of cholinergic, anticholinergic, or sympathetic nervous-system stimulation. The patient's pharynx and skin should be examined for signs of irritation. A complete cardiopulmonary exam is important in patients at risk for arrhythmias or cardiac conduction defects. The patient's abdomen should be assessed for tenderness, and flank tenderness, jaundice, or alterations in mental status should be noted.

Laboratory studies are rarely helpful in identifying the type of plant ingested. Their use should be guided, therefore, by the patient's clinical status. In the case of mushroom ingestion, however, laboratory studies may have a higher yield and should include a complete blood count, electrolytes, BUN, creatinine, glucose, and urinalysis. If symptoms are suggestive of ingestion of a cytotoxic mushroom, serum amylase and liver-function tests should be obtained. An ECG is appropriate for patients with hemodynamic compromise. If a sample of the plant or mushroom is available, it should be sent to a botanist or mycologist for identification.

Emergency Department Care and Disposition

Initial treatment is supportive, including airway management, ventilation, and fluid resuscitation with isotonic saline as indicated. Patients with altered mental status should be assessed for hypoglycemia. **Diazepam** can be used to control seizures and agitation. Acid-base and electrolyte abnormalities should be corrected. **Activated charcoal** (0.5 to 1 g/kg orally or by NG tube) should be administered. In the absence of spontaneous diarrhea, a cathartic such as sorbitol should be administered. If ingestion of a cytotoxic mushroom is suspected, **whole-bowel irrigation** (0.5 to 2 L/h of Colyte or Golytely, orally or by NG tube) within 24 h of ingestion should be considered. Patients with potential amatoxin, gyromitrin, or orellanine/orelline poisoning, or those with refractory symptoms, should be admitted. Other patients may be discharged if symptom-free after 4 to 6 h of observation or treatment. They should be instructed to return at once if they develop vomiting, abdominal pain, diarrhea, or hallucinations.

Specific interventions in amatoxin poisoning include forced diuresis and **charcoal hemoperfusion.** Penicillin G (0.3 to 1 million units/kg per day in divided doses) may inhibit liver uptake of amatoxin. Seizures and hyperkalemia are possible complications of this high-dose therapy. Cimetidine (600 mg intravenously) may inhibit amatoxin-induced liver damage. This effect may be enhanced by oral or IV administration of ascorbic acid (10–40 mg/kg per day in divided doses). A regimen of N-acetylcysteine similar to that used in acetaminophen poisoning may also be effective.

With gyromitrin poisoning, pyridoxine (25 mg/kg intravenously over 15 to 30 min) may reverse neurologic toxicity. Benzodiazepines are used to treat agitation and neuromuscular hyperactivity. Maintenance of a normal urine output may prevent hemolysis-induced renal dysfunction. Methemoglobinemia is treated with intravenous methylene blue (0.1 to 0.2 mL/kg of a 1% solution).

The treatment of orellanine/orelline toxicity consists of fluid and electrolyte support and temporary or chronic dialysis. **Charcoal hemoperfusion** may enhance toxin elimination. Patients suffering from coprine–ethanol reactions may require pressor support for hypotension unresponsive to fluid resuscitation. Beta-blockers can be used for control of tachyarrhythmias. Neuromuscular hyperactivity and seizures due to ibotenic acid/muscimol poisoning are treated with benzodiazepines and barbiturates. Physostigmine (1 to 2 mg in adults, 0.5 mg in children) may be administered as a slow intravenous bolus over several min for refractory agitation, but only in the presence of peripheral anticholinergic findings and an ECG showing sinus tachycardia and normal PR, QRS, and QT intervals.

Patients with muscarine poisoning are treated with intravenous **atropine** (0.5–1.0 mg in adults, 0.01 mg/kg in children), inhaled bronchodilators, and antihistamines. Psilocin/psilocybin poisoning is treated with reassurance, a quiet environment, and sedation. Standard cooling measures are used for hyperthermia. Poisoning by miscellaneous unidentified mushroom toxins is treated with supportive care.

For further reading in *Emergency Medicine: A Comprehensive Study Guide*, 4th edition, see Chapter 174, Mushroom Poisoning, by Christopher H. Linden and Robert P. Dowsett; and Chapter 175, Poisonous Plants, by David C. Michener, Rodger Keller, and Robert F. Kowalski.

14 | ENDOCRINE EMERGENCIES

Michael P. Kefer

HYPOGLYCEMIA

Glucose is the main energy source of the brain. Severe hypoglycemia can cause brain damage and death. Diabetics on insulin therapy are especially at risk.

Clinical Features

Typical symptoms include sweating, shakiness, anxiety, nausea, dizziness, confusion, slurred speech, blurred vision, headache, lethargy, and coma. Other major neurologic manifestations noted are cranial-nerve palsies, hemiplegia, seizure, and decerebrate posturing. Understandably, unsuspected hypoglycemia can easily be misdiagnosed as a primary neurologic, psychiatric, or cardiovascular condition.

Diagnosis and Differential

The actual blood glucose level that defines hypoglycemia is arbitrary. Some people with low glucose levels are asymptomatic, and some people with normal levels are symptomatic. The diagnosis, therefore, is based on glucose level in conjunction with the clinical presentation. The history usually gives important clues to the cause of hypoglycemia. Consider the patient, for example, who presents with hypoglycemia and depression who is or has a family member being treated with an oral hypoglycemic agent.

As suggested by the clinical features, the differential diagnosis is extensive, in part, due to the wide variety of possible presentations.

Emergency Department Care and Disposition

Treatment is **glucose** administration, oral or IV, as patient condition warrants. Often diabetics with insulin reactions will require a continuous infusion of a 5%, 10%, or 20% glucose solution to maintain a blood glucose of > 100 mg/dL. If there is not a prompt response to glucose infusion, hydrocortisone (100 mg) and glucagon (1 mg) should be added to each additional 1 of glucose solution. Glucagon (0.5 to 2.0 mg IV, IM, or SQ) is used in select cases.

Hypoglycemia secondary to the sulfonylureas may require adjunctive treatment with Diazoxide (300 mg IV over 30 min q 4 h prn).

Most diabetics with insulin reactions respond rapidly and can be discharged with instructions to continue oral intake of carbohydrates. All patients with sulfonylurea-induced hypoglycemia should be admitted because of prolonged half-life and risk of recurrence from these agents.

DIABETIC KETOACIDOSIS

Diabetic ketoacidosis results from a relative insulin deficiency and counter-regulatory hormone excess causing hyperglycemia and ketonemia. Diabetic ketoacidosis is precipitated by noncompliance with insulin therapy, infection, stroke, MI, trauma, pregnancy, and many other physiologic stresses.

Clinical Features

Clinical manifestations are directly related to metabolic derangements. Hyperglycemia causes an osmotic diuresis with dehydration, hypotension, and tachycardia. Ketonemia causes an acidosis with myocardial depression, vasodilation, and compensatory Kussmaul respiration. Nausea, vomiting, and abdominal pain, and tenderness are also common. Inappropriate normothermia is seen, so infection must be excluded by other means.

Laboratory investigation reveals elevated levels of serum glucose and ketones and decreased levels of sodium, chloride, calcium, phosphorus, and magnesium from osmotic diuresis. Pseudohyponatremia is common; for each 100 mg/dL increase in blood glucose, the sodium decreases by 1.6 mEq/l. Serum potassium may be low from osmotic diuresis and vomiting, normal, or high from acidosis. Note, in acidosis, potassium is driven extracellularly, therefore, the acidotic patient with normal or low potassium has marked depletion of total body potassium.

An anion-gap metabolic acidosis results from formation of ketone bodies. Acetone, formed from oxidation of ketone bodies, causes a characteristic fruity order of the patient's breath.

In diabetic ketoacidosis, formation of beta-hydroxybutyrate from acetoacetate is favored. The patient therefore may have low levels of acetoacetate and high levels of beta-hydroxybutyrate. If the nitroprusside test is used to detect serum or urine ketones, it may be falsely low or negative as it only detects acetoacetate and not beta-hydroxybutyrate.

Diagnosis and Differential

Diagnosis of diabetic ketoacidosis is suspected based on clinical presentation and laboratory values of a glucose > 300 mg/dL, HCO_3 < 15 mEq/l, and a pH < 7.3.

Differential diagnosis includes other causes of an anion-gap metabolic acidosis, easily recalled by the acronym MUDPILES (see Table 118-1). Hypoglycemia and nonketotic hyperosmolar coma are two other causes of metabolic coma that should be considered in a diabetic patient.

Emergency Department Care and Disposition

Basic lab investigation consists of serum glucose, electrolytes, BUN, creatinine, phosphorus, ABG, CBC, UA (and pregnancy, if indicated),

EKG, and chest x-ray to assess the severity of diabetic ketoacidosis and search for the underlying cause. The goal of treatment is to correct the volume deficit, acid-base imbalance, and electrolyte abnormalities, administer insulin, and treat the underlying cause.

The average patient in diabetic ketoacidosis has a body water deficit of 5 to 10 L. Rapid administration of **isotonic fluid** is the most important initial step to restore intravascular volume and tissue perfusion. The first L is administered over 30 to 60 min. Once intravascular volume is restored, or if the serum sodium is > 155 mEq/l, hypotonic solution is infused to provide free water for intracellular volume replacement. Patients with heart disease may need invasive monitoring to avoid CHF.

Insulin is required to shut off ketosis and restore cellular glucose stores. Low-dose IV insulin has the advantage of allowing close control of the amount of insulin given compared to IM or SQ where absorption may be erratic or delayed in an unstable patient. The half-life of insulin given IV is 5 min; given IM is 2 h. Continuous IV infusion of insulin (5–10 units/h) is recommended with or without a loading dose of 10 units IV bolus. If there is no response within the first h of treatment, insulin resistance is suggested and the infusion rate is doubled each h until a response is obtained. Hyperglycemia is controlled much more rapidly with insulin than is ketoacidosis. To reverse ketoacidosis, insulin treatment must continue despite decreasing blood glucose. Glucose infusion will therefore be necessary when the blood glucose falls to 250 mg/dL to prevent hypoglycemia.

Potassium is administered to maintain normal serum levels during the acute phase of treatment. When treatment for diabetic ketoacidosis begins, potassium levels will fall due to dilution from volume replacement, correction of acidosis, renal excretion, and insulin effect of driving potassium intracellularly. To avoid the dangerous effects of hypokalemia, potassium replacement should begin early. If the urine output is adequate, potassium chloride (20 mEq), may be added to each L of IV fluid, as required by close monitoring of serum potassium. Potassium phosphate (20 mEq) may be used if phosphorus supplementation is also required.

Phosphorus has an important role in energy production (ATP), oxygen delivery (2,3-DPG), and enzymatic reactions. Acute deficiency has been associated with all types of muscle dysfunction. Phosphorus replacement is recommended if the serum level is < 1 mg/dL. Potassium phosphate (20 mEq IV) may be used if the patient still requires potassium.

Bicarbonate therapy remains controversial as to when the benefits of correcting the effects of acidosis (vasodilation, depression of cardiac contractility and respiration, CNS depression) outweigh the risk of bicarbonate treatment (paradoxical CSF acidosis, hypokalemia, impaired oxyhemoglobin dissociation, rebound alkalosis sodium overload). Current recommendations, however, favor administration of bicarbonate when the pH is < 6.9.

All patients on insulin infusion will require close monitoring to avoid complications of treatment. Development of cerebral edema during treatment is a continual problem, predominantly in young patients. The blood glucose, anion gap, potassium, and bicarbonate should be monitored every 1 to 2 hours until recovery is well established.

NONKETOTIC HYPEROSMOLAR COMA

Nonketotic hyperosmolar coma is characterized by hyperglycemia, hyperosmolality, and dehydration. It is distinguished from diabetic ketoacidosis by the absence of ketosis. It is thought marked hyperglycemia develops because ketoacidosis does not, possibly because there is enough endogenous insulin to inhibit lipolysis, but not hyperglycemia. It is a relatively common presentation of new-onset diabetes. Similar to diabetic ketoacidosis, precipitating factors include noncompliance, MI, CVA, infection, and trauma. Drugs such as thiazide diuretics and steroids also predispose to this condition.

Clinical Features

Decreased responsiveness is the main reason patients are brought in for medical care. Metabolic changes occur over days to weeks, and symptoms may not be obvious. Physical exam reveals signs of profound dehydration with hypotension and tachycardia. Kussmaul's respiration and the smell of acetone on the breath are not present. Mental status changes range from confusion to coma. Focal deficits and focal or generalized seizures also occur.

Blood glucose levels are usually $> 1,000$ mg/dL and serum osmolality > 350 mOsm/kg. Electrolyte abnormalities and prerenal azotemia are similar to those in diabetic ketoacidosis. Pseudohyponatremia is more prominent. Serum and urine ketones are absent, however, metabolic acidosis may be present from lactic acid or azotemia.

Diagnosis and Differential

Diagnosis is based on clinical and laboratory findings. Nonketotic hyperosmolar coma must be distinguished from diabetic ketoacidosis. This is done by lab investigation. In comparison to the values mentioned above for nonketotic hyperosmolar coma, in diabetic ketoacidosis serum glucose is usually < 600 mg/dL, serum osmolality is < 350 mOsm/kg, and serum ketones are strongly positive.

Emergency Department Care and Disposition

Treatment is aimed at correction of volume deficit, electrolyte imbalance, and hyperosmolality. **Fluid treatment** consists of restoring intravascular volume and providing free water with hypotonic fluids to restore intracellular volume. The average fluid deficit is 8 to 12 L. One half the deficit is replaced over 12 h, the other half over the next 24 h. Along with large volume losses are sodium and potassium losses. As with diabetic ketoacidosis, potassium replacement should be initiated as soon as renal function is determined adequate. Glucose should be added to IV fluids when the blood glucose level approaches 250 mg/dL. Rapid lowering below this level poses an increased risk of cerebral edema.

An infusion of **insulin** 5 to 10 units per hour can be initiated. Alternatively, a bolus dose of insulin (10–20 units IV or IM) may be used. Insulin should be stopped as the blood glucose approaches 300 mg/dL.

For further reading in *Emergency Medicine: A Comprehensive Study Guide*, 4th edition, see Chapter 176, Hypoglycemia, Chapter 177, Diabetic Ketoacidosis; and Chapter 179, Hyperosmolar Nonketotic Coma, by Gene Ragland.

Michael P. Kefer

Alcoholic ketoacidosis results from heavy alcohol intake, either acute or chronic, and minimal or no food intake. Alcohol and body-fat metabolism generate ketoacids, with a resultant anion-gap metabolic acidosis.

Clinical Features

The patient with alcoholic ketoacidosis typically presents with complaints of nausea, vomiting, orthostasis, and abdominal pain 24 to 72 h after the last alcohol intake. Physical exam reveals the patient to be acutely ill and dehydrated with a tender abdomen. Abdominal tenderness is either diffuse and nonspecific or is a result of other causes associated with the use of alcohol, such as gastritis, hepatitis, or pancreatitis. Further, presentation may be confounded by other common complications of alcoholism, such as infection or alcohol withdrawal.

Laboratory investigation reveals an anion-gap (Na − [Cl + HCO_3] > 12 ± 4 mEq/L) metabolic acidosis. The serum pH may be low, normal, or high, however, as these patients often have mixed acid-base disorders, such as a metabolic acidosis from alcoholic ketoacidosis and a metabolic alkalosis from vomiting and volume depletion. Blood glucose ranges from low to mildly elevated. The alcohol level is usually low to normal, as vomiting and abdominal pain limit intake. Serum ketones, acetoacetate, and beta-hydroxybutyrate, are elevated. Serum and urine ketones are measured by the nitroprusside test, which detects acetoacetate but not beta-hydroxybutyrate. Although serum ketones are usually detected in significant amounts, the redox state may be such that most or all detectable acetoacetate is converted to beta-hydroxybutyrate, resulting in a falsely negative or falsely low estimate of the severity of ketoacidosis.

Diagnosis and Differential

The diagnosis of alcoholic ketoacidosis is established in the patient with a history of recent heavy alcohol consumption, decreased food intake, vomiting, abdominal pain, and laboratory findings of an anion-gap metabolic acidosis, a positive nitroprusside test for ketones, and a low or mildly elevated glucose.

Differential includes other causes of an anion-gap metabolic acidosis, commonly recalled by the acronym MUDPILES (Table 118-1). These can be excluded by clinical and lab data.

Emergency Department Care and Disposition

Treatment of alcoholic ketoacidosis consists of infusion of a crystalloid solution containing glucose. The **crystalloid** solution restores intravas-

TABLE 118-1. Differential Diagnosis of an Anion-Gap Metabolic Acidosis

Methanol
Uremia
Diabetic ketoacidosis
Paraldehyde
Iron, isoniazid, inhalants
Lactic acidosis
Ethanol, ethylene glycol
Salicylates

cular volume, and glucose administration stimulates insulin release, which inhibits ketosis. **Thiamine** (50–100 mg IV) also should be given.

Unlike treatment for diabetic ketoacidosis, insulin administration is not necessary, as endogenous insulin secretion occurs normally with restoration of volume and glucose administration. Sodium bicarbonate administration is controversial but is considered for a pH < 7.1. Reversal of alcoholic ketoacidosis usually occurs in 12 to 18 h but may occur sooner or later depending on the severity.

For further reading in *Emergency Medicine: A Comprehensive Study Guide*, 4th edition, see Chapter 178, Alcoholic Ketoacidosis, by Gene Ragland.

Michael P. Kefer

Lactic acidosis is the most common metabolic acidosis. Classification is based on oxygen supply to tissues. Type-A lactic acidosis is associated with hypoperfusion or severe hypoxia, as occurs with shock states. Type-B lactic acidosis includes all other form: there is no evidence of tissue anoxia; cardiovascular function is not impaired; BP is not decreased. Type-B lactic acidosis results from any condition affecting the liver's ability to clear lactate, such as cirrhosis, drugs that inhibit hepatic enzymes, or conditions leading to increased lactate production, such as leukemia or ethanol metabolism.

Clinical Features

Clinical findings in lactic acidosis are nonspecific and depend on the cause and degree of acidosis. The patient appears ill; hyperventilation or Kussmaul respiration as a compensatory response is the most constant feature. The level of consciousness varies from lethargy to coma. Vomiting and abdominal pain may be seen. Patients who present with a type-A lactic acidosis, by definition, are in shock with hypotension or severe hypoxia. Lab investigation reveals an anion gap (Na − [Cl + HCO_3] > 12 ± 4 mEq/L) metabolic acidosis with elevated lactate levels.

Diagnosis and Differential

Diagnosis of lactic acidosis requires the presence of an anion-gap metabolic acidosis with a serum lactate level > 5 mEq/L. Differential diagnosis includes other causes of an anion-gap metabolic acidosis again recalled by the acronym MUDPILES (see Table 118-1).

Emergency Department Care and Disposition The treatment of lactic acidosis is to identify the underlying cause and to counteract the adverse physiologic effects of the acidosis. **Bicarbonate** is generally recommended if the pH is > 7.1 to counteract the associated depressed myocardial contractility, arterial dilation, and impaired hepatic clearance of lactate. The dose is approximated as follows: HCO_3 deficit = (25 mEq/L HCO_3 − measured HCO_3) × 0.5 body weight in kg.

When large amounts of bicarbonate are required, an infusion can be prepared by adding 3 to 4 ampules of sodium bicarbonate to 1 liter D_5W. Administration of a loop diuretic to maintain a brisk diuresis may be needed to prevent hyperosmolarity and volume overload. If the patient is oligemic, hemodialysis will be necessary. Admission to the ward or ICU will depend on the clinical status of the patient.

For further reading in *Emergency Medicine: A Comprehensive Study Guide*, 4th edition, see Chapter 180, Lactic Acidosis, by Gene Ragland.

Stephen W. Meldon

Thyroid storm is a rare life-threatening complication of hyperthyroidism. It is most often seen in patients with antecedent Grave's disease and is usually precipitated by infection or some other stressful event.

Clinical Features

The clinical presentation is extremely variable; however, clues to the diagnosis include a history of Graves' disease, exophthalmos, a widened pulse pressure, and a palpable goiter. Earliest signs are fever, tachycardia, diaphoresis, and emotional lability. CNS disturbance occurs in 90% of patients and varies from restlessness, manic behavior, and psychosis to mental confusion and coma. Cardiovascular abnormalities are seen in 50% of patients, with sinus tachycardia common. Other arrhythmias include atrial fibrillation and PVCs. GI symptoms, such as diarrhea and hyperdefecation, occur in most patients. Apathetic thyrotoxicosis is a distinct presentation seen in elderly patients, in which the characteristic symptoms are absent, and lethargy, slowed mention, and apathetic facies is seen. Goiter, weight loss, and proximal muscle weakness are present. Atrial fibrillation and CHF may occur.

Diagnosis and Differential

Thyroid storm is a clinical diagnosis, since no laboratory tests distinguish it from thyrotoxicosis. Diagnostic criteria include a temperature higher then 37.8°C; tachycardia out of proportion to fever; dysfunction of the CNS, cardiovascular, or GI systems; and exaggerated peripheral manifestations of thyrotoxicosis. In this clinical setting, an elevated T_4 and a suppressed TSH confirms the diagnosis. The differential diagnosis includes sepsis, pulmonary or enteric infections, and meningitis; other causes of CHF; stroke; complications of diabetes (diabetic ketoacidosis, hypoglycemia); heat stroke; and sympathomimetic drug overdose. The diagnosis is complicated by the fact that any of these entities may precipitate thyroid storm.

Emergency Department Care and Disposition

The importance of early treatment of thyroid storm based upon the clinical impression must be emphasized. Therapeutic goals can be divided into five areas: general supportive care; inhibition of thyroid hormone synthesis; retardation of thyroid hormone release; blockade of peripheral thyroid hormone effects; and identification and treatment of precipitating events.

1. Supplemental **oxygen,** IV fluids, and cardiac monitoring are indicated. Fever should be controlled by the use of acetaminophen and

a cooling blanket. Intravenous glucocorticoids such as **dexametha-sone** (10 mg IV) should be given.

2. The antithyroid drugs **propylthiouracil (PTU)** and methimazole act by blocking thyroid hormone synthesis. They must be given orally or by NG tube. The initial loading dose of PTU is 900 to 1200 mg po, followed by 300 to 600 mg daily. Methimazole (90 to 120 mg po, followed by 30 to 60 mg daily) is an acceptable alternative.

3. **Iodide** retards thyroid release of stored hormones. Iodide should be administered 1 h after PTU. The dose is 10 drops of potassium iodide (1 g/mL) every 4 to 6 h, or sodium iodide (1 g every 8–12 h by slow IV infusion).

4. Adrenergic blockade is a mainstay of therapy. **Propranolol** (1 mg IV every 10 min to a total dose of 10 mg) is the drug of choice. The lowest possible dose required to control the cardiac and psychomotor symptoms should be used and can be repeated every 3 to 4 h as needed. Propranolol should be used with caution in the setting of severe bronchospastic disease, heart block, or CHF. Guanethidine (1 to 2 mg/kg orally per day) and reserpine (1 to 5 mg IM, followed by 1 to 2.5 mg every 4 to 6 h) are alternatives to propranolol.

5. Precipitating causes should be sought. Appropriate cultures and anti-biotics may be indicated. CHF may be refractory to standard therapy. All patients should be monitored closely and admitted to the ICU.

If Standard Treatment Fails

If conventional therapy is not successful, alternative treatments to re-move circulating thyroid hormone and control storm include peritoneal dialysis, charcoal hemoperfusion or plasmapheresis.

HYPOTHYROIDISM AND MYXEDEMA COMA

Myxedema coma is a rare life-threatening expression of severe hypothy-roidism. It is most often seen during the winter months in elderly women with undiagnosed or undertreated hypothyroidism. Precipitating events include pulmonary infections, CHF, and exposure to a cold environment.

Clinical Features

The typical symptoms of hypothyroidism include fatigue, weakness, cold intolerance, constipation, weight gain, menstrual irregularities, and deepening of voice. Cutaneous signs include dry, scaly, yellow skin, puffy eyes, and thinning eyebrows. A nonpitting, dry, waxy edema of the skin—termed myxedema—may occur, resulting in a puffy face and extremities. Paresthesia, ataxia, and prolongation of the deep tendon reflexes are characteristic neurological findings. Delusions and psycho-sis (myxedema madness) may occur. Cardiac findings include bradycar-dia, enlarged heart, and low-voltage ECG. A thyroidectomy scar may be present, but a goiter is uncommon. The patient with myxedema coma will present with several additional findings: hypothermia (in 80% of cases), hyponatremia, hypotension and bradycardia, and a paralytic ileus and acquired megacolon. Respiratory failure with hypoventilation, hypercapnia, and hypoxia is common. Neurologic dysfunction, such as psychiatric disorders or seizures, may precede coma.

Diagnosis and Differential

The diagnosis of myxedema coma must be suspected, based on the clinical presentation and characteristic laboratory abnormalities previously mentioned. Confirmatory thyroid tests will typically show low free T_4 and elevated TSH levels. Patients suspected of myxedema coma should be evaluated with a low-reading thermometer, arterial blood gases, chest x-ray, EKG, and serum electrolytes. Differential diagnosis includes coma secondary to respiratory failure, hyponatremia, hypothermia, CHF, stroke, or drug overdose.

Emergency Department Care and Disposition

Patients with myxedema coma are critically ill, and initial treatment must be supportive. Specific treatment requires large doses of thyroid hormone, which could be fatal to a euthyroid comatose patient. Other causes of coma must be considered and ruled out. All patients require IV fluids, cardiac monitoring, and Foley and NG catheters. Respiratory failure should be treated with supplemental oxygen and mechanical ventilation, if needed. Hypothermic patients should be gradually rewarmed. Hyponatremia may require hypertonic saline and furosemide in addition to fluid restriction. Vasopressors are usually ineffective in this setting and should be used only for severe hypotension. Sedating drugs, such as phenothiazines, generally should be avoided. Antibiotics are indicated for underlying infection and hydrocortisone (300 mg) should be given.

Thyroid hormone is the most critical and specific therapy for myxedema coma. IV **thyroxine** in an initial dose of 400 to 500 μg should be given by slow infusion, followed by 50 to 100 μg IV daily. Alternative treatment consists of L-triiodothyronine initial dose 25–50 μg IV, followed by 65 to 100 μg per day in 3 or 4 divided doses. L-triiodothyronine dosage should be halved in patients with cardiovascular disease. Overall clinical improvement should be seen in 24 to 36 h with either regimen.

If Standard Treatment Fails

If standard therapy for myxedema coma fails, the diagnosis must be reconsidered. In addition, precipitating causes must be sought and treated, and drugs which might induce coma must be avoided. Mortality is greater than 50%, however, even with optimum treatment.

For further reading in *Emergency Medicine: A Comprehensive Study Guide*, 4th edition, see Chapter 181, Thyroid Storm and Chapter 182, Hypothyroidism and Myxedema Coma, by Gene Ragland.

Adrenal insufficiency may manifest clinically as a chronic disorder or as an acute, life-threatening emergency. Etiologies include primary dysfunction of the adrenal gland (Addison's disease), secondary and tertiary insufficiency due to pituitary and hypothalamus hypoactivity, respectively, adrenal suppression by chronic steroid administration, abrupt withdrawal of chronically administered steroids, and acute stress in patients with underlying adrenal disease.

Clinical Features

Chronic adrenal insufficiency. The clinical manifestations of chronic adrenal insufficiency develop gradually with subtle signs and symptoms. The presentation of Addison's disease can be explained on the basis of a deficiency of cortisol and aldosterone and a lack of feedback inhibition of adrenocorticotropic hormone (ACTH) and melanocyte-stimulating hormone (MSH). Cortisol deficiency presents with anorexia, nausea, vomiting, diarrhea, abdominal pain, weight loss, lethargy, stress-related shock, symptoms associated with hypoglycemia, and inability to excrete free water resulting in water intoxication. Aldosterone deficiency manifests with dehydration, hypotension, postural syncope, and decreased cardiac size and output, with associated diminished heart sounds on auscultation. Excess ACTH and MSH secretion results in brownish hyperpigmentation over exposed body areas, such as the face, neck, arms, and over friction or pressure points, such as the elbows, knees, and nipples. Pigmentation of mucous membranes, a darkening of hair, and longitudinal pigmented bands in the nails may also be seen. Women may exhibit decreased growth of axillary and pubic hair. Mental-status changes can be seen, as can enhancement of the senses of olfaction, taste, and hearing. Paralysis due to hyperkalemia is a rare, emergent complication.

Secondary and tertiary adrenal insufficiency The clinical manifestations of secondary adrenal insufficiency are due to deficiency of cortisol, adrenal androgens, and growth, thyroid, and gonadotropic hormones. Aldosterone is largely unaffected. Patients are therefore less prone to developing shock in the setting of salt deprivation than are patients with Addison's disease. In contrast, patients are more likely to develop hypoglycemia because of the growth hormone deficit associated with hypopituitarism. Hyperpigmentation is not seen. Both men and women may shows signs of androgen deficiency. Tertiary adrenal insufficiency has similar manifestations but is usually seen in patients on chronic steroid therapy who are exposed to increased stress.

Adrenal crisis Adrenal crisis is an acute, life-threatening emergency with manifestations of cortisol and aldosterone insufficiency, usually in response to a specific physiologic stressor. Patients look acutely ill, with weakness, mental status changes, seizures, distant heart sounds, tachycardia, orthostatic hypotension, circulatory collapse, and fever, often due to precipitating underlying infection. Patients almost universally have anorexia, nausea, vomiting, and abdominal pain, mimicking an acute abdomen. Symptoms associated with hypoglycemia may be severe.

Diagnosis and Differential

Primary adrenal insufficiency is diagnosed by demonstrating a low baseline plasma cortisol level that does not increase in response to exogenous ACTH. In a rapid screening test, plasma is drawn for determination of the cortisol level and 25 units of corticotropin administered IV, SQ, or IM. A followup cortisol level is drawn 30 to 60 min later. Normal persons should respond with a doubling of the baseline cortisol level, with a peak level of greater than or equal to 20 mg/dL. Patients with primary adrenal insufficiency show no increase in plasma cortisol levels.

Common laboratory abnormalities include mild to moderate hyponatremia (>120 mEq/ L), mild hyperkalemia (<7 mEq/L), azotemia, and in some cases hypoglycemia. Electrocardiographic changes include flat or inverted T waves, prolongation of the PR, QRS, or QT intervals, and ST depression. ECG changes reflective of hyperkalemia may be seen. The chest x-ray often reveals a small cardiac silhouette due to decreased intravascular volume. A flat plate of the abdomen may show adrenal calcification due to hemorrhage or to tuberculosis or other infections.

Secondary adrenal insufficiency is diagnosed by a low plasma cortisol level and urinary metabolite levels that increase with repetitive ACTH stimulation. Laboratory abnormalities are less common in secondary adrenal insufficiency than in Addison's disease. Hyponatremia, hyperkalemia, and azotemia are not prominent features, however, hypoglycemia is a frequent finding.

Adrenal crisis is usually associated with mild hyponatremia. Serum potassium may be normal or mildly elevated. Rarely, profound hyperkalemia with associated cardiac arrhythmias or hyperkalemic paralysis is seen. Hypoglycemia is a common finding and may be life-threatening. Confirmatory diagnostic testing of adrenal insufficiency can be performed during patient resuscitation. A baseline plasma cortisol level is drawn, and the patient is given over the first h a 1 l intravenous infusion of D_5NS containing 4 mg of dexamethasone and 25 units of corticotropin. A repeat cortisol level is obtained. Additional corticotropin is added to subsequent IV solutions so that the patient receives at least 3 units/

h for 8 h. A third cortisol level is obtained between the 6th and 8th h of IV therapy. A 24-h urine collection is obtained for measurement of 17-hydroxycorticosteroid (17-OHCS). If the patient has primary adrenal insufficiency, all plasma levels are <15 mg/dL and the urine 17-OHCS is also low.

Emergency Department Care and Disposition

Primary adrenal insufficiency is managed with cortisol and aldosterone replacement and, at times, supplemental estrogen in female patients. The usual maintenance dose for glucocorticoid replacement varies from 20 to 37.5 mg of cortisol per day. A generally accepted regimen is 5 mg **prednisone** in the morning and 2.5 mg in the afternoon. Large, active men may require a total of 10 mg per day. Mineralocorticoid replacement in patients with primary adrenal insufficiency can be achieved by administration of the synthetic mineralocorticoid **fludro-cortisone acetate** (Florinef, 0.05 to 0.2 mg/day orally). The dose should be decreased in patients with hypertension. Supplemental oral androgen replacement with 2 to 5 mg of fluoxymesterone (Halotestin) can be administered to women with decreased growth of axillary and pubic hair.

Secondary adrenal insufficiency is managed differently than primary disease in that patients do not generally require mineralocorticoid replacement and can maintain salt and fluid balance with dietary sodium chloride. Supplementary oral fludrocortisone acetate, 0.05 to 0.1 mg/day, can be given to patients prone to hypotension. Thyroid hormone replacement is usually necessary. Androgen replacement in females can be achieved with 2 to 5 mg of fluoxymesterone orally per day. Larger doses of this medication or long-acting testosterone (Depo-Testosterone) may be required in males.

Adrenal crisis must be treated aggressively. Management should not be delayed for confirmatory tests of adrenal function. Therapy involves fluid resuscitation, administration of glucocorticoids, and correction of hyponatremia, hypoglycemia, and hyperkalemia. Potential underlying precipitants should be sought.

1. A rapid intravenous infusion of D_5NS should be started immediately. The first l should be given over 1 h, and 2 to 3 l may be required during the first 8 h of therapy. The patient should be observed for evidence of fluid overload.
2. As soon as the diagnosis of adrenal crisis is entertained, 100 mg of **hydrocortisone sodium succinate** (Solu-Cortef) or phosphate should be given as an IV bolus. An additional 100 mg is added to the IV solution. Usually 200 mg of hydrocortisone is given every 6 h for the first 24 h.
3. Mineralocorticoid therapy is not required during initial treatment of adrenal crisis. After the dose of glucocorticoid administered is re-

duced to less than 100 mg/24 h, however, mineralocorticoid replacement may be warranted, provided as desoxycorticosterone acetate (Percorten), 2.5 to 5.0 mg IM, once or twice daily.
4. Vasopressors may be required if hypotension persists despite adequate fluids and corticosteroid replacement.

The adrenal crisis should begin to resolve within a few h after initiation of therapy. Intensive treatment and monitoring should continue for 24 to 48 h. Once stabilized, the patient can be put on oral maintenance therapy.

For further reading in *Emergency Medicine: A Comprehensive Study Guide,* 4th edition, see Chapter 183, Adrenal Insufficiency and Adrenal Crisis, by Gene Ragland.

HEMATOLOGIC AND ONCOLOGIC EMERGENCIES

122

Evaluation of the Bleeding Patient

C. Crawford Mechem

Most bleeding seen in the ED occurs in patients with normal hemostasis and results from local wounds, such as lacerations or other structural lesions. Patients who present with spontaneous bleeding from multiple sites, bleeding from untraumatized sites, delayed bleeding several h after injury, or bleeding into deep tissues or joints should be evaluated for the presence of bleeding disorders.

Clinical Features

The site of hemorrhage can help to elucidate the underlying hemostatic abnormality in patients with bleeding disorders. Patients with qualitative or quantitative platelet disorders present with mucocutaneous bleeding, including petechiae, ecchymoses, purpura, epistaxis, or gastrointestinal, genitourinary, or heavy menstrual bleeding. Deficiency of coagulation factors may present with delayed bleeding or bleeding into joints and potential spaces, such as between fascial planes and into the retroperitoneum. Patients with combined abnormalities of platelets and coagulation factors, such as in disseminated intravascular coagulation, may present with both mucocutaneous and deep-space bleeding.

Diagnosis and Differential

Laboratory studies used to diagnose bleeding disorders can be divided into three categories: (1) those that test the initial formation of a platelet plug (primary hemostasis); (2) those that assess the formation of cross-linked fibrin (secondary hemostasis); and (3) tests of the fibrinolytic system, which is responsible for limiting the size of the fibrin clots formed. These tests are detailed in Table 122–1. Basic lab studies that should be obtained in patients with suspected bleeding disorders are a CBC with platelet count, PT, and PTT. Further testing will be guided by the clinical situation.

Historical information also can be of value in diagnosing the etiology of bleeding disorders. For example, a wide variety of medications can induce thrombocytopenia and associated impairment of coagulation (Table 122-2). A detailed medication history, therefore, including use of over-the-counter products, should be obtained from all patients with suspected bleeding abnormalities.

For further reading in *Emergency Medicine: A Comprehensive Study Guide,* 4th edition, see Chapter 184, Evaluation of the Bleeding Patient, by Mary E. Eberst.

TABLE 122-1. Tests of Hemostasis

Screening tests	Normal value	Measures	Clinical correlations
Platelet count	150,000–300,000/ mm^3	Number of platelets per mm^3	Decreased platelet count (thrombocytopenia) Bleeding usually not a problem until platelet count <50,000; high risk of spontaneous bleeding, including CNS with count < 10,000/mm^3 Causes Decreased production—viral infections (measles); marrow infiltration; drugs (thiazides, ETOH, estrogens, interferon-α) (see Table 122-2) Increased destruction—viral infections (mumps, varicella, EBV, HIV); ITP, TTP, DIC, HUS; drugs heparin, protamine (see Table 122-2) Splenic sequestration (hypersplenism, hypothermia). Loss of platelets (hemorrhage, hemodialysis, extracorporeal circulation). Pseudothrombocytopenia—platelets are clumped but not truly decreased in number, examine blood smear to recognize this. Elevated platelet count (thrombocytosis)—commonly reactive to inflammation or malignancy, or in polycythemia vera; can be associated with hemorrhage or thrombosis
Bleeding time (BT)	2.5–10 min (template BT)	Interaction between platelets and the subendothelium	Prolonged BT caused by: Thrombocytopenia (platelet count < 50,000/mm^3) Abnormal platelet function (vWD, ASA, NSAIDs, uremia, liver disease) Collagen abnormalities (congenital abnormality or prolonged use of steroids)

		Secondary hemostasis	
Prothrombin time (PT)	10–12 s, but laboratory variation	Extrinsic system and common pathway—factors VII, X, V, prothrombin, and fibrinogen	*Prolonged PT*—most commonly caused by: Use of coumadin/warfarin (inhibits vitamin K dependent factors II, VII, IX and X) Liver disease and decreased factor synthesis Antibiotics, some cephalosporins, (moxalactam, cefamandole, cefotaxime, cefoperazone) that inhibit vitamin K-dependent factors.
Activated partial thromboplastin time (aPTT)	Depends on type of thromboplastin used; activated with Kaolin	Intrinsic system and common pathway including factors XII, XI, IX, VIII, X, V, prothrombin, and fibrinogen	*Prolongation of aPTT* most commonly caused by: Heparin therapy Factor deficiencies; factor levels have to be < 30% of normal to cause prolongation Note: high doses of heparin or warfarin can cause prolongation of both the PT and aPTT due to their activity in the common pathway
Thrombin clotting time (TCT)	10–12 s	Conversion of fibrinogen to fibrin monomer	*Prolonged TCT* caused by: Low fibrinogen level (DIC) Abnormal fibrinogen molecule (liver disease) Presence of heparin, FDPs or a paraprotein (multiple myeloma); these interfere with the conversion Very high fibrinogen level (acute phase reactant)
Mixes	Variable	Performed when one or more of the above screening tests is prolonged; the patients plasma (abnormal) is mixed with normal plasma and the screening test is repeated	*If the mix corrects the screening test, one or more factor deficiencies are present* *If the mix does not correct the screening test, an inhibitor is present*

(Table continues)

TABLE 122-1. Continued

		Other Hemostatic Tests
Fibrin degradation products and D-dimer (evaluate fibrinolysis)	Variable	*FDPs* measure breakdown products from fibrinogen and fibrin monomer; *D-dimer* measures breakdown products of cross-linked fibrin	Levels of these are elevated in DIC, thrombosis, pulmonary embolus, liver disease
Factor level assays	60–130% (0.60–1.30 units/mL)	Measures the % activity of a specified factor compared to normal	Used to identify specific factor deficiencies and in therapeutic management of patients with deficiencies
Inhibitor screens	Variable	Verifies the presence or absence of antibodies directed against one or more of the coagulation factors	*Specific inhibitors*—directed against deficiencies factor, most commonly against factor VIII; can be in patients with congenital or acquired deficiency. *Nonspecific inhibitors*—directed against more than one of the coagulation factors; example is lupus-type anticoagulant

ASA, aspirin; CNS, central nervous system; DIC, disseminated intravascular coagulation; EBV, Epstein–Barr virus; ETOH, ethanol; FDPs, fibrin degradation products; HIV, human immunodeficiency virus; HUS, hemolytic uremic syndrome; ITP, idiopathic thrombocytopenic purpura; NSAIDs, nonsteroidal anti-inflammatory drugs; TTP, thrombotic thrombocytopenic purpura; vWD, von Willebrand disease.

TABLE 122-2. Commonly Used Drugs Associated with Platelet Dysfunction

Aspirin, NSAIDs	Calcium channel blockers
Heparin and thrombolytics	Propranolol
Penicillins and cephalosporins	Nitroprusside
Nitrofurantoin	Nitroglycerin
Prostaglandins	Tricyclic antidepressants
Dextran	Phenothiazines
Chemotherapeutics	Antihistamines

NSAIDs, nonsteroidal anti-inflammatory drugs

C. Crawford Mechem

Acquired bleeding disorders result from platelet abnormalities, coagulation factor deficiencies, endogenous anticoagulants, drugs, and systemic illnesses. Early recognition of these disorders is required for prompt, etiology-specific treatment.

Platelet Abnormalities

Etiologies include uremia, splenectemy, polycythemia vera, inflammatory reactions, HIV infection, liver disease, DIC, TTP, antiplatelet antibodies, cardiopulmonary bypass, malignancy, von Willebrand disease, and drugs (Table 123-1).

Emergency Department Care and Disposition Management of patients with thrombocytopenia and bleeding involves hemorrhage control and maintenance of adequate intravascular volume to assure tissue perfusion.

1. **Platelet transfusion** is warranted in patients with a platelet count $< 50,000/mm^3$ and active bleeding and in all patients with a platelet count $< 10,000/mm^3$.
2. Therapy is also directed at correcting the underlying etiology.

TABLE 123-1. Drugs Associated with Thrombocytopenia

		Relative incidence		Relative incidence
Heparin	4+	Thiazides	2+
Gold salts	4+	Furosemide	2+
Sulfa-containing antibiotics	4+	Procainamide	2+
Quinine/quinidine	4+	Digoxin/digitoxin	2+
Amrinone	3+	Cimetidine/ranitidine	2+
Ethanol (chronic use)	3+	Phenytoin	1+
Aspirin	3+	Penicillins/cephalosporins	1+
Indomethacin	3+	Estrogens	1+
Valproic acid	3+	Protamine sulfate	1+
Heroin	3+	Interferon-α	1+

Relative incidence based on number of case reports: 4+ equivalent to at least 50–100 reports; 3+ is 20 or more reports; 2+ is 10–20 reports; 1+ is 10 or less case reports.

Warfarin and Vitamin-K Deficiency

Patients taking warfarin or certain antibiotics, such as third-generation cephalosporins, may develop hemorrhagic complications due to deficiencies of vitamin-K-dependent clotting factors.

Emergency Department Care and Disposition Management depends on the severity of clinical manifestations. In the absence of bleeding, stopping the medication may be sufficient.

1. Active bleeding may be treated with **fresh frozen plasma** (FFP).
2. **Vitamin K** (10 mg SQ or IM) will reverse bleeding within 12 to 24 h. Hemorrhage due to socalled superwarfarins may require 50 to 100 mg/day for several wks.

Liver Disease

Liver disease predisposes to bleeding due to thrombocytopenia, anemia, increased fibrinolysis, and deficiencies of coagulation factors and vitamin K.

Emergency Department Care and Disposition Patients with active bleeding require aggressive stabilization of the airway, breathing, and circulatory status, while addressing the underlying disease process.

1. **Packed red blood cells** (RBCs) are given in the presence of significant blood loss.
2. **Vitamin K** (10 to 15 mg SQ or IM) should be administered to all patients.
3. **FFP** can be given to temporarily replace coagulation factors.
4. Platelets can be transfused in cases of severe bleeding, but their effect is transient.
5. **Desmopressin** (DDAVP, 0.3 mg/kg SQ or IV q12 h), will shorten bleeding time.

Renal Disease

The bleeding tendency in renal patients is related to the degree and duration of uremia. Contributing factors include platelet dysfunction, chronic anemia, coagulation-factor deficiency, and thrombocytopenia. Spontaneous bleeding is common.

Emergency Department Care and Disposition Management is both preventative and directed at the acute bleeding episode.

1. Packed RBCs are transfused to optimize the hematocrit.
2. **DDAVP** (0.3 mg/kg SQ or IV) is used to reduce the bleeding time.
3. Conjugated estrogens decrease bleeding time in 80% of uremic patients.
4. Platelet transfusions are generally not effective, because platelets quickly acquire the uremic defect. Platelets and cryoprecipitate are only indicated for life-threatening bleeding, used in combination with packed RBCs, DDAVP, and estrogens.
5. Dialysis improves platelet function transiently, lasting 1 to 2 days.

Disseminated Intravascular Coagulation (DIC)

DIC results from activation of both the coagulation and fibrinolytic systems and has many causes, including infection, carcinoma, trauma, shock, liver and vascular disease, and pregnancy.

Clinical Features   Bleeding occurs in up to 75% of patients and presents as petechiae, ecchymoses, purpura, epistaxis, bleeding from venipuncture sites and surgical wounds, and GI or GU hemorrhage. Thrombosis predominates in some patients and presents with altered mental status, focal ischemia, oliguria, renal cortical necrosis, and ARDS.

Diagnosis and Differential   Characteristic laboratory abnormalities include a prolonged PT and PTT; elevated fibrinogen degradation products and D-dimer; and decreased platelets, clotting factors, and fibrinogen.

Emergency Department Care and Disposition   Management involves stabilizing the patient hemodynamically while addressing the underlying disease process. Further therapy depends on whether bleeding or thrombosis predominates.

1. **FFP** is used if there is active bleeding and the PT is prolonged by more than 2 to 3 s. Two units are transfused initially while watching for evidence of fluid overload.
2. **Cryoprecipitate** is used to replace fibrinogen. Ten bags are typically administered.
3. **Platelet replacement** is indicated if the platelet count is $< 50,000/mm^3$ in the presence of bleeding or $< 20,000/mm^3$ regardless of bleeding. Typically 6 units are given.
4. **Vitamin K** and folate should be administered to all patients.
5. The use of heparin to treat microthromboses in DIC is controversial. It should be considered in patients with carcinoma, promyelocytic anemia, retained uterine products, or purpura fulminans, at a low-dose infusion of 5 to 10 units/kg/h. Patients with large thromboses should receive full-dose heparin.
6. The use of antibiotics and removal of fetal tissue may be indicated in pregnancy.

Heparin and Thrombolytic Therapy

Bleeding occurs in up to 33% of patients treated with heparin. Patients with underlying renal failure, GI bleeding, head injury, ethanol abuse, malignancy, recent trauma or surgery, hemorrhagic disorders, or who use aspirin, warfarin, steroids, or NSAIDs are at especially high risk. Heparin use results in thrombocytopenia, both a benign form in which the platelet count remains $> 100,000/mm^3$, and a life-threatening form in which platelets drop below $50,000/mm^3$, with associated arterial thromboses. Thrombolytics may also cause bleeding complications, felt to be due to dissolution of hemostatic plugs at sites of recent vascular injury.

Emergency Department Care and Disposition Patients with hemorrhagic complications of heparin or thrombolytics may require aggressive stabilization of their oxygenation and perfusion.

1. When there is significant bleeding, heparin, or thrombolytics are stopped immediately.
2. **Protamine** neutralizes heparin at a dose of 1 mg IV per 100 units of heparin infused.
3. In the setting of hemorrhage due to thrombolytic agents, cryoprecipitate can be given to replete fibrinogen, and Amicar may reverse the thrombolytic state.

Circulating Anticoagulants

Circulating anticoagulants are acquired antibodies directed against one or more of the coagulation factors. These include factor-VIII-specific inhibitors and the lupus anticoagulant, which affects several factors and, despite its name, is rarely seen in patients with lupus.

Clinical Features Patients with factor-VIII inhibitors present with massive spontaneous bruises, ecchymoses, and hematomas. Patients with the lupus anticoagulant may present with arterial or venous thromboses or recurrent fetal loss. Bleeding abnormalities in patients with the lupus anticoagulant are uncommon.

Diagnosis and Differential Lab studies in patients with factor-VIII inhibitors include a normal PT and thrombin-clotting time (TCT) and a greatly prolonged PTT. A factor VIII-specific assay will show very low or absent activity. Patients with the lupus anticoagulant will have a normal or slightly prolonged PT, moderate prolongation of the PTT, and a normal TCT. Factor specific assays will show a decrease in all factor levels.

Emergency Department Care and Disposition Patients are resuscitated with attention to the airway, breathing, and circulatory status.

1. Patients with factor VIII inhibitors who present with active bleeding should be managed in consultation with a hematologist. Options include the use of factor-VIII concentrates, prothrombin complex concentrates, and porcine factor VIII.
2. Patients with the lupus anticoagulant and venous thrombosis are treated with long- term anticoagulation. Those with arterial thrombosis are treated with low-dose ASA.

For further reading in *Emergency Medicine: A Comprehensive Study Guide*, 4th edition, see Chapter 185, Acquired Bleeding Disorders, by Mary E. Eberst.

Hemophilias and Von Willebrand Disease

C. Crawford Mechem

Hemophilias are hereditary bleeding disorders resulting from deficiency of factor VIII (hemophilia A) or factor IX (hemophilia B, Christmas disease). Von Willebrand disease is the most common inherited bleeding disorder and results from a deficiency of von Willebrand factor, a portion of the factor-VIII complex.

HEMOPHILIAS

Clinical Features

The clinical classification of the hemophilias is based on the severity of factor deficiency. A mild deficiency corresponds to 6% to 60% of normal factor-VIII activity. Moderate deficiency indicates 1% to 5% activity, and severe deficiency involves less than 1% activity.

Common bleeding manifestations include hemarthroses, hematomas, and mucocutaneous bleeding. Spontaneous or traumatic bleeding into the neck, retropharynx, or pharynx can result in airway compromise. Retroperitoneal hemorrhage may present with back, thigh, groin, or abdominal pain and is potentially life-threatening. Patients with bleeding into the fascial spaces of the extremities may develop signs and symptoms of compartment syndrome. CNS bleeding may present with new headache or other neurologic symptoms. These symptoms warrant urgent evaluation, since intracranial bleeding is the most common cause of bleeding death in hemophiliacs. Other manifestations of hemophilia include hematuria and potentially life-threatening bleeding from sites of arterial or venous-line placement. In general, hemophiliacs do not have problems with minor cuts and abrasions.

Among hemophiliacs who received blood products before the mid-1980s, 90% have serologic evidence of hepatitis B, 85% to 100% have hepatitis C antibodies, and 60% to 90% have HIV infection. Hemophiliacs may present with a constellation of signs and symptoms related to these diseases.

Diagnosis and Differential

Patients with hemophilia are usually identified in childhood or adolescence. Coagulation tests typically show a normal prothrombin time (PT) and thrombin clot time (TCT), but a prolonged aPTT. If factor-VIII activity is greater than 30% normal, the aPTT may be normal. Hemophilias A and B can only be distinguished by specific assays of factors VIII and IX.

Hemophiliacs also may possess circulating inhibitors or antibodies directed against factor VIII or factor IX, whichever they are missing.

The quantity of inhibitor present is measured by the Bethesda inhibitor assay (BIA) and affects the type of factor-replacement therapy the patient receives.

Emergency Department Care and Disposition

All hemophiliacs who present with bleeding should be aggressively evaluated and managed, with initial attention to stabilization of the airway, breathing, and circulatory status.

Hemophilia A

1. **DDAVP** is indicated in patients with mild to moderate hemophilia A, at a dose of 0.3 mg/kg IV or SQ.
2. Patients with moderate or severe hemophilia A and significant bleeding will require factor-VIII replacement, preferably with virally safe factor-VIII concentrate. **Factor VIII concentrates** are dosed by units, where one unit will raise the factor-VIII level by 2%. Table 124-1 outlines specific recommendations for factor replacement.
3. When factor-VIII concentrate is unavailable, cryoprecipitate or fresh frozen plasma (FFP) may be used, however, these carry the risk of viral transmission. Each bag of cryoprecipitate contains 100 units of factor VIII, while each ml of FFP contains 1 unit.
4. Ancillary therapy for bleeding episodes includes rest, immobilization, analgesia, and antifibrinolytic agents, such as amicar and tranexamic acid.
5. The management of bleeding in patients with hemophilia A and inhibitors is guided by the inhibitor titer (in BIA units) and is outlined in Table 124-2.

Hemophilia B

1. Highly purified **factor-IX concentrates** are the replacement therapy of choice, when available. One unit per kg raises the factor-IX level by 1%.
2. **FFP** can be used to raise the factor-IX level when concentrates are not available. Because of the risk of viral transmission, FFP should only be used in emergencies. One unit of FFP will raise the factor IX level by 3% in an average-sized patient.
3. Products available for management of bleeding in patients with hemophilia B and inhibitors are outlined in Table 124-3.

Indications for hospital admission of patients include potentially life-threatening bleeding involving the CNS, neck, pharynx, retropharynx, or retroperitoneum, or patients at risk for developing compartment syndrome. Patients who are not capable of administering factor replacement at home should be admitted, as should patients requiring treatment for several days or those requiring close monitoring or parenteral analgesia.

TABLE 124-1. Factor-VIII Replacement Therapy for Patients with Hemophilia A (No Inhibitor)

Type of hemorrhage	Factor-VIII level required for hemostasis, % of normal	Factor-VIII dose in units/kg (initial dose)	Dosing interval, h*	Duration of therapy, days
Minor				
Hemarthroses	30–50	15–25	24	1–2
Superficial muscular or soft tissue	30–50	15–25	24	1–2
Moderate				
Epistaxis	30–50	15–25	12	Until resolved
Dental extractions	50	25	12–24	1–2
Muscular or soft tissue with dissection	50–100	25–50	12	Variable
GI bleeding	50–100	25–50	12	7–10
Hematuria	50–100	25–50	12	Until resolved
Life threatening				
Central nervous system	75–100	50	12	10–14
Retropharynx/phamyx	75–100	50	12	10–14
Retroperitoneum	75–100	50	12	10–14
Surgery	75–100	50	12	Variable

*Continuous infusion of factor-VIII concentrate may be used in hospitalized patients; a typical dose after the loading dose is 150 units/h; this is adjusted based on factor-VIII levels. GI, gastrointestinal.

TABLE 124-2. Replacement for Hemophilia A Patients with Inhibitors

Type of product (trade name)	Used for	Dose	Frequency, h	Comments
Factor-VIII concentrates	Inhibitor titer less than 5–10 BIA units	5,000–10,000 unit bolus	Continuous infusion at about 1000	If patient is a high responder, in about 3 days the inhibitor titer will rise
Prothrombin complex concentrates PCCs contian II, VII, IX, X (Bebulin VH, Proplex T, Profilnine HT, and Konyne-80	Inhibitor titer > 10 units; known good response to these products	75–100 units/kg of bodyweight	Repeat dose every 8–12 h	Complications of use include development of thromboembolic disease, include development of DIC, low risk of hepatitis transmission
Activated prothrombin complex concentrates aPCCs contain II, VII, IX, and X with variable amounts of activated factors VII$_a$, IX$_a$, and X$_a$ (Autoplex, FEIBA)	Patients who do not respond to PCCs	Same as with PCCs	Repeat dose every 12–24 h	Same as with PCCs
Porcine factor VIII	Patients with high inhibitor titers not responsive to the above products	Variable	Variable	Patients will often develop an inhibitor to the procine product
Recombinant factor VII$_a$	Not yet commercially available	Variable	Variable	Less thrombogenic risk than PCCs and no risk of viral transmission

TABLE 124-3. Products Used for Replacement Therapy in Patients with Hemophilia B with Inhibitors

Type of product	Used for	Initial dose
Highly purified factor-IX concentrations	Bethesda inhibitor titer < 10 units	Variable
Prothrombin complex concentrates	Bethesda inhibitors titer < 10 units	75 units/kg
Activated prothrombin complex concentrates	Bethesda inhibitors titers > 10 units or unresponsive to the above	Variable, about 75 units/kg
Recombinant factor VII$_a$	Not yet commercially available	Variable

VON WILLEBRAND DISEASE

Clinical Features

Von Willebrand disease (vWD) is divided into three types, based on the severity of bleeding and on laboratory testing. The hemorrhagic tendency is highly variable. Mild bleeding from mucocutaneous surfaces is most characteristic and manifests as epistaxis, easy bruising, bleeding after dental extractions, menorrhagia, and gastrointestinal bleeding. Patients with the most severe form, type III, may develop spontaneous hematomas and hemarthroses similar to patients with hemophilia.

Diagnosis and Differential

Coagulation screening tests will show a normal PT, normal TCT, and usually a normal aPTT. In moderate or severe disease, the aPTT may be prolonged. Other laboratory findings include a prolonged bleeding time, low von Willebrand factor (vWF) activity, and low or normal factor VIII activity.

Von Willebrand disease may be very difficult to distinguish from mild hemophilia A. The bleeding time in hemophilia should be normal, whereas in vWD it is usually prolonged. Factor VIII activity will be low in hemophilia, but may be only mildly decreased or normal in vWD. Von Willebrand factor antigen and factor activity will be normal or elevated in hemophiliacs, but low or normal in patients with vWD

Emergency Department Care and Disposition

The treatment of vWD depends on the type of disease present and the severity of bleeding.

1. Patients with type I vWD are treated with **DDAVP** (0.3 mg/kg SQ or IV).
2. Patients with types II and III vWD are treated with factor-VIII concentrate or cryoprecipitate. Each bag of cryoprecipitate contains

about 100 units of vWF activity. Its use is associated with a small risk of viral transmission.

3. Women are often treated with estrogens or progesterones, which cause an increase in vWF activity.

4. Bleeding associated with dental procedures is often managed with antifibrinolytic agents, such as amicar and tranexamic acid.

For further reading in *Emergency Medicine: A Comprehensive Study Guide*, 4th edition, see Chapter 186, Hemophilias and Von Willebrand Disease, by Mary E. Eberst.

C. Crawford Mechem

Hemolytic anemias can be divided into acquired and hereditary types. Acquired anemias may be antibody-mediated or result from fragmentation, direct toxicity, mechanical injury, or hypersplenism. Hereditary anemias include sickle cell anemia, glucose-6-phosphate dehydrogenase deficiency, and hereditary spherocytosis.

ACQUIRED HEMOLYTIC ANEMIAS

Clinical Features

Antibody-mediated hemolytic anemias include warm and cold antibody types. The warm type is more common in elderly, female patients with underlying medical conditions. In children it may develop after acute infections or immunizations. The presentation ranges from mild anemia and splenomegaly to life-threatening anemia, splenomegaly, pulmonary edema, mental status changes, and venous thromboses.

Cold antibody hemolytic anemia may present as an acute disease in younger people following infections such as *Mycoplasma* pneumonia. Anemia is usually mild. Paroxysmal cold hemoglobinemia is another acute form in patients with untreated syphilis or viral illnesses and presents with fever, chills, hemoglobinuria, and pain in the back, legs, and abdomen. The chronic form is seen in elderly patients with underlying lymphoid neoplasms and involves hemolysis in parts of the body exposed to cold.

Autoimmune hemolytic anemia also can be drug-induced, involving alpha-methyldopa, penicillin, sulfa drugs, and quinidine. Hemolysis ceases after discontinuation of the drug.

Fragmentation hemolysis involves damage to RBCs from passage through artificial heart valves, calcified aortic valves, or through arterioles damaged by thrombotic thrombocytopenia purpura (TTP), hemolytic uremic syndrome (HUS), or pregnancy.

TTP more commonly affects women and presents with fever, neurologic changes, hemorrhage, and renal insufficiency. HUS is a disease of early childhood and presents with fever, acute renal failure, and neurologic deficits following a prodromal infection. Fragmentation hemolysis in pregnancy is seen in pre-eclampsia, eclampsia, and abruption.

Direct toxic effects causing hemolysis may result from infection, copper exposure, and the venoms of bees, wasps, certain spiders, and cobras. Oxidative hemolysis of RBCs results from methemoglobin-producing drugs, such as lidocaine and sulfonamides.

Mechanical damage to RBCs can result in hemolysis and hemoglobinuria. Etiologies include extensive burns and strenuous physical activity. Patients who have been on cardiopulmonary bypass can develop post-perfusion syndrome, with hemolysis, fever, and leukopenia, thought to be due to passage of blood through the oxygenator.

Hypersplenism, as seen in portal hypertension, infiltrative disease, or infections, leads to hemolysis following sequestration and destruction of RBCs in the spleen.

Diagnosis and Differential

CBC will reveal anemia. Patients with TTP may have platelet counts < 20,000/mL. The reticulocyte count is the best indicator of a normal bone marrow in the setting of hemolysis and may be as high as 30% to 40%. The peripheral smear may reveal schistocytes from direct trauma and spherocytes in patients with warm antibody immune hemolysis and hereditary spherocytosis. Other lab abnormalities include an elevated indirect bilirubin and LDH. The direct Coombs test will be positive in patients with immune-mediated hemolysis. The BUN and creatinine will be markedly elevated in HUS. Patients with the HELLP syndrome demonstrate hemolysis, elevated LFTs, and low platelets in the setting of pre-eclampsia.

Emergency Department Care and Disposition

Treatment is directed at stabilization of vital signs and correction of the underlying disease process.

1. Prednisone (1.0 mg/kg per day) is used in the treatment of warm antibody hemolytic anemia and TTP. Azathioprine and cyclophosphamide are sometimes administered, and splenectomy may be required.
2. **Plasma exchange transfusion** is the foundation of therapy for TTP. If unavailable, plasma can be infused while arranging transfer to a tertiary-care center. Platelet transfusions should be avoided because they can aggravate the thrombotic process. Antiplatelet therapy consisting of aspirin or dipyridamole also is initiated.
3. Transfusion of RBCs is indicated for angina, CHF, mental status changes, or hypoxia.
4. Patients with cold antibody hemolytic anemia should be kept in a warm environment.
5. Management of HUS involves early dialysis.
6. Patients with HELLP syndrome are managed with prompt delivery of the infant.
7. Patients with traumatic hemolysis due to artificial heart valves are given iron and folate. If hemolysis is severe, the defective valve may need to be replaced.
8. Methemoglobin levels greater than 20% to 30% of total hemoglobin are treated with methylene blue, (1–2 mg/kg in a 1% solution IV over 5 min).

HEREDITARY HEMOLYTIC ANEMIAS

Sickle-Cell Disease (SSD)

Clinical Features

The presentation is highly variable and can involve virtually every organ system. Patients may have flow murmurs, CHF, cardiomegaly, cor pulmonale, lower extremity ulcerations, icterus, and hepatomegaly. Painful vaso-occlusive crises are the most common reason for ED visits and are precipitated by cold exposure, dehydration, high altitude, and infections, particularly with encapsulated organisms such as *Haemophilus* or *Pneumococcus*. Patients may present with joint, muscle, or bone pain, or diffuse abdominal pain without peritoneal signs.

Pulmonary manifestations include pleuritic chest pain, fever, a sudden decrease in pulmonary function, and hypoxia. Neurologic manifestations include cerebral infarction in children, cerebral hemorrhage in adults, TIA, headache, seizure, and coma. Hematologic crises present with weakness, dyspnea, fatigue, worsening CHF, or shock, in the setting of a precipitous drop in hemoglobin. This may result from splenic sequestration of blood or bone marrow suppression, the socalled aplastic crisis.

Other clinical presentations of SCD include priapism; swelling of the hands or feet due to vaso-occlusion; and infarction of the renal medulla, with flank pain, and hematuria.

Diagnosis and Differential

ED evaluation is guided by the patient's symptoms. CBC should be obtained in most patients with a severe crisis. A drop in hemoglobin by 2 g/dL from the patient's baseline suggests a hematologic crisis or blood loss. A reticulocyte count should be obtained in all such patients. A count less than the baseline of 5% to 15% may reflect aplastic crisis. WBC above baseline, or a left shift, may indicate infection. Electrolytes should be obtained in patients with evidence of dehydration and a urinalysis in patients with urinary symptoms. LFTs are indicated in patients with abdominal pain. Radiology studies may include chest radiograph for patients with pulmonary symptoms, abdominal CT or ultrasound for abdominal pain, head CT or MRI for neurologic complaints, and plain radiographs for patients with focal bone pain.

Differential diagnosis for complaints related to SCD is extensive and includes osteomyelitis, acute arthritides, surgical abdomen, pancreatitis, hepatitis, PID, pyelonephritis, pneumonia, pulmonary embolus, and meningitis.

Emergency Department Care and Disposition

Management is primarily supportive, with close attention to possible precipitants of acute crises.

1. Patients with evidence of dehydration or acute pain should be rehydrated either orally or with IV solutions, such as 0.5 NS at $1\frac{1}{2}$ times maintenance.
2. **Narcotics** should be administered promptly for severe pain. Patients who present to the ED frequently will benefit from a protocol treatment plan.
3. Supplemental oxygen is only necessary when the patient is hypoxic.
4. Cardiac monitoring is appropriate for patients with cardiopulmonary symptoms.
5. Patients with infectious symptoms or a temperature $> 38°C$ should be cultured and given IV antibiotics, generally Cefuroxime or ceftriaxone.
6. Heparinization is indicated in pulmonary crisis with evidence of pulmonary embolus.
7. Exchange transfusion may be indicated in patients with significant cardiopulmonary decompensation, an acute CNS event, or priapism.
8. Priapism is managed with hydration, analgesia, and immediate urologic consultation.
9. Patients with bone pain and the possibility of osteomyelitis should be given antibiotics covering *S. aureus* and *S. typhimurium* after needle aspiration for culture.

Admission criteria include pulmonary, neurologic, aplastic, or infectious crises; splenic sequestration; inadequate pain control; persistent nausea and vomiting; or patients with an uncertain diagnosis. Discharged patients should have a supply of oral analgesics, close followup, and instructions to return at once for fever $>38°C$ or worsening symptoms.

Glucose-6-Phosphate Dehydrogenase (G-6-PD) Deficiency

African-American males are most commonly affected and may present with acute hemolytic crises, hemoglobinuria, and vascular collapse due to infections, exposure to oxidant drugs, metabolic acidosis, and ingestion of fava beans. The diagnosis is made by decreased G-6-PD activity on quantitative assay. There is no specific treatment; prevention involves early treatment of infection and avoidance of oxidant stress.

Hereditary Spherocytosis (HS)

HS is seen in people of northern European descent and is characterized by mild hemolytic anemia, splenomegaly, and intermittent jaundice. Laboratory features include mild anemia, spherocytes on peripheral smear, a normal MCV, and an increased MCHC ($>36\%$). Splenectomy is the treatment of choice.

For further reading in *Emergency Medicine: A Comprehensive Study Guide*, 4th edition, see Chapter 187, Acquired Hemolytic Anemias; and Chapter 188, Hereditary Hemolytic Anemias, by Mary E. Eberst.

126 | Blood Transfusions and Component Therapy

Judith E. Tintinalli

This chapter will review component therapy, immediate and delayed complications of transfusions, emergency transfusion, and massive transfusion.

AVAILABLE BLOOD PRODUCTS

Whole Blood

Whole blood simultaneously provides volume and oxygen-carrying capacity. This is better accomplished by the use of packed red blood cells (PRBCs) and crystalloid solution. Disadvantages to the use of whole-blood transfusion include the following: clotting factors are present in low levels; whole blood often contains elevated levels of potassium, hydrogen ion, and ammonia; the patient is exposed to a large number of antigens; and volume overload can occur before the needed components are replenished. A unit of whole blood contains about 500 mL of blood plus a preservative and anticoagulant, usually CPDA-I (citrate phosphate dextrose adenine).

Packed Red Blood Cells

Each unit of PRBCs transfused should raise the hemoglobin by 1 g/dL or the hematocrit by 3%. The clinical impact of blood loss depends on the underlying cause, the rate of loss, underlying health status, cardiopulmonary reserve, and the activity level of the patient. Major indications for transfusion of PRBCs include:

1. Acute hemorrhage—In otherwise healthy patients, the loss of up to about 1500 mL of blood (about 25% to 30% of the blood volume in a 70-kg person) can be replaced entirely with crystalloid solutions. Blood losses greater than this usually require the transfusion of PRBCs to replace oxygen-carrying capacity and crystalloid solution to replace volume.
2. Surgical blood loss—Most patients will require transfusion of PRBCs and crystalloid when blood loss exceeds 2L.
3. Chronic anemia—Patients with chronic stable anemia may require transfusion of PRBCs if the hemoglobin falls to less than 7 g/dL or if they are symptomatic or have underlying cardiopulmonary disease.

Red blood cells are available as leukocyte-poor, frozen, or washed, when required for certain patients. Leukocyte-poor RBCs have 70% to 85% of the leukocytes removed. They are indicated for transplant recipients, transplant candidates, and in patients who have a history of previous febrile nonhemolytic transfusion reactions. Frozen RBCs can provide a supply of rare blood types, and reduces antigen exposure for transplant candidates. Washed RBCs are used for patients who have hypersensitive reactions to plasma, for neonatal transfusions, and in patients with paroxysmal nocturnal hemoglobinuria.

Platelets

Generally, ABO- and Rh-compatible platelets are given 6 at a time (6–pack), totaling 250 to 350 mL with about 4×10^{11} platelets, and should raise the platelet count by 50,000/mL in an average-sized adult. The post-transfusion platelet count should be checked 1 h and 24 h after platelet infusion. Transfused platelets should survive 3 to 5 days unless there is platelet consumption or refractoriness.

General principles for platelet transfusion in adults include:

1. When the platelet count is above 50,000/mL, excessive bleeding due to thrombocytopenia is unlikely unless there is platelet dysfunction.
2. The platelet count should be maintained at 50,000/mL or greater in patients undergoing major surgery or in those with ongoing bleeding.
3. When the platelet count is between 10,000 and 50,000/mL, there is an increased risk of bleeding with trauma or invasive procedures and an increased spontaneous bleeding risk in those with platelet dysfunction.
4. When the platelet count is below 10,000/mL, there is high risk of spontaneous hemorrhage and platelets should be transfused prophylactically.
5. When the patient has thrombocytopenia due to the presence of anti-platelet antibodies, platelet transfusion is generally futile.

Fresh-frozen Plasma (FFP)

Each bag of FFP contains 200 to 250 mL and, by definition, contains 1 unit of each coagulation factor per milliliter of FFP and 1 to 2 mg of fibrinogen per milliliter of FFP. Transfused FFP should be ABO-compatible. The desired dose to be transfused can be estimated from the plasma volume and the desired incremental increase in factor activity. A typical starting dose is 8 to 10 mL/kg, or approximately 2 bags of FFP. After infusion, the patient should be re-evaluated for clinical bleeding and post-transfusion coagulation studies obtained. The indications for transfusion of FFP are as follows:

1. Acquired factor(s) deficiency from liver disease, warfarin, or DIC, with active bleeding or prior to invasive procedures 1.5x prolongation of the prothrombin time (PT) or activated partial thromboplastin time (aPTT), or a specific coagulation factor assay less than 25% of normal.
2. Patients with congenital isolated factor deficiencies when specific virally safe replacement products are not available; those with iso-

lated deficiencies of fibrinogen, factor VIII, or factor XIII are probably better treated with cryoprecipitate.
3. Patients with thrombotic thrombocytopenic purpura (TTP) in the process of plasma exchange.
4. Some patients who receive massive transfusion and have evidence of a coagulapathy and active bleeding.
5. Patients with antithrombin-III deficiency, when antithrombin III concentrates are not available. FFP is *not* indicated for patients who require volume expansion.

Cryoprecipitate

Cryoprecipitate is the cold precipitable protein fraction derived from FFP. It contains about 100 units of Factor VIII-C; 80 units of von Willebrand Factor; 250 mg of fibrinogen; and 50 units of Factor XIII. The typical dose of ABO-compatible cryoprecipitate given is 2 to 4 bags per 10 kg usually 10 to 20 bags at a time. The indications for transfusion of cryoprecipitate are as follows:

1. Fibrinogen level less than 100 mg/dL.
2. Patients with von Willebrand disease and active bleeding, when desmopressin (DDAVP) is not available or does not work and factor-VIII concentrates containing von Willebrand factor are not available.
3. Patients with hemophilia A, only when virally-inactivated factor VIII concentrates are not available.
4. Use as fibrin-glue surgical adhesives.
5. Fibronectin replacement.

Albumin

Albumin replacement products are available as 5% or 25% solutions in saline. Plasma protein fraction (PPF) is a similar product; it is a 5% solution containing 88% albumin and 12% globulins. These products are not known to transmit viral disease. The clinical indications for albumin infusion are controversial, and its use is becoming less common.

Antithrombin III (ATIII)

Antithrombin III is a serum protein that inhibits coagulation factors, activated factor II (thrombin), and activated factors IX, X, XI, and XII. Deficiency of ATIII can be congenital or acquired. Its main use is for patients with hereditary deficiency of ATIII with acute thromboembolism or the prophylaxis of thrombosis in these patients.

COMPLICATIONS OF TRANSFUSIONS

Up to 20% of all transfusions may lead to some type of adverse reaction, but most are mild. Transfusion reactions can be immediate or delayed.

TABLE 126-1. ABO Blood Group System Compatibility

Phenotype	Antigens on RBCs	Antibodies in serum	Can receive blood type
A	A	Anti-B	A, O
B	B	Anti-A	B, O
AB	A and B	None	A, B, O
O	None	Anti-A; anti-B	O

The detection of delayed complications is important because outpatient transfusion therapy is becoming more common.

Immediate Transfusion Reactions

1. Acute Hemolytic Transfusion Reactions—An acute hemolytic reaction occurs when the incompatible donor transfused cells are immediately destroyed by host antibodies (Table 126-1).

   Symptoms include fever, chills, low back pain, breathlessness, or a burning sensation at the site of infusion. If the reaction progresses, the patient may develop hypotension, bleeding, respiratory failure, and acute tubular necrosis. Treatment is the immediate discontinuation of the transfusion, and hydration and furosemide to urine output at 100 mL/hr for 24 h. The donor unit should be sent to the blood bank, and a host blood sample sent for free hemoglobin, haptoglobin, bilirubin, direct and indirect Coombs test, CBC, renal and coagulation studies.

2. Febrile Nonhemolytic Transfusion Reaction—During the transfusion or within a few hours, the patient develops fever and chills, usually because of an antigen–antibody reaction involving plasma, platelets, or WBCs that are passively transfused to the recipient along with the RBCs. The first step is to stop the transfusion. Clinically, it is important to distinguish initially between a febrile nonhemolytic reaction and an acute hemolytic transfusion reaction. Thus, management includes serologic evaluation, hydration, and diuresis and, possibly, treatment of suspected injection. Patients with a known history of febrile reactions can be pretreated with acetaminophen or aspirin and meperidine or be given leukocyte-depleted blood components.

3. Allergic Transfusion Reaction—Allergic reactions are felt to be due to exposure to plasma proteins. Typical symptoms are skin erythema, urticaria, pruritus, bronchospasm, vasomotor instability and, rarely, anaphylaxis. When an apparent allergic transfusion reaction occurs, the infusion should be discontinued while the patient is evaluated and treated with diphenhydramine. If the patient improves with this therapy, the transfusion can be restarted. Some clinicians routinely premedicate patients who have a history of allergic transfusion reactions.

Delayed Reactions

1. Infections—Although small, the risk of disease transmission from blood products is still present for HIV, Hepatitis B and C, HTLVI/II, and CMV. Rarer still is the transmission of EBV, syphilis, malaria, babesiosis, toxoplasmosis, and trypanosomiasis.

2. Delayed Hemolytic Reaction—This reaction occurs 7 to 10 days after transfusion as a result of an antigen–antibody reaction that develops after the transfusion. Laboratory studies reflect a slowly falling hemoglobin, and a previously negative Coombs test becomes positive.

3. Hypervolemia—Transfusion results in the rapid expansion of intravascular volume. Such expansion may not be well tolerated by patients with limited cardiovascular reserve, infants, and the elderly. Patients may complain of headaches and shortness of breath; on examination, they will have signs of CHF. Treatment consists of slowing the rate of infusion and diuresis.

4. Hypothermia—Hypothermia may develop in patients who receive rapid infusion of large quantities of refrigerated blood. This is generally only a problem if three or more units are given rapidly. PRBCs are stored at 4 C, platelets at 20 to 24 C, and FFP at -18 C. Electric blood warmers may be used but should not raise the temperature to more than 40°C or hemolysis can occur. The easiest method for warming blood is to infuse it along with warmed (39 to 43 C) normal saline, which will warm and dilute the blood.

5. Noncardiogenic Pulmonary Edema—Noncardiogenic pulmonary edema is rare, and is thought to be due to incompatibility of passively transferred leukocyte antibodies. Clinically, the patient develops respiratory distress, fever, chills, and tachycardia within four hours, and a chest radiograph shows diffuse patchy infiltrates without cardiomegaly. There is no evidence of fluid overload. The pulmonary infiltrates resolve over a few days and supportive care is needed.

6. Electrolyte Imbalance—Citrate is a component of the preservative solution and functions as an anticoagulant by chelating calcium. Significant hypocalcemia is rare because patients with normal hepatic function metabolize citrate to bicarbonate. Even with massive transfusion, calcium replacement is rarely needed. Hypokalemia can develop when citrate is metabolized to bicarbonate. The blood becomes alkalotic, and potassium is driven intracellularly. Hyperkalemia is rare, even though potassium increases in stored blood.

EMERGENCY TRANSFUSIONS

While the administration of type-O blood or type-specific, incompletely crossmatched blood may be life-saving, its use is limited to the early resuscitation from hemorrhagic shock. Whenever possible, ABO group and Rh-type specific blood should be given. Typing can be done in 10 to 15 min. Fully crossmatched blood can typically be obtained in 30 to 60 min. Most hospitals use Rh-negative blood when it has not been fully crossmatched. PRBCs are the only blood product that can be given for emergency transfusion. Plasma products contain too many antibodies. Subsequent crossmatching will become more difficult as increasing amounts of uncrossmatched blood are transfused.

Blood products are generally infused through large-bore IV tubing (16-gauge or greater) to prevent hemolysis and to permit rapid infusion. Normal saline is the only crystalloid fluid compatible with PRBCs. If multiple units of blood are to be given or are being given rapidly, warmed saline can be given concurrently (warmed to 39°–43°C) or the blood itself can be warmed in an electric blood warmer. Blood will hemolyze if warmed to more than 40°C. Except in emergency settings, the infusion of blood is started slowly over the first 30 min, when reactions are most likely to occur. Patients without cardiovascular disease can be given a unit of PRBCs over 1 to 2 h. Those with a risk of hypervolemia should receive each unit over 3 to 4 h. Micropore filters should be used when giving any blood product in order to filter microaggregates of platelets, fibrin, and leukocytes. Rapid infusion of blood in the emergency setting may be facilitated by the use of pressure infusion devices that apply pneumatic pressure (up to 300 mmHg) to the blood unit.

MASSIVE TRANSFUSION

Massive transfusion is defined as the replacement of a volume equivalent to the patient's normal blood volume within a 24–h period. Potential complications of this procedure are bleeding, citrate toxicity, and hypothermia. Bleeding is the most frequent complication and is related to platelet and factor deficiencies. Actual thrombocytopenia does not regularly occur in this setting because even after the replacement of one blood volume, most patients still have about 35% to 40% of their original platelet count, about 100,000/mL. Bleeding is due to mild thrombocytopenia combined with platelet dysfunction from renal or liver disease, DIC, and coagulation factor deficiencies. Coagulation factor deficiencies can develop because stored blood has low levels of coagulation factors, especially factors V and VIII. The coagulopathy may be worsened by hypothermia, shock, sepsis, underlying liver disease, or DIC. In current practice, the routine use of platelet transfusions and FFP in massive transfusion is unwarranted, costly, and dangerous. Platelet transfusions should be given only if there is thrombocytopenia with oozing or excess bleeding. FFP should be given only when there is documented coagulopathy and bleeding.

Citrate toxicity is rarely a problem in modern blood banking unless whole blood is being transfused. Patients receiving more than 5 units of whole blood, neonates, or patients with liver disease are at risk of hypocalcemia. An ionized calcium level should be obtained. The QT interval is not a reliable indicator of hypocalcemia in this setting. If calcium needs to be repleted, 5 to 10 mL of calcium gluconate given slowly IV is recommended.

For further reading in *Emergency Medicine: A Comprehensive Study Guide*, 4th edition, see Chapter 189, Blood Transfusions and Component Therapy, by Mary Eberst.

Emergency Complications of Malignancy

Judith E. Tintinalli

Patients with malignancy can develop the same medical emergencies as the general population. However, the presence of localized or metastatic disease, or the myelosuppressive effects of chemotherapy, can cause unique problems.

ACUTE SPINAL CORD COMPRESSION

Clinical Features

Spinal cord compression can result from bleeding, infection, or fracture. It is generally suspected in individuals with previously documented malignancy who develop paraparesis, paraplegia, sensory deficits, urinary incontinence, or acute urinary retention. All patients with acute urinary retention should have a careful neurologic examination, including assessment of reflexes, motor and sensory function, rectal sphincter tone, and gait, to rule out spinal cord compression. Pain localized to involve vertebrae may be present and intensified by local percussion during the physical examination. As is often the case in lymphomas, however, if lytic bony lesions are not present, local pain is absent and the patient may have only a sensory-level or distal flaccid paralysis. Hypoesthesia, lower extremity weakness, or gait disturbance are early symptoms and should alert the ED physician.

Emergency Department Care and Disposition

Early treatment may avert progression to paraplegia and prevent sphincter loss. Management includes assessment of fluid status, clotting parameters, anemia, cardiorespiratory systems, and expeditious neurologic consultation. MRI scanning of the thoracolumbar spine can demonstrate the level of compression. **Decadron** (10 mg IV) or **Solumedrol** (30 mg/kg IV), as recommended for acute traumatic spinal cord injury, should be given. Emergency surgical decompression or emergency radiotherapy is necessary to prevent irreversible neural damage.

UPPER AIRWAY OBSTRUCTION

Clinical Features

Malignancy-related obstruction to airflow is usually insidious and often attended by voice change. This is generally a late manifestation of tumors arising in the oropharynx, neck, and superior mediastinum. Acute compromise is uncommon unless infection, hemorrhage, or inspissated secretions supervene. Rapidly growing tumors such as Burkitt lymphoma and anaplastic carcinoma of the thyroid are capable of compromising airflow within weeks and should be suspected in afebrile individuals with laryngeal stridor and palpable anterior neck masses.

Emergency Department Care and Disposition

The emergency physician must rapidly assess the patency of the patient's airway. **Orotracheal intubation** or **cricothyroidotomy** should be performed in the patient who is in respiratory distress or who has impending compromised airway. Urgent otolaryrgologic surgery consultation is necessary to establish a definitive surgical airway in the controlled environment of the OR.

MALIGNANT PERICARDIAL EFFUSION

Clinical Features

Malignant pericardial effusion can result from tumor invasion, infection, secondary hemorrhage, or from chemotherapeutic agents. The hemodynamic consequences of malignant pericardial effusions are a function of the volume and speed of accumulation. Even collections greater than 500 mL may be well-tolerated if development is slow. Sudden intrapericardial bleeding is associated with dyspnea, chest pain, and hypotension. If the myocardium is also involved with metastatic disease, cardiac dysfunction will result in a decrease in cardiac output as well.

The classic clinical features of cardiac tamponade are (1) hypotension and a narrowed pulse pressure; (2) jugular venous distension; (3) diminished heart sounds; (4) pulsus paradoxus greater than 10 mmHg; (5) low QRS voltage; and (6) cardiomegaly without evidence of congestive heart failure on chest x-ray. Diagnosis is confirmed by echocardiography.

Emergency Department Care and Disposition

Emergency percutaneous **pericardiocentesis** may be lifesaving. It can be done blindly or under fluoroscopic guidance. Definitive treatment consists of pericardiectomy, establishment of a pericardial window, radiation, or intrapericardial chemotherapy.

SUPERIOR VENA CAVA SYNDROME

Clinical Features

Obstruction to blood flow in the superior vena cava elevates venous pressure in the arms, neck, face, and cerebrum. Patients with moderate obstruction complain of headache, edema of the face and arms, or a nondescript feeling of head congestion and fullness in the neck and face. As venous pressure rises, intracranial pressure also rises and syncope may ensue. Critical intracranial pressure elevations are a true

medical emergency and are usually associated with bilateral papilledema.

On physical exam, neck vein and upper chest vein distension may
be apparent. Facial plethora and telangiectasia often are prominent,
but edema of the face and arms is generally subtle. Papilledema on
fundoscopic exam indicates critical intracranial pressure and justifies
early diuretic therapy. When tumefaction is located in the superior
mediastinum, a palpable mass due to direct tumor extension can occasionally be appreciated in the supraclavicular space. Chest x-ray will
demonstrate an enlarged mediastinum and, possibly, an isolated primary
lesion in the lung parenchyma.

Emergency Department Care and Disposition

Furosemide (Lasix), 40 mg IV, and methylprednisolone (Solumedrol),
80 to 120 mg IV, should be given to reduce intracerebral edema.
Radiotherapy to improve cardiodynamics is frequently necessary before
tissue diagnosis can be obtained.

HYPERCALCEMIA OF MALIGNANCY

Clinical Features

When serum calcium levels rise rapidly or exceed ionic thresholds,
cardiac, neural, and muscular electrophysiology may be greatly altered,
and sudden death can occur. Hypercalcemia from any cause may induce
hypertension, constipation, and an altered sensorium. Elevated ionic
(nonbound) calcium is responsible for neuromuscular dysfunction and,
therefore, serum calcium levels should be interpreted in concert with
phosphorous, serum albumin, and blood pH determinations. The Q-T
interval of the ECG may shorten as the serum calcium rises.

Emergency Department Care and Disposition

The majority of patients will improve with **saline infusion and IV
furosemide** (1–2 L saline load and 80 mg of IV furosemide), as long
as renal function is adequate. For severe hypercalcemia or in the presence of renal failure, hemodialysis or peritoneal dialysis against a low-
or no-calcium dialysate may be necessary. The use of IV inorganic
phosphate is controversial because of the associated adverse effects.
Serum calcium may fall within min and decline in calcium levels may
continue for several days. Oral phosphate, given as 1-g of sodium
acid phosphate daily, produces maximum effect after several days.
Glucocorticoids can be given empirically in comatose or obtunded
patients with serum calcium levels greater than 13 mg/dL. The dose is
100 mg of prednisone or equivalent, but the hypocalcemic effect takes
several days to develop. **Mithramycin** acts by inhibiting bone resorp-

tion. The dose is 25 mg/kg delivered as IV infusion. Its effect is usually evident in 24 to 48 h.

SYNDROME OF INAPPROPRIATE ADH

Clinical Features

Ectopic secretion of antidiuretic hormone (ADH) may come from a variety of malignancies, but in any case the end result is the syndrome of inappropriate ADH (SIADH), which consists of serum hyponatremia, less than maximally dilute urine, excessive urine Na excretion (> 30 mEq/L), and normal renal, adrenal, and thyroid functions.

Emergency Department Care and Disposition

Treatment is aimed at removing the source of ADH secretion. **Water restriction** usually raises the serum sodium over a period of several days. The intravenous infusion of 100 to 250 mL of **hypertonic saline solution** (3%) may be necessary in the face of hyponatremic-induced seizures.

HYPERVISCOSITY SYNDROME

Clinical Features

Fatigue, headache, anorexia, and somnolence are early nonspecific symptoms. Microthromboses may occur, with the advent of local symptoms, such as deafness, visual disturbances, and seizures. The most readily appreciated physical findings are in the ocular fundi and include sausage-linked retinal vessels, hemorrhages, and exudates. Lab evaluation should include coagulation, renal, and electrolyte profiles. Rouleaux may be seen on peripheral blood smear. Hypercalcemia can develop, and when M-component protein concentrations are high, factitious hyponatremia may also be present. A clue to the presence of hyperviscosity may be the laboratory's inability to perform chemical tests because of the serum stasis in the analyzers, undoubtedly due to *too thick* blood.

Emergency Department Care and Disposition

Initial therapy is rehydration followed by emergency plasmapheresis. When coma is present and the diagnosis is rapidly established, a temporizing measure may be a two-unit **phlebotomy** with saline infusion and replacement of the patient's red cells.

ADRENAL INSUFFICIENCY AND SHOCK

Clinical Features

Adrenal insufficiency may be related to adrenal gland replacement by metastic tumors or to adrenocortical suppression by therapeutic glucocorticoid administration. In either case, maximal adrenal function may be inadequate to support the individual when stressed by infection, dehydration, surgery, or trauma.

Emergency Department Care and Disposition

Adrenal crisis is less common than bleeding and sepsis, but the steroid-dependent patient should be empirically given IV glucocorticoids. The initial dose of **hydrocortisone** (Solucortef) is 250 to 500 mg intravenously.

GRANULOCYTOPENIA, IMMUNOSUPPRESSION, AND INFECTION

Clinical Features

Overwhelming infection is a common cause of death in the immunocompromised host. Both the frequency of infection and the mortality rate increase significantly when the circulating granulocyte pool is below 1000 to 1500 per cubic mm. Cancer patients are at risk for a variety of bacterial, viral, and fungal infections. Frequently encountered infections include pneumococcal sepsis and pneumonia; *Staphylococcus aureus* infection; enteric gram-negative pneumonia or sepsis, including *Pseudomonas* infections; and localized or disseminated varicella zoster viral and cytomegaloviral infections. Opportunistic infections include *Pneumocystis carinii* pneumonia (protozoal), disseminated candidiasis, aspergillosis, cryptococcal meningitis, pulmonary nocardiosis, and histoplasmosis.

Emergency Department Care and Disposition

For fever in the presence of malignancy or a history of chills and rigor, assume an infectious etiology and initiate appropriate lab studies and cultures. Life-threatening gram-negative sepsis with hypotension should be aggressively treated after appropriate cultures. **Fluids, broad-spectrum antibiotics,** and intravenous glucocorticoids are advised. Few bacterial organisms would be missed with regimens containing a second- or third-generation cephalosporin (cefazolin, cefoxitin, cefoperazone, cefotaxime) and an aminoglycoside (gentamicin, tobramycin, amikacin). Anaerobic coverage may be added (clindamycin) if peritonitis or abdominal symptomatology exists. Other choices include piperacillin/lazobactam (3.375 g IV q 6 h) or ampicillin/sulbactam (3.0 g IV q 6 h), or ticarcillin clavulanate (3.1 g IV q 6 h).

HEMATOLOGIC SYNDROMES

Clinical Features

Thromboembolism is not uncommon in cancer patients and is due to a number of factors such as a hypercoagulable state; decreased proteins

C, S, and antithrombin III; and the effect of metastases on activation of the coagulation pathway. Cancer patients are at increased risk for both deep venous thrombosis and pulmonary embolism. Anticoagulation may result in bleeding at sites of metastatic disease, however, so that treatment options are more complex and may include placement of a filter in the inferior vena cava.

Polycythemia is enhanced production of red cells due to increases in sensitivity of erythropoietin. Any organ system can be affected by resultant thrombosis, bleeding, or hyperviscosity, but CNS affects are the most devastating. Celiac or mesenteric vessel ischemia or Budd–Chiari syndrome are is seen when GI vessels are involved. If the hematocrit is > 60% and symptoms are present, emergency phlebotomy is necessary.

Either acute or chronic leukemias can result in WBC counts > 100,000 per mL. A leukocrit of > 10% is often associated with clinically significant hyperviscosity, and CNS dysfunction and respiratory distress can occur from capillary leukostasis.

Emergency Department Care and Disposition

Diuretics worsen symptoms because they will increase the leukocrit. Treatment is directed at the underlying malignancy, and allopurinol should also be administered in anticipation of massive tumor lysis to prevent acute gouty arthropathy.

For further reading in *Emergency Medicine: A Comprehensive Study Guide*, 4th edition, see Chapter 190, Emergency Complications of Malignancy, by Mary Eberst.

Kent N. Hall

HEADACHE

Headache is a ubiquitous complaint, with 40% of Americans suffering from significant headache at some time, 10% seeking care from a physician for headache, and 23 million suffering from migraine headaches. Headache pain can arise from extracranial or intracranial structures; the brain parenchyma, most of the dura, arachnoid, and pia cannot produce pain.

Clinical Features

Clinical features of headache depend on the cause. Migraine headaches can occur with or without aura, the latter being more common. Table 128-1 lists the criteria to be met for an individual headache to be classified as a migraine headache. Because migraine headaches are recurrent phenomena, the patient must have at least 2 attacks before the diagnosis of migraine with aura is made, 5 before the diagnosis of migraine without aura is made. Factors that may precipitate a migraine headache in susceptible people are listed in Table 128-2.

TABLE 128-1. Diagnosis of Migraine Headache

For a headache to be classified as a migraine headache, the following must be present: Duration of 4–72 h (without treatment), and at least 2 of the following:
 Unilateral position
 Pulsating quality
 Moderate or severe intensity (inhibits or prohibits daily activities)
 Aggravation by walking stairs or similar routine physical activity
And at least one of the following:
 Nausea, vomiting, or both
 Photophobia and phonophobia

In addition, to be classified as a migraine with aura, the following must be satisfied:
 One or more fully reversible aura symptoms indicating brain dysfunction
 At least one aura symptom developing gradually over more than min, or 2 or more symptoms in succession
 No single aura symptoms lasts more than 60 min
 Headache follows aura with a free interval of less than 60 min

Cluster headache is relatively uncommon, predominantly affects men, and has its onset in the late 20's. It is an episodic headache, occurring more frequently in spring and autumn. There is no associated aura, peak pain occurs 10 to 15 min after onset and lasts 45 to 60 min. Pain is unilateral (often felt behind the eye and in the temple), excruciating, penetrating, and non-throbbing. Associated findings include ipsilateral

TABLE 128-2. Factors Known to Provoke Migraine Headaches

Changes in the body's internal milieu
  Menstruation, sleep disturbances (too little and too much), fasting
Foods
  Alcoholic beverages, chocolate, hard cheeses, herring, citrus fruits,
  processed meats, monosodium glutamate, caffeine
Medications
  Contraceptive estrogens, nitroglycerin

lacrimation, conjunctival injection, and nasal stuffiness or rhinorrhea. Ptosis and miosis may occur. Attacks tend to be nocturnal, often occurring at a particular time. Alcohol, nitroglycerin, and histamine may trigger an attack.

Tension-type headache is the most common type of headache. To be diagnosed as a tension-type headache, at least two of the following should be present: (1) pressing/tightness quality; (2) mild or moderate intensity; (3) bilateral location; (4) no aggravation by mild physical activity. Associated symptoms include anorexia, photophobia, and phonophobia. Nausea or vomiting are rare; pain usually progresses throughout the day.

Postlumbar puncture headache occurs in 5% to 30% of patients receiving a lumbar puncture. It occurs within hours of the procedures, lasts 1 to 2 days, is bicranial, pulsatile, and is exacerbated by the upright position. Usually the pain is cervical and suboccipital in location.

Diagnosis and Differential

The most important tool in making the diagnosis in the patient with headache is the history. The differential diagnosis of the patient with headache is seen in Table 128-3, along with associated historical and physical findings. A thorough physical exam, especially the neurologic examination, can rule out significant underlying pathology in the majority of patients with headache. Areas to concentrate on include the fundoscopic exam, palpation of the temporal region, sinuses, teeth, and distribution of the fifth cranial nerve, stiffness of the neck, and unilateral drift in an outstretched, supinated arm.

Ancillary tests are required only if the diagnosis of a benign condition causing the headache cannot be made with the history and physical exam. When the diagnosis is unclear, a computed tomography (CT) scan is indicated. Lumbar puncture is necessary to identify small subarachnoid hemorrhages and intracranial infections. Further lab tests may be indicated depending on the clinical differential diagnosis (i.e., ESR in possible temporal arteritis)

Emergency Department Care and Disposition

Care of the patient with migraine headache consists of general comfort measures, abortive medications, and prophylactic therapy. General com-

TABLE 128-3. Differential Diagnosis of the Patient With Headache

Type of headache	History/physical findings
Migraine headache	Young at onset; lasts longer than 60 min; unilateral, pulsating, throbbing; +/- visual aura; nausea and vomiting; precipitated by foods, drugs, alcohol, exercise or orgasm; + family history
Cluster headache	Onset in 20s; predominantly male; brief episodes of pain (45–60 min); orbital/retro-orbital pain; periodic and seasonal (spring/autumn); nasal congestion and conjunctival injection/tearing associated; − family history
Tension-type headache	Onset at any age; dull, nagging, persistent pain; progressively worse throughout day
Subarachnoid headache	Sudden onset, *worst headache ever*; loss of consciousness; meningismus; vomiting
Hypertensive headache	Throbbing, occipital
Meningitis	Entire head; fever; meningismus
Mass lesions	
Subdural hematoma	Depressed mental status; variable quality headache
Epidural hematoma	History of trauma, consciousness with headache followed by unconsciousness; fracture across groove of middle meningeal artery
Brain tumor	Pain on awakening or with valsalva; new headache associated with nausea or vomiting
Brain abscess	Findings similar to those of mass lesions; fever
Sinusitis	Stabbing or aching pain, worse by bending or coughing, decreased in supine position
Toxic/metabolic headache	Bicranial; headache remits after removal from offending agent/environment
Postconcussion headache	History of trauma within h to days; vertigo, nausea, vomiting, mood alterations, concentration difficulty associated
Pseudotumor cerebri	Obese, young female; irregular menstrual cycles/amenorrhea; papilledema; slit ventricles on CT
Acute glaucoma	Nausea, vomiting, orbital pain; Edematous/cloudy cornea; mid-position pupil; conjunctival injection; increased intraocular pressure

TABLE 128-4. Agents Used in the ED Management of Migraine Headache

Agent	Route	Considerations
Ergotamine	Inhalation, rectal	Contraindicated in coronary artery disease, hypertension, pregnancy
Chlorpromazine	0.1 mg/kg IV	May cause extrapyramidal effects, excellent antiemetic
Prochlorperazine	10 mg IV	May cause extrapyramidal effects, excellent antiemetic
Metoclopramide	10–20 mg IV	May cause extrapyramidal effects, excellent antiemetic
DHE	0.75–1.0 mg IV over 2 min	Contraindicated in coronary artery disease, hypertension, pregnancy
Sumatriptan	6 mg SQ	Contraindicated in coronary artery disease, hypertension, pregnancy
Ketoralac	60 mg IM	Moderately effective only

fort measures include placing the patient in a darkened, quiet room and providing a cool, damp cloth for the forehead.

Abortive medications used in the treatment of the patient with migraine headache include ergotamine, **phenothiazine derivatives,** and serotonin agonists, such as dihydroergotamine mesylate **(DHE),** and **sumatriptan.** Doses and considerations in the use of these agents are seen in Table 128-4. For cluster headaches, inhaled **oxygen** at 5 to 8 L/min for 10 min may be effective in up to 70% of patients, as is 4% intranasal lidocaine in the ipsilateral nostril. Tension headaches usually require only mild analgesics (acetaminophen, aspirin, and other NSAIDs). The best treatment of postlumbar puncture headache is preventive. Patients should avoid lifting for 3 days. Successful medications include simple analgesics, narcotic analgesics, ergots, barbiturates, and caffeine. If these fail, epidural blood patch can be placed.

Discharge instructions should include avoidance of use of machinary or driving for patients who have received mentation-altering medications. Referral to a primary care physician is important, as headache is often a chronic problem requiring ongoing care not best delivered in the ED. Discharge with combination analgesics that combine different mechanisms of action, thus leading to a lower dose of both analgesics is recommended. These include acetaminophen or aspirin plus butalbital, with or without caffeine. This combination is also available with or without codeine. Ergotamine is available sublingually, if not contraindicated.

If Standard Treatment Fails

Admission for management of pain associated with headache is rare. Reasonable indications for admission include:

1. Migraine lasting for days associated with vomiting and dehydration.
2. Headache complicated by overuse of abortive medications.
3. Chronic headache unresponsive to outpatient therapy.
4. Headache secondary to suspected intracranial pathology (SAH, tumor, meningitis).
5. Underlying significant medical or surgical pathology.
6. Intractable cluster headache.
7. Headache that significantly interferes with activities of daily living.

FACIAL PAIN

Temporal Arteritis

Temporal arteritis is a vasculitis affecting branches of the external carotid artery. Women are affected 4 times more frequently than men. It occurs in people over 50 years old, and is often associated with polymyalgia rheumatica. The pain is usually unilateral and has a piercing or burning quality, which is often worse at night. The artery is tender. Systemic signs and symptoms are often present and include fever, malaise, weight loss, anorexia, diploplia, blurred vision, and polymyalgia. Differential diagnosis includes other causes of headache mentioned above. This condition is distinguished by tenderness over the involved artery, elevated ESR (usually > 50 mm/hr), and the frequently associated systemic signs and symptoms. Biopsy of the artery is diagnostic. Emergency treatment includes prednisone at a dose of 60 to 80 mg/d to prevent blindness secondary to ischemic papillitis. NSAIDs are beneficial in relieving associated pain. Close followup is required and should be arranged prior to discharge from the ED. Prednisone can be vision-saving, even if the patient has already lost vision in the ipsilateral eye, as 75% of patients will lose vision in the contralateral eye in 1 to 20 days without this therapy.

Trigeminal Neuralgia

Trigeminal neuralgia is characterized by brief, intermittent pain that often has an *electric* quality. It rarely occurs before the 5th decade of life, and women are affected slightly more often than men. Less than 4% of cases occur bilaterally, and the right side of the face predominates. The V1 segment is rarely affected. Inciting maneuvers include eating, talking, washing the face, or applying cosmetics. The most sensitive areas are the ala nasi, the lower lip of one of the molar or premolar teeth, or the central or medial portion of the eyebrow. Conditions included in the differential diagnosis include postherpetic neuralgia, dental and maxillary sinus problems, cluster headaches, and atypical facial pain. History provides the key to diagnosis. The physical exam, including the neurologic examination are normal. ED treatment with parenteral narcotic analgesics is usually required. Discharge instructions should include close followup with the primary care physician. Chronic medications used for pain control include carbamazepine, phenytoin, and baclofen, alone or in combination.

Temporomandibular Joint Syndrome (TMJ)

Patients with TMJ present with unilateral or bilateral pain in the TMJ. The area may be tender to palpation and clicking or sticking of the joint with limitation of opening of the mouth may be seen. Deviation of the mandible to the affected may be present, as may a sense of fullness, popping, and tinnitus in the ear. Differential diagnosis includes temporal arteritis, trigeminal neuralgia, cluster headache, and pain of dental origin. The history and physical examination should effectively exclude these diagnoses. Treatment with NSAIDs, with appropriate referral to a dentist or oral surgeon at the time of discharge from the ED, is usually all that is required. Definitive treatment consists of occlusal splint or bite guard.

For further reading in *Emergency Medicine: A Comprehensive Study Guide*, 4th edition, see Chapter 192, Headache and Facial Pain, by Gwendolyn L. Hoffman.

Stroke is the third leading cause of death and is a major cause of disability in the U.S. It affects 500,000 Americans annually and costs $20 billion a year in medical costs and lost wages.

Clinical Features

There are two main mechanisms of stroke: (1) blood-vessel occlusion leading to neuronal ischemia and death (85% of all strokes); and (2) blood-vessel rupture leading to hemorrhage, direct cell trauma, mass effect, elevated intracranial pressure and release of biochemical toxins (15% of all strokes).

Ischemic strokes are most often caused by large-vessel thrombosis, although they can also be caused by embolism or hypoperfusion. Causes of thrombosis include atherosclerotic disease, vasculitis, dissection, polycythemia, hypercoagulable states, and infectious diseases (syphilis, trichinosis). Common sources of emboli in embolic strokes are the heart (valvular vegetations, mural thrombi, paradoxical emboli, cardiac tumor) and major vessels.

Hemorrhagic strokes have a 30-day mortality of 30% to 50%, occur in a younger patient population than ischemic strokes, and are divided into intracerebral (ICH) and subarachnoid (SAH) hemorrhages. Risk factors for an ICH include hypertension, older age, and prior stroke. Bleeding diathesis, vascular malformations, and cocaine use can cause ICH. Subarachnoid hemorrhages are due to berry aneurysm rupture and arteriovenous malformations.

Diagnosis and Differential

In obtaining a history, it is important to ask if there is any recent history of TIA-like symptoms. Aspects of the stroke itself, including timing of onset, presence of headache, nausea, vomiting, and recent neck trauma are important.

Physical exam should include a general physical examination and a neurologic examination. The general exam should look for underlying causes (infections, signs of embolization). It includes a complete evaluation of skin, fundi, heart, and lungs.

Neurologic exam is done to assess the patient's baseline level of function and to localize the brain lesion. Six areas of the neurologic examination are: (1) level of consciousness, (2) visual assessment, (3) motor function, (4) sensation and neglect, (5) cerebellar function, and (6) cranial nerves. These are incorporated into the NIH stroke scale, and are used to monitor the patient's progress over time.

Integration of information from the history and physical exam allows the physician to determine the area of brain involvement. Specific stroke

693

TABLE 129-1. Stroke Syndromes

Ischemic Stroke Syndromes
   Dominant hemispheric infarction—contralateral weakness/numbness, contralateral visual field cut, gaze preference, dysarthria, aphasia
   Nondominant hemispheric infarction—contralateral weakness/numbness, visual field cut, constructional apraxia, dysarthria
   Middle cerebral artery infarcts—contralateral weakness/numbness (arm/face more than leg)
   Anterior cerebral artery infarcts—contralateral weakness/numbness (leg more than arm), dyspraxia
   Vertebrobasilar syndrome—dizziness, vertigo, diplopia, dysphagia, ataxia, cranial nerve palsies, bilateral limb weakness, crossed neurologic deficits
   Basilar artery occlusion—quadriplegia, coma, locked-in syndrome
   Transient ischemic attach (TIA)—resolves within 24 h, 5% to 6% risk of stroke per yr
   Lacunar infarct—pure motor or sensory deficits
Hemorrhagic Syndromes
   Intracerebral hemorrhage—similar to cerebral infarction with lethargy, headache, nausea, vomiting
   Cerebellar hemorrhage—dizziness, vomiting, truncal ataxia, inability to walk, rapidly progress to coma, herniation, and death
   Subarachnoid hemorrhage—severe headache, vomiting, decreased LOC

syndromes are seen in Table 129-1. Table 129-2 lists the differential diagnosis of patients with stroke syndromes.

Emergency Department Care and Disposition

Diagnostic tests that should be immediately obtained include a blood sugar, head CT, and ECG. Other tests that may be helpful include a CBC, coagulation studies, toxic screen, and cardiac enzymes.

There are few proven treatment modalities for patients with stroke. The patient should be placed on oxygen and a cardiac monitor, the head of the bed should be slightly elevated, and IV access should be

TABLE 129-2. Differential Diagnosis of Acute Stroke

Hypoglycemia
Postictal paralysis (Todd paralysis)
Bell's palsy
Hypertensive encephalopathy
Epidural/subdural hematoma
Brain tumor/abscess
Complicated migraine
Encephalitis
Diabetic ketoacidosis
Hyperosmotic coma
Meningoencephalitis

secured. Assess and manage the hydration status of the patient carefully. Dehydration can result in decreased perfusion of areas around the infarction. Overhydration can cause cerebral edema and increased neuronal damage. **Avoid glucose containing solutions** because of increased neuronal damage in hyperglycemia. Only severe hypertension (SBP ≥ 220 or DBP ≥ 120 mm Hg) should be treated. Hypotension should be treated with fluid therapy and vasopressors if needed.

Patients with TIAs should be given **heparin** if they have known high-grade stenosis, a cardioembolic source, increasing frequency of TIAs (crescendo TIAs), or TIAs despite antiplatelet therapy. Similarly, patients with known embolic strokes and minor deficits should be anticoagulated immediately. If the deficit is large, heparin should be withheld for 3 to 4 days. Treatment for stable completed thrombotic stroke is supportive. Early neurosurgical consultation is needed for patients with cerebellar infarction.

Patients with intracerebral hemorrhage and hypertension should have their BP lowered only if their SBP is ≥200 mm Hg or their DBP is ≥120 mm Hg. **Labetalol** or **nitroprusside** are the agents of choice. Therapy to lower BP should be done over 12 to 24 h. The desired endpoint is the prehemorrhage level of blood pressure, if it is known. Hyperventilation, mannitol, and furosemide are recommended if increased intracranial pressure is suspected.

In patients with subarachnoid hemorrhage, mean arterial pressure should be maintained at 110 mm Hg to prevent rebleeding. **Nimodipine,** (60 mg every 6 h) should be given to prevent vasospasm related to the SAH. Prophylactic dilantin should be given to all patients with SAH, and nausea and vomiting should be treated promptly.

Patients with new-onset strokes should be admitted to the hospital, as should patients with new onset TIAs. Patients with a prior history of anterior circulation stroke who present with a completed (>24 h old) stroke and have reliable support may be discharged home after appropriate consultation and with close followup. Clear instructions to return for worsening symptoms should be emphasized to the patient and family.

For further reading in *Emergency Medicine: A Comprehensive Study Guide*, 4th edition, see Chapter 193, Management of Stroke, by Rashmi U. Kothari and William Barsan.

Keith L. Mausner

Dizziness is one of the most common presenting complaints in the ED. A careful history is the most important aspect of its evaluation. The ED physician must distinguish between vertigo (an illusion of spinning or motion), weakness or lightheadedness, disequilibrium (a feeling of imbalance), and syncope or near syncope.

Clinical Features

Vertigo is classified as *peripheral*, involving structures peripheral to the brain stem (8th nerve, vestibular apparatus), and *central*, involving the brain stem or cerebellum. Peripheral vertigo commonly has an abrupt onset with intense symptoms and is aggravated by movement or changes in posture. Central vertigo tends to be less intense, associated with brain stem or cerebellar findings, and not affected by movement. Table 130-1 lists the major characteristics of central and peripheral vertigo.

Diagnosis and Differential

The majority of vertiginous patients seen in the ED have peripheral vertigo. Vestibular neuronitis is characterized by abrupt onset of peripheral vertigo without hearing loss. Symptoms are worsened by changes in head position. There may have been an upper respiratory infection in the preceding 2 to 3 wks. It usually resolves over days to wks. This may be a viral illness, although the exact etiology is not known.

Labyrinthitis causes peripheral vertigo with hearing loss. It may be associated with a viral infection or, rarely, a bacterial infection. Bacterial labyrinthitis is associated with chronic otitis media, mastoiditis, meningitis, dermoid tumors, or postsurgical infections.

Meniere's disease usually presents with recurrent episodes of severe peripheral vertigo with vomiting. It is associated with progressive deafness and tinnitus in one or both ears over a period of mo to yrs. It occurs equally in men and women, typically after the age of 50. The etiology is not known, but it is associated with dilation of the endolymphatic system.

Benign positional vertigo is a form of recurrent peripheral vertigo precipitated by sudden movements of the head. There is no hearing loss or tinnitus. Attacks may last sec to min, and usually resolve within wks. It is the most common cause of vertigo in the elderly. It may be due to calcium carbonate crystals that have detached from the utricle and fallen against the posterior semicircular canal.

Eighth-nerve acoustic schwannomas or meningiomas may produce peripheral vertigo, usually of gradual onset and preceded by hearing

TABLE 130-1. Characteristics of Vertigo

Peripheral origin
  Intense spinning, swaying, or impulsion
  Nausea, vomiting, possibly diarrhea
  Diaphoresis
  Aggravated by change of position, movement
  Possible tinnitus, hearing loss
  Acute onset
  Fatiguable, unidirectional nystamus
  Nystagmus inhibited by ocular fixation
Central origin
  Ill-defined, less intense vertigo
  Not positionally related, concomitant brain stem or cerebellar signs
    and symptoms (diplopia, dysphagia, facial numbness or weakness,
    ataxia, hemiparesis)
  Nystagmus not inhibited by ocular fixation
  Nonfatiguable, multidirectional nystagmus

loss. Unsteadiness rather than vertigo may be the primary complaint. Cerebellopontine (CP) angle tumors may present with chronic deafness, disequilibrium, and peripheral vertigo. They also may have associated cranial nerve deficits (especially 5th and 7th) and cerebellar signs on the same side.

Other miscellaneous causes of peripheral vertigo include post-traumatic vertigo and benign paroxysmal vertigo of childhood. Foreign bodies or cerumen impaction, as well as middle ear disease, can cause vertigo. A number of drugs affect the inner ear and can cause vertigo or hearing loss. Examples are listed in Table 130-2.

TABLE 130-2. Drugs and Chemicals Affecting the Inner Ear

Antibiotics	Anticonvulsants
Aminoglycosides	Phenytoin
Erythromycin	Barbiturates
Minocycline	Carbamazepine
Diuretics	Ethosuccinimide
Ethacrinic acid	Others
Furosemide	Quinine
Bumetanide	Chloroquine
Nonsteroidal anti-inflammatory agents	Propylene glycol
Salicylates	Ethanol
Ibuprofen	Methanol
Naproxen	Mercury
Indomethacin	
Cytotoxic agents	
Vinblastine	
Cisplatin	
Nitrogen mustard	

Central vertigo is caused by lesions of the brain stem and cerebellum. In conditions affecting the brain stem, there are typically other findings, including dysphagia, dysarthria, ataxia, diplopia, facial numbness, bilateral limb weakness, or bilateral visual blurring. Hearing is usually unaffected, and tinnitus is rare. A brain stem transient ischemic attack may produce brief central vertigo but, by definition, it must be associated with other brain stem neurologic findings. Multiple sclerosis with lesions in the brain stem, as well as neoplasms of the fourth ventricle can produce central vertigo.

Cerebellar hemorrhage or infarction typically presents with acute central vertigo and ataxia. There may or may not be associated nausea, vomiting, or headache. The patient may not be able to sit without support, but cursory neurologic exam on the supine patient may reveal no focal abnormality.

Nonvertiginous dizziness and lightheadedness can have a number of etiologies. Disequilibrium syndrome is due to multiple sensory abnormalities and is typically seen in elderly patients with poor vision, hearing, proprioception, or peripheral neurologic function. Ill-defined lightheadedness is by definition difficult to characterize. It may be associated with fatigue, aches, and generalized weakness. Frequently, no specific etiology can be found for these complaints. Hyperventilation syndrome can produce lightheadedness. Anxiety can produce a sensation of disequilibrium.

Near-syncope can present as dizziness. Careful history can usually identify these patients. (See Chap. 12 for discussion of syncope.)

History should include how rapidly the symptoms developed, their duration, and their relationship to posture or movement. Inquire about associated nausea, vomiting, blurred vision, visual loss, diplopia, tinnitus, focal or general weakness, paresthesias, palpitations, or loss of consciousness. A history of medication use, trauma, and prior episodes should be obtained.

Physical exam should focus on the ear and the neurologic and cardiovascular systems. Listening to a softly whispered voice while covering the opposite ear is a good bedside test of hearing. Weber's and Rinne's tests distinguish between conductive and sensory–neural hearing loss. Assess the extraocular motions and note the presence or absence of nystagmus. Cranial nerve testing, in addition to the eighth nerve, should focus on closely associated nerves: 5th-nerve function, including corneal reflex, 7th-nerve function, and 9th- and 10th-nerve function (gag reflex, swallowing). Coordination (finger-to-nose testing, rapid alternating movements), gait, and ability to sit without support should be evaluated. Peripheral vertigo can often be precipitated by having the patient turn his head while standing with eyes open or making a sudden turn while walking. The etiology of vertigo can be clarified further through the Nylen–Barany maneuver, as explained in Table 130-3.

Orthostatic vital signs are not reliable unless there are marked changes

TABLE 130-3. Nylen–Barany (Hallpike) Maneuver

Test: Patient is in sitting position on a stretcher. Clinician supports head and has patient rapidly assume supine position, first with head straight, then with head turned 45° left, then 45° right.

Findings with peripheral vertigo:
  Vertigo and nystagmus produced, latency 2–20 s
  Duration less than 1 min
  Unidirectional nystagmus
  Nystagmus and vertigo fatigue with repeated testing
  Even straight head position may elicit vertigo (Barany's)
Findings with central vertigo
  Latency of nystagmus, none
  Nystagmus nonfatiguing, multidirectional
  Duration greater than 1 min

and the patient experiences identical symptoms. During the cardiac exam note the rate and rhythm and any evidence of valvular heart disease. Other exam techniques that may reproduce and clarify symptoms include the Valsalva maneuver and 3 min of hyperventilation.

Thorough history and physical exam are usually sufficient to make diagnosis, or they may point to the need for selected lab and diagnostic tests. Glucose testing may diagnose diabetes mellitus, which may cause disequilibrium secondary to poor peripheral neurologic function or near-syncope secondary to hypoglycemia Serologic screening for syphilis may be useful in evaluating long-term hearing loss and vestibular dysfunction. If a cardiac etiology is suspected, echocardiography, ambulatory cardiac rhythm monitoring, or other diagnostic tests may be indicated. CT scanning is indicated for suspected cerebellar hemorrhage or infarction. MRI is more sensitive than CT for tumors at the CP angle.

Emergency Department Care and Disposition

The key to evaluation, treatment, and disposition is to determine the etiology of the patient's symptoms. Peripheral vertigo may be effectively treated by the medications listed in Table 130-4. Not all antihistamines and antiemetics are effective. The antihistamines with anticholinergic properties are the most effective. The antiemetics hydroxyzine and promethazine have strong antihistaminic properties and are effective at relieving vertigo, whereas chlorpromazine and chlorperazine are not effective. Peripheral vertigo also may be suppressed by visual fixation on a nearby object. Resting in a comfortable position and slowing movements that can precipitate attacks is helpful. Benign positional vertigo may respond to repeated head movements, which provoke an attack and then fatigue the response. Bacterial labyrinthitis requires antibiotic therapy and ENT consultation. It is important to reassure patients that peripheral vertigo is usually a benign and self-limited condition.

TABLE 130-4. Drugs used for Vertigo of Peripheral Origin

Antihistamines	
Diphenhydramine	25–50 mg PO q6h
Dimenhydrinate	50 mg PO q4h
Cyclizine	50 mg PO q4h*
Metclizine	25 mg PO q6h
Promethazine	25–50 mg PO q4–6h
Anticholinergics	
Atropine	1 mg IM or IV
Scopolamine	0.5 mg patch behind ear q3d
Antiemetics	
Hydroxyzine	0.5 mg/kg up to 25–50 mg PO q4–6h
Promethazine	25–50 mg PO q4–6h
Sedatives	
Diazepam	2–10 mg PO q6–8h
Chlordiazepoxide	5–25 mg PO q6–8h

*Not to exceed 200 mg in 24 h.

Patients who may have central vertigo require an urgent imaging study and neurologic consultation. An urgent imaging study is not necessary in most patients with apparent peripheral vertigo, as long as there is no suspicion of a CP angle tumor or 8th-nerve lesion.

It is important to remember that patients with disequilibrium syndrome and ill-defined lightheadedness may experience a worsening of their symptoms on vertigo medications. These patients may benefit from withdrawing sedating medications or addressing sensory deficits by improving ambient lighting.

If Standard Treatment Fails

Patients who cannot keep hydrated or with disabling symptoms who may be at risk for injury from falls, require admission for symptomatic treatment and more urgent evaluation.

For further reading in *Emergency Medicine: A Comprehensive Study Guide*, 4th edition, see Chapter 194, Vertigo and Dizziness, by Neal Little.

131 | Seizures and Status Epilepticus in Adults

Keith L. Mausner

A seizure is a period of altered neurologic function caused by abnormal neuronal electrical discharges. Approximately 1% to 2% of the general population has recurrent seizures.

Clinical Features

Seizures are primary, or idiopathic, when there is no apparent cause, and they are secondary, or symptomatic, when they are due to a discernible structural, metabolic, or other etiology. Table 131-1 summarizes the most widely accepted classification scheme for seizures. Generalized seizures begin with an abrupt loss of consciousness. If motor activity is present, it symmetrically involves all four extremities. Generalized seizures may be preceded by prodromal symptoms, such as irritability, tension, or myoclonic jerks; this is not an aura, which is only associated with focal seizures. Absence seizures are generalized but there is no motor activity. They usually last for several seconds, during which the patient is unresponsive to external stimuli and may stare and twitch the eyelids. The patient usually does not fall or experience incontinence. The seizure stops abruptly and the patient resumes activity, unaware of the event. Absence seizures usually occur in school-age children and may occur up to 100 times per day.

Partial (focal) seizures are due to localized neuronal discharge and may suggest the presence of a structural or focal lesion in the brain. Unilateral extremity movements imply a motor cortex lesion, and tonic deviation of the head and eyes (usually away from the side of the seizure) point to a frontal lobe focus. An aura is a focal sensory seizure. Occipital foci produce visual disturbances; temporal lobe discharges may produce olfactory or gustatory hallucinations; and sensory cortex foci produce paresthesias.

Partial (focal) seizures are either simple or complex. In simple partial seizures there is no impairment of consciousness. In complex partial seizures, the level of consciousness is impaired. Simple partial seizures may progress to complex partial seizures. Simple or complex partial seizures may progress and become secondarily generalized.

In complex partial seizures there may be alterations in cognition and behavior, and the patient may be misdiagnosed as having a psychiatric illness. These patients often experience distortions in visual perception and may perceive time as passing slowly or quickly. Memory disturbances such as *deja vu* (familiarity in unfamiliar a place) or *jamais vu* (strangeness or unfamiliarity in a familiar place) may occur, as well as automatisms such as lip smacking or picking at clothing. Emotions such as fear, paranoia, or depression may be seen.

TABLE 131-1. Classification of Seizures

Generalized seizures (consciousness always lost)
  Absence seizures (petit mal)
  Myoclonic seizures
  Tonic seizures
  Clonic seizures
  Tonic–clonic seizures
  Atonic seizures
Partial (focal) seizures
  Simple (elementary), no alteration of consciousness
    Motor seizures
    Sensory seizures
    Autonomic seizures
  Complex (psychomotor or temporal lobe seizures) consciousness
  impaired
    With psychic, cognitive, or affective symptoms
    With automatisms
    Partial seizures (elementary or complex) with secondary
    generalization
    Unclassified (due to inadequate information)

Diagnosis and Differential

The differential diagnosis of seizures includes syncope, narcolepsy, cataplexy, movement disorders, hyperventilation syndrome, psychogenic seizures, paroxysmal vertigo, rage attacks, transient ischemic attacks, and migraine syndromes. Differentiating a seizure from a seizurelike episode can be difficult, and a careful history from the patient and witnesses is essential. Occasionally extensive neurologic workup with repeat EEGs is necessary to establish or exclude the presence of seizures.

Several important historical points may be helpful in establishing a diagnosis. Most seizures begin abruptly; episodes that develop over min to h are less likely to be seizures. Most seizures only last 1 to 2 min, but witnesses tend to exaggerate the duration of an episode. Occurrence of a sensory aura is consistent with a focal seizure, but the absence of an aura does not rule one out. Patients with seizure disorders tend to have stereotyped, or similar, seizures with each episode and are unlikely to have inconsistent or highly variable attacks. Motor activity during seizures, except complex partial seizures, is usually purposeless or inappropriate. True seizures are usually not provoked by emotional distress. Except in simple partial seizures, patients do not remember details of their attacks. Most seizures, except for absence or simple partial seizures, are followed by a postictal state with lethargy and confusion.

In patients with previously diagnosed seizures, a typical attack may not require any further evaluation. If the patient is on anticonvulsant medication, inquire about recent changes in dose, missed doses, or a change from brand name to generic medication. Also inquire about sleep deprivation and alcohol or drug use.

Patients with first-time seizures require a much more detailed evaluation. Inquire about previous neurologic symptoms, head trauma, and family history. A search for reversible and secondary causes of seizures is indicated. Table 131-2 lists major causes of secondary seizures.

Physical exam should focus on uncovering injuries sustained during the seizure, as well as systemic conditions that may have caused the seizure. Look for bruises, fractures, tongue lacerations, and broken teeth. Posterior shoulder dislocations may occur and often are overlooked. The neurologic exam should evaluate the level of consciousness and look for evidence of elevated intracranial pressure, focal weakness, or other asymmetry.

Patients with known seizure disorders who have an isolated seizure may not require any lab tests, although anticonvulsant levels may be helpful. A therapeutic anticonvulsant level is any level that controls seizures without unacceptable side-effects; it does not always correspond with the conventional ranges reported by the lab. Depending on the clinical context, patients with first-time seizures may benefit from more extensive lab evaluation, especially if they are at risk for electrolyte disturbances or the history is unclear. Glucose is easily evaluated with a rapid test at the bedside. Electrolytes, BUN, creatinine, calcium, magnesium, and toxicology screening may be useful. If it is unclear

---

TABLE 131-2. Some Causes of Secondary Seizures

Intracranial etiologies
  Trauma (recent or remote)
  Infection (meningitis, encephalitis, abscess)
  Vascular lesion (stroke, arteriovenous malformation, vasculitis)
  Mass lesions (neoplasms, subdural hematoma)
  Degenerative disease
Extracranial etiologies
  Anoxic–ischemic injury (e.g., cardiac arrest, severe hypoxemia)
  Endocrine/electrolyte disorders
    Hypoglycemia
    Hyperosmolar states
    Hyponatremia
    Hypocalcemia, hypomagnesemia (rare)
  Toxins and drugs
  Cocaine, lidocaine
  Antidepressants
  Theophylline
  Alcohol withdrawal
  Barbiturate withdrawal
  Benzodiazepine withdrawal
  Anticonvulsant withdrawal and *many* others
  Eclampsia of pregnancy (may occur postpartum)
  Hypertensive encephalopathy

whether a seizure occurred, an ABG may show metabolic acidosis, and there may be elevation of creatine kinase.

Patients with known seizure disorders who have a typical seizure do not require routine CT scanning. Emergent CT scanning is necessary in patients with deteriorating condition or evidence of a structural lesion. CT scans with contrast are more sensitive at detecting tumors and vascular abnormalities but are not usually performed in the ED. MR scanning is even more sensitive than CT. In a stable patient with a self-limited seizure and no evidence of a focal lesion, it is reasonable to obtain an MR scan later and not perform an ED CT scan. Consultation with a radiologist and neurologist to determine the most appropriate test and to arrange followup is indicated.

Emergency Department Care and Disposition

Assess and stabilize airway, breathing, and circulation. During a seizure, protect the patient from injury and prevent falls. If possible turn the patient on one side to decrease the risk of aspiration. It is usually not possible to ventilate acutely seizing patients or to safely place a bite block. Most seizures are brief and self-limited, and suctioning and airway measures can be performed after the seizure. Start an IV line as soon as possible. A postictal state may persist for min to h. An abnormally prolonged postictal state or lack of improvement of level of consciousness over time should prompt further evaluation.

In patients with known seizure disorders, if the anticonvulsant level is low from noncompliance, a supplemental dose and resumption of the medication may be all that is indicated. If the level is therapeutic, the patient may have had an isolated breakthrough seizure and not require any additional treatment. The anticonvulsant dose should only be increased after consultation with the patient's neurologist, since small increases may lead to dramatic rises in serum levels.

Anticonvulsant therapy is not necessary in all patients with first-time self-limited seizures. The decision to treat can often be made on followup with the private physician or neurologist, when more data, such as an EEG is available. If treatment is started, Table 131-3 summarizes current drug recommendations.

Upon discharge, all seizure patients should be cautioned about swimming, operating hazardous machinery, and driving. All ED physicians should be aware of their state's regulations concerning driving privileges for seizure patients and physician reporting of seizures to the motor vehicle division.

Alcohol withdrawal seizures are usually self-limited and respond to treatment of the withdrawal state with benzodiazepines. alcohol withdrawal may unmask an underlying seizure disorder, however, and alcoholics may be more likely to be hypoglycemic or have another underlying cause of seizures. Patients with prolonged seizures or status epilepticus require further anticonvulsant therapy.

TABLE 131-3. Anticonvulsant Drugs: Indications

Generalized seizures	
Absence seizures	Ethosuximide (1st)
	Valproic acid (2nd)
Myoclonic seizures	Valproic acid
Tonic–clonic seizures	Carbamazepine or phenytoin (1st)
	Phenobarbital or primidone (2nd)
	Valproic acid (3rd)
Partial seizures (simple or complex, with or without generalization)	Carbamazepine or phenytoin (1st)
	Phenobarbital or primidone (2nd)
	Valproic acid (3rd)

STATUS EPILEPTICUS

Clinical Features and Emergency Department Care

Status epilepticus is defined as continuous seizure activity for 30 min or more, or 2 or more seizures without full recovery of consciousness between attacks. Status epilepticus should be presumed in any patient with prolonged seizures whether or not the 30-min criteria has been met. Status epilepticus is obvious in patients with generalized convulsive seizures. Simple and complex partial seizures may also present in status epilepticus, in which case the diagnosis may not be obvious. In generalized convulsive status epilepticus, motor activity may diminish over time, and the patient may appear to be in a postictal state while having ongoing seizure activity. The diagnosis of status epilepticus requires high suspicion and, occasionally, bedside EEG monitoring. Without appropriate treatment, irreversible neuronal damage may occur in 30 to 60 min. The mortality rate of convulsive status epilepticus is as high as 30%.

Status epilepticus may be caused by medication noncompliance or changes, CNS infections, trauma, anoxia, stroke, hemorrhage, toxins or overdose, or metabolic disturbances.

Management includes assessment and stabilization of airway, breathing, and circulation, with endotracheal intubation if indicated. Protect the patient from injury. Establish a large-bore IV line. NG tube placement to empty the stomach is recommended. Check glucose, electrolytes and, if indicated, anticonvulsant levels and toxicology screening. Administer glucose and thiamine if indicated. In prolonged seizures, check creatine kinase and urine myoglobin to assess for rhabdomyolysis. ABGs are not usually helpful acutely. If meningitis is suspected, empiric antibiotic therapy is indicated, and lumbar puncture can be performed after stabilization. CT scanning is usually delayed until the seizures are controlled. A rapid search for and correction of reversible causes is essential.

Table 131-4 is a protocol for the management of status epilepticus. IV phenytoin may produce hypotension, decreased myocardial contractility and atrioventricular (AV) block. It is contraindicated in patients

TABLE 131-4. Management of Status Epilepticus

General measures
  Establish/maintain airway
  Thiamine 100 mg IV
  Dextrose 25–50 g IV
Standard regimen
  Diazepam 5 mg IV (repeat as necessary q 5 min to total of 20 mg) or
  lorazepam up to 0.1 mg/kg) and
  Phenytoin 18 mg/kg IV at 25 min mg/min
  If not effective, then
  Phenobarbital IV 100 mg/min to total of 10 mg/kg or seizures are
  controlled
  If not effective, then
  Phenobarbital 50 mg/min to total (including previous doses) of
  20 mg/kg or seizures are controlled
  If not effective, then
  Phenobarbital 50 mg/min to total (including previous doses) of
  30 mg/kg or seizures are controlled
  If not effective, then
  Consider barbiturate coma, general anesthesia, or diazepam drip.
Alternative regimen
  Phenobarbital 100 mg/min IV to total of 10 mg/kg or seizures are
  controlled
  If not effective, then
  Phenytoin 18 mg/kg IV (at dose of 25–50 mg/min) and phenobarbital
  50 mg/min to total dose of 20 mg/kg or seizures are controlled
  If not effective, then
  Phenobarbital 50 mg/kg to total dose (including previous doses) of 30
  mg/kg or seizures are controlled
  If not effective, then
  Consider barbiturate coma or general anesthesia

with second- or third-degree AV block. It should not be infused faster than 50 mg/min; 25 mg/min is safer in elderly patients. Phenytoin is incompatible with glucose-containing fluids. Phenobarbital may produce respiratory depression and hypotension. All patients should be monitored closely.

If Standard Treatment Fails

If the above measures are ineffective, consider lidocaine (2–3 m/kg IV, followed by an infusion at 2–4 mg/min, or a diazepam infusion at 8–10 mg/h). Rectal paraldehyde has also been used. General anesthesia with pentobarbital (5–15 mg/kg IV, followed by an infusion at 0.5 to 3 mg/kg/h) may be necessary in refractory cases. In this case anesthesia and neurology should be consulted, and EEG monitoring should be employed to assess response.

Neuromuscular blocking drugs (vecuronium or pancuronium) will eliminate muscular activity and may be helpful in ventilating the patient, lessening acidosis, and decreasing the risk of rhabdomyolysis. There is no effect on CNS neuronal activity, however, and EEG monitoring is necessary to guide treatment.

A special case of refractory status epilepticus occurs with isoniazid overdose. This may be unresponsive to all treatment except pyridoxine administration.

For further reading in *Emergency Medicine: a Comprehensive Study Guide,* 4th edition, see Chapter 195, Seizures and Status Epilepticus in Adults, by Thomas R. Pellegrino.

A systematic approach to the evaluation of acute neurologic symptoms of the extremities consists of: (1) differentiation between acute and chronic symptoms; (2) separation of central and peripheral origin; (3) reflex assessment; (4) and close followup. This chapter will concentrate on both common and acute entities.

ACUTE NEUROPATHIES

Diphtheria

Clinical features are characterized by rapid onset of symptoms, exudative pharyngitis, high fever, and malaise. The most commonly observed paralyses involve the intrinsic and extrinsic muscles of the eye, producing ptosis, strabismus, and problems in accommodation. The critically ill patient may have bilateral flaccid weakness or paralysis accompanied by absent deep tendon reflexes. Urinary retention, incontinence, and incompetent anal sphincter tone may be present. ED treatment involves endotracheal intubation for **airway protection,** support of hemodynamic status, and administration of the **serum diphtheria antitoxin** in consultation with an infectious disease specialist.

Botulism

This disease, which is caused by a toxin from the organism *C. botulinum*, occurs in three forms: food-borne, wound, and infantile. The principal source of botulism in the U.S. is food that has been improperly prepared. In infantile botulism, organisms in the gut, arising from ingested spores, produce toxin that is systemically absorbed. Wound botulism should be considered in any patient with a wound or a chronic history of IV drug abuse associated with a progressive descending symmetric paralysis. Clinical features include neurologic symptoms that usually appear 24 to 48 h after ingestion and may or may not be preceded by nausea, vomiting, and diarrhea. The most common early presenting neurologic complaints are related to the eyes and bulbar musculature, which is followed by a descending symmetric muscle weakness and respiratory insufficiency. Good mental status is maintained until the terminal stages. Symptoms of infantile botulism are poor suck, constipation, listlessness, regurgitation, and generalized weakness. ED treatment involves **respiratory support** and removal of the remaining offending agents by gastric lavage, activated charcoal, and instillation of cathartics. Administration of **botulinum antitoxin** should be made in consultation with an infectious-disease specialist. Surgical consultation for wound debridement is mandatory in wound botulism.

Neuropathy of Guillain–Barré

The clinical features of this syndrome usually follows an acute febrile episode, upper respiratory infection, or an acute metabolic problem by days or wks and may be rapidly progressive. The typical pattern of presentation is that of an ascending motoneuron involvement. The lower extremities are usually affected initially and more severely than the upper extremities. Both motor and sensory symptoms may be present, and the bulbar musculature may be partially or totally involved. Although the ED diagnosis of Guillain–Barré is difficult, any patient who presents with lower extremity weakness and loss of lower extremity reflexes should be considered to have this entity until proven otherwise. The differential diagnosis would include diphtheria, botulism, lead poisoning, and porphyria. ED treatment centers around **respiratory support,** admission into an intensive care setting, and neurologic consultation.

ACUTE MYOPATHIES

Polymyositis Syndrome

There is little value in the ED physician subclassifying acute polymyositis into its multiple causes. This clinical syndrome is characterized by rapidly evolving signs and symptoms of severe weakness, muscular pain, arthralgia, dysphagia, fever, and Raynaud phenomenon. The differential diagnosis includes endocrinopathies, adrenal–cortical lesions, and parathyroid lesions. Steroids, which are used in treating many forms of polymyositis, can actually exacerbate the problem. Since there is no specific ED therapy, steroids should be administered in consultation with a neurologist.

Alcoholic Myopathy

This clinical syndrome, which develops during prolonged periods of heavy alcohol intake, is characterized by the chronic alcoholic patient who presents with severe muscle tenderness and swelling, muscle cramps, and severe weakness. Signs and symptoms may be generalized or focal. This syndrome represents an acute diffuse necrosis of skeletal muscle fibers or acute rhabdomyolysis. Muscle degeneration can lead to life-threatening hyperkalemia or hypocalcemia, and myoglobinuria can cause renal failure. In the alcohol-abusing patient with acute muscle pain and weakness, serum electrolyte levels, muscle enzymes, and urinalysis are necessary. These patients should be admitted for observation and supportive therapy.

Acute Periodic Paralysis

There are three basic types or primary forms of this acute weakness syndrome: hyperkalemic, hypokalemic, or normokalemic. Cold weather, large meals, trauma, and surgery may provoke an attack. The patient also may describe being awakened from sleep by weakness. The typical history is one of rapid onset of extreme weakness without associated pain. Patients will give a history of being normal before and after the attack. The ED physician should maintain a high index of suspicion for this syndrome when evaluating a patient presenting with unexplained weakness. ED management entails respiratory support, if needed, obtaining a serum potassium level, and timely referral to a neurologist.

Specific Isolated Peripheral Nerve Lesions

Herpes Zoster

Elderly and immunocompromised patients are at greatest risk of developing herpes zoster. Extreme pain, generally in a dermatomal distribution, usually precedes the infection by several days. The dermatomes most commonly affected are the thoracic, followed by the trigeminal nerve, lumbar plexus and, finally, the cervical plexus. Herpes produces principally sensory involvement. Tympanic membrane and corneal involvement may be seen as part of the Ramsey–Hunt syndrome. ED treatment consists of **acyclovir** (800 mg 5 times a day for 10 days). Patients do not require admission unless the disease is disseminated, or unless patients are immunocompromised or receiving steroids or chemotherapy. Ophthalmologic consultation is appropriate if corneal lesions are suspected.

Tic Douloureux

The clinical features of tic douloureux, or trigeminal neuralgia, are severe pain, usually confined to the area of distribution of the 3rd portion of the trigeminal nerve. Bilateral involvement is unusual. ED treatment includes acute pain relief with analgesics and initiating long-term therapy, such as carbamazepine, in consultation with a neurologist.

Bell's Palsy

The clinical feature of this entity is dysfunction of the 7th cranial nerve. The patient presents with weakness of the forehead, around the eyes, and lower face. No other focal deficits are noted on thorough neurologic exam. Idiopathic Bell's palsy is a diagnosis of exclusion. Disease processes such as Lyme disease, parotid tumors, lesions of the middle ear, cerebellopontine angle tumors, 8th cranial nerve lesions, and vascular disease can all present with Bell's palsy. It is vital to localize the level of involvement to distinguish between a structural process and idiopathic Bell's palsy. If the patient retains muscle strength in the forehead and upper face but is weak in the lower face, then the lesion is probably central (i.e., in the brainstem or above). CT scanning of the head and admission are required for patients with suspected central lesions. Once idiopathic Bell's palsy is determined, ED therapy involves starting the patient on a short course of high-dose **steroids**, along with close followup with a neurologist or otolaryngologist.

For further reading in *Emergency Medicine: A Comprehensive Study Guide*, 4th edition, see Chapter 196, Acute Peripheral Neurological Lesions, by Gregory L. Henry.

133 | Multiple Sclerosis

O. John Ma

Multiple sclerosis (MS) is the leading cause of neurologic morbidity and mortality among young adults. The average age of onset is in the third and fourth decades, and females are affected more commonly than males.

Clinical Features

MS presents as recurrent attacks of a focal neurologic disease. The presence of clinical remissions remains the clinical rule. The first episode of MS presents as more than one symptom or sign in the majority (55%) of cases; the remaining cases become evident as a single sign or symptom.

Symptomatic fatigue is the most common symptom of MS patients, occurring in approximately 70% of cases. Simple tasks, such as dressing, may be exhausting to patients, even when the individual has normal or near-normal strength. This symptomatic fatigue usually takes place over a day's activities and can be exacerbated by exercise or hot weather.

Symptoms and signs of neurologic dysfunction in MS arise from lesions in the optic nerve, posterior visual pathways, brainstem, cerebellum, and spinal cord. More than one third of patients with MS present with sensory or motor visual symptoms, and they occur at some stage of the disease in nearly all MS patients.

The first symptom of MS in 10% to 30% of patients is optic neuritis. It often begins with pain around the eye, which is increased by eye movement. Blurring of vision may precede or follow the ocular pain. Various degrees of visual loss may occur over a wk. Eye examination reveals variable loss of visual acuity. Fundal examination, which is normal in half the patients, may reveal swelling of the disk (papillitis) that may be indistinguishable from papilledema.

Other common visual findings associated with MS include diplopia, nystagmus, and internuclear ophthalmoplegia (INO). Patients with acute INO have horizontal diplopia on lateral gaze in either direction, with minimal or no diplopia on primary gaze. This is due to an inability to adduct the eye ipsilateral to the lesion and to nystagmus in the abducting eye.

Lesions in the brainstem, affecting the 5th, 7th, and 8th cranial nerves, can occur in MS. Unilateral facial numbness, paresthesia, or pain is associated with the descending root of the 5th cranial nerve. Paroxysmal unilateral facial pain, indistinguishable from trigeminal neuralgia without concomitant sensory loss, occurs in approximately 2% of MS patients. A unilateral central facial nerve palsy is associated with the 7th cranial nerve. Deafness, though rare in MS, may be the initial presenting symptom.

Lesions involving the cerebellum in MS may produce truncal or limb ataxia, intention tremor, saccadic dysmetria, acquired pendular nystagmus, and isolated ocular motor nerve palsies.

When spinal cord lesions are involved in MS, most patients may demonstrate upper motoneuron dysfunction characterized by paresis, spasticity, hyperreflexia, clonus, upgoing toes, and loss of abdominal reflexes. Sensation of diminished pain and temperature, decreased vibratory sensation, urinary tract dysfunction, severe constipation, and sexual dysfunction also indicate spinal cord involvement.

Diagnosis and Differential

Clinical diagnostic criteria remain the standard method of diagnosis of MS and require that a patient of an appropriate age has had at least two episodes of neurologic disturbances that implicate two distinct sites in the white matter. MRI is the recommended imaging technique for supporting the diagnosis. Typical abnormalities of MS are multiple discrete lesions located in the supratentorial white matter, especially in the periventricular areas. Lesions are less commonly detected in the cerebellum and brainstem. The MRI detects abnormalities consistent with MS in 70% to 95% of MS patients. The cerebrospinal fluid (CSF) of most MS patients has a normal cell number. Whereas slight increases in cell counts have been reported, cell counts greater than 50 cells/μL are rare. The cells in the CSF are usually T lymphocytes. The protein concentration of the CSF is elevated in approximately 25% of patients. The most characteristic CSF finding in MS is an increase in immunoglobulin (IgG) caused by synthesis of IgG in the CNS.

ED physicians should suspect the diagnosis of MS by a careful history and physical exam. Since there is not a single diagnostic test, and since many of the tests needed to help make the diagnosis—such as MRI, evoked-potential, and CSF studies—are not readily available in the ED, referral to a neurologist for serial neurologic exams and completion of the diagnostic tests is essential. The differential diagnosis of MS includes systemic lupus erythematosus, Lyme disease, sarcoidosis, neurosyphilis, and HIV disease.

Emergency Department Care and Disposition

Exacerbations often develop over h to days. If the exacerbation is severe with significant motor or cerebellar dysfunction, the patient may be treated with **steroids.** A short-term (5 days), high-dose (1 g) course of pulsed IV methylprednisolone, followed by an oral tapering course of prednisone for 2 to 3 wks, is beneficial in the acute exacerbation of MS.

Preservation of the integrity of the upper urinary tract is of primary importance in the management of MS urinary dysfunction. The treatment of this problem depends on the magnitude of postvoiding residual

(PVR), as well as the patient's symptoms. If the MS patient has symptomatic voiding or evidence of bacteriuria, a PVR urine determination is indicated. When the amount of residual urine is either greater than 100 mL or more than 20% of the voided volume, the treatment of choice is intermittent catheterization.

Acute urinary tract infection (UTI) may be asymptomatic, produce nonspecific symptoms, or produce classic symptoms. Since occult UTIs may aggravate seemingly unrelated neurologic symptoms, such as lower-extremity weakness or spasticity, in MS patients prompt diagnosis and treatment of UTIs is important.

Small increases in body temperature can worsen existing signs and symptoms, as well as produce additional neurologic manifestations. It is therefore important to lower the body temperature in the febrile MS patient.

New agents for MS treatment include interferon and immunosuppressive therapy. Prompt neurologic consultation is necessary to set up this therapy.

For further reading in *Emergency Medicine: A Comprehensive Study Guide*, 4th edition, see Chapter 197, Multiple Sclerosis, by Richard F. Edlich and Marie Louise Hammarskjold.

Although uncommon, myasthenia gravis (MG) remains the most common disorder of neuromuscular transmission, producing varying degrees of muscle weakness. It is an autoimmune disease where the cause for weakness is an antibody-mediated depletion of acetylcholine receptors at the muscle endplate.

Clinical Features

The clinical hallmark of MG is muscle weakness, usually with some component of fatigability. The patient typically will see their strength improve after a period of resting, but weakness of a particular muscle group will increase after sustained and repetitive use. Increasing weakness may be due to a variety of causes, including an acute exacerbation of the disease precipitated by an underlying infection, thyroid disease, hypokalemia, and under- or over-medication with acetylcholinesterase inhibitors, such as pyridostigmine bromide.

Most frequently, the first muscles to become weak are the extraocular muscles, although weakness in other muscle groups, such as the bulbar muscles, may be the presenting symptom. Either diplopia or ptosis may be the initial symptoms. Bright light may exacerbate ptosis or diplopia, and heat may increase muscle weakness. When limb muscles become symptomatic, proximal muscles are typically weakest.

The most severe manifestation of the disease produces weakness of the respiratory muscles, precipitating the life-threatening myasthenic crisis. This condition occurs in a severe MG patient who is either not being treated or who is undertreated because of insufficient medication or drug resistance. Overmedication with cholinesterase inhibitors, however, can also lead to the development of muscle weakness. This cholinergic crisis may be indistinguishable from myasthenic crisis in the ED.

Diagnosis and Differential

The diagnosis of MG in the ED can be strongly suspected on clinical grounds. The combination of ocular, bulbar, and limb weakness, which fluctuates during the day and decreases with resting, is highly typical of MG. The patient who presents with isolated ocular symptoms or mild to moderate weakness in various muscle groups can be difficult to diagnose with certainty.

Diagnosis of MG can be confirmed at bedside through the use of the edrophonium test. Edrophonium is an acetylcholinesterase inhibitor that prevents rapid breakdown of acetylcholine at the myoneural junction. Edrophonium is administered as an IV bolus while the patient's muscle strength is tested. It acts within a few seconds and its effects last 5 to 10 min. The pharmacologic effect of improved muscle strength is dramatic but transient. A positive edrophonium test is a definite increase in motor strength of a previously weak muscle that lasts for 5 to 10 min. Muscle weakness then slowly returns.

The differential diagnosis includes mitochondrial myopathy, oculopharyngeal muscular dystrophy, inflammatory myopathies, amyotrophic lateral sclerosis, periodic paralysis syndromes, and neurasthenia. Discussion of these entities goes beyond the scope of this chapter.

Emergency Department Care and Disposition

The patient with MG who presents to the ED complaining of worsening weakness should be admitted to the hospital. The MG patient can rapidly develop respiratory insufficiency or bulbar dysfunction leading to an inability to handle secretions. For the patient who presents in myasthenic crisis, administering supplemental **oxygen** and securing the airway through **endotracheal intubation** are the top priorities. Patients with MG are sensitive to long-acting nondepolarizing paralytic agents, but intermediate-acting agents, such as vecuronium, can be titrated to achieve adequate neuromuscular blockade without producing prolonged paralysis. In addition, other drugs that should be used cautiously in MG patients are listed in Table 134-1.

High-dose steroid therapy should be initiated for the MG patient suffering from a severe exacerbation of the disease. Any MG patient who receives steroids in the ED should be admitted to an ICU, since steroids can worsen the weakness in the MG patient. Neurologic consultation should be made for admission and to arrange for plasmapheresis therapy, which has been shown to help dramatically improve strength after several sessions.

LAMBERT-EATON MYASTHENIC SYNDROME

The Lambert–Eaton myasthenic syndrome (LEMS) is a disorder in which there is an antibody-mediated decrease in the number of presynaptic calcium channels, which mediate the release of acetylcholine at motor-nerve terminals.

Clinical Features

The clinical hallmark of LEMS is proximal muscle weakness, particularly of the lower extremities, which may resolve with repetitive activation of the muscle. The patient rarely experiences weakness of the respiratory or extraocular muscles. Deep tendon reflexes may be markedly diminished or absent. The patient also may complain of autonomic symptoms, particularly a dry mouth, as a consequence of decreased cholinergic transmission at peripheral autonomic synapses.

TABLE 134-1. Drugs That Should Be Used With Caution in Myasthenia Gravis

Steroids	Colchicine
ACTH*	Chloroquine
Methylprednisolone*	*Cardiovascular*
Prednisone*	Quinidine*
Anticonvulsants	Procainamide*
Dilantin	Beta blockers
Lathosuximide	Propranolol
Inmethadione	Oxprenolol
Paraldehyde	Practolol
Magnesium sulfate	Pindolol
Barbiturates	Sotalol
Antimalarials	Lidocaine
Chloroquine*	Dilantin
Quinine*	Trimethaphan
IV Fluids	*Local Anesthetic*
Salactate solution	Lidocaine*
Antibiotics	Procaine*
Aminoglycosides	*Analgesics*
Neomycin*	Narcotics
Streptomycin*	Morphine
Kanamycin*	Dilaudid
Gentamicin	Codeine
Tobramycin	Pantopon
Dihydrostreptomycin*	Meperidine
Amikacin	*Endocrine*
Polymyxin A	Thyroid* replacement
Polymyxin B	*Eyedrops*
Bacitracin	Tinolol*
Sulfonamides	Ecothiopate
Viomycin	*Others*
Colistin	Amantadine
Colistimethate*	Diphenhydramine
Lincomycin	Emetine
Clindamycine	Diurotico
Ietracycline	Muscle relaxants
Oxytetracycline	CNS depressants
Rolitetracycline	Respiratory depressants
Psychotropics	Sedatives
Chlorpromazine*	Procaine*
Lithium carbonate*	Tranquilizers
Amitriptyline	*Neuromuscular blocking agents*
Droperidol	Tubocurarine
Haloperidol	Pancuronium
Imipramine	Gallamine
Paraldehyde	Dimethyl tubocurarine
Trichlorethanol	Succinylcholine
Antirheumatics	Decamethomium
D-Penicillamine	

*Case reports implicate drugs in exacerbations of MG.
Modified table from Adam SL, Matthews J, Grammer LC. Drugs that may exacerbate myasthenia gravis. *Ann Emerg Med* Vol. 3, p. 532, 1984. Used by permission.

Approximately 30% to 50% of LEMS patients have a malignant neoplasm, most commonly oat-cell carcinoma of the lung.

Diagnosis and Differential

The diagnosis of LEMS in the ED can be suspected based on clinical findings in the history and physical exam. Referral to a neurologist for EMG studies should be initiated.

Emergency Department Care and Disposition

In consultation with a neurologist, admission to the hospital should be made based on the degree of symptoms and findings on the physical exam. The most effective treatment of non-neoplastic cases of LEMS is combined therapy with prednisone and azathioprine.

For further reading in *Emergency Medicine: A Comprehensive Study Guide*, 4th edition, see Chapter 198, Disorders of Neuromuscular Transmission, by Lawrence H. Phillips and Richard F. Edlich.

Meningitis, Encephalitis, and Brain Abscess

O. John Ma

MENINGITIS

The primary goal in the ED management of bacterial meningitis is prompt recognition and empiric treatment.

Clinical Features

In classic and fulminant cases of bacterial meningitis, the patient presents with fever, headache, stiff neck, photophobia, and altered mental status. Seizures may occur in up to 25% of cases. The presenting picture, however, may be more nonspecific in the very young and elderly. Confusion and fever may be signs of meningeal irritation in the elderly. It is important to inquire about recent antibiotic use, which may cloud the clinical picture in a less florid case. Physical exam must include assessment for meningeal irritation with resistance to passive neck flexion, Brudzinski's sign (flexion of hips and knees in response to passive neck flexion), and Kernig's sign (contraction of hamstrings in response to knee extension while hip is flexed). The skin should be examined for the purpuric rash characteristic of meningococcemia. Paranasal sinuses should be percussed and ears examined for evidence of primary infection in those sites. Focal neurologic deficits, which are present in 25% of cases, should be documented.

Diagnosis and Differential

When bacterial meningitis is considered, performing a lumbar puncture (LP) is mandatory. At a minimum, cerebrospinal fluid (CSF) should be sent for gram stain and culture, cell count, protein, and glucose. Typical CSF results for meningeal processes are listed in Table 135-1. Additional studies to be considered are latex agglutination or counterimmune electrophoresis for bacterial antigens in potentially partially treated bacterial cases: India ink and latex agglutination assay for fungal antigen in cryptococcal meningitis; acid-fast stain and culture for mycobacteria in tuberculous meningitis; Borrelia antibodies for possible Lyme disease; and viral cultures in suspected viral meningitis. Other lab tests should include complete blood count, blood cultures, partial thromboplastin and prothrombin times, as well as serum glucose, sodium, and creatinine.

The differential diagnosis includes subarachnoid hemorrhage, meningeal neoplasm, brain abscess, viral encephalitis, and cerebral toxoplasmosis.

TABLE 135-1. Typical Spinal Fluid Results for Meningeal Processes

Parameter (Normal)	Bacterial	Viral	Neoplastic	Fungal
O.P. (< 170 mm CSF)	> 300 mm	200 mm	200 mm	300 mm
WBC (< 5 mononuclear)	> 1000/μL	< 1000/μL	< 500/μL	< 500/μL
% pmns (0)	≥ 80%	1–50%	1–50%	1–50%
Glucose (> 40 mg/dL)	< 40 mg/dL	< 40 mg/dL	< 40 mg/dL	< 40 mg/dL
Protein (< 50 mg/dL)	> 200 mg/dL	> 200 mg/dL	> 200 mg/dL	> 200 mg/dL
Gram stain (−)	+	−	−	−
Cytology (−)	−	−	+	+

O.P., opening pressure; WBC, white blood cells; pmns, polymorphonuclear cells.

Emergency Department Care and Disposition

Emergent respiratory and hemodynamic support remains the top priority. On presentation of the patient with suspected bacterial meningitis, LP should be performed expeditiously if the patient has no focal neurologic deficits or evidence of intracranial mass and coagulopathy on clinical grounds. Antibiotics can be administered during or immediately after LP. If the patient has focal neurologic deficits or papilledema, however, a head CT scan should be performed prior to LP in order to determine the possible risks for transtentorial or tonsillar herniation associated with LP. In these cases, antibiotic therapy must be administered prior to patient transport to the radiology suite for CT scanning. Antibiotic therapy should always be initiated in the ED and never be delayed for CT scanning or other studies.

Presently, the antibiotic therapy of choice is a **third-generation cephalosporin,** such as ceftriaxone or cefotaxime. A dose of 2 gm IV should be administered and will cover the most common organisms (*S. pneumoniae, H. influenzae, N. meningitidis*). Additionally, it is recommended that **ampicillin** (2 gm IV) be administered to cover for *L. monocytogenes.* For the patient who is severely penicillin-allergic, the combination of chloramphenicol and trimethoprim–sulfamethoxazole is recommended. Steroid therapy is controversial in adults and, if initiated, should be given prior to the first dose of antibiotics.

Other general management measures also are important. Hypotonic fluids should be avoided. Serum sodium levels should be monitored to detect the syndrome of inappropriate antidiuretic hormone or cerebral salt-wasting. Hyperpyrexia should be treated with acetaminophen. Coagulopathies need to be corrected using specific replacement therapies. Seizures should be treated with benzodiazepines and, if needed, phenytoin loading. Evidence of marked intracranial pressure should be treated with hyperventilation, head elevation, and mannitol.

Viral meningitis, without evidence of encephalitis, can be managed on an out-patient basis provided the patient is nontoxic in appearance and has reliable followup. It remains a diagnosis of exclusion, however, and unless the diagnosis of viral meningitis is obvious, admission is warranted.

ENCEPHALITIS

Viral encephalitis is a viral infection of brain parenchyma producing an inflammatory response. It is distinct from, although often coexists with, viral meningitis.

Clinical Features

Encephalitis should be considered in patients presenting with any or all of the following features: new psychiatric symptoms, cognitive deficits (aphasia, amnestic syndrome, acute confusional state), seizures, and movement disorders. Signs and symptoms of headache, photophobia, fever, and meningeal irritation may be present. Assessment for neurologic findings and cognitive deficits is crucial. Encephalitides may show special regional trophism. Herpes simplex virus (HSV) involves limbic structures of the temporal and frontal lobes, with prominent psychiatric features, memory disturbance, and aphasia. Some arboviruses predominantly affect the basal ganglia, causing chorea-athetosis and parkinsonism.

Diagnosis and Differential

ED diagnosis can be suggested by findings on MRI and LP. MRI not only excludes other potential lesions, such as brain abscess, but may display findings highly suggestive of HSV encephalitis if the medial temporal and inferior frontal gray matter are involved. On LP, findings of aseptic meningitis are typical.

The differential diagnosis includes brain abscess; Lyme disease; subarachnoid hemorrhage; bacterial, tuberculous, fungal, or neoplastic meningitis; bacterial endocarditis; postinfectious encephalomyelitis; toxic or metabolic encephalopathies; and primary psychiatric disorders.

Emergency Department Care and Disposition

The patient suspected of suffering from viral encephalitis should be admitted. Of the viruses causing encephalitis, only HSV has been shown by clinical trial to be responsive to antiviral therapy. The agent of choice is **acyclovir** (10–14 mg/kg IV). Potential complications of encephalitis—seizures, disorders of sodium metabolism, increased intracranial pressure, and systemic consequences of a comatose state—should be handled in standard ways.

BRAIN ABSCESS

A brain abscess is a focal pyogenic infection. It is composed of a central pus-filled cavity, ringed by a layer of granulation tissue and an outer fibrous capsule.

Clinical Features

Since patients typically are not acutely toxic, the presenting features of brain abscess are nonspecific. For this reason, the initial diagnosis can be difficult in the ED. The most common symptom is headache. Approximately 50% of the time, the patient will have fever, vomiting, confusion, or obtundation. Meningeal signs and focal neurologic findings, such as hemiparesis, seizures, and papilledema, are present in less than half the cases.

Diagnosis and Differential

Classically, brain abscess can be diagnosed by CT scan of the head with contrast, which demonstrates one or several thin, smoothly contoured rings of enhancement surrounding a low-density center and, in turn, surrounded by white-matter edema. LP is contraindicated when brain abscess is suspected and after the diagnosis has been established. Other studies, such as blood work and EEG, are nonspecific. Blood cultures should be obtained.

The differential diagnosis includes cerebrovascular disease, meningitis, brain neoplasm, subacute brain hemorrhage, and other focal brain infections, such as toxoplasmosis.

Emergency Department Care and Disposition

Decisions on antibiotic therapy for brain abscess should depend on the likely source of the infection. In a suspected otogenic case, initial therapy should consist of a **third-generation cephalosporin** or trimethoprim–sulfamethoxazole with chloramphenicol or metronidazole. In a suspected sinogenic or odontogenic case, initial therapy should consist of high-dose **penicillin with chloramphenicol** or metronidazole. In a suspected cardiac case, initial therapy should consist of **vancomycin with chloramphenicol** or metronidazole. When communication with the exterior is suspected, as in penetrating trauma or postneurosurgical procedure, initial therapy should consist of vancomycin. Ceftazidime should be added if gram-negative aerobes are suspected. Finally, in cases where no clear etiology exists, initial empiric therapy should consist of a third-generation cephalosporin and metronidazole.

Neurosurgical consultation and admission are warranted, since many cases will require neurosurgery for diagnosis and bacteriology, if not for definitive treatment.

For further reading in *Emergency Medicine: A Comprehensive Study Guide*, 4th edition, see Chapter 199, Meningitis, Encephalitis, and Brain Abscess, by David C. Anderson and Alan J. Kozak.

Neuroleptic malignant syndrome (NMS) is a rare disorder characterized by hyperthermia, muscular rigidity, altered mental status, and autonomic dysfunction, it is primarily found in young and middle-aged adults who use neuroleptic agents.

Clinical Features

A history of psychiatric illness is common, and phenothiazine use is almost always noted in patients with NMS. Withdrawal from anti-Parkinson medications and recreational drug use also can be associated with NMS. Hyperthermia is present in 98% of reported cases; 40% have a temperature greater than 40°C. Generalized rigidity is reported in 97% of patients and can lead to myonecrosis. Increased muscular rigidity is the primary cause of the hyperthermia. Akinesia, tremor, dysarthria, and dysphagia also may be present. Mental status changes are noted in 97% of patients and can range from confusion to stupor or coma. Autonomic instability is noted in 95% of patients, which is manifested as tachycardia, fluctuations in BP, or cardiac dysrhythmias.

Symptoms usually develop 1 to 7 days after exposure to a neuroleptic agent and may occur up to 4 wks after exposure. Once use of the neuroleptic agent has been stopped, symptoms will last approximately 10 days. Death may occur from respiratory failure or cardiac arrest.

Diagnosis and Differential

Major criteria for NMS include fever, rigidity, and elevated CPK; minor criteria include tachycardia, abnormal blood pressure, tachypnea, altered mental status, diaphoresis, and leukocytosis. To make the diagnosis, three major or two major and four minor findings should be present, along with a history of neuroleptic agent use.

Diagnostic evaluation should include a CBC with differential, chemistry panel, ABG, calcium, urinalysis, urine myoglobin, coagulation studies, EKG, chest x-ray, and CSF analysis. Leukocytosis is present in 98% of patients; metabolic acidosis or hypoxemia on ABG analysis is present in 75%; CPK elevation is present in 95%; urine myoglobin can be present in 66% of patients. The lumbar puncture is critical in helping to exclude meningitis.

Other causes of the patient's clinical picture should be ruled out. The differential diagnosis of NMS is found in Table 136-1.

Emergency Department Care and Disposition

The treatment of NMS is based on cessation of neuroleptic medications, institution of rapid cooling, fluid replacement, support of the cardiovas-

TABLE 136-1. Differential Diagnosis of Neuroleptic Malignant Syndrome

Endocrine
  Hyperthyroidism
Environmental
  Heat stroke
Infections
  Meningitis
  Encephalitis
  Sepsis
  Tetanus
  Rabies
Neuromuscular
  Malignant hyperthermia
  Parkinson disease
  Severe dystonia
Psychiatric
  Lethal catatonia
Rahabdomyolysis
Toxic
  Cocaine
  Amphetamines
  Strychnine
  Anticholinergics
  Monoamine oxidase inhibitors

cular and pulmonary systems, and prevention of complications. Patients should be placed on a cardiac and pulse oximetry monitor, and have an IV line started.

1. **Oxygen** should be administered. Intubation should be performed, as needed, to support the patient's respiratory status.
2. **Crystalloid IV fluids** should be given initially for hypotension. A urine output of 30 ml/h or greater should be maintained. This should be monitored with a Foley catheter.
3. **Rapid cooling** should be undertaken using evaporation with a mist fan, cooling blankets, ice packs, and antipyretics (acetaminophen).

Patients with NMS should be admitted to the ICU. Aggressive monitoring of vital signs, urine output, respiratory and mental status are required. Nontoxic patients with an unclear diagnosis may be followed closely on an outpatient basis after a thorough ED evaluation. Along with close followup, a short course of bromocriptine (2.5 mg PO tid) and dantrolene (50 mg PO bid) may be given until symptoms resolve.

If Standard Treatment Fails

Fever unresponsive to cooling measures may respond to bromocriptine (Parlodel). An initial dose of 5 mg, followed by 2.5 to 10 mg orally tid, should be used. Patients with severe vasoconstriction contributing to hyperthermia may benefit from nitroprusside. Muscular rigidity and hyperthermia may respond to dantrolene (Dantrium, 0.8 to 3 mg/kg IV every 6 h, max dose 10 mg/kg per 24 h). Oral dosing of dantrolene is 50 to 100 mg bid. Benzodiazepines may be effective for muscular rigidity as well. Patients with a history of withdrawal from Parkinson-disease medications may benefit from a combination of levodopa and carbidopa (Sinemet), with or without amantadine (Symmetrel).

For further reading in *Emergency Medicine: A Comprehensive Study Guide,* 4th edition, see Chapter 200, Neuroleptic Malignant Syndrome, by Philip L. Henneman.

17 | EYE, EAR, NOSE, THROAT, ORAL EMERGENCIES

BLUNT TRAUMATIC OCULAR EMERGENCIES

Subconjunctival hemorrhage This injury represents a disruption of blood vessels within the normally clear conjunctiva and will resolve spontaneously. A dense, circumferential subconjunctival hemorrhage (bloody chemosis) requires further investigation to rule out occult globe rupture.

Corneal abrasions Traumatic abrasions may cause superficial or deep epithelial defects resulting in tearing, blepharospasm, and severe pain. A topical anesthetic (proparacaine or tetracaine) will facilitate the exam. A small amount of fluorescein is used to stain the tear film and dye uptake (green color) is seen wherever epithelial cells are disrupted. Consider treating corneal abrasions with a cycloplegic (1% cyclopentolate or 5% homatropine) unless the patient is at risk for narrow-angle glaucoma; cycloplegia relaxes ciliary spasm to provide pain relief. Simple, clean abrasions are treated with a layer of topical antibiotic ointment (erythromycin, tobramycin, gentamycin, or bacitracin/polymyxin), followed by placement of a light-pressure eye patch. Dirty abrasions with a high potential for infection are left unpatched and treated with antibiotic drops every 1 to 2 h while awake. Broad-spectrum choices include ciprofloxacin, norfloxacin, tobramycin, and gentamicin. All patients may be discharged with oral analgesics, but topical anesthetics are absolutely contraindicated, since repeated use may cause permanent corneal damage. All but the simplest of abrasions should be re-examined in 24 h when the patch is removed.

Contact lens-related injuries These corneal injuries may be caused by ill-fitting lenses, foreign matter trapped under the lens, lens overuse, or trauma during lens placement or removal. Simple abrasions are treated in the standard manner, but corneal ulcerations and infections must be ruled out. An ulcer will appear as a fluorescein-stained epithelial defect with a local corneal infiltrate (white spot or haze). Emergency ophthalmologic consultation is required since *Pseudomonas* is a leading cause and can rapidly destroy the cornea. Hourly use of quinolone eye drops (ciprofloxacin or norfloxacin), avoidance of patching, and meticulous followup are required.

Traumatic iritis and iridocyclitis Mild inflammation of the iris (iritis) or iris and ciliary body (iridocyclitis) is commonly seen after blunt trauma to the eye. Symptoms include a deep, aching pain with photophobia. Signs include injection at the corneoscleral limbus (ciliary flush), as well as WBC and protein in the anterior chamber (cell and flare). Treatment consists of topical cycloplegics (1% cyclopentolate or 5%

homatropine applied t.i.d.) and ophthalmologic consultation to consider topical steroids.

Traumatic miosis and mydriasis   The ciliary body may respond to blunt trauma with either mydriasis (pupillary dilation) or miosis (constriction). Small triangular defects at the pupillary margin result from tears of the sphincter. None of these injuries require specific treatment, although they should be followed by an ophthalmologist.

Iridodialysis   Blunt trauma may cause iridodialysis, a separation of the iris peripherally at the ciliary body. This serious injury creates a lentiform defect (accessory pupil) at the limbus, and there is often an associated hyphema. Ophthalmologic consultation must be obtained.

Hyphema   Hyphema is blood in the anterior chamber. The volume ranges from minimal amounts seen only with a slit lamp to massive amounts filling the entire chamber. Rebleeds often occur between 2 and 5 days following the initial injury and are associated with a high rate of complications. Management consists of a Fox shield to prevent further injury, placement of the patient at 45° to keep red cells from staining the cornea and emergent ophthalmologic consultation to consider various treatment options. Patients with sickle-cell disease tolerate hyphemas poorly, and emergent consultation should be sought.

TRAUMATIC RETINOPATHIES AND OTHER INJURIES

Commotio retinae   Blunt ocular trauma may result in transient retinal edema that appears as patchy white areas. Consultation should be obtained.

Traumatic retinal detachments   Traction on the retina is painless and causes a sensation of flashing lights as the retina is stimulated. Detachment of the retina may occur acutely, although it is sometimes delayed by mo to y. Depending on the location of the injury, a visual field defect may be identified and the actual billowy gray detached retina may be seen. Urgent consultation is required.

Vitreous and retinal hemorrhages   Hemorrhage into the vitreous often results in floaters, clumps of red blood cells that are seen by the patient as specks or strands floating in the visual field. Retinal hemorrhages, often visible with the ophthalmoscope, are frequently asymptomatic unless they involve the macula. Both retinal and vitreous hemorrhage require ophthalmologic referral.

Ruptured globe   Globe rupture is a catastrophic injury that must be immediately identified. Suggestive findings include teardrop-shaped pupil, bloody chemosis, extrusion of globe contents, and a streaming appearance to fluorescein instilled onto the tear layer. Once identified, any further manipulation of the eye must be avoided. Place a Fox shield over the eye to protect it from direct pressure, start broad-spectrum parenteral antibiotics, and consult an ophthalmologist emergently.

Optic nerve trauma Traumatic damage to the optic nerve results in an afferent pupillary defect with variable fundoscopic findings depending on the nature and extent of the injury. Elevated intraorbital pressure may result from hematomas and cause ischemic injury to the optic nerve unless decompressed with a lateral canthotomy. Optic nerve injury requires immediate ophthalmologic consultation.

EXTERNAL FOREIGN BODIES

Conjunctival foreign bodies Foreign bodies of the conjunctiva are removed under topical anesthesia using a moistened sterile swab. Eversion of the upper lid is performed to rule out foreign matter in the superior conjunctival fornix.

Corneal foreign bodies Foreign bodies of the cornea are removed under topical anesthesia using a slit lamp. They may be approached with a moistened sterile swab, fine needle tip, or special eye spud. Metallic foreign bodies often leave an epithelial rust ring that may be removed immediately with an eye burr. Alternatively, it may be easier to remove at followup if allowed to soften for 1 to 2 days. A corneal abrasion will result from foreign body removal and is treated in the standard manner, even if a rust ring is present.

Cyanoacrylate glue removal Cyanoacrylate glue (Super-Glue, Krazy-Glue) readily adheres to the eyelids and corneal surface but causes no permanent damage. The lids and ocular surface should be irrigated for 15 min with warm water. Mineral oil may be applied to eyelid adhesions to further soften the glue. Resultant corneal abrasions should be treated in the standard manner, and all cases should be referred to an ophthalmologist for followup.

PENETRATING OCULAR TRAUMA

Lid lacerations All eyelid and adnexal lacerations require meticulous evaluation to rule out ocular and nasolacrimal injury. Lid margin lacerations require closure under magnification by an ophthalmologist. For medial lid lacerations, injury to the lacrimal canaliculi and puncta must be ruled out. Fluorescein instilled into the tear layer that appears in an adjacent laceration confirms the injury. All suspected or proven nasolacrimal injuries require ophthalmologic evaluation. Upper lid lacerations that involve the levator mechanism and all through-and-through lid lacerations must be repaired in the OR.

Corneal and scleral lacerations Full thickness lacerations are differentiated from partial-thickness lacerations by Seidel's test, the appearance of fluorescein streaming from a full-thickness wound. Either lesion requires emergent ophthalmologic consultation and placement of a Fox shield to avoid any pressure on the eye.

Retained intraocular foreign body Foreign bodies may enter the globe and leave no obvious evidence of penetration. Maintain a high index of suspicion and perform a thorough history and exam. Consider the use of direct visualization (slit lamp, ophthalmoscope), skull radiographs, CT/MRI scanning, and ultrasound. Removal requires immediate ophthalmologic consultation.

CHEMICAL BURNS

All corrosive burns, whether acid or alkali, are managed in a similar manner. *The eye should be immediately flushed at the scene and at least 1 to 2 additional l of normal saline should be continued in the ED.* A topical anesthetic and a Morgan lens will facilitate flushing. Inspect the fornices for retained matter and continue irrigation until the pH is 7.4 to 7.6. Wait 10 min and recheck the pH to make sure no additional corrosive is leaking out from the tissues. Record intraocular pressures, especially in alkali burns. Apply a cycloplegic (1% cyclopentolate or 5% homatropine) to alleviate ciliary spasm and coat the eye with a broad-spectrum antibiotic ointment. Most patients will need generous pain medications. An ophthalmologist should be consulted to arrange immediate followup.

LIGHT-INDUCED OCULAR TRAUMA

Ultraviolet keratitis and laser-induced scotomas UV keratitis is a corneal sunburn that may result from tanning booths, welding flashes, or prolonged sun exposure. Severe pain and photophobia take 4 to 8 h to develop. Conjunctival hyperemia and punctate corneal fluorescein uptake are easily identified. Treatment consists of cycloplegia (1% cyclopentolate or 5% homatropine), antibiotic ointment, eye patching, and pain medication. No permanent sequelae should be anticipated. Conversely, laser light that strikes the retina has the potential to permanently scar the tissue and cause a scotoma. There is no treatment for this injury.

NONTRAUMATIC OCULAR EMERGENCIES

Conjunctivitis

Conjunctivitis is inflammation of the normally clear conjunctiva. It is important to separate infectious from noninfectious conjunctivitis and to differentiate simple conjunctivitis from more ominous causes of reddened eye.

Viral conjunctivitis The majority of patients who present with *pink eye*, have viral conjunctivitis, often with concurrent viral upper respiratory infection. The patient may complain of excessive tearing (epiphora) and discomfort. Epidemic keratoconjunctivitis (EKC) is a particularly contagious viral infection that causes greater pain and redness, often with photophobia and eventual contralateral involvement. Subepithelial corneal infiltrates are often visible and may significantly reduce visual acuity. Viral conjunctivitis is self-limited in about 10 days, although EKC may last up to 3 wks. Cases are generally treated with a topical antibiotic to prevent superinfection, and because bacterial causes can not always be distinguished clinically. Ophthalmologic consultation for topical steroids in severe EKC may be considered.

Bacterial conjunctivitis Bacterial conjunctivitis presents with eyelash matting, mucopurulent discharge, and minimal pain. Treatment consists of topical antibiotic drops (e.g., sulfacetamide, tobramycin, or gentamicin) up to 6 times daily for 7 days. Extremely purulent conjunctivitis should prompt culture and treatment for *Neisseria gonorrhea*. Ceftriaxone (1 g IM), topical tetracycline drops, frequent saline washes, and close followup are required.

Chlamydial conjunctivitis This infection may appear like viral or bacterial conjunctivitis, but there is also a marked follicular response on the palpebral conjunctiva. Treatment requires both oral and topical antibiotics for 3 wks. Oral regimens include doxycycline or erythromycin; topical choices are tetracycline or sulfonamide drops.

Allergic conjunctivitis This is a noninfectious seasonal conjunctivitis that causes stringy white discharge, redness, chemosis, and intense pruritus. Treatment includes topical antihistamines such as levocobastine (Livostin) or topical antihistamine/decongestant combinations such as naphazoline/antizoline. Cool compresses and avoidance of contact lens wearing will promote comfort.

Keratitis

Keratitis refers to inflammation of the cornea.

Bacterial keratitis and corneal ulcers Bacterial keratitis typically presents with a white corneal infiltrate and an overlying epithelial defect (i.e., corneal ulcer). An associated iritis is often seen. Treat once with a topical cycloplegic and use ciprofloxacin or norfloxacin hourly while awake. All cases require emergent followup.

Viral keratitis Herpes simplex keratoconjunctivitis is a primary infection of the eye that causes herpetic vesicles and characteristic dendrites on the cornea. Herpes zoster keratitis is distinguished from primary herpes infections by the concurrent cutaneous eruption along the ophthalmic division of the trigeminal nerve. Both infections require immediate ophthalmologic consultation for specific antiviral therapy. Topical steroid use in patients with herpes simplex keratoconjunctivitis may be catastrophic.

Episcleritis Episcleritis is a benign, self-limited inflammation of the tissue at the junction of the conjunctiva and sclera known as the episclera. Patients present with discomfort, localized hyperemia, and swelling. Topical decongestants (e.g., naphazoline HCL), topical steroids, and oral NSAIDs may help but should be used in consultation with an ophthalmologist.

Scleritis Scleritis presents with violaceous scleral injection and deep orbital pain. Full medical evaluation is required to rule out associated systemic disease. Immediate ophthalmologic consultation is required.

Acute Angle Closure Glaucoma (AACG)

Shallow anterior chambers may block aqueous outflow and predispose the patient to an attack of AACG. In severe episodes, patients may present with ocular injection, corneal haziness, iritis, minimal to nonreactive pupils, and intraocular pressures (IOP) of 40 to 70 mm Hg (normal is 10 to 20). Intense orbital pain with nausea and blurry vision is common. Treatment to decrease the IOP must be started emergently. Pilocarpine (2%) is a miotic that promotes aqueous outflow; use 1 drop every 15 min in the affected eye, and one drop every 6 h on the contralateral side for prophylaxis. Topical timolol (Timoptic) directly lowers IOP and may facilitate the action of pilocarpine; use one drop in the affected eye immediately. Carbonic anhydrase inhibitors decrease aqueous formation; use acetazolamide (Diamox, 500 mg IV). Hyperosmotic agents may also be initiated. Oral regimens include 50% glycerol (1 cc/kg), or 45% isosorbide (1.5 g/kg or about 220 cc). Both drugs are poured over ice to decrease their sweetness, and glycerol is relatively contraindicated in diabetics. Alternatively, mannitol 20% (0.5 to 2.0 g/kg) may be given IV. All cases require immediate ophthalmologic consultation.

Uveitis and Iritis

Uveitis is inflammation of the iris, ciliary body, and choroid. Most commonly, anterior uveitis is seen, and this is known as iritis. This disorder may result from traumatic, infectious, and autoimmune causes. Symptoms may include blurred vision, deep orbital aching, photophobia, and redness. Slit lamp examination will identify cells in the anterior chamber (cell) with suspended proteins causing a fogginess of the slit lamp beam (flare). Treatment consists of topical steroids, topical cycloplegics, and ophthalmologic consultation.

Amaurosis Fugax

Amaurosis fugax is a transient, monocular ischemic attack from an embolic event involving the retinal artery or arterioles. It causes a painless graying or blurring of the visual field often described as a descending nightshade. Focal arteriole obstructions (Hollenhorst plaques) are occasionally seen with the ophthalmoscope. Thorough evaluation to uncover the embolic source is required.

Central Retinal Artery Occlusion (CRAO)

CRAO is an acute, painless, monocular loss of vision. Occlusion of the CRA itself will cause complete visual loss; branch obstruction will only cause loss in the involved field. Physical exam confirms the visual loss and may show an afferent pupillary defect, narrowed arterioles with segmented flow (boxcarring), and a bright red macula (cherry red spot). This is a true ophthalmologic emergency and treatment must begin instantaneously once the diagnosis is suspected. A moderate pressure massage is applied to the globe for 5 sec, rapidly released for 5 sec, and then repeated as necessary for the next 30 min. Breathing Carbogen, a 95:5 mixture of O_2 and CO_2 for 10 min each h may also promote vasodilation and relief. An ophthalmologist should be consulted immediately to consider surgical decompression and anticoagulation.

Central Retinal Vein Occlusion (CRVO)

CRVO causes acute, painless visual loss, although not quite as abruptly as in CRAO. Examination reveals retinal hemorrhages, cotton wool spots, and edema in a dramatic pattern previously described as retinal apoplexy. There is no immediate treatment for CRVO, but ophthalmologic followup is required.

Optic Neuritis (ON)

Optic neuritis refers to inflammation at any point along the optic nerve. The primary causes are infection (often viral), demyelination (frequently the presenting symptom of multiple sclerosis), and autoimmune disorders. ON results in a reduction or dimness of vision, often with poor color perception. Over half of patients have pain, mainly during extraocular movement. Visual field cuts with an afferent pupillary defect are the usual findings. In anterior ON, the optic disc appears swollen; there are no ophthalmoscopic findings in retrobulbar cases. Evaluation and treatment should be directed by an ophthalmologist.

For further reading in *Emergency Medicine: A Comprehensive Study Guide*, 4th edition, see Chapter 201, Ocular Emergencies, by Alvina M. Janda.

OTOLOGIC EMERGENCIES

Otalgia

Ear pain may result from any pathologic process that affect the ear itself. It may also arise as pain referred from the proximal cervical region, temporomandibular joint, mandible, teeth, tongue, tonsil, larynx, or cervical esophagus. Treatment consists of addressing the underlying cause, providing analgesia, and providing ENT referral when appropriate.

External Otitis

External otitis (EO) and malignant external otitis are diseases at the extremes of the spectrum progressing from dermatitis of the external auditory canal (EAC), to cellulitis, chondritis, and finally to osteomyelitis of the temporal bone and base of the skull. Malignant external otitis is more correctly known as necrotizing external otitis (NEO). EO occurs frequently in swimmers, and NEO occurs primarily in diabetics and immunocompromised patients.

Patients with EO have ear pain exacerbated by movement of the pinna or tragus. The EAC may be erythematous, or may be suppurative with edema, exudate, and debris that often completely obstructs the EAC and causes a conductive hearing loss. In NEO, the disease has spread to involve the pinna and periauricular structures. As NEO progresses, patients may develop trismus, fever, sepsis, cranial nerve palsies, meningitis, or brain abscess. The diagnosis of EO and NEO is strictly clinical.

EO is treated with hydrocortisone and neomycin mixed with either polymyxin B (Cortisporin Otic) or colistin sulfate (Coly-Mycin S Otic). Cortisporin Otic solution is preferred over the suspension but may irritate the middle ear if the tympanic membrane (TM) is perforated. If the TM is perforated or not visualized, use the suspension. The EAC should first be cleansed of debris with light suction, irrigation, or curettage. A gauze wick will facilitate antibiotic penetration for EACs with moderate obstruction. Four drops of medication should be placed in the ear 4 times daily until the EO resolves. If the TM is not visualized, the patient should be treated presumptively with additional oral antibiotics for concurrent otitis media. Patients with only mild erythema of the pinna who are not a risk for NEO may be closely followed as outpatients. Patients with NEO require urgent ENT consultation and treatment with either an antipseudomonal cephalosporin or an antipseudomonal penicillin plus an aminoglycoside.

Otitis Media

Acute otitis media (AOM) is a common infection often heralded by acute otalgia. Fever frequently occurs, but findings may be much less specific, especially in infants. The diagnosis requires direct visualization of the TM, which may appear erythematous, opacified, or bulging. In otitis media with effusion, an air-fluid level or bubbles may be seen. Loss of mobility on insufflation during pneumatic otoscopy is a sensitive sign of AOM. Bullous myringitis (BM) is a variant of AOM that includes bullae or vesicles on the TM. The causative organisms are often the same, although some cases of BM are secondary to *Mycoplasma*.

Patients with AOM are prescribed a 10-day course of antibiotic therapy with out-patient followup at the completion of treatment. Antibiotic treatment is usually started with amoxicillin; trimethoprim–sulfamethoxazole or erythromycin–sulfisoxazole may be used for the penicillin-allergic patient. Macrolides effective against Mycoplasma are the best choice for patients with BM. Failure to respond to 2 to 3 days of therapy warrants an antibiotic change to include coverage of β-lactamase-producing species (e.g., amoxicillin–clavulanate). Complications of AOM may include TM perforation, cholesteatoma, hearing loss, mastoiditis, meningitis, or brain abscess.

Mastoiditis

Mastoiditis is a serious complication of inadequately treated otitis media and occurs most often in the pediatric age group. Frequently, there is a history of otitis media, antibiotic use, persistent otalgia, or otorrhea. Clinical deterioration in the otitis media patient should always prompt concern for suppurative complications, including mastoiditis.

Clinical findings of suspected mastoiditis may include mastoid tenderness and erythema, loss of the postauricular crease, inferolateral displacement of the pinna, or local fluctuance. The TM is often erythematous, edematous, or perforated, although 10% of TMs may be normal. CBC may show a leukocytosis and plain radiographs occasionally reveal mastoid opacification. All patients should have a CT scan to help confirm the diagnosis and to rule out other intracranial processes.

Emergent ENT consultation for surgical drainage is required. Antibiotic therapy should be started with either ampicillin–sulbactam, ceftriaxone and metronidazole, or imipenem–cilastatin. Complications of mastoiditis may include facial palsies, extension of the abscess into the neck, meningitis, intracranial abscess, or septic thrombophlebitis.

Sudden Hearing Loss

Sudden hearing loss is categorized as either conductive or sensory. Conductive deficits occur when sound waves are not conducted to the inner ear, such as in cerumen impaction, foreign body obstruction, external otitis, TM perforation, tympanosclerosis, disruption of the ossicular chain, or middle-ear fluid. Sensorineural deficits are a consequence of disruption of the neural pathway and may result from viral neuronitis, acoustic neuroma, Ménière's disease, autoimmune disorders, and idiopathic causes.

Two forms of hearing loss can be evaluated by the Weber and Rinne tests. In Weber's test, for cases of sensorineural hearing loss, sound lateralizes to the normal ear; in conductive loss, sound lateralizes to the abnormal ear. In the Rinne's test, the tuning fork will be inaudible if there is a conductive deficit.

Trauma

Seromas and hematomas of the ear present as a firm, painful swelling of the auricle. These lesions require needle aspiration, followed by placement of a periauricular packing and a firm mastoid dressing.

Thermal injury to the auricle may be caused by either excessive heat or cold. Superficial injury is treated with cleansing and topical antimicrobial agents. Full-thickness lesions require ENT consultation for debridement. Frostbite is treated with rapid rewarming using saline soaked gauze at 38°C to 42°C; subsequent ENT referral is required.

Perichondritis and chondritis often occur if a traumatized ear becomes infected and may result in severe destruction of the ear cartilage. The patient has pain and fever with erythema, warmth, and swelling localized to the perichondral region. Parenteral antibiotics active against *Pseudomonas, Proteus*, and *Staphylococcus* are required. ENT consultation for surgical drainage must be obtained.

Foreign Bodies in the Ear

On examination, the foreign body (FB) is usually visualized, and signs of infection or TM perforation should be sought. Live insects are particularly distressing to the patient and should be immobilized immediately with 2% lidocaine instilled into the ear canal prior to removal. Patient cooperation is essential in order to avoid lodging the FB more medially. Options for removal depend on the size and composition of the FB. Irrigation is often useful for small objects, although organic matter may absorb the water and swell. Small FBs can be grasped with microforceps, whereas larger objects can be hooked from behind and removed with traction. Cyanoacrylate glue on the tip of a probe may allow the probe to be attached to a hard, smooth FB for removal. ENT consultation is required in cases of TM perforation, ossicular damage, caustic substances, and if an impacted FB cannot be safely and easily removed.

Tympanic Membrane (TM) Perforations

Perforation of the TM may result from several diverse causes, including trauma, infection, or lightning. The patient may have slight hearing loss and pain. Vertigo and deafness signifies injury to the ossicles, labyrinth, or temporal bone and requires urgent consultation. Antibiotics are not useful in uncomplicated TM perforation, but standard antibiotics are used when there is coexistent otitis media. All perforations require ENT followup.

SALIVARY GLAND PROBLEMS

Sialoadenitis

Mumps is the most common cause of painful parotid swelling in the pediatric age group. Symptoms progress from fever and malaise to increasing pain with parotid swelling. Bilateral parotitis occurs in 70% of patients, although there is no discharge from Stenson's duct. The diagnosis is clinical and the treatment is symptomatic.

Bacterial parotiditis sometimes occurs in people with a decreased flow of saliva. This includes debilitated patients, the elderly, postoperative patients, and patients on anticholinergic medications. The parotid is swollen and tender with pus often expressed at Stenson's duct. Progression is heralded by fever, trismus, and involvement of the face and neck. Treatment consists of hydration, massage, local heat, sialagogues (e.g., lemon drops), and β-lactamase-resistant antibiotics. Severe cases and treatment failures require ENT consultation.

Salivary Calculi

Sialolithiasis presents with unilateral pain and swelling, with over 80% of cases involving the submandibular glands. The stone is often palpable and visible on intraoral radiographs. Treatment consists of analgesics, sialagogues; antibiotics are given if an infection is present. Easily located calculi may be milked from the duct or removed after dilation or incision of the ductal orifice. Complicated cases and intraglandular sialoliths require ENT referral.

POSTADENOTONSILLECTOMY BLEEDING

This is a rare but potentially fatal complication of tonsillectomy. Management consist of ensuring an adequate airway and suctioning for clot removal. Active bleeding requires direct pressure with a ring forceps and oxidized cellulose, thrombin packing, or gauze moistened with 1:000 epinephrine and 4% lidocaine. Further resources include silver nitrate cautery and local injection of lidocaine with epinephrine. Massive hemorrhage may require resuscitation, posterior nasal packing, and emergency surgery.

ACUTE UPPER AIRWAY OBSTRUCTION

Airway foreign bodies may present in a straightforward manner, or they may have an insidious presentation such as progressive stridor or recurrent pneumonia. Upper airway FBs may cause stridor and odyno-phagia with subsequent respiratory arrest. Lower airway FBs, commonly on the right side, may present as cough, wheezing, dyspnea, pneumonia, or respiratory distress.

The stable patient is a candidate for direct inspection of the oropharynx, possibly aided by a laryngoscope and topical anesthesia. Soft-tissue radiographs and endoscopy are further diagnostic adjuncts. Equipment for definitive management of the airway must be available, and extreme care is taken to avoid destabilizing a partial obstruction. Unstable patients may have the Heimlich maneuver performed in the prehospital setting, but once in the ED, a quick attempt at removal with direct laryngoscopy is indicated. Failure at removal may require a surgical airway or a deeply placed, double-lumen endotracheal tube to attempt unilateral ventilation of the unaffected lung while preparation is made for emergent bronchoscopy.

LARYNGEAL TRAUMA

Laryngeal injuries may result from blunt or penetrating trauma and have significant morbidity and mortality. Patients may present with hoarseness, hemoptysis, dyspnea, dysphagia, aphonia, stridor, or respiratory distress. Physical signs include laryngeal swelling, tenderness, anterior neck contusion, altered laryngeal contour, tracheal deviation, or subcutaneous emphysema.

Emergent ENT consultation is warranted for all patients with signs and symptoms consistent with laryngeal injury. Initially minor laryngeal injuries may progress due to edema and expanding hematomas, and close observation is required. Stable patients may be placed on humidified oxygen while awaiting ENT consultation. The unstable patient requires aggressive airway management with tracheostomy. If this cannot be performed, gentle endotracheal intubation or cricothyroidotomy may be required. Antibiotics active against respiratory flora (e.g., ampicillin/sulbactam are given when there is mucosal violation or subcutaneous emphysema.

HEAD AND NECK INFECTIONS

Epiglottitis

Epiglottitis is an acute, life-threatening supraglottic infection occurring in all age groups, although predominantly in children ages 1 to 5. Pediatric epiglottitis progresses over a 12- to 24-h period, and may include fever, anxiety, sore throat, dysphagia, drooling, toxic appearance, or respiratory arrest. Adult epiglottitis often presents with h to days of dysphagia and throat pain out of proportion to the clinical exam.

In toxic patients, especially children, all diagnostic procedures are deferred until the patient is in the operating room with an ENT specialist.

Cooperative, stable adult patients with suspected epiglottitis should undergo indirect laryngoscopy; on occasion, the epiglottis of a calm older child can be visualized with a tongue blade alone. A soft tissue lateral neck radiograph may show an edematous (thumbprint) epiglottis with ballooning of the hypopharynx and loss of the vallecula.

Treatment consists of oxygen, aggressive airway management, and antibiotics. The unstable patient may be temporized with a bag–valve mask, but a definitive airway should be secured emergently in the OR. If intubation is unsuccessful, children under 8 years old may require needle cricothyroidotomy, and those over 8 may need standard open cricothyroidotomy. An ENT physician must be consulted for emergent tracheostomy. The stable pediatric patient is treated with endotracheal intubation in the operating room. Stable adults may be managed in the ICU without intubation. Parenteral antibiotics (cefuroxime, cefotaxime, ceftriaxone) should cover *H. influenzae*. Aztreonam or chloramphenicol can be used in penicillin-allergic patients. Steroid therapy to decrease airway edema is controversial.

Peritonsillar Abscess

Peritonsillar abscess occurs predominantly in teenagers and young adults, and is often preceded by a throat infection. Presenting symptoms may include fever, sore throat, drooling, muffled voice, trismus, dysphagia, otalgia, or foul breath. Classic physical signs include a unilaterally enlarged tonsil with swelling of the anterior tonsillar pillar and contralateral deviation of the uvula. Advanced cases may have airway obstruction, pulmonary aspiration, or mediastinitis.

In stable patients, ENT consultation for needle aspiration is both diagnostic and therapeutic and provides immediate resolution of trismus and odynophagia. These patients are then discharged on broad-spectrum antistaphylococcal antibiotics such as amoxicillin–clavulanate. Patients who are toxic, uncooperative, or unable to be successfully aspirated require parenteral antibiotics and drainage under general anesthesia.

Retropharyngeal Abscess

Retropharyngeal abscess is a disease predominantly of children less than 5 years old, although it also occurs in adults. Signs include fever, odynophagia, neck swelling, drooling, torticollis, meningismus, and possibly stridor. The lateral neck radiograph frequently shows prevertebral soft-tissue swelling that exceeds one half the width of the adjacent vertebral body. CT scanning is useful in differentiating cellulitis from abscess.

ED treatment consists of meticulous airway control and parenteral antibiotics (high-dose penicillin G and metronidazole). Emergent ENT consultation for operative drainage is required.

Parapharyngeal Abscess

The parapharyngeal space extends lateral to the pharynx from the base of the skull to the hyoid. Abscesses in this area may result from local infection, trauma, or dental procedures. Presenting complaints may include fever, pain on neck movement, sore throat, dysphagia, or drooling. Physical exam often finds cervical adenopathy, pharyngitis, torticollis, and bulging of the pharyngeal wall. Lateral neck radiographs may show retropharyngeal swelling, and CT scanning helps to confirm involvement of the parapharyngeal area.

All patients require parenteral broad-spectrum antibiotics such as ampicillin-sulbactam. Emergent ENT consultation is mandatory for possible operative drainage. Patients in respiratory distress should be orally intubated with extreme care, although it is preferable to establish a surgical airway in the OR.

Masticator Space Abscess

The masticator space consists of four contiguous spaces bounded by the muscles of mastication. Abscesses in this space often extend from infections in the buccal, submandibular, and sublingual areas. Signs and symptoms vary depending on the location of the abscess, and may include trismus, facial swelling, fever, dysphagia, or sepsis. Radiographs may show mandibular osteomyelitis and CT scanning may define the extent of the abscess, but neither is required for the management of the stable patient.

Well-appearing patients with only minimal symptoms, slight trismus, and no palpable abscess, are candidates for outpatient treatment. Therapy includes analgesics, oral antibiotics (e.g., penicillin, erythromycin, or clindamycin) and followup in 24 h. Patients with significant trismus, airway compromise, palpable abscess, diffuse cellulitis, or sepsis require parenteral antibiotics and emergent ENT consultation for operative drainage.

Ludwig's Angina

Ludwig's angina is an extensive bilateral cellulitis of the submandibular space that commonly evolves from infection of the lower molars. Patients present with a febrile illness and painful edema of the submandibular area. Neck motion is restricted and there may be drooling, trismus, dysphagia, dysphonia, or displacement of the tongue in a posterior and superior direction. Severe cases may have progressive respiratory distress with complete airway obstruction, involvement of the carotid artery and jugular vein, and mediastinitis. Direct laryngoscopy can provoke laryngospasm and should be avoided. Lateral neck radiographs are extremely useful and frequently show airway narrowing, soft-tissue swelling, and subcutaneous emphysema. CT scanning is diagnostic, although it is often impossible to perform in the stridorous patient who is unable to lie supine.

Treatment consists of parenteral antibiotics and emergent ENT consultation for possible operative drainage. Antibiotic choices include penicillin, clindamycin, or chloramphenicol. Equipment for airway control must be readily available, and all patients are admitted to an intensive care unit.

For further reading in *Emergency Medicine: A Comprehensive Study Guide*, 4th edition, see Chapter 202, Otolaryngologic Emergencies, by Frank Peacock IV.

EPISTAXIS

Clinical Features

Epistaxis is classified as either anterior or posterior. Anterior epistaxis arises from the anterior nasal septum, and the site of hemorrhage is often easily visualized. Posterior epistaxis arises from more posterior locations and usually requires endoscopic instruments for localization. Posterior epistaxis is suspected when:

1. An anterior source is not identified once bleeding has stopped, or.
2. Bleeding occurs from both nares, or.
3. Blood is seen draining into the posterior pharynx after anterior sources have been controlled.

Both anterior and posterior epistaxis require an initial evaluation to identify and control the source:

1. A quick history should determine the duration and severity of the hemorrhage, as well as contributing factors (trauma, anticoagulant use, infection, bleeding diathesis, etc.).
2. The patient should blow his nose to dislodge any clots.
3. A quick inspection is made to identify obvious anterior sources. A Frazier suction catheter will help to keep the passage clear.
4. A pledget moistened with a topical vasoconstrictor–anesthetic is inserted into the nasal cavity with bayonet forceps. Acceptable agents include 4% cocaine, 4% lidocaine with 1:1000 epinephrine, 4% lidocaine with 1% phenylephrine (Neo-Synephrine), or 4% lidocaine with 0.05% oxymetazoline (Afrin).
5. Direct external pressure is then applied for 5 to 10 min. Active bleeding into the pharynx despite direct pressure suggests either inadequate pressure, drainage from a clot in the posterior nasal cavity, or true posterior epistaxis.
6. Following compression, the pledgets are removed and the nasal cavity is inspected with a speculum. If anterior hemorrhage is controlled and the site of mucosal disruption is identified, the area may be locally cauterized. If anterior bleeding continues, direct pressure should be attempted twice more. If this fails, an anterior pack should be placed. If the anterior pack fails to control bleeding, then the diagnosis of posterior epistaxis should be considered, and the nasal cavity should be packed both anteriorly and posteriorly. At this point, an IV line is started and blood is sent for CBC, PT, PTT, and cross typing. Close monitoring is required and an ENT physician must be consulted.

Emergency Department Care and Disposition

Chemical cautery with **silver nitrate** is the standard of care for ED cautery of anterior epistaxis; thermal techniques are no longer recommended. After hemostasis is achieved, the mucosa is cauterized by firmly rolling the tip of a silver nitrate applicator over the area until it turns silvery-black. A small surrounding area should also be cauterized to control local arterioles. Overzealous use of cautery is discouraged since it may cause septal perforation and unintended local tissue necrosis.

Anterior nasal packing may be performed either with gauze or with newer commercial devices. The technique for placement of a standard gauze pack requires skill and experience; an improperly placed pack is a frequent cause of treatment failure:

1. Hemorrhage should be maximally controlled, as outlined above.
2. Using a nasal speculum and bayonet forceps, a strip of petrolatum-impregnated gauze is inserted all of the way into the posterior limit of the nasal cavity.
3. The speculum is then withdrawn and replaced so that the packing is firmly pressed against the nasal floor.
4. The bayonet forceps then grabs another loop of gauze and layers it in an accordion fashion onto the first layer.
5. The process of using the forceps to place the next layer, then reintroducing the speculum to compress the preceding layer is repeated until the entire nasal cavity is tightly packed. When applied correctly, the folded end of each layer will be visible at the nostril, the end of the strip will extend from the nostril for easy removal of the pack, and anterior bleeding will be controlled. Generally, the pack is removed in 2 to 3 days at a followup appointment with an ENT physician.

There are several commercial nasal packs that have nearly the same efficacy as standard gauze packs but are more comfortable and easier to use. One popular device is the Merocel **nasal sponge** (Merocel Corp., Mystic, CT), a compactly dehydrated sponge available in several lengths in order to control both anterior and posterior epistaxis. The sponge is rapidly inserted into the nasal cavity and will expand upon contact with blood and secretions. Expansion may be slowed by first coating the sponge with a film of antibiotic ointment, or it may be hastened by rehydrating the sponge with sterile water from a catheter-tipped syringe after the sponge has been inserted. The longer sponges used to control posterior hemorrhages have been associated with some morbidity and should only be used when indicated, and not for the control of isolated anterior epistaxis. All nasal packs are removed in 2 to 3 days by an ENT physician.

Posterior epistaxis may be treated with either a dehydrated posterior sponge pack (Merocel), as outlined above, or with a commercial balloon tamponade device. The balloon devices use independently inflatable anterior and posterior balloons to quickly control refractory epistaxis at these sites (instructions for insertion are included in the catheter kit). To protect against potentially serious complications, all patients with posterior packs require ENT consultation for possible hospital admission. Posterior packs are removed 2 to 3 days after placement.

Complications of nasal packing include dislodgment of the pack, recurrent bleeding, sinusitis, and toxic shock syndrome. All patients with nasal packs should be started on **antibiotic prophylaxis** with either cephalexin (250 to 500 mg QID) or amoxicillin–clavulanate (250 to 500 mg TID). Penicillin-allergic patients may be given clindamycin (150 to 300 mg QID) or trimethoprim–sulfamethoxazole (BID).

NASAL FRACTURES

Clinical Features

Nasal fracture should be suspected in all cases of facial trauma. Findings may include swelling, tenderness, crepitance, gross deformity, periorbital ecchymosis, epistaxis, or rhinorrhea. Radiographs are generally not indicated in the ED, although they may be obtained at the followup appointment.

Emergency Department Care and Disposition

A simple, nondisplaced nasal fracture only requires oral analgesics, protection from further injury, decongestant sprays if necessary, and elevation of the head with local ice therapy to reduce swelling. Uncomplicated anterior epistaxis may require a nasal pack. ENT referral is not mandatory unless there is nasal congestion or cosmetic deformity after the swelling diminishes in 2 to 5 days. When soft-tissue swelling is severe, it may be impossible to acutely determine if a displaced fracture exists. These patients are treated in the same manner as patients with nondisplaced fractures, but they require followup with a specialist in 2 to 5 days. This time period allows the swelling to resolve so that the nasal bones can be re-evaluated and reduced if necessary.

Perhaps the most important step in the evaluation of nasal trauma is to **rule out serious associated injuries,** particularly septal hematoma and fracture of the cribriform plate. A septal hematoma is a collection of blood beneath the perichondrium of the nasal septum easily identified on physical examination by the presence of a bluish, fluid-filled sac overlying this location. If left untreated, a septal hematoma may result in abscess formation or necrosis of the nasal septum. Treatment is local incision and drainage, with placement of an anterior nasal pack to prevent reaccumulation of blood. A fracture of the cribriform plate may violate the subarachnoid space and cause cerebrospinal fluid (CSF) rhinorrhea. This injury should be suspected in any patient who presents with clear nasal drainage following facial trauma, even if the trauma occurred days to wks earlier. The most accurate method to diagnose CSF rhinorrhea is with a highly specialized procedure known as metrizamide computed tomography cisternography (MCTC). If positive, immediate neurosurgical consultation must be obtained.

NASAL FOREIGN BODIES

Clinical Features

Nasal foreign bodies may present with a straightforward history, but they should be suspected in any case of unilateral nasal obstruction, foul rhinorrhea, or persistent unilateral epistaxis. They are often directly visible, but radiographs will occasionally demonstrate radiopaque foreign bodies that are not otherwise seen.

Emergency Department Care and Disposition

In cooperative children, nasal foreign bodies may be removed in the ED, as follows:

1. The nasal mucosa is prepared with a topical spray of a vasoconstrictor and anesthetic agent; 0.25% phenylephrine (Neo-Synephrine) mixed with 4% lidocaine is an effective combination.
2. Using a nasal speculum, the object is directly visualized.
3. Loose objects may be removed with a suction catheter. Small, irregular objects may be grasped with bayonet or alligator forceps.
4. Small or round objects may be removed if a small hooked instrument is passed behind them, rotated, and withdrawn. Care must be exercised to avoid lodging the object further into the nasopharynx.
5. Difficult objects may also be withdrawn once a #4-Fogarty-vascular catheter is passed behind them. The balloon is inflated and the object is withdrawn. Alternatively, the balloon may act as a buttress while frontal approaches are tried again.

If unsuccessful, ENT consultation is required. Immediate consultation is sought for ill-appearing children and for those whose foreign bodies are at risk of aspiration; all other patients may be seen in 24 h.

SINUSITIS

Clinical Features

Maxillary sinusitis presents with pain in the infraorbital area, whereas frontal sinusitis causes pain in the supraorbital and lower forehead regions. Ethmoid sinusitis, which is especially serious in children because of its tendency to spread to the CNS, often produces a dull, aching sensation in the retro-orbital the area. Sphenoid sinusitis is extremely uncommon and has vague signs and symptoms. Chronic sinusitis often produces local discomfort and a chronic, purulent exudate.

Physical findings are neither sensitive nor specific. They may include local erythema and warmth, tenderness to palpation and percussion, swollen nasal mucosa with purulent discharge, and diminished transillumination. Radiographs may show sinus opacification, air-fluid levels, or mucosal thickening (≥ 6 mm).

Emergency Department Care and Disposition

Treatment of sinusitis includes nasal decongestant sprays such as oxymetazoline (Afrin) or phenylephrine (Neo-Synephrine) used twice daily for no longer than 3 days. Antibiotic choices for a 10-day regimen include **ampicillin, amoxicillin–clavulanate,** or **cephalexin.** Penicillin-allergic patients may use erythromycin or trimethoprim–sulfamethoxazole. Cool-mist vaporizers, warm facial compresses, and analgesic medications may help to alleviate symptoms. Toxic patients, and those with spread of the infection beyond the sinus cavity, require admission. Treated patients whose symptoms last more than 7 days and those with chronic sinusitis require followup with their physician or ENT specialist.

For further reading in *Emergency Medicine: A Comprehensive Study Guide*, 4th edition, see Chapter 203, Nasal Emergencies and Sinusitis, by James Smith.

SOFT-TISSUE INJURIES

Facial Abrasion and Laceration

Clinical Features

Examination of all facial soft-tissue injuries resulting from blunt trauma requires not only attention to the specific wound but also an assessment of the adjacent anatomic structures, such as the bony framework and articulations, various neurovascular elements, and the salivary ducts and glands. Adequate examination of the wound may necessitate pretreatment with anesthesia; complete exploration of the wound is mandatory to rule out injury to deeper structures, as well as the retained foreign body.

Emergency Department Care and Disposition

Management of such injuries begins with proper **wound cleansing.** Facial abrasions should be cleaned with a dilute soap solution followed by pulsatile irrigation with normal saline. Debridement of all devitalized structures is encouraged. Antibiotic ointment is then applied. Facial lacerations, after anesthetic application, wound exploration, thorough cleaning with irrigation, and debridement, may be closed with interrupted, nonabsorbable, 4-0 to 6-0 monofilament nylon sutures. Larger or deeper wounds may require multilayered closure with both absorbable and nonabsorbable suture. Primary closure of facial lacerations may occur up to 24 h after occurrence of the injury. Sutures should be removed within 3 to 5 days of placement

The use of antibiotics in most facial abrasions and lacerations is unnecessary. Situations in which antibiotic therapy (first-generation cephalosporin, penicillinase-resistant penicillin, erythromycin, or clindamycin) may be warranted include the following: dirty or contaminated wounds; wounds with large devitalized areas; older wounds (greater than 24 h); and wounds with suspected or obvious infection at presentation. Tetanus prophylaxis, ranging from booster administration to primary immunization with both passive (tetanus immune globulin) and active (tetanus toxoid) means, must also be addressed.

Lip Laceration

Clinical Features

Lacerations involving the lip, in particular those injuries violating the vermilion border (the junction between the skin and lip mucosa), may result in significant cosmetic deformity. As such, careful attention to proper closure is mandatory. The examination must address several issues, including integrity of the vermilion border, involvement of the

749

orbicularis oris muscle, retained foreign body within the lip (particularly tooth fragment), and injury to underlying osseous and dental structures.

Emergency Department Care and Disposition

Anesthetic agent is best applied using the mental field block, providing adequate anesthesia with minimal medication to the anterior mandibular teeth, associated gingiva, and lip to the midline. Local infiltration of lidocaine into the wound margin is possible but may distort local anatomy and impair proper alignment of vermilion border and other structures. After adequate anesthesia is achieved, wound cleaning, copious irrigation, and exploration are undertaken. Debridement of devitalized tissues is performed if necessary. Approximately 30% of the lower lip may be removed during debridement or lost as a result of the initial injury and still produce satisfactory cosmetic healing; the upper lip, due to its intimate association with various anatomic structures, does not cosmetically tolerate similar tissue loss.

The wound should be closed in layers with the initial placement of two landmark-preserving sutures using nonabsorbable 5-0 monofilament nylon: the initial suture at the vermilion border (vitally important for cosmetic result), followed by a second suture at the wet-dry interface of the lip and intraoral mucosa. Lacerations involving the orbicularis oris muscle must be repaired to restore function using 4-0 to 5-0 absorbable gut or polyglycolic acid suture. Through-and-through lip lacerations are closed starting with the oral cavity using 5-0 absorbable suture and progressing externally. The skin and external lip mucosa are closed last with 5-0 nonabsorbable suture. Antibiotic ointment is applied externally and the patient is encouraged to perform mouth rinses with a dilute saline solution for 3 to 5 days. The absorbable sutures are removed 3 to 5 days after placement. Antibiotic prophylaxis for 5 days is indicated using penicillin or, in the penicillin-allergic patient, clindamycin. Attention to tetanus prophylaxis is indicated.

Intraoral and Lingual Lacerations

Clinical Features

Intraoral injuries involving the mucosa or tongue must be considered as potential airway threats until proven otherwise. Airway compromise may result from hemorrhage, subsequent edema, fracture, or airway obstruction from foreign body. Fractured teeth must be accounted for; fragments may be found within the wound upon exploration or in the respiratory or gastrointestinal tracts with radiographic analysis. Wounds potentially involving either the gland or ductile structures of the salivary system must be addressed by an oral surgeon with either sialography or open exploration followed by repair of associated ducts using a stent.

Emergency Department Care and Disposition

Wounds of the oral mucosa less than 1 to 2 cm in length and lingual wounds less than 1 cm most often do not require closure. Mucosal and lingual wounds requiring closure should be irrigated with normal saline after adequate anesthesia is obtained using local infiltration in most cases or nerve block (mental, inferior alveolar, infraorbital, or lingual nerves) in selected instances. Young children or other particularly anxious patients may require parenteral conscious sedation for adequate exploration and closure. Debridement is usually not indicated. Oral mucosal wounds are repaired using 4-0 or 5-0 absorbable suture. Lacerations of the tongue requiring repair should be performed with 4-0 absorbable, interrupted suture (gut or polyglycolic acid). Forward traction is maintained on the tongue using either gauze pads or the placement of 2-0 silk suture through the tip of the tongue after adequate anesthesia. Antibiotic prophylaxis is encouraged using similar agents recommended for lip lacerations; tetanus prophylaxis is also addressed. Patients are encouraged to use a soft diet for 3 to 5 days as well as frequent rinsing with chlorhexidine gluconate or dilute saline solutions.

Mandibular Dislocation

Clinical Features

Temporomandibular joint (TMJ) dislocation is most often due to blunt trauma to the chin when the mouth is open or, less commonly, because of aggressive yawning, laughing, or mastication. Dislocation occurs when the mandibular condyle becomes locked anterior to the articular eminence of the temporal bone and is maintained in place by spasm of the adjacent muscles. Dislocation occurs unilaterally or bilaterally.

The patient is unable to close the mouth, presenting with an anterior open bite and pronounced malocclusion. Talking and swallowing are extremely difficult; mastication is impossible. Patients with unilateral dislocation present with the mandible displaced toward the unaffected side. An obvious anterior open bite is noted with bilateral dislocation. A palpable deformity (the displaced head of the condyle) may be noted anterior to the ear and immediately below the zygomatic arch. Radiographic study with a mandibular series, at times supplemented by the panoramic view or panorex (actually a tomogram), is required in all cases to aid in distinguishing between TMJ dislocation and mandibular fracture.

Emergency Department Care and Disposition

The majority of cases of acute TMJ dislocation can be successfully reduced using an IV benzodiazepine to assist in reducing patient anxiety and to aid in muscle relaxation; a parenteral narcotic will reduce discomfort. If needed, local infiltration of the muscles of mastication with 1%

lidocaine further reduces muscular spasm. The patient is then seated with the physician standing on the side of the dislocation. The physician's thumb, wrapped in gauze to protect against forceful occlusion when successful reduction occurs, is placed on the occlusal surfaces of the posterior teeth and the fingers are stationed around the inferior border of the mandible at the angle. Downward, posteriorly directed pressure is exerted as the mandible is opened. Patience—not extreme pressure—is needed to accomplish reduction. The chin is then forced gently backwards. In bilateral TMJ dislocations, the process is repeated on the other side. The patient is encouraged to avoid wide excursions of the mandible and to use a soft diet for 1 wk.

Medial Canthal Ligament Disruption

Blunt injury to the naso-orbital area may result in medial canthal ligament disruption (MCLD). Physical findings suggestive of MCLD include: the presence of a nasal fracture; a widened bridge of the nose; telecanthus (an intercanthal distance greater than 3.5 cm); and an almond-shaped medial palpebral fissure (in contrast to the normal elliptical shape). Immediate treatment of MCLD is not necessary; management is accomplished by consultation with an ophthalmologist or facial surgeon as an outpatient.

FRACTURES

Mandibular Fractures

Clinical Features

The signs and symptoms associated with mandibular fracture include: pain with focal tenderness; soft tissue swelling with ecchymosis; focal pain at the fracture site(s) with occlusion on a tongue blade; external deformity with palpable stepoff and crepitance; malocclusion; an anterior open bite; disruption of the alveolar arch and an interruption in the continuity of the mandibular teeth; deviation to the unaffected side with unilateral subcondylar fracture; ecchymosis of the floor of the mouth; and mental nerve hypoesthesia. Other issues to consider include: inability to maintain an adequate seal with potential bag-valve-mask ventilation; airway compromise from sublingual hematoma; intraoral laceration resulting in open mandibular fracture; and dental and alveolar ridge trauma. As in other ring- or partial ring-like bony structures, multiple fractures are not uncommon. The most common site of mandibular fracture is the condyle followed by the body, angle, symphysis, ramus, and coronoid regions. Radiographic analysis is accomplished with the traditional three-view mandibular series (PA and the two lateral oblique views detailing the condylar areas) or the panorex view. Fractures of the condyle are difficult to visualize at times with conventional plain films; with high clinical suspicion and a negative radiograph, a CT scan should be obtained.

Emergency Department Care and Disposition

Treatment includes admission to the hospital followed by reduction with fixation (intermaxillary, dental or intraoral, and internal). With intraoral lacerations, wound care and exploration, as well as tetanus prophylaxis and systemic antibiotic therapy, are essential.

Maxillary Fractures

Clinical Features

Maxillary fractures, characterized by varying degrees of craniofacial separation, result most often from blunt, high-velocity vehicular trauma and are best described by the Le Fort classification. Le Fort type-I fracture is noted with a transverse fracture line running above the maxillary teeth from the lateral nasal apertures through the lateral wall of the maxillary sinuses and across to the lateral pterygoid plates. The type-II, or pyramidal, fracture is characterized by bony disruption through the facial aspects of the maxilla extending upward to the nasal and ethmoid bones; the fracture also involves the maxillary sinuses, infra-orbital rims, and the bridge of the nose. The type-III fracture extends through the fronto-zygomatic suture bilaterally across the orbits involving the base of the nose and ethmoid region. The orbital rim is often damaged with separation laterally and fracture inferiorly. The zygoma may be involved, and a pyramidal fracture may be noted. Complex variations of these three fractures are encountered. Physical findings include: midfacial and orbital soft-tissue swelling; blood in the nares (types II and III); varying degrees of midfacial mobility; cerebrospinal fluid (CSF) rhinorrhea indicating a cribriform plate fracture (types II and III); subconjunctival hemorrhage; anterior open bite and other malocclusive presentations; and the dishface deformity with retroposition of the entire midface relative to the base of the skull (at a 45° angle). Segments of the midface demonstrate mobility when the examiner exerts a gentle, anterior–posterior pressure on the maxillary teeth, including the following anatomic portions: maxillary (type I), nasomaxillary (type II), and zygonasomaxillary (type III). Plain view films of the facial bones may not demonstrate the fracture (type I); the Waters' view often reveals the fracture in types II and III. Additional radiographic studies include bilateral orbital tomograms and CT scan of the midface.

Emergency Department Care and Disposition

With soft-tissue injuries complicating Le Fort fractures, proper wound care, tetanus prophylaxis, and antibiotic administration are essential.

After hospital admission, surgical correction is required to restore normal cosmetic appearance as well as proper function.

Zygoma Fractures

Clinical Features and Emergency Department Care

Direct trauma to the zygomatic prominence is unlikely to result in isolated fracture of the zygoma. Rather, the fracture may occur in any of the following areas: frontozygomatic suture, zygomaticomaxillary suture, infraorbital rim, lateral wall of the maxillary sinus, or the zygomatic arch. The central portion of the orbital floor may also fracture along with the zygomaticomaxillary complex.

Examination may reveal edema of cheek and periorbital area; facial flattening of the upper cheek area immediately after injury (within 1 to 2 h) or after initial edema resolves (in 3 to 5 days); periorbital ecchymosis and subconjunctival hemorrhage in the lateral scleral area; unilateral epistaxis; anesthesia of cheek, upper lip to the midline, maxillary teeth, and gingiva (infraorbital nerve distribution); tenderness with step-off deformity of inferior orbital margin, frontozygomatic suture, zygomatic arch, and lateral wall of maxillary sinus; diplopia with entrapment and other extraocular movement abnormalities; limitation of mandibular movement due to mechanical compression of the condyle by the depressed zygomatic arch; and emphysema of associated soft tissues. Radiographs include plain film views (Waters' and the basal skull), facial tomograms, and CT scan. Management is at the subspecialist level involving surgical fixation of the fracture.

Nasal Fractures

Clinical Features and Emergency Department Care and Disposition

The nasal fracture, which occurs either laterally or posteriorly, is the most common facial fracture encountered. Specific injuries include fracture of the nasal bone, nasal spine, and the nasoethmoid complex. Physical examination may reveal soft-tissue swelling, crepitation with focal tenderness, hypermobility of the nose, deformity ranging from minimal edema to marked lateral deviation, epistaxis, CSF rhinorrhea, and septal hematoma. Failure to recognize a septal hematoma may result in abscess formation, destruction of cartilage, and chronic saddle-nose deformity. Radiographic diagnosis—via lateral soft tissue and AP occlusal views—is often unnecessary acutely and is misleading in that frequent false negative and false positive results are recorded. Immediate treatment considerations include **aspiration of the septal hematoma,** reduction of a markedly deviated nose with lateral pressure from the examiner's finger, nasal packing to control epistaxis, and pain medication. Facial surgery consultation should be arranged for 5 to 7 days postinjury. Additionally, patients with nasoethmoid fracture should be admitted with neurosurgical consultation and antibiotic prophylaxis.

Orbital Fractures

Clinical Features and Emergency Department Care and Disposition

Fracture of the orbital floor may occur along with injury to the zygomaticomaxillary complex as a result of direct trauma to the zygomatic prominence. Alternatively, blunt trauma to the soft-tissue structures of the orbit produces a pressure wave that is transmitted to the relatively weak orbital floor, resulting in the isolated blow-out fracture. Patients may complain of double vision due to soft-tissue entrapment of the inferior rectus or inferior oblique muscles into the maxillary sinus, disruption of extraocular muscular attachments, interruption of innervation, or associated hemorrhage and edema. Examination findings include enophthalmos, limitation of upward gaze, infraorbital hypoesthesia, and diplopia. Complete evaluation of the globe and visual ability is essential. Radiographs include Waters's and AP facial views, in addition to orbital tomography and CT scan. Plain film findings include opacification of the maxillary sinus, air-fluid level in the sinus, disruption of the orbital floor or rim, and orbital emphysema. Urgent surgical consultation is indicated if entrapment is noted; otherwise, outpatient management aimed at reconstruction of the orbit is accomplished by either an ophthalmologist or a facial surgeon.

For further reading in *Emergency Medicine: A Comprehensive Study Guide*, 4th edition, see Chapter 204, Maxillofacial Fractures, by Barry H. Hendler.

ORAL AND FACIAL PAIN

Tooth Eruption

Eruption of primary teeth in infants and children is often associated with pain, low-grade fever ($\geq$38°C), diarrhea, and refusal to eat. Adequate hydration along with oral analgesics (e.g., acetaminophen) or topical anesthetics (e.g., benzocaine) will usually control the symptoms. Adults may experience pain and local inflammation (i.e., pericoronitis) with the eruption of the third molars. Oral antibiotics (e.g., penicillin or erythromycin) and frequent rinsing of the mouth will temporize symptoms until an oral surgeon can remove the teeth in 1 to 2 days. Superficial incision and drainage is required for abscesses.

Dental Caries

The most common cause of toothache is a carious tooth. Examination sometimes finds a grossly decayed tooth, although frequently there is no visible pathology. Localization is easily accomplished by percussing individual teeth with a tongue blade. Treatment includes oral analgesics and referral to a dentist. Fluctuant oral abscesses from infected teeth require local incision and drainage, oral antibiotics, frequent saline rinses, and followup within 24 h.

Postextraction Pain

Pain experienced within 24 h of a tooth extraction, termed periosteitis, responds well to analgesics. Severe pain with foul odor and taste 2 to 3 days after an extraction is termed alveolar osteitis (dry socket). Treatment consists of irrigation of the socket followed by packing the socket with medicated dental packing or 1″ of iodoform gauze dampened with eugenol (oil of cloves). Immediate followup should be arranged.

Periodontal Abscess

A periodontal abscess results from plaque and debris entrapped between the tooth and gingiva. Most cases resolve with oral antibiotics and saline irrigation. Larger abscesses may require a stab incision for drainage.

Acute Necrotizing Ulcerative Gingivitis (ANUG or *Trenchmouth*)

ANUG is the only periodontal disease in which bacteria actually invade nonnecrotic tissue. It occurs mainly in adolescents and young adults who complain of gingival pain, halitosis, malaise, and fever. Examination may find regional lymphadenopathy with edematous and inflamed gingiva. The hallmark is ulceration and blunting of the interdental papilla with a gray pseudomembrane. Treatment requires oral antibiotics (**tetracycline** may be preferable to penicillin) and **dilute hydrogen-peroxide rinses;** topical anesthetics (2% viscous lidocaine) may provide relief. Symptomatic improvement is dramatic, but dental followup is required.

Oral Lesions

Patients frequently present with pain from oral lesions. It is often difficult to distinguish primary herpetic lesions from herpangina, herpes zoster, and other etiologies. Such ulcerations are best treated symptomatically with topical anesthetics (2% viscous lidocaine) and saline rinses, although definite primary herpetic lesions may be additionally treated with oral acyclovir. Most lesions are at risk for secondary infection so penicillin or erythromycin is often appropriate.

A pyogenic granuloma is a commonly encountered benign gingival lesion. It results from nonspecific infection or irritation and appears as a pedunculated or sessile mass of vascular tissue. It may also appear during pregnancy and is then referred to as pregnancy tumor. Referral is required to rule out other etiologies and to consider definitive excision.

DENTOALVEOLAR TRAUMA

Dental Fractures

In all cases of tooth fracture, lacerated adjacent tissue should be palpated for missing tooth fragments and radiographed if necessary. Regardless of how minor a dental injury may appear, all patients with dental trauma should be warned that there may be occult injury to the neurovascular supply and that the tooth may subsequently be lost. A painless dental injury may suggest this neurovascular disruption. The Ellis system is used to classify the anatomy of fractured teeth (Fig. 141-1).

Ellis Class 1 fractures involves only the enamel of the tooth. These injuries may be smoothed with an emery board or referred to a dentist for cosmetic repair. *Ellis Class 2* fractures expose the underlying pale yellow or pink dentin. These are serious fractures in patients less than 12 years old, since incorrect management increases the chance of infecting the dental pulp. In these patients, the dentin should be thoroughly dried and **calcium hydroxide paste (Dycal)** placed over the exposed dentin. The area is then covered with gauze, aluminum foil, or adhesive-backed dental foil. Dental referral is needed within 24 h. Patients over 12 should be given oral analgesics, and told to avoid extremes of temperature and seek dental care within 24 h. *Ellis Class 2* fractures with a large amount of exposed dentin should be treated with a calcium hydroxide dressing regardless of the patient's age. *Ellis Class 3* fractures expose the dental pulp and are true dental emergencies. They are identified by a red blush of the dentin or a drop of frank blood. If a dentist

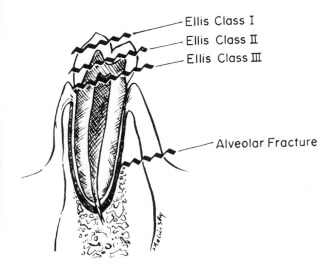

FIG. 141-1.   Ellis classification for fractures of anterior teeth.

is not immediately available, the tooth may be covered with **aluminum foil** or sealed with cavet, a temporary root canal sealer. Oral analgesics may be needed, but topical anesthetics are contraindicated since they may cause sterile abscesses. Referral to a dentist is needed emergently.

Subluxated, Intruded, and Avulsed Teeth

Dental trauma may result in loosening of a tooth, termed *subluxation*. Blood in the gingival crevice is also a subtle indicator of trauma. Minimally subluxated teeth heal well in 1 to 2 wks if the patient maintains a soft diet. Grossly mobile teeth require stabilization by a dentist. The patient may gently bite on gauze to stabilize the tooth while awaiting further evaluation.

Dental intrusion occurs when a tooth is forced below the gingiva. Intruded primary (baby) teeth are allowed to erupt for 6 wks before considering repositioning. Intruded permanent teeth require surgical repositioning. Failure to diagnose dental intrusion may result in infection and cosmetic deformity.

Dental avulsion describes a tooth that has been completely removed from the socket; this is a true dental emergency. If the missing tooth is not located, a radiograph must be obtained to rule out dental intrusion. Primary teeth in children 5 years old or younger are not replaced, since they may ankylose and cause facial deformity. Permanent teeth that have been avulsed for less than 3 h must be immediately reimplanted. A percentage point for successful reimplantation is lost for each min that the tooth is out of the socket. If a patient with an avulsed tooth is being transported, the tooth should be held only by the crown, gently rinsed under running water, and replaced into the socket. If reimplantation is not possible, the best transport medium is **Hank's solution,** available commercially in the Save-A-Tooth kit. Other options, in descending order of preference, include placing the tooth in the patient's mouth to bathe in saliva, placing the tooth in a glass of milk, or wrapping the tooth in wet gauze. Once in the ED, the tooth should be gently rinsed; scrubbing damages the delicate periodontal ligaments. If available, the tooth should be placed in Hank's solution for 30 minutes to restore cell viability. As soon as possible, gently clean the socket and reimplant the tooth. Once replaced, the patient may gently bite on gauze until seen by a dentist, who will perform permanent stabilization. Alternatively, teeth may be left in Hank's solution and the patient can be referred directly to a dentist or oral surgeon.

Oral Lacerations

Lacerations of the lips, oral mucosa, and gingiva are often associated with dentoalveolar trauma. Since stabilization of the dental injury will often require stretching of the soft tissues, it is preferable to repair soft tissues after repair of the dental injury. All oral lacerations require adequate tetanus prophylaxis. **Prophylactic penicillin therapy** is indicated.

Intraoral mucosal lacerations tend to heal poorly and become infected if they are gaping open. Smaller lacerations (< 1.5 cm) may be left alone. The wound should be inspected for foreign matter (including tooth fragments), debrided as necessary, irrigated, and closed with 4-0 chromic sutures. Laceration of the frenulum alone does not usually require repair. Tongue lacerations greater than 1 cm should be closed with 4-0 silk or chromic sutures.

Palate lacerations may involve the soft or hard palate. Soft palate injuries occur commonly in children who fall with a pointed object in their mouth. These may be treated as puncture wound and left open to drain. Gaping edges should be loosely approximated and injuries to the retropharynx and neighboring vascular structures must be considered. Lacerations to the hard palate are difficult to close since the tissue is not very mobile. Closure may be attempted with 4-0 chromic or silk on a fine needle.

Lip lacerations require meticulous closure. The subcutaneous tissues must be closed with resorbable deep sutures to prevent premature separation when the superficial sutures are removed in 4 to 5 days. The skin is then closed with 6-0 monofilament material. Failure to exactly reapproximate the edges of the lip at the vermilion border will lead to a noticeable cosmetic deformity. When the vermilion border has been lacerated, therefore, the first suture should be meticulously placed to align the cut edges. Lip wounds should be cleansed daily with dilute hydrogen peroxide and covered with antibiotic ointment.

Hemorrhage Secondary to Extraction and Surgery

Bleeding following dental extraction is usually controlled by direct pressure applied by biting on gauze. Negative pressure from smoking, spitting, and use of straws will increase the amount of hemorrhage.

If bleeding persists, the socket should be suctioned free of clot and direct pressure should be tried again. If this is unsuccessful, 2% lidocaine with epinephrine should be locally infiltrated into the area of the socket and gingiva followed by reapplication of pressure. A small absorbable gelatin sponge can also be packed into the socket and sutured with 3-0 silk. Failure of the above measures warrants a screening coagulation profile and consultation with an oral surgeon. Bleeding following periodontal surgery requires immediate consultation with the periodontist since incorrect placement of periodontal packs can result in treatment failure.

For further reading in *Emergency Medicine: A Comprehensive Study Guide,* 4th edition, see Chapter 205, General Dental Emergencies, by James T. Amsterdam.

18 | SKIN AND SOFT-TISSUE EMERGENCIES

TOXICODENDRON DERMATITIS

Toxicodendron dermatitis (TD), caused by the antigenic compound oleoresin found in poison ivy, poison oak, and poison sumac, occurs throughout the continental United States. Patients may come in contact with oleoresin directly from any portion of the plant or indirectly from another person, animal, clothing, tools, sports equipment, and smoke-laden particles from partially incinerated vegetation. The dermatitis is not spread by contact with blister fluid. Significant variation is found throughout the population regarding the sensitivity, extent of involvement, and progression of disease; factors impacting on this variation include differing degrees of patient sensitivity, amount of plant material exposed to, age of plant (season), and regional differences in oleoresin content.

Clinical Features

Dermatitis usually begins 48 h after plant sap exposure, with a range of 8 h to 10 days. Symptoms include redness, pain, and pruritus. Signs include erythema, papules, vesicles, and bullae; a linear configuration of erythema or other skin lesions is highly suggestive of TD. Healing is complete within 10 days (mild) to 3 wks (severe). Cutaneous hyperpigmentation is a rare sequela.

Diagnosis and Differential

The diagnosis is made based on the appropriate skin lesions in a patient who has been exposed to, or has had potential for exposure to, members of the *Toxicodendron* species. Syndromes to consider in the differential include other contact dermatitides, phytodermatitis due to lime, parsley, or celery, erythema multiforme, primary blistering disorders, herpes zoster infection, and drug reactions.

Emergency Department Care and Disposition

Treatment is governed by disease severity.
  Mild (localized disease):

1. Calamine lotion
2. Topical steroids
3. Cold tap water soaks
4. Oral antihistamines

  Moderate/severe (facial, perineal, or widespread vesiculobullous disease):

1. Cool Domeboro solution (diluted 1:10 aluminum sulfate) soaks

2. Potassium permanganate baths
3. Oatmeal baths
4. Oral or parenteral antihistamines
5. Systemic corticosteroid (with 2–3 wk taper)

Admission is recommended in the following situations: extensive involvement with vesiculobullae, upper airway compromise, or severe debilitating disease. To prevent disease development, all sap must be thoroughly removed from the skin within 30 min of contact.

EXFOLIATIVE DERMATITIS

Exfoliative dermatitis, a cutaneous reaction to a drug, chemical, or underlying disease state, occurs when most or all of the skin is involved with a scaling erythema leading subsequently to exfoliation. Men are affected more often than women; the majority of patients are over age 40. Etiologies responsible for exfoliative dermatitis include (in decreasing order of incidence) generalized flares of pre-existing skin disease (psoriasis, atopic and seborrheic dermatitides, lichen planus, pemphigus foliaceus, etc.), contact dermatitis, malignancy, and medications or chemicals.

Clinical Features

Patients may present with either acute, acute/chronic, or chronic disease. The acute form is encountered most often in cases involving medications, contact allergens, or malignancy, whereas the chronic variety usually is related to an underlying cutaneous disease. Patients may complain of pain, pruritus, tightening of the skin, a chilling sensation of the skin, fever, nausea, vomiting, weight loss, and fatigue. The physical examination may show generalized warmth and erythroderma, scaling with desiccation, and exfoliation of the skin, as well as fever and other signs of systemic toxicity. High-output congestive failure may be noted due to extensive cutaneous vasodilation in poorly compensated individuals. Chronic findings include dystrophic nails, thinning of body hair, alopecia, and hypo-/hyperpigmentation. Acute complicating factors include fluid and electrolyte losses, secondary infection, and excessive heat loss with hypothermia. Chronic malnutrition may occur due to protein loss and negative nitrogen balance.

Diagnosis and Differential

Diffuse erythema with desiccation or exfoliation must be considered exfoliative dermatitis until proven otherwise. The diagnosis is confirmed with dermatologic consultation and skin biopsy. A careful search for etiologic factors is mandatory. Dermatologic syndromes to consider in the differential include acute generalized exanthematous pustulosis, toxic epidermal necrolysis, primary blistering disorders, and the toxic–

infectious erythemas as well as the general ichthyoses (dry-skin conditions).

Emergency Department Care and Disposition

ED management includes attention to the ABCs with appropriate correction of any life-threatening abnormality. After resuscitation is completed, treatment of secondary infection, correction of electrolyte disorder(s), control of body temperature, and management of CHF are clinical issues to address. Dermatologic treatment includes **oral antihistamines, steroids** (topical or systemic), oatmeal baths, and bland lotions. For patients with a new presentation of, or a significant recurrence of, exfoliative dermatitis, admission with dermatologic consultation is advised. For patients with chronic disease with mild recurrence who are not systemically ill, outpatient treatment with prompt dermatologic followup is reasonable.

ERYTHEMA MULTIFORME

Erythema multiforme (EM) is an acute inflammatory skin disease with significant associated morbidity and mortality. EM presents across a spectrum of disease, ranging from a mild papular eruption (EM minor) to the severe vesiculobullous form with mucous membrane involvement and systemic toxicity (EM major, or the Stevens–Johnson syndrome). EM strikes all ages, with the highest incidence in young adults, affects males twice as often as females, and occurs commonly in the spring and fall. Etiologies include infection, drugs, malignancy, rheumatologic disorders, physical agents, and pregnancy. Medications (adults) and infections (children) are the major etiologic factors.

Clinical Features

Symptoms include malaise, arthralgias, myalgias, fever, diffuse pruritus, and a generalized burning sensation, which may be noted many days prior to skin abnormalities. Signs noted on exam primarily involve the skin and mucosal surfaces, including erythematous papules or maculopapules, target (iris) lesion, urticarial plaques, vesicles, bullae, vesiculobullous lesions, and mucosal (oral, conjunctival, respiratory, and genitourinary) erosions. Significant systemic toxicity may also be noted on initial presentation. Patients are at risk for significant fluid and electrolyte deficiencies, as well as secondary infection. Sequelae include hypo- or hyperpigmentation and blindness. Recurrence is noted especially involving cases where infection or medication were involved. Mortality is 10%.

Diagnosis and Differential

The diagnosis of EM is based upon the simultaneous presence of lesions with multiple morphologies, at times with mucous membrane involvement. The target lesion is highly suggestive of EM. Urticarial plaques are frequently misdiagnosed as allergic reaction. The differential diagnosis includes herpetic infections, vasculitis, toxic epidermal necrolysis, primary blistering disorders, and toxic–infectious erythemas.

Emergency Department Care and Disposition

Patients may present in extremis; as such, attention to the standard resuscitative therapies is required. Patients with localized papular disease without systemic manifestation and mucous membrane involvement may be managed as outpatients with dermatologic consultation. Topical steroids to noneroded skin, as well as oral analgesics and antihistamines, are recommended. For patients with extensive disease or systemic toxicity, inpatient therapy in a critical-care setting with immediate dermatologic consultation is advised. In addition to intensive management of potential fluid, electrolyte, infectious, nutritional, and thermoregulatory issues, parenteral **analgesics** and **antihistamines** are required. Systemic steroids are recommended by some authorities. Diphenhydramine and lidocaine rinses are useful for painful oral lesions; cool Burow's solution (aqueous aluminum sulfate/calcium acetate) compresses are applied to blistered regions. Ophthalmologic care is advised if any eye complaints or findings are noted.

TOXIC EPIDERMAL NECROLYSIS

Toxic epidermal necrolysis (TEN) is an explosive, potentially fatal, inflammatory skin disease, striking all age and gender groups equally. Potential etiologies include medications, chemicals, infections, and immunologic factors. Medications are by far the major etiologic group; infectious triggers are much less commonly involved compared to EM.

Clinical Features

Patients may complain of malaise, anorexia, myalgias, arthralgias, fever, painful skin, and upper respiratory infection symptoms; these symptoms may be present prior to the development of skin abnormality. Physical exam findings include a warm, tender erythema, flaccid bullae, a positive Nikolsky's sign, erosions with exfoliation, mucous membrane (oral, conjunctival, respiratory, and genitourinary) lesions, and systemic toxicity. Acute and chronic complications are similar to those encountered in EM major patients. Mortality is 30%.

Diagnosis and Differential

The clinical diagnosis is often possible at presentation based on the following features: diffuse, tender erythema; mucous membrane involvement; areas of denuded skin with adjacent large bullous lesions; a positive Nikolsky's sign; and systemic toxicity. Ultimate diagnosis is made by skin biopsy. The differential includes toxic–infectious erythemas, exfoliative drug eruptions, primary blistering disorders, Kawasaki syndrome, and EM major (Stevens–Johnson syndrome).

Emergency Department Care and Disposition

Management of all patients with TEN is best performed in a critical-care setting such as a **burn unit.** In fact, much of the care of the TEN patient is similar to that of the burn patient. Attention to adequate cardiorespiratory function is essential; correction of fluid, electrolyte, and infectious complications are early treatment considerations. Immediate dermatologic consultation is required.

For further reading in *Emergency Medicine: A Comprehensive Study Guide*, 4th edition, see Chapter 206, Toxicodendron Dermatitis; Chapter 207, Exfoliative Dermatitis; Chapter 208, Erythema Multiforme; and Chapter 209, Toxic Epidermal Necrolysis and the Staphylococcal Scalded Skin Syndrome, by Thomas Chapel and Johanna Chapel.

Subcutaneous Abscesses and
Soft-Tissue Infections

Andrew T. Guertler

Cutaneous abscesses and infections are common in patients presenting
to the ED. The bacteriology may involve the patient's normal flora, as
well as many other organisms. Immunocompromised patients may have
unusual organisms isolated from cutaneous abscesses, whereas any
traumatic injury may introduce unusual bacteria into the tissue.

CUTANEOUS ABSCESSES

Clinical Features

Patients with abscesses complain of localized pain and swelling and
have fluctuance, induration, and erythema at the affected site. A retained
foreign body should be considered if the history is suggestive. Abscesses
seen in the ED include: *Furuncles*—Infected hair follicle usually caused
by *Staphylococcus sp*; *Carbuncle*—Staphylococcal abscess of the neck
with a honeycomb system, which does not adequately drain spontaneously; *Pilonidal abscess*—Occurs in the gluteal fold over the coccyx,
with skin flora (staphylococcus) being most common, *Bartholin abscess*—Unilateral swelling of the labia resulting from Bartholin-duct
obstruction and composed of mixed vaginal flora but may contain *N.
gonorrhoeae* or *C. trachomatis*; *Hydradenitis suppurativa*—Chronic
suppurative abscesses of the apocrine sweat glands of the groin and
axilla. (*S. Aureus*, *Streptococcus viridans*, and *Proteus sp*. are common
pathogens); *Paronychia*—Superficial abscess of the lateral nail fold
commonly involving *S. Aureus*, *Candida*, and anaerobes. *Perirectal
abscess*—Abscesses originating in the anal crypts and extending through
the ishiorectal space via fistulous tracts. (*B. Fragilis* is the predominant
anaerobe, and most abscesses contain mixed flora); *Infected sebaceous
cyst*—Sebaceous cysts result from sebaceous gland duct obstruction
and may become infected with abscess formation.

Emergency Department Care and Disposition

Therapy for cutaneous abscesses is **incision and drainage (I&D).**
Needle aspiration may be helpful in locating the abscess or distinguishing an abscess from cellulitis. Failure to aspirate pus indicates treatment
with warm soaks and antibiotics whereas aspiration of pus indicates
the need for I&D. Most abscesses can be treated in the ED if adequate
anesthesia or sedation and analgesia can be provided. Local infiltration,
field block, or nerve block may be sufficient, but parenteral sedation
and analgesia with benzodiazepines, narcotics, and nitrous oxide may
be required. Deep abscesses, those near neurovascular bundles, on the

palm, or in which sufficient anesthesia cannot be provided in the ED are best handled in the OR.

The area is prepped and draped, and an incision (following natural skin folds and creases when possible) is made through the entire length of the abscess. Blunt probing with a hemostat to break up loculations is followed by copious irrigation and packing with gauze. Patients with abscesses of the face or hands or have impaired health (e.g., DM) should be seen again in 24 h whereas everyone else is seen in 48 h. Surgical referral is indicated for patients with pilonidal abscesses for more extensive excision to minimize recurrence and with infected sebaceous cysts for cyst capsule excision. Bartholin abscess treatment is maximized by placement of iodoform gauze or a Word catheter and sitz baths to help drainage.

Antibiotic therapy is used for patients at high risk for infection (immunocompromised, DM, collagen vascular disease), those with facial abscesses, and those with evidence of systemic spread (fever, lymphangitis). Antibiotic regimens for soft-tissue infections based on organism are listed in Table 143-1. Patients at risk for endocarditis should receive prophylactic parenteral antibiotics prior to I&D.

SOFT TISSUE INFECTIONS

Cellulitis and Erysipelas

Clinical Features

Cellulitis, a localized bacterial infection of the skin with associated soft-tissue inflammation, presents with local tenderness, warmth, induration, and erythema. Lymphangitis or lymphadenitis indicates a more serious infection whereas high fever and chills indicate bacteremia.

TABLE 143-1. Oral Therapy of Superficial Soft-Tissue Infections

Streptococcus, group A	
Penicillin V (phenoxymethyl penicillin)	250–500 mg qid
Erythromycin	500 mg–1 g q 6 h
Staphylococcus aureus	
Cloxacillin	250–500 mg q 8 h
Dicloxacillin	125–500 mg q 6 h
Erythromycin	500 mg–1 g q 6 h
Clindamycin	150–450 mg q 6 h
Cephradine	250–500 mg q 6 h
Cephalexin	250–500 mg q 6 h
Amoxicillin/clavulanate	250–500 mg q 8 h
Haemophilus influenzae	
Cefaclor	250–500 mg q 8 h
Cephradine	250–500 mg q 6 h
Cephalexin	250–500 mg q 6 h
Amoxicillin/clavulanate	250–500 mg q 8 h
Trimethoprim/sulfamethoxazole	160 mg TMP/800 mg SMX bid

Erysipelas is a specific type of cellulitis with lymphatic involvement, usually caused by group *A Streptococcus*. Abrupt onset of high fever, chills, nausea, and malaise with subsequent development of localized erythema with a burning sensation. Infection progresses to a red, shiny, hot plaque, which is tense with painful induration and sharply demarcated from surrounding normal tissue. Lymphangitis and lymphadenopathy are common and purpura, bullae, and necrosis may be seen.

Diagnosis and Differential

The diagnosis is based on physical findings. In otherwise healthy patients, attempts to isolate the causative organism are not warranted. Evidence of bacteremia dictates the need for blood cultures. In erysipelas, blood cultures are rarely positive (5%) and serologic tests to determine ASO and anti-DNAase B titers are acutely unhelpful. Differentiating DVT from lower extremity cellulitis may be difficult, requiring Doppler studies or venogram.

Emergency Department Care and Disposition

Healthy adults with simple cellulitis and well-localized erysipelas are treated as outpatients with **oral antibiotics** directed at the likely organism (see Table 143-1). Patients with face or neck cellulitis should be treated as inpatients with IV antibiotics, such as cephalosporins, penicillinase-resistant penicillins, vancomycin, ampicillin/sulbactam, or ticaricillin/clavulanate. Patients with evidence of bacteremia, underlying diseases (DM, alcoholism) or other immunosuppresive disorders, and serious cases of erysipelas should be **admitted for IV antibiotics.** Emperic therapy is begun with one of the antibiotics listed above and changed based on culture results. Erysipelas responds well to Penicillin G, 4 to 6 million units daily in divided doses.

Sporotrichosis

Clinical Findings

Sporotrichosis is a fungal infection caused by *Sporothrix schenckii*, which is found on plants, vegetation, and in soil. Infection, caused by traumatic inoculation, remains in the local soft tissue and lymphatics. An average incubation of 3 wks precedes one of three types of infection. The fixed cutaneous type is restricted to the site of inoculation and is a fixed crusted ulcer or verrucous plaque. The local cutaneous type remains localized but presents as a subcutaneous nodule or pustule, which may ulcerate and have associated local lymphadenitis. The lymphocutaneous type is most common and is characterized by an initial painless nodule or papule at the inoculation site and development of subcutaneous nodules with clear skip areas along lymphatic channels.

Diagnosis and Differential

History and physical are the key to diagnosis, but fungal cultures and tissue biopsy are often diagnostic as well. The differential diagnosis includes TB, tularemia, cat-scratch disease, leishmaniasis, staphylococcal lymphangitis, and nocardiosis.

Emergency Department Care and Disposition

The treatment of choice is **potassium iodide** (SSKI, 3 to 4 g PO tid) continued 1 mo after symptom resolution. Oral ketoconazole can be used for those not tolerating SSKI. IV amphotericin B use is limited due to the side-effect profile. Basic wound-care instructions for open lesions are included in discharge instructions.

GAS GANGRENE

Clinical Features

Clostridial myonecrosis is a rapidly progressive life- and limb-threatening soft tissue infection caused by *C. Perfringens* or *C. septicum.* Pain out of proportion to physical findings and a sensation of heaviness are the most common presentations. Tissue may have a brawny, woody edema with crepitance and be cool to the touch. Brown discoloration of the skin with bullae and a malodorous serosanguinous discharge develops. The patient may have altered mental status and laboratory findings of metabolic acidosis, leukocytosis, anemia, thrombocytopenia, coagulopathy, myoglobinemia/uria, or liver or kidney dysfunction. Gram-stain of the bullae show pleomorphic gram-positive bacilli, with or without spores, and few WBCs. Radiographs may demonstrate gas within soft tissue, fascial planes, or peritoneal and retroperitoneal spaces.

Diagnosis and Differential

Early diagnosis is achieved by familiarity with the disease and an awareness of the subtle findings. Pain out of proportion to exam, low-grade fever, and significant tachycardia are indicative signs. Crepitance may be absent or a late finding. A gram-stain of exudate showing gram-positive rods with a paucity of leukocytes is diagnostic. The differential diagnosis includes gas-forming infections, such as necrotizing fasciitis, streptococcal myositis, acute streptococcal hemolytic gangrene, crepitant cellulitis, and synergistic necrotizing cellulitis. Crepitance should be differentiated from that caused by pneumothorax, pneumomediastinum, and fracture of the larynx or trachea.

Emergency Department Care and Disposition

Resuscitation using crystalloid, plasma, and red cells is directed by vital signs, laboratory analysis, and response to therapy. Vasopressors should be avoided. **Penicillin G,** 10–40 million units daily in divided doses is recommended in combination with aminoglycosides, vancomycin, or penicillinase-resistant penicillin due to the polymicrobial nature of the infection. Clindamycin, metronidazole, and chloramphenicol may be substituted for penicillin G. **Surgical consultation** for debridement is mandatory.

TETANUS

Clinical Features

Tetanus results from local wound contamination by C. tetani which produces a toxin, tetanospasmin, responsible for the disease manifestations. In the U.S., this is frequently a disease of the elderly who lack adequate immunization. Generalized tetanus presents as trismus due to masseter spasm, nuchal rigidity, or dysphagia. General muscular rigidity progresses to reflex spasm precipitated by external stimuli (noise, touch), which may last sec to min. Opisthotonus flexion, adduction of arms with clenched fists over the thorax, and lower extremity extension may occur with resulting vertebral and long-bone fractures and tendon avulsions. Autonomic instability may cause labile hypertension, tachycardia, arrhythmias, diaphoresis, hyperpyrexia, and hypotension. Local tetanus is a clinical form in which symptoms are initially limited to muscles closely related to the wound. Cephalic tetanus (following a head injury or otitis media) involves the muscles innervated by one or more of the cranial nerves (facial nerve most common). These often progresses to generalized tetanus.

Diagnosis and Differential

The diagnosis is based on clinical grounds, since cultures are positive in only 30% of cases. Serum antitoxin levels of 0.01 IU/ml are protective and make the diagnosis unlikely. The differential includes parotitis, peritonsillar abscess, mandible fracture, TMJ dysfunction, dystonic reactions, strychnine poisoning, hypocalcemia, and hysterical reaction.

Emergency Department Care and Disposition

Human tetanus immunoglobulin (3000–5000 units IM) neutralizes circulating tetanospamin. Active immunization is initiated with IM tetanus toxoid in a separate site. **Surgical cleansing and debridement** to a 2–cm margin of normal-appearing tissue around the wound edge should follow high-dose penicillin or metronidazole therapy. Cephalosporins, imipenem, tetracycline, or erythromycin are other options. Patients are admitted to the ICU for hemodynamic monitoring and minimization of external stimuli. Muscle rigidity is treated with IV benzodiazepines. Neuromuscular blockade with vecuronium (minimal CV profile) and mechanical ventilation is instituted for airway-threaten-

TABLE 143-2. Summary Guide to Tetanus Prophylaxis in Routine
Wound Management, 1991

	Clean, Minor Wounds		All Other Wounds	
	Td	TIG	Td	TIG
Uncertain of <3 doses	Yes	No	Yes	Yes
3 or more doses and < 5 y since last dose	No	No	No	No
3 or more doses and 5–10 y since last dose	No	No	Yes	No
3 or more doses and >10 y since last dose	Yes	No	Yes	No

Adapted from: Summary of recommendations of ACIP for tetanus prophylaxis in routine wound management—United States, 1991. MMWR, vol.
41, No. SS-8, 1–9, December 11, 1992.

ing laryngospasm. Autonomic instability should be treated with short-
acting titrateable medications.

Tetanus prevention rests on active immunization and proper wound
care. Tetanus-prone wounds are older than 6 h, have crushed, necrotic,
or ischemic edges, or are contaminated with dirt or other debris. Wounds
are cleansed, irrigated, and debrided, and local infection is treated
with antibiotics. Careful review of immunization status is important to
determine if the patient requires tetanus prophylaxis (Table 143-2).

If Standard Treatment Fails

Patients with cutaneous abscesses or soft-tissue infections who do not
respond to standard therapy should be evaluated for the presence of
a foreign body, an inadequately drained or deep abscess, inadequate
antibiotic regimen, or an underlying immunocompromising disorder
(DM, HIV, connective-tissue disease).

For further reading in *Emergency Medicine: A Comprehensive Study
Guide*, 4th edition, see Chapter 210, Cutaneous Abscesses, by E. Jackson
Allison and John E. Gough; and Chapter 211, Soft Tissue Infections,
by Steven G. Folstad.

19 | TRAUMA

Trauma

Charles J. Havel, Jr.

Trauma is a major health concern in the U.S. and the leading cause of death up to the age of 44. All ED physicians must be skilled in trauma resuscitation and initiating a team approach to patient management in concert with the ED staff and the surgeon on call.

Clinical Features

Many trauma patients will present with obviously abnormal vital signs, neurologic deficit, or other gross evidence of trauma. These signs must prompt a thorough search for the specific underlying injuries and rapid interventions to correct the abnormalities. Nonspecific signs, such as tachycardia, tachypnea, or mild alterations in consciousness, must similarly be presumed to signify serious injury until proven otherwise and these aggressively evaluated and treated. Furthermore, without signs of significant trauma, the mechanism of injury may suggest potential problems, and these also should be pursued assiduously.

Diagnosis and Differential

The diagnosis in trauma begins with a history that includes the mechanism and sites of apparent injury. Other pertinent details are blood loss at the scene, damage to vehicles or types of weapons involved, as applicable. The primary survey (A-B-C-D-E) is then initiated, characterized by the orderly identification and concomitant treatment of the most life-threatening conditions. First, *A*irway patency is assessed and secured. *B*reathing is assessed by means of examination of the head and neck for tracheal deviation, quality of breath sounds, flail chest, crepitation, sucking chest wounds, and fractures of the sternum. Problems such as tension pneumothorax, pneumothorax, hemothorax, and misplacement of the endotracheal tube are identified and immediately treated before proceeding further. Next, the patient's *C*irculatory status is addressed. Two large-bore IVs are placed for fluid resuscitation, as appropriate, and blood is obtained for laboratory evaluation. Cardiac monitoring is initiated and the rhythm documented. Heart sounds are evaluated, and the presence or absence of neck vein distention is noted. Cardiac tamponade, evidenced by Beck's triad (hypotension, muffled heart sounds, and elevated venous pressure), is relieved if present. Emergent echocardiography, available in some EDs, can replace diagnostic pericardiocentesis in the identification of tamponade. Finally, the primary survey concludes with a brief neurologic examination for *D*isability, consisting of assessment of consciousness by the Glasgow Coma Scale, pupil size and reactivity, and motor function. Vital signs are recorded, including rectal temperature, response to fluid replacement is evaluated, and the patient is completely *E*xposed and prepared for secondary survey.

The secondary survey is a rapid but thorough head-to-toe examination to identify all injuries and set priorities for care. Resuscitation and frequent monitoring of vital signs continue throughout this process. Evidence for significant head injury (e.g., skull and facial fractures) is sought, and the pupils are rechecked. The neck, chest, and abdominal examinations are completed and the stability of the pelvis is assessed. Then X-rays of the lateral cervical spine, chest, and pelvis are ordered. The GU system is evaluated by external inspection, a rectal exam is done, and a urethrogram is ordered for suspected urethral injury (meatal blood present, the prostate boggy or displaced); otherwise, a urinary catheter is placed and the urine obtained is checked for blood and a pregnancy test is ordered for females of childbearing age. Vaginal blood on a bimanual exam is an indication for a speculum exam. Patients must be log-rolled maintaining cervical spine stabilization for examination of the back. Extremities are checked for soft-tissue injury and fracture. A more thorough neurologic exam is done.

On completion of the secondary survey, lab studies are ordered as needed. Additional radiologic studies, such as a cystogram, IVP, aortogram, or CT scan of the head or abdomen are considered. Diagnostic peritoneal lavage is suggested rather than CT scan to evaluate the unstable patient for intra-abdominal bleeding. If resuscitation has not been achieved by this time through crystalloid or blood administration, transfer to the OR for exploration should be considered.

Emergency Department Care and Disposition

ED management of the trauma patient begins before patient arrival. A team captain and assistants with defined roles are assigned, a prehospital history is acquired, and two units of O-negative blood are obtained in cases of known hypotension. Equipment for monitoring, airway management, IV fluid administration, and lab evaluation should be ready.

At the outset of the primary survey, **Airway** patency is assured. A chin lift may initially help in opening the airway; suctioning may remove foreign material, blood, and loose tissue or avulsed teeth. Nasopharyngeal or oropharyngeal airways can be useful adjuncts. Tracheal intubation is indicated for patients with altered mental status or those who for any reason are unable to maintain an open airway on their own; agitated patients may require rapid sequence intubation. In cases of extensive facial trauma or when tracheal intubation is indicated but not able to be accomplished in another way, cricothyrotomy is the procedure of choice. During the evaluation of **Breathing,** 100% O_2 is administered by mask or endotracheal tube. Suspected tension pneumothorax is treated immediately with needle decompression followed by tube thoracostomy. For large hemothoraces, consideration may be given to autotransfusion and immediate operative exploration for initial chest tube output of ≥1500 ccs of blood. For patients already intubated who are noted to have unilateral (especially right-sided), decreased, or absent breath sounds, proper tube placement must be confirmed and consideration given to withdrawal of the endotracheal tube a short distance. The presence of a flail chest may mandate tracheal intubation to ventilate the patient adequately. Sucking chest wounds require placement of an occlusive dressing followed by chest-tube placement. Management of **Circulation** requires placement of at least two large-bore peripheral IVs; central lines are used initially only if adequate peripheral access cannot be accomplished. Two l of warm crystalloid is administered as rapidly as possible to treat shock followed by O-negative or type-specific blood as required. Severe external hemorrhage should be managed with compression at the bleeding site. Patients with **Disability** and evidence for intracranial injury on examination may benefit from tracheal intubation and hyperventilation. **Exposure** of the patient facilitates the remainder of the management with the provision that measures to prevent hypothermia are taken.

Interventions are undertaken during the secondary survey to control problems as they are discovered. Bleeding from scalp lacerations can be controlled with Raney clips. Tamponade of severe epistaxis can be achieved with balloon compression devices. Reduction of fractures with signs of distal neurovascular compromise may be therapeutic; all fractures should be splinted. A gastric tube should be inserted (orally in the setting of facial fractures) and a urinary catheter placed, if not contraindicated. Tetanus prophylaxis must be assured; IV antibiotics are indicated for possible ruptured abdominal viscus, vaginal or rectal lacerations, and open skeletal fractures. IV mannitol should be available and considered for acute neurologic deterioration. Potential closed spinal-cord injuries are treated with IV steroids. Patients with pelvic fractures and signs of persistent hemorrhage may benefit from pelvic arteriography and embolization.

Upon completion of the secondary survey, options for disposition of the patient are to move to the OR, admit to the hospital, or transfer to another facility. Ideally, the surgeon on call is present for the secondary survey and can at that point assume primary responsibility for the patient. If transfer is to be made, the resuscitating physician must relay all pertinent findings and occurrences to the accepting physician. Complete records including flow sheets documenting vital signs, intake and output, and neurologic status, laboratory study results, and X-rays, should be sent with the patient. Personnel trained to monitor vital signs and neurologic status and administer IV fluids must accompany the patient during transport.

If Standard Treatment Fails

For patients who fail initial resuscitation or who deteriorate during the ED course, the physician must return to the starting point by repeating the ABCs and proceeding back through the primary and secondary surveys. It must be emphasized that aggressive and rapid evaluation and resuscitation, systematic thoroughness, and a high degree of suspicion for injury based upon mechanism are essential. Additional diagnostic testing or therapeutic procedures may be necessary, including emergency thoracotomy. The primary indication for ED thoracotomy is cardiac arrest in the patient with a penetrating wound to the chest and signs of life at the scene who subsequently sustains cardiac arrest or displays signs of severe cardiac tamponade despite aggressive management, including pericardiocentesis. Less clear indications for thoracotomy include cardiac arrest in blunt trauma and persistent, severe hypotension.

For further reading in *Emergency Medicine: A Comprehensive Study Guide*, 4th edition, see Chapter 212, Trauma, by Ernest Ruiz.

145 | Pediatric Trauma

Charles J. Havel, Jr.

Trauma is the most common cause of death in children more than 1 year old. Although the priorities are similar for the trauma management of both adults and children, important differences in anatomy, physiology, and psychology dictate some modification to the evaluation and treatment of injured pediatric patients. An additional factor to be considered in the evaluation of these patients is the possibility of nonaccidental trauma (child abuse).

Clinical Features

Be aware of subtle variations in the presentation of injured children versus injured adults. As obligate nose breathers, infants less than 6 mo old with facial trauma or bleeding into the nasopharynx will evidence significant respiratory distress. A difference in the mechanics of breathing in children results in early tachypnea and accessory muscle use in dyspneic patients. Nasal flaring, grunting, and retractions also are signs that should be noted in the evaluation of respiratory status. The physiology of shock in children causes tachycardia to be the most sensitive and earliest sign of volume loss; conversely, hypotension is a late and therefore ominous finding. Other important signs of hemorrhage are increased capillary refill time, decreased degree of responsiveness, decreased urine output, narrowed pulse pressure, and decreased skin temperature. The ratio of surface area to mass is greater than in adults, putting pediatric patients at greater risk for hypothermia following injury.

Diagnosis and Differential

The process of evaluation for adult and pediatric trauma patients is the same; the primary survey (A-B-C-D-E) and the secondary survey are completed in a systematic fashion. *A*irway patency and adequacy of *B*reathing are assessed. Definitive airway management and treatment of pneumothorax or hemothorax are accomplished before continuing further. The *C*irculatory status is evaluated, hemodynamic and cardiac monitoring is initiated, vascular access is secured, and fluid resuscitation is begun. A brief neurologic examination for *D*isability must include modification of the Glasgow Coma Score, based upon age and examination of the fontanelle in infants, for indications of changes in intracranial pressure. To complete the primary survey, the patient is *E*xposed in preparation for the secondary survey, vital signs are recorded, and response to fluid administration noted.

The secondary survey proceeds from head to toe while resuscitation and monitoring of vital signs continue. Head and neck are examined for signs of injury, specifically for evidence of basilar skull fracture, facial bone fractures, and cervical spine fracture. Evaluation of the chest is performed recognizing that, due to the more compliant chest wall of the child, serious intrathoracic injury may exist without obvious external signs. As a corollary to this principle, external evidence of trauma such as a rib fracture is a sensitive indicator of serious underlying injury. The abdomen, pelvis, and perineum are examined, and a rectal examination is performed. Cervical spine, chest, and pelvis x-rays are obtained, a naso- or oro- gastric tube is placed to decompress the stomach, and a urinary catheter inserted. The patient must be log-rolled to examine the back, and the extremities must be checked for soft-tissue injury and fractures. Lastly, a thorough neurologic examination is done in the context of the appropriate developmental stage of the patient and considering the typical heightened apprehension of the pediatric patient.

On completion of the secondary survey, additional diagnostic studies are ordered. Routine lab studies are CBC with differential, electrolytes, BUN and creatinine, urinalysis, and liver enzymes (in abdominal trauma), along with type and crossmatch for blood products. In the evaluation of pediatric abdominal injury, the physical exam has both a high false-positive and relatively high false-negative rate. Therefore, either CT scanning or diagnostic peritoneal lavage (primarily for hemo-dynamically unstable patients) is utilized frequently. The imaging modality of choice for evaluation of head injury is the CT scan; indications for ordering this test include significant loss of consciousness, deteriorating level of consciousness, apparent skull fracture on physical examination, repeated and persistent emesis, and seizure. High clinical suspicion must be maintained for cervical spine injury in the younger child, to include spinal-cord injury without radiographic abnormality (SCIWORA). Physical findings consistent with spinal-cord injury or abnormalities on spine x-rays are strong indications for CT scanning or standard tomography. Burn patients must have accurate documentation of the depth and extent of the injury and consideration given to evaluation for carbon monoxide poisoning.

Emergency Department Care and Disposition

Many problems identified in pediatric trauma patients during the primary and secondary surveys are managed similarly to adults. Several issues deserve special discussion. Airway management in children can be particularly challenging. Anatomic differences responsible for this include a relatively larger tongue and more cephalad location of the larynx. All patients should initially be administered 100% oxygen. Suctioning, jaw-thrust, or chin-lift maneuvers, and placement of either a nasal or an oral airway are more aggressive measures to be considered. In patients requiring tracheal intubation, **orotracheal intubation** is the route of choice; nasotracheal intubation should be avoided due to potential swelling and injury to the nasopharynx. In children less than 8 years old, the narrowest portion of the airway is subglottic, and a tube that fits through the vocal cords may not pass through this region. Choosing an appropriate endotracheal tube size is done by using the following formula:

$$\text{Internal Diameter (in mm)} = \frac{16 + \text{age of patient in years}}{4}$$

Patients in this age range should also have an uncuffed endotracheal tube placed. Rapid sequence intubation using pretreatment with 100% oxygen, IV lidocaine at 1.0 mg/kg, IV atropine (0.02 mg/kg—min dose 0.1 mg, max dose 1.0 mg), and appropriate sedation and pharmacologic paralysis can be useful for patients with head injuries or those who are uncontrollably combative. Securing an airway in the setting of severe facial trauma is best achieved by transtracheal catheter ventilation. Identification of the cricothyroid membrane can be difficult and the cricoid cartilage is easily damaged, so cricothyrotomy is not recommended in small children. Having achieved transtracheal catheter placement through the cricoid membrane, however, and if prolonged ventilation is required before surgical creation of a tracheostomy, a tracheostomy tube or shortened endotracheal tube can be placed over a guide wire using the catheter in a Seldinger-type procedure.

Vascular access can be difficult in children, especially with accompanying hypotension. Strong consideration must be given to early use of interosseous cannulation, particularly in young children and infants. Resuscitative fluids should be administered in **20 cc/kg boluses of crystalloid;** if there is no improvement, or deterioration occurs after an initial response, 10 cc/kg boluses of packed RBCs or whole blood are indicated. Fluids should be warmed and used in conjunction with warming lights to prevent hypothermia.

Neurologic injuries in children deserve individual discussion. Spinal immobilization must be achieved in infants and younger children with allowance for their relatively larger head by placement of padding behind the shoulders. Evaluation of mental status may be difficult due to developmental stage and heightened anxiety. Consequently, more liberal use of sedation in children is appropriate after completion of the neurologic examination. Children tend to recover better from head injury than adults, but aggressive treatment of hypoxia and hypotension is important to facilitate a good outcome. Severe head injury should be treated with tracheal intubation and hyperventilation, elevation of the head of the bed to 30°, and maintaining the head and neck in neutral position. Intravenous mannitol at 0.5 to 1.0 g/kg and lasix at 1.0 mg/kg may be useful in treating cerebral edema. Post-traumatic seizures are more common in children than adults and consideration is warranted for prophylaxis with phenytoin loading at 18 mg/kg.

For further reading in *Emergency Medicine: A Comprehensive Study Guide*, 4th edition, see Chapter 213, Pediatric Trauma, by Marte E. Baro and Gary C. Fifield.

With the rapid growth in the size of the elderly population, the incidence of geriatric trauma is expected to increase as well. ED physicians need to stay abreast of the unique injury mechanisms and clinical features associated with geriatric trauma patients, and apply special management principles when caring for them.

Clinical Features and Diagnosis and Differential

Common mechanisms of injury: (1) Falls are the most common accidental injury in patients over 75 years old and the second most common injury in the 65 to 74 age group. Syncope has been implicated in many cases, which may be secondary to dysrhythmias, venous pooling, autonomic derangement, hypoxia, anemia, and hypoglycemia. (2) Motor vehicle-related injuries rank as the leading mechanism of injury to bring elderly patients to trauma centers in the U.S. (3) The 65-year and older age group accounts for 22% of pedestrian–automobile fatalities in the U.S. (4) The overall increase in violent crimes in the U.S. has not spared the elderly. Violent assaults account for 4% to 14% of trauma admissions in this age group. Just as in pediatric trauma cases, ED physicians should have heightened suspicion for elder or parental abuse in the geriatric trauma patient.

Special attention should be paid to anatomical variation that may make airway management more difficult. These include the presence of dentures, cervical arthritis, or TMJ arthritis. A thorough secondary survey is essential to uncover less serious injuries. These injuries, which include various orthopaedic and minor head trauma, may not be severe enough to cause problems during the initial resuscitation but cumulatively may cause significant morbidity and mortality. Seemingly stable geriatric trauma patients can deteriorate rapidly and without warning.

History

Since elderly patients may have a significant past medical history that impacts their trauma care, obtaining a precise history is vital. Often, the time frame for obtaining information about the traumatic event, past medical history, medications, and allergies is quite short. Family members, medical records, and the patient's primary physician may be helpful in gathering information regarding the traumatic event and the patient's previous level of function.

Vital Signs

Early assessment and frequent monitoring of vital signs is essential. ED physicians should be wary of a normal heart rate in the geriatric trauma victim. A normal tachycardic response to pain, hypovolemia, or anxiety may be absent or blunted in the elderly trauma patient. Medications such as β-blockers may mask tachycardia and delay appropriate resuscitation.

Head Injuries

When evaluating the elderly patient's mental status during the neurologic exam, it would be a grave error to assume that alterations in mental status are due solely to any underlying dementia or senility. Elderly persons suffer a much lower incidence of epidural hematomas than the general population. There is, however, a higher incidence of *sub*dural hematomas in elderly patients. More liberal indications for CT scanning are justified.

Cervical Spine Injuries

The pattern of cervical spine injuries in the elderly is different than in younger patients, as there is an inceased incidence of C-1 and C-2 fractures with the elderly. When the elderly trauma patient presents with neck pain, ED physicians need to place special emphasis on maintaining cervical immobilization until the cervical spine is properly assessed. Because underlying cervical arthritis may obscure fracture lines, the elderly patient with persistent neck pain and negative plain radiographs should undergo CT scanning of the neck.

Chest Trauma

In blunt trauma, there is an increased incidence of rib fractures due to osteoporotic changes. The pain associated with rib fractures, along with any decreased physiologic reserve, may predispose patients to respiratory complications. More severe thoracic injuries, such as hemopneumothorax, pulmonary contusion, flail chest, and cardiac contusion, can quickly lead to decompensation in elderly individuals whose baseline oxygenation status may already be diminished. Frequent arterial blood gas analysis may provide early insight into elderly patients' respiratory function and reserve.

Abdominal Trauma

The abdominal exam in elderly patients is notoriously unreliable compared to younger patients. Even with an initially benign physical exam, ED physicians must be highly suspicious of intra-abdominal injuries in patients who have associated pelvic and lower rib-cage fractures. For older patients, adhesions associated with previous abdominal surgical procedures may increase the risk of performing diagnostic peritoneal lavage in the ED. CT scanning with contrast, therefore, is a valuable diagnostic test. It is important to ensure adequate hydration and baseline assessment of renal function prior to the contrast load for the CT scan. Some patients may be volume depleted due to medications, such as diuretics. This hypovolemia coupled with contrast administration may exacerbate any underlying renal pathology.

Orthopaedic Injuries

Hip fractures occur primarily in four areas: intertrochanteric, transcervical, subcapital, and subtrochanteric. Intertrochanteric fractures are the most common, followed by transcervical fractures. ED physicians must be aware that pelvic and long-bone fractures are not infrequently the sole etiology for hypovolemia in elderly patients. Timely orthopaedic consultation, evaluation, and treatment with open reduction and internal fixation should be coordinated with the diagnosis and management of other injuries.

Long-bone fractures of the femur, tibia, and humerus may produce a loss of mobility with a resulting decrease in the independent lifestyle of elderly patients. Early orthopaedic consultation for intramedullary rodding of these fractures may result in increased early mobilization.

The incidence of Colles's fractures and humeral head and surgical neck fractures in elderly patients are increased by falls on the outstretched hand or elbow. Localized tenderness, swelling, and ecchymosis to the proximal humerus are characteristic of these injuries. Early orthopaedic consultation and treatment with a shoulder immobilizer or surgical fixation should be arranged.

Emergency Department Care and Disposition

As in all trauma patients, the ABCDEs of the primary survey should be assessed expeditiously.

1. The main therapeutic goal is to aggressively maintain adequate oxygen delivery. Prompt **tracheal intubation** and use of mechanical ventilation should be considered in patients with more severe injuries, respiratory rates greater than 40 breaths per min, or when the PaO_2 is <60 mmHg or $PaCO_2$ > 50 mmHg. Whereas nonventilatory therapy helps to prevent respiratory infections and is always desirable, early mechanical ventilation may avert disastrous results associated with hypoxia.
2. Geriatric trauma patients can decompensate with over-resuscitation just as quickly as they can with inadequate resuscitation. Elderly patients with underlying coronary artery disease and cerebrovascular disease are at a much greater risk of suffering the consequences of ischemia to vital organs when they become hypotensive after sustaining trauma. During the initial resuscitative phase, crystalloid, while the primary option, should be administered judiciously, since elderly patients with diminished cardiac compliance are more susceptible to volume overload. Consideration should be made for early and more liberal use of **RBC transfusion.** Transfusion early in

resuscitation would enhance oxygen delivery and help minimize tissue ischemia.

3. **Early invasive monitoring** has been advocated to help physicians assess elderly hemodynamic status. One major study found that urgent invasive monitoring provides important hemodynamic information early, aids in identifying occult shock, limits hypoperfusion, helps prevent multiple organ failure, and improves survival. Survival was improved because of enhanced oxygen delivery through the use of adequate volume loading and inotropic support.

4. If the insertion of invasive monitoring lines is impractical in the ED, every effort should be made to expedite care of elderly trauma patients and prevent unnecessary delays. In the ED evaluation of blunt trauma patients, the chest radiograph, cervical spine series, and pelvic radiographs are necessary diagnostic tests during the secondary survey. Although it is vital to be thorough in the diagnosis of occult orthopaedic injuries, taking a great deal of time in radiology may compromise patient care. Only a few radiologic studies, such as emergent head and abdominal CT scans, should take precedence over obtaining vital information from invasive monitoring. Elderly trauma patients will benefit most from an expeditious transfer to the ICU for invasive monitoring so that their hemodynamic status can be further assessed. Invasive monitoring in the intensive-care environment may provide clues to subtle hemodynamic changes that may compromise geriatric patients with limited physiologic reserve.

For further reading in *Emergency Medicine: A Comprehensive Study Guide*, 4th edition, see Chapter 214, Geriatric Trauma, by O. John Ma and Daniel J. DeBehnke.

O. John Ma

Head injuries account for approximately half of all trauma-related deaths. An initial impact injury to the brain produces varying degrees of mechanical neuronal and axonal injury which, at the present stage of medical science, cannot be treated. Secondary brain injury occurs from potentially treatable factors such as intracranial hemorrhage, cerebral edema, ischemia, hypoxia, hypercarbia, and increased intracranial pressure (ICP). Optimal ED management is paramount in helping to minimize secondary brain injury, thus decreasing the overall mortality and morbidity.

Clinical Features

General Out-of-hospital medical personnel often may provide critical parts of the history, including mechanism and time of injury, loss of consciousness, mental status, respiratory effort, seizure activity, verbalization, and movement of extremities. An elevated systolic blood pressure can reflect a rise in ICP and be part of the Cushing reflex (hypertension and bradycardia). Serial neurologic examinations are essential in establishing the severity of the head injury and its clinical course. The pupillary examination should be recorded for size in mm, symmetry, and reactivity to light. Checking the corneal reflex with a wisp of cotton provides insight into brainstem function. The Glasgow Coma Scale (GCS) (Table 147-1) is a highly reproducible system of examination. The GCS ranges from a maximum score of 15 to a low score of 3. In general, severe head injury is associated with a GCS of 8 or less, moderate head injury with 12 to 15, and mild head injury 13 to 15.

Skull fractures Isolated linear nondepressed fractures with intact scalp do not require treatment. Life-threatening intracranial hemorrhage may result, however, if the fracture causes disruption of the middle meningeal artery or a major dural sinus. Depressed skull fractures are classified as open or closed, depending on the integrity of the overlying scalp. Although basilar skull fractures can occur at any point in the base of the skull, the typical location is in the petrous portion of the temporal bone. Findings associated with a basilar skull fracture include hemotympanum, otorrhea or rhinorrhea, periorbital ecchymosis (raccoon eyes), and retroauricular ecchymosis (Battle sign).

Brain concussion Concussion is a diffuse head injury associated with transient loss of consciousness that occurs immediately following a nonpenetrating blunt impact to the head. It generally occurs when the head, while moving, strikes or is struck by an object. The duration of unconsciousness is typically brief (sec–min). Complete recovery is typical, although persistent headache and problems with memory, anxi-

TABLE 147-1. The Glasgow Coma Scale

	EYES	
Open	Spontaneously	4
	To verbal command	3
	To pain	2
No response		1
	BEST VERBAL RESPONSE	
	Oriented and converses	5
	Disoriented and converses	4
	Inappropriate words	3
	Incomprehensible sounds	2
	No response	1
	BEST MOTOR RESPONSE	
To verbal command	Obeys	6
To painful stimulus	Localizes pain	5
	Flexion-withdrawal	4
	Abnormal flexion (decorticate rigidity)	3
	Extension (decerebrate rigidity)	2
	No response	1
Total		3–15

ety, insomnia, and dizziness can continue in some patients for wks after the injury.

Brain contusion Common locations for contusions are the frontal poles, the subfrontal cortex, and the anterior temporal lobes. Contusions may occur directly under the site of impact or on the contralateral side (contrecoup lesion). The contused area is usually hemorrhagic with surrounding edema and is occasionally associated with subarachnoid hemorrhage. Neurologic dysfunction may be profound and prolonged, with patients demonstrating mental confusion, obtundation, or coma. Focal neurologic deficits may be present.

Intracerebral hemorrhage Parenchymal hemorrhage result from lacerated blood vessels. Combination of parenchymal hemorrhage and contusion can produce an expanding mass lesion; when present in the anterior temporal lobe, uncal herniation can occur without a diffuse increase in ICP. Physical findings are often similar to patients with severe contusions.

Epidural hematoma Epidural hematoma results from an acute collection of blood between the inner table of the skull and dura. Approximately 80% of the time, it is associated with a skull fracture that lacerates a meningeal artery, most commonly the middle meningeal artery. Underlying injury to the brain may not necessarily be severe. In a classic scenario, the patient may present with clear mentation, signifying the lucid interval, and then begin to develop mental status deterioration in the ED. A fixed and dilated pupil on the side of the lesion with contralateral hemiparesis are classic late findings.

Subdural hematoma A subdural hematoma, a collection of venous blood between the dura and overlying the arachnoid and brain, results from tears of the bridging veins that extend from the subarachnoid space to the dural venous sinuses. A common mechanism is sudden acceleration–deceleration. Patients with brain atrophy, such as alcoholics or the elderly, are more susceptible to a subdural hematoma. Acute subdural hematomas become symptomatic within 24 h of injury. Symptoms may range from a headache to lethargy or coma. It is important to distinguish between acute and chronic subdural hematomas by history, physical exam, and CT scan.

Herniation Diffusely or focally increased ICP can result in herniation of the brain at several locations. Transtentorial (uncal) herniation occurs when a subdural hematoma or temporal lobe mass forces the ipsilateral uncus of the temporal lobe through the tentorial hiatus into the space between the cerebral peduncle and the tentorium. This results in compression of the oculomotor nerve and parasympathetic paralysis of the pupil on the same side, causing it to become fixed and dilated. The cerebral peduncle is simultaneously compressed, resulting in contralateral hemiparesis. The increased ICP and brainstem compression result in progressive deterioration in the level of consciousness. Occasionally the contralateral cerebral peduncle is forced against the free edge of the tentorium on the opposite side, resulting in paralysis ipsilateral to the lesion—a false localizing sign. The posterior cerebral artery can be compressed against the free edge of the tentorium, resulting in infarction of the occipital lobe. If the herniation continues untreated, there is progressive brainstem deterioration leading to hyperventilation, decerebration, and to apnea and death. Cerebellar tonsillar herniation through the foramen magnum occurs much less frequently. Resultant medullary compression causes bradycardia, respiratory arrest, and death. Cingulate or subfalcial herniation occurs when one cerebral hemisphere is displaced underneath the falx cerebri into the opposite supratentorial space. This is rarely clinically diagnosed.

Penetrating injuries Gunshot wounds and penetrating sharp objects can result in penetrating injury to the brain. The degree of neurologic injury will depend on the energy of the missile, whether the trajectory involves a single or multiple lobes or hemispheres of the brain, the amount of scatter of bone and metallic fragments, and whether a mass lesion is present.

Diagnosis and Differential

Approximately 5% of patients suffering severe head injury will have an associated cervical spine fracture. Cervical spine radiographs should be obtained in all patients who present with altered mental status, neck pain, neurologic deficit, severe distracting injury, or if the mechanism of injury is serious enough to potentially produce cervical spine injury.

Main indications for CT scanning in the assessment of head-injured patients are: (1) persistent decrease in level of consciousness; (2) clinical neurologic deterioration; (3) persistent focal neurologic or mental status deficit; and (4) skull fractures in the vicinity of the middle meningeal artery or major venous sinuses. The CT scan can: (1) define the location and extent of hemorrhage; (2) distinguish intraparenchymal hemorrhage from cerebral edema; and (3) determine the amount of midline shift.

Anteroposterior and lateral skull radiographs may be obtained for penetrating wounds of the skull or for suspected depressed skull fracture. Skull radiographs help localize the position of a foreign body within the cranium and may determine the amount of bony depression. If a CT scan of the head will be obtained, bone windows can be obtained, eliminating the need for skull films. Routine skull radiographs are not necessary in patients who have not lost consciousness, have no neurologic deficit, no evidence of depressed skull fracture, and no indwelling shunt.

Lab work for significant head injury patients should include immediate type and crossmatching, CBC, electrolytes, glucose, arterial blood gas, directed toxicologic studies, partial thromboplastin time, prothrombin time, platelets, fibrinogen level, and urinalysis.

Emergency Department Care and Disposition

Mild and moderate head injury A period of **observation** in the ED is essential. Disposition depends on the findings of serial neurologic exams, reliability of the patient, and availability of friends or family to observe the patient after discharge. Hospital admission is indicated for patients with persistent diminished level of consciousness, deterioration in neurologic function, focal neurologic deficit, seizures, penetrating cranial injury, open or depressed skull fractures, or lack of reliable friends and family to observe the patient after ED discharge.

Severe head injury Supplemental 100% oxygen, cardiac monitoring, and two IV lines should be secured. **Endotracheal intubation** to protect the airway and provide for mechanical **hyperventilation,** if desired, is the top priority. Should rapid sequence intubation be utilized, it is imperative to provide adequate cervical immobilization and use a sedation/induction agent. Following intubation, in order to reduce ICP, patients should be artificially hyperventilated to maintain an arterial pCO_2 between 25 and 30.

Since hypotension can lead to depressed cerebral perfusion pressure, restoration of an adequate BP is vital. Once adequate BP is achieved, IV fluids should be administered cautiously to prevent cerebral edema. Hypotonic and glucose-containing solutions should be avoided.

In patients with focal neurologic deficits, pupillary size inequality, neurologic deterioration, or a GCS score 8, IV **mannitol** (0.5–1.0 g/kg) should be administered to further reduce ICP. Since mannitol acts as an osmotic diuretic, Foley-catheter insertion is necessary, and hypotension is a relative contraindication. Since an intracranial hematoma can expand somewhat as the cerebral edema resolves, mannitol should only be administered when a definitive study and definitive neurosurgical referral are in order. Also, in order to reduce ICP, the head of the bed should be elevated 30°, provided the patient is not hypotensive.

Post-traumatic seizures Prophylactic phenytoin use in severe head injuries is controversial and should be administered in consultation with the neurosurgeon. Seizures should be treated with benzodiazepines, such as lorazepam or diazepam, and phenytoin at a loading dose of 18 mg/kg IV, infused at a rate no faster than 50 mg/min.

Head injury referral In hospitals where neurosurgical care is not available, head injury patients who should be referred to a neurosurgeon at another institution include those with persistent altered mental status, neurologic deficits or deterioration, intracranial hemorrhage, basilar skull fractures, and depressed skull fractures.

Prior to transfer, direct communication between the referring physician and the receiving physician must occur. A plan for the best mode of transport, the need for artificial ventilation, the administration of significant drugs, and the potential need for blood transfusion, especially in the pediatric patient, should be determined before the patient leaves the referring institution.

For further reading in *Emergency Medicine: A Comprehensive Study Guide*, 4th ed., see Chapter 215, Head Injury, by Gaylan L. Rockswold.

Spinal Injuries

Charles J. Havel, Jr.

Spinal cord injuries cause catastrophic sequelae both in human terms and in health-care dollars expended. There were approximately 13,000 new spinal cord injury patients in the U.S. in 1994 alone.

Clinical Features

Not all patients with spinal injuries present with an obvious neurologic deficit; unstable bony injury may exist without actual spinal cord or nerve root trauma. Some patients may complain of paresthesias, dysesthesias, or other sensory disturbances, with or without specific physical findings. More severely injured patients will have obvious neurologic deficits on physical examination. Patients with severe acute spinal cord injuries typically present with spinal shock; that is, with flaccid hemiplegia or quadriplegia, arreflexia, and mild hypotension. The hypotension is neurogenic in origin and due to a loss of sympathetic tone. As opposed to hypovolemic shock, neurogenic shock is characterized by warm, pink, dry skin; adequate urine output; and relative (paradoxical) bradycardia. Other signs of autonomic dysfunction may also accompany spinal shock, such as GI ileus, urinary retention, fecal incontinence, priapism, and loss of normal ability to regulate body temperature.

Diagnosis and Differential

The history is useful in defining the mechanism of injury, allowing the clinician to anticipate specific potential injuries (Table 148-1).

Any neurologic complaints from the patient, even if transitory, must raise suspicion for a spinal injury. As part of a complete primary and secondary survey, the evaluation for a potential spinal injury should focus on examination of the spine itself and the neurologic exam.

The neurologic examination should include the following assessments; pain perception, light touch and proprioception (to evaluate the posterior columns), motor strength and tone, reflexes, rectal tone, perianal sensation and wink, bulbocavernosus reflex, and priapism.

Patients with any one of the following characteristics must have (at the least) plain film radiography of the traumatized portion of their spine:

1. Midline bony spinal tenderness, crepitus, or stepoff.
2. Physical findings of a neurologic deficit.
3. Altered mental status.
4. The presence of additional painful or distracting injuries.
5. Patient complaint of paresthesias or numbness.

As for cervical spine x-rays, a minimum of three views is required to evaluate for fracture or other bony abnormality—a lateral view, an

TABLE 148-1. Cervical Spine Injuries: Mechanism of Injury

Flexion
  Anterior subluxation (hyperflexion sprain)
  Bilateral interfacetal dislocation
  Simple wedge (compression) fracture
  Clay-shoveler (coal-shoveler) fracture
  Flexion teardrop fracture
Flexion–Rotation
  Unilateral interfacetal dislocation
Extension–Rotation
  Pillar fracture
Vertical Compression
  Jefferson bursting fracture of atlas
  Burst (bursting, dispersion, axial loading) fracture
Hyperextension
  Hyperextension dislocation
  Avulsion fracture of anterior arch of atlas
  Extension teardrop fracture of axis
  Fracture of posterior arch of atlas
  Laminar fracture
  Traumatic spondylolisthesis (hangman's fracture)
  Hyperextension fracture–dislocation
Lateral flexion
  Uncinate process fracture
Diverse or Imprecisely Understood Mechanisms
  Atlantooccipital disassociation
  Odontoid fractures

odontoid view, and an AP view. A complete and systematic survey of the x-ray must be completed such as follows:

1. Determine that all 7 cervical vertebral bodies and the superior margin of T1 are visible.
2. Check for alignment of the 4 lordotic curves—the anterior longitudinal line, the posterior longitudinal line, the spinolaminar line, and the tips of the spinous processes.
3. Check for abrupt angulation of greater than 11° at a single interspace.
4. Check for fanning of spinous processes.
5. Check each vertebra for fracture.
6. Examine the atlanto-occipital relation for dislocation.
7. Determine the width of the pre-dental space—greater than 3 mm in adults or 4 mm in children may suggest cruciform ligament instability.
8. Check the AP diameter of the spinal canal.
9. Examine the width of the prevertebral soft tissues.
10. Look for fracture of the odontoid in the open mouth view.
11. Examine the AP film for alignment of the spinous processes or any other sign of rotation.

Additional imaging may be indicated for patients with positive findings on initial plain films or those for whom spinal injury is still suspected despite a negative initial x-ray. These studies include: flexion and extension views (for the cervical spine), looking for ligamentous instability; standard tomography; CT scan with or without contrast myelography; or MRI (for evaluation of neural elements).

Once a bony abnormality is identified, a key part of the differential is the degree of stability associated with that particular type of injury (Table 148-2). Apart from the cervical fractures listed, thoracic and lumbosacral fractures have differing degrees of stability depending on the type. Wedge or compression fractures may be unstable if there is loss of greater than 50% of vertebral body height and failure of the posterior ligaments. Burst fractures result from axial loading and may be responsible for retropulsion of fragments causing spinal cord compression. Distraction fractures are associated with auto crashes; a severe and unstable variant is the Chance fracture, with horizontal fracture from the spinous process through the vertebral body. Thoracolumbar fracture–dislocations are grossly unstable and have a significant incidence of associated spinal cord injury. Only occasionally do sacral fractures result in a neurologic deficit, usually related to sacral nerve impingement.

For patients with obvious spinal cord injuries, the differential includes complete lesions and a number of incomplete lesions or syndromes. Anterior cord syndromes involve the loss of motor function and pain and temperature sensation distal to the level of injury with preservation of light touch, vibration, and proprioception. Hyperextension injuries

---

TABLE 148-2 The Spectrum of Acute Instability in Cervical Spine Injuries

Most Unstable
  Rupture of transverse atlantal ligament
  Fracture of dens
  Burst fracture with posterior ligamentouts disruption (flexion teardrop)
  Bilateral facet dislocation (or equivalent posterior disruption)
  Burst fracture of vertebral body without posterior ligamentous disruption
  Hyperextension fracture dislocation
  Hangman's fracture
  Extension teardrop fracture (stable in flexion)
  Jefferson fracture (burst of C1)
  Unilateral facet dislocation (or equivalent posterior disruption)
  Anterior subluxation
  Simple wedge compression fracture without posterior disruption
  Pillar fracture
  Fracture of the posterior arch of C1
  Spinous process fracture (clay-shoveler)
Least Unstable

in older patients typically produce the central cord syndrome, with motor weakness more prominent in the arms than legs and with variable sensory loss. The Brown-Sequard syndrome most often results from penetrating trauma and causes hemisection of the spinal cord. The findings in this instance are ipsilateral loss of motor function, proprioception, and vibratory sensation and contralateral loss of pain and temperature sensation. Final determination of complete versus incomplete lesions, however, must await the resolution of spinal shock.

Emergency Department Care and Disposition

There are three priorities in the care of the patient with a potential spinal injury:

1. Overall trauma care by addressing the ABCs and completion of the primary and secondary surveys. Airway management involves in-line stabilization (not traction), cricoid pressure, and appropriate intubation for patients unable to protect their own airway. Fluid resuscitation also facilitates spinal cord resuscitation; occult hemorrhage should be controlled or ruled out.
2. Stabilization of the injured spine, thereby avoiding secondary injury and preserving residual spinal cord function. Patients must have constant **full-spine immobilization,** including cervical stabilization with a hard collar and sandbags or similar devices, and they must remain on a long backboard until the potential of fracture is ruled out.
3. Initiating treatments to promote the highest possible chance for spinal cord recovery. Besides adequate fluid resuscitation and oxygenation, closed spinal cord injuries are treated with IV high-dose **methylprednisolone.** Current recommendations are for a loading dose of 30 mg/kg over 15 min, followed by initiation of a drip 45 min later at 5.4 mg/kg/h for 23 h.

Disposition is as important for patients who, after evaluation, are found not to have significant spinal injury, as it is for those with major spinal cord injuries. Any patient with an unstable spine, nerve root injury, uncontrollable pain, or intestinal ileus (common with lumbar fractures) should be admitted to the hospital. Patients with significant vertebral or cord trauma should be managed at a regional trauma or spinal cord injury center. For patients evaluated and able to be discharged, analgesia and anti-inflammatory medications, cold packs, and relative rest is reasonable first line treatment. Followup should be arranged within 3 wks for a re-evaluation, specifically to look for signs of subacute instability, particularly for patients with cervical trauma.

If Standard Treatment Fails

Failure to respond in a patient with known or potential spine injury implies a failure of resuscitative measures. Spinal shock is a diagnosis of exclusion, and hemorrhage—occult or otherwise—must be presumed, identified, and controlled. Persistent hypotension can often be treated successfully with a low-dose dopamine infusion (5–10 mcg/kg/min).

For further reading in *Emergency Medicine: A Comprehensive Study Guide*, 4th edition, see Chapter 216, Spinal Injuries, by Brian D. Mahoney.

Charles J. Havel, Jr.

Neck injuries due to either blunt or penetrating trauma can result in significant morbidity and mortality. Deep vital structures at risk include airway; major blood vessels; a variety of neural elements, including the cervical spinal cord; and the upper portion of the GI tract.

Clinical Features

Due to the different structures with potential for injury, patients with neck trauma demonstrate a variety of clinical presentations, which range from nearly asymptomatic to full cardiopulmonary arrest. Laryngeal or pharyngeal trauma can cause dysphonia, hemoptysis, hematemesis, dysphagia, neck emphysema, and dyspnea progressing to respiratory arrest. Acute hemorrhage can be visible externally or may occur internally, leading to hematoma formation with tracheal deviation or bleeding into the pharynx. In both situations, tachycardia, hypotension, and other signs of shock indicate significant blood loss; airway compromise may result from the mass effect of an expanding hematoma. Neurologic symptoms and signs range from complaints of paresthesias to hemiplegia, quadriplegia, and coma. GI injury tends to be asymptomatic, although patients may complain of dysphagia and hematemesis may be observed.

Diagnosis and Differential

The patient with neck trauma generally is approached in the same fashion as other trauma patients. The primary survey addresses the ABCs, and the secondary survey identifies and treats injury to specific structures. Penetrating wounds are classified as to the zone of injury (Table 149-1) and are evaluated for possible violation of the platysma muscle. No further probing of such wounds is warranted in the ED; full exploration awaits surgical consultation and the capability for proximal and distal vascular control in the OR. Lab testing (CBC, electrolytes and other blood chemistries, blood typing) is indicated for all patients in whom there is even the suspicion of serious injury. Plain film radiography can identify cervical spine injury, the presence of any penetrating foreign body, air in the soft tissues, and soft-tissue swelling. A chest x-ray is warranted for any suspected thoracic cavity penetration. Additional diagnostic procedures that should be ordered, as appropriate, in

TABLE 149-1. Regions of the Neck

Zone I	Base of the neck to the cricoid cartilage
Zone II	Cricoid cartilage to the angle of the mandible
Zone III	Angle of the mandible to the base of the skull

conjunction with surgical consultation include contrast imaging of the esophagus, endoscopy of the airway and esophagus, arteriography, and CT scanning of the larynx or cervical spine.

The differential diagnosis relates to the various structures at risk for injury. Airway injury, common in blunt trauma (generally due to a direct blow), can be seen with penetrating wounds as well. Vascular injury is most common with penetrating trauma, although major vessel injury can come from blunt trauma and may simulate acute stroke. Neurologic injuries include spinal cord trauma, nerve root damage, and peripheral nerve trauma. Cervical spine injury may present without neurologic deficit, but the spine can be cleared clinically in selected blunt trauma and gunshot wound victims. Other patients must have their cervical spine cleared radiographically. GI injuries are often occult and generally require evaluation by endoscopy or contrast radiography.

Emergency Department Care and Disposition

Management of neck injuries proceeds according to the same algorithms as generally apply to the trauma patient. Hemodynamic and cardiac monitoring, IV access, and 100% oxygen with pulse oximetry are required initially for all patients.

1. Airway management is particularly important and made critical by the potential for direct injury and resulting potential for compromise. Tracheal intubation is indicated for patients unable to maintain airway patency secondary to structural disruption, edema, secretions, bleeding, enlarging hematoma, or impending respiratory arrest. In cases where oral or nasal intubation is not possible or is contraindicated, cricothyrotomy or transtracheal jet insufflation may be performed.
2. The chest must be evaluated for pneumothorax and hemothorax secondary to vascular injury, primarily in the setting of penetrating trauma. Needle decompression relieves tension pneumothorax, and tube thoracostomy is performed for pneumothorax and hemothorax.
3. External hemorrhage is controlled with direct pressure; blind clamping of bleeding vessels is contraindicated due to the complex vital anatomy compressed into a relatively small space and the danger of causing further injury with a misguided surgical instrument. Vascular access and fluid resuscitation are achieved, first with crystalloid, then with blood products, if needed.
4. The cervical spine is secured and cleared clinically or radiographically, as appropriate.
5. The full extent of injuries is assessed in the secondary survey, and additional diagnostic studies are ordered, depending on what specific injuries are suspected.

Penetrating wounds that violate the platysma muscle mandate surgical consultation. Further evaluation and management are somewhat contro-

TABLE 149-2. Indications for Neck Exploration

Vascular
  Continued hemorrhage
  Unstable vital signs
  Diminished or absent pulses
  Large or expanding hematoma
Airway
  Difficulty breathing
  Voice change
Visceral
  Difficulty swallowing
  Subcutaneous emphysema
  Coughing, spitting, or vomiting blood
Neurologic

versial and involve a selective operative approach versus mandatory surgical exploration (Table 149-2). Blunt trauma may initially present with subtle signs of injury. Hoarseness, dysphagia, and dyspnea are indications for more in-depth evaluation. Symptoms of airway, vascular, or neurologic injury demand aggressive evaluation and stabilization paired with urgent surgical consultation.

If Standard Treatment Fails

For any trauma patient, deterioration requires the clinician to *return to the beginning with the ABCs and reassess the patient.* A high degree of suspicion for occult injury is necessary to avoid missed pathology. Early consultation and a low threshold for transfer or admission to surgical care for observation can guard against sudden delayed deterioration in uncontrolled circumstances.

For further reading in *Emergency Medicine: A Comprehensive Study Guide*, 4th edition, see Chapter 217, Penetrating and Blunt Neck Trauma, by Robert A. Swor.

Thoracic trauma is directly responsible for 25% of trauma deaths and is a contributing factor in an additional 25%. Patients who do not manifest hypotension or severe respiratory distress in the ED usually do very well. In patients with systolic BP less than 80 mm Hg or requiring urgent endotracheal intubation, resuscitative measures that have shown the most benefit include adequate ventilation and oxygenation, rapid fluid resuscitation, and insertion of one or more chest tubes.

GENERAL PRINCIPLES AND CHEST-WALL INJURIES

Clinical Features and Diagnosis and Differential

The first step is to evaluate the patient's effort to breathe; no effort indicates a probable CNS problem, whereas significant effort signals an airway obstruction. The most common causes of airway obstruction in comatose patients is a foreign body (including the tongue) in the hypopharynx, larynx, or trachea. If a laryngeal injury is suspected, careful endoscopic evaluation of the airway is required. If the patient is attempting to breathe and the airway is clear, thoracic injuries (flail chest, hemopneumothorax, diaphragmatic injury) should be considered.

The most frequent symptoms associated with thoracic trauma are chest pain and shortness of breath. Physical exam begins with inspection of the chest wall, looking for open (sucking,) chest wounds, flail segments, and contusions. The neck is examined for the presence of distended neck veins, which are associated with pericardial tamponade, tension pneumothorax, air embolus, and cardiac failure. Swelling and cyanosis of the face and neck often signal a superior mediastinal injury resulting in superior vena cava blockage. Subcutaneous emphysema from a bronchial injury or pulmonary laceration can result in severe swelling of the face and neck. The contour of the abdomen should be evaluated; a scaphoid abdomen may indicate a diaphragmatic injury. Palpation of the trachea to determine its normal position, of the chest to localize areas of tenderness or crepitation, and of the abdomen for the position of abdominal contents is important. Auscultation should be done systematically and thoroughly. The quality and equality of breath sounds should be documented. The presence of bowel sounds in the chest may be the first indication of a diaphragmatic injury. Inequality of breath sounds may suggest pneumothorax, hemothorax, or an improperly inserted endotracheal tube.

Simple rib fractures should be suspected in the patient with point tenderness over a rib. The goal of evaluating these injuries is to look for complications, such as pneumothorax, pulmonary contusion, or major vascular injury. Pain from rib fractures can decrease ventilation, possibly resulting in atelectasis or pneumonia. First and second rib fractures not due to direct trauma may be associated with significant underlying injuries, including myocardial contusions, pulmonary contusions, bronchial tears, and major vascular injuries. Multiple rib fractures, especially the 9th, 10th and 11th, are often associated with intra-abdominal injuries. In addition, the presence of hypotension should alert the physician to evaluate for tension pneumothorax or hemopneumothorax.

Segmental fractures of three or more adjacent ribs produces a flail segment of the chest, which can increase the work of breathing. Flail chest is recognized by paradoxical movement of the segment during the respiratory cycle (outward during expiration, inward during inspiration).

Traumatic asphyxia, caused by an inability to breathe due to added weight on the chest wall, results in subconjunctival hemorrhage or petechiae and vascular engorgement, edema, and cyanosis of the head, neck, and upper extremities. Neurologic impairment is often temporary, and long-term morbidity is usually due to associated injuries.

Emergency Department Care and Disposition

If a tension pneumothorax is suspected (severe respiratory distress, decreased breath sounds, and hyperresonance on one side of the chest; distended neck veins or deviation of the trachea away from the involved side), a **large-bore needle or IV catheter** should be inserted in the 2nd intercostal space at the midclavicular line for decompression. A **chest tube** can then be inserted for definitive treatment. If a hemothorax or nontension pneumothorax is suspected in a patient with severe respiratory distress, a chest tube should be inserted before obtaining a chest x-ray. Indications for ventilatory support are seen in Table 150-1. Continuous pulse oximetry is mandatory in any patient with severe chest trauma.

Although adequate ventilation is being ensured, restoration of adequate tissue perfusion should be achieved. Forty percent of patients in shock have extrathoracic injuries contributing to the shock state.

TABLE 150-1. Indications for Ventilatory Support

Impaired ventilation in spite of an open airway
Shock
Multiple injuries
Coma
Flail chest
Hypoxia ($pO_2 < 50$ mm Hg on room air)
Drainage of hemopneumothorax
Pre-existing pulmonary disease
Respiratory rate > 30 bpm
Relief of chest-wall pain
Multiple transfusions required
Elderly

Management of these patients includes the insertion of two large-bore IV catheters with rapid infusion of large volumes of crystalloid. If peripheral veins are not accessible, subclavian catheterization on the same side as the injury is recommended. Monitoring chest tube drainage is also important. If vital signs deteriorate as a large amount of blood is being evacuated from a chest tube, the tube should be clamped, and the patient should have an emergency thoracotomy, either in the OR or the ED.

The patient with penetrating thoracic trauma who loses vital signs just prior to or in the ED may require **open cardiac massage.** An incision is made in the left 5th intercostal space, anterolateral position. The pericardial sac is inspected for blood; the pericardium is opened vertically, being careful to avoid the phrenic nerve. The heart, lung hilum, and aorta are inspected for injuries that can be repaired primarily. Patients sustaining blunt traumatic arrest, penetrating abdominal or head injuries, or prolonged arrest times receive little if any benefit from a resuscitative ED thoracotomy.

Bleeding from chest-wall injuries is best controlled by **direct pressure.** Probing of these wounds is not recommended. Open (sucking) chest wounds indicate invasion into the pleural space and can act as one-way valves, potentially creating a tension pneumothorax. These should be covered with a sterile, air-tight dressing, followed immediately by tube thoracostomy. When subcutaneous emphysema is present, an underlying pneumothorax should be presumed. If the patient is to be intubated for any reason, therefore, a chest tube should be inserted.

In the treatment of rib fractures, adequate analgesia—orally if the patient is to be discharged, IV or through the intercostal nerve block if the patient is to be admitted—and pulmonary toilet are the mainstays of therapy. Patients with multiple rib fractures should be admitted for observation and serial examination if they cannot cough and clear secretions, if they are elderly, or if they have pre-existing pulmonary disease.

Flail chest management consists of stabilizing the flail segment, either external using sandbags, or internally by endotracheal intubation and mechanical ventilation. Indications for ventilatory support are seen in Table 150-2. Patients with a flail chest should be suspected of having an underlying pulmonary contusion. Adequate analgesia and

TABLE 150-2. Indications for Endotracheal Intubation in the Presence of a Flail Segment

Presence of shock
Three or more associated injuries
Severe head injury
Previous severe pulmonary disease
Fracture of 8 or more ribs
Age > 65

frequent pulmonary toilet are very important in the management of these patients.

Sternal fractures should alert the physician to the possible presence of underlying soft-tissue injuries, especially of the heart and great vessels. Therapy for these fractures includes adequate analgesia and pulmonary toilet. Admission based solely on the presence of sternal fractures is controversial.

LUNG INJURIES

Clinical Features and Diagnosis and Differential

Pulmonary contusions are usually seen as opacifications of the lung on chest x-ray within 6 h of injury.

Pneumothorax is a collection of air in the pleural space. It does not usually cause significant symptoms unless a tension pneumothorax develops, the pneumothorax occupies more than 40% of one hemithorax, or the patient has pre-existing shock or cardiopulmonary disease. Pneumothoraces are readily seen on expiratory chest x-rays.

Hemothorax should be considered in the severely traumatized patient with unilateral decreased breath sounds and dullness to percussion. Volumes in excess of 1 l of blood may be missed on supine chest radiographs because of its appearance as diffuse haziness without a distinct air-fluid level.

Emergency Department Care and Disposition

Treatment of pulmonary contusions involves maintenance of **adequate ventilation,** with the use of mechanical ventilation and positive end-expiratory pressure (PEEP) to optimize ventilation–perfusion matching. With severe unilateral lung injury, synchronous independent lung ventilation through a double-lumen endobronchial catheter prevents overinflation of the normal lung and provides better overall oxygenation. Pulmonary hematomas are caused by pulmonary parenchyma tears, and generally resolve spontaneously over a few wks. The major concern with these is the risk of developing lung abscesses. Intrabronchial bleeding is poorly tolerated and can result in death from drowning with small amounts of blood. Adequate pulmonary toilet with frequent suctioning is mandatory. Selective intubation of the bronchi to ensure proper ventilation of the nonbleeding lung may be life-saving in severe cases.

Aspiration after severe trauma is common. Radiologic changes associated with aspiration are often delayed 12 to 24 hrs. If recognized promptly, immediate bronchoscopy with irrigation of the tracheobronchial tree with buffered saline or a bicarbonate solution may reduce the severity of pneumonitis.

If tension pneumothorax is suspected, a needle thoracostomy in the 2nd intercostal space at the midclavicular line will provide temporary relief until a chest tube can be inserted. Small pneumothoraces that have not expanded on serial chest x-rays taken 6 to 12 h apart do not require chest-tube insertion. Admission of these patients for observation and serial examinations is important. An occult pneumothorax (seen on CT, but not on plain x-rays) does not require chest-tube insertion unless the patient is on a ventilator. Insertion of a small (24F or 28F) chest tube is adequate if no hemothorax is present. Failure to completely evacuate a pneumothorax is usually related to equipment problems (improper connection or leak in the water-seal apparatus or tubing), anatomic problems (occlusion of bronchi by secretions or foreign body, tear of a large bronchus, large tear of the lung parenchyma), or tube problems (improper position of the chest tube). A chest x-ray should be immediate in all patients after insertion of a chest tube.

Small hemothoraces should be carefully observed. If the hemothorax is large, a chest tube should be inserted. Serial examinations of the chest, including chest x-rays, and monitoring of the ongoing blood loss through the chest tube are important Indications for thoracotomy for intrathoracic bleeding are seen in Table 150-3.

TABLE 150-3. Indications for Thoracotomy for Continuing Hemorrhage in Chest Trauma

Systolic BP < 90 mm Hg with no other source found
Deterioration of vital signs associated with insertion of the chest tube and a large amount of blood (>1000 mL) evacuated
More than 1500 mL of blood is lost in the first 12 h, with continued bleeding
Drainage exceeds 300 mL/h for 3 h
Chest remains more than ½ full of blood after chest-tube placement

TRACHEOBRONCHIAL INJURY

Clinical Features and Diagnosis and Differential

Injuries to the lower trachea and bronchi are usually caused by severe deceleration forces. Common presenting signs and symptoms include dyspnea, hemoptysis, subcutaneous emphysema, Hamman sign, and sternal tenderness. On chest x-ray, a large pneumothorax, pneumomediastinum, deep cervical emphysema, or an endotracheal tube balloon that appears round all suggest tracheobronchial injury.

Emergency Department Care and Disposition

Management includes assuring adequate ventilation and referral for immediate **bronchoscopy** to fully evaluate and treat the injury. Intrathoracic tracheal injury is usually associated with other intrathoracic injuries and is almost invariably fatal. Injuries of the cervical trachea usually occur at the junction of the trachea and cricoid cartilage and are caused by direct trauma, such as from a steering wheel. Inspiratory stridor is common in these patients and indicates a 70% to 80% obstruction. Oral intubation should be attempted first. If gentle intubation is not possible, a formal tracheostomy should be performed. Blind cricothyroidotomy is relatively contraindicated in the patient with cervical tracheal injury.

DIAPHRAGMATIC INJURY

Clinical Features and Diagnosis and Differential

The majority of diaphragmatic injuries are caused by penetrating trauma. When blunt injury causes a diaphragmatic injury, it is usually leftsided. The diagnosis of diaphragmatic injury is often made intraoperatively due to the paucity of physical findings. An entrance wound in the abdomen, with the missile located in the chest cavity, should alert the physician to probable injury to the diaphragm. In the setting of blunt trauma, any abnormality of the diaphragm or lower lung fields on chest x-ray should make the physician consider the possibility of diaphragmatic injury. Peritoneal lavage is insensitive in diagnosing diaphragmatic injuries.

PENETRATING INJURY TO THE HEART

Clinical Features and Diagnosis and Differential

All patients with hypotension and penetrating thoracic injury between the midclavicular line on the right and anterior axillary line on the left should be considered as having a penetrating cardiac injury until proven otherwise. Beck's triad (distended neck veins, hypotension, and muffled heart tones) suggests a pericardial tamponade, although most patients with this type of injury do not have distended neck veins until volume resuscitation has occurred. Chest x-rays are rarely of help in diagnosing acute cardiac injury, and electrocardiographic changes are usually nonspecific. Echocardiography is a sensitive test in practiced hands for the detection of pericardial fluid. Pericardiocentesis has limited value in the evaluation of the patient with possible cardiac injury due to the high incidence of false positive and false-negative aspirates. In the hemodynamically stable patient when echocardiography is not available a subxiphoid pericardial window can be performed.

Emergency Department Care and Disposition

Management of the patient with cardiac injury includes attention to the airway, assurance of breathing, and adequate fluid resuscitation. Two large-bore IV lines should be placed, with one flowing into the venous system draining into the inferior vena cava. Patients in shock who do not respond to adequate fluid resuscitation and who are suspected of having a cardiac injury should undergo an **emergent thoracotomy.**

BLUNT INJURY TO THE HEART

Clinical Features and Diagnosis and Differential

The most common mechanism of injury causing cardiac trauma is a deceleration injury. In addition, compression between the sternum and vertebrae, a sudden increase in intrathoracic pressure or abdominal compression forcing abdominal contents against the heart can all cause cardiac injury. Any history or physical finding suggestive of moderate to severe chest or upper abdominal trauma should make the physician consider cardiac injury.

Cardiac rupture results in immediate death in 80% to 90% of cases. Patients with cardiac rupture who arrive at the hospital alive usually have a right atrial tear. Shock out of proportion to the degree of recognized injury and shock that persists despite control of hemorrhage elsewhere and volume expansion should make one consider the possibility of cardiac rupture. Immediate left anterior thoracotomy may be lifesaving in these cases. Septal defects and valve injuries are rare after blunt trauma but should be considered if a murmur exists in the setting of possible cardiac damage. Signs of a ventricular septal defect include severe early hypoxemia with a relatively normal chest x-ray, heart murmur, and an injury pattern on ECG. Rupture of the aortic valve is the most common valvular lesion.

Most patients with myocardial contusion have few if any problems. The most common clinical features associated with a significant myocardial contusion are tachycardia out of proportion to blood loss, arrhythmias (especially premature ventricular contractions and atrial fibrillation), and conduction defects. The chest x-ray is most useful in detecting associated injuries. ECG changes, especially ST–T wave abnormalities, new atrial fibrillation, multiple PVCs or conduction disturbances are commonly found in patients with myocardial contusion, although a normal ECG does not exclude the diagnosis. Cardiac enzymes, including SGOT, LDH, and CPK, are of little help in making this diagnosis. Radionuclide angiography evaluates the wall motion of the right and left ventricles. Two-dimensional echocardiography is useful in evaluating the patient with suspected myocardial contusion. The most common finding seen with myocardial contusion is right ventricular free-wall dyskinesia.

Emergency Department Care and Disposition

Blunt cardiac injuries rarely cause death, and the incidence of clinically significant dysrhythmias and other cardiac complications is low. Patients with normal left and right ventricular ejection fractions and no other significant problems may be observed in the ED and discharged if no abnormalities occur in 4 to 6 hrs. Management of the patient with significant myocardial contusion calls for the administration of supplemental oxygen and analgesics, treatment of significant cardiac dysrhythmias, and the administration of fluids or inotropes for hypotension. The presence of a myocardial contusion does not preclude surgical procedures, however, the pulmonary artery wedge pressure and cardiac rhythm should be monitored closely.

PERICARDIAL INJURY

A pericardial effusion may develop acutely or over time. The rate of fluid collection influences the onset and severity of symptoms. Evidence of acute pericardial injury is usually seen on the ECG as diffuse ST-segment elevation. Most patients are asymptomatic, and no specific therapy is required. A tear of the parietal pericardium at the apex of the heart may result in sudden severe shock and cardiac arrest if the heart herniates through the hole.

POSTPERICARDIOTOMY SYNDROME

This is seen in patients 2 to 4 wks after heart surgery or trauma. Classically, patients will have chest pain, fever, and pleural or pericardial effusions. Friction rubs, arthralgia and pulmonary infiltrates may also be seen. The ECG will often show diffuse ST–T wave changes consistent with pericarditis. Management is symptomatic, with salicylates and rest often the only therapy required. Occasionally glucocorticoids are required.

PENETRATING TRAUMA TO THE GREAT VESSELS OF THE CHEST

Clinical Features and Diagnosis and Differential

Only 5% to 15% of patients with penetrating trauma who require hospital admission will need a thoracotomy, but 25% of these will have injury to a great vessel. When injury is caused by a stab wound, survival is generally much higher than when caused by a gunshot wound. Simple lacerations of the great vessels can lead to exsanguination, tamponade, hemothorax, air embolism, or development of an AV fistula.

Specific historical facts about the injury can be very helpful. Information such as the amount of time the patient spent at the scene and in transit, the size, depth and angle of penetration of the weapon, and the number of gunshots heard should be sought. It is important to thoroughly inspect the chest, remembering to look in the axilla, in thick chest hair, and in skin folds for possible occult entrance and exit wounds. In general, these wounds should not be probed. Assessment of bilateral upper extremity pulses for equality is important, as a large mediastinal hematoma may compress the subclavian vessels. The entire chest should be auscultated for bruits that may indicate a false aneurysm or AV fistula.

Radiographic evaluation starts with plain chest x-rays. In addition to evaluation for pneumothoraces, widening of the upper mediastinum may indicate injury to brachiocephalic vessels. A fuzzy foreign body may indicate motion artifact caused by the foreign body being located within or adjacent to pulsatile structures. CT scans are rarely performed immediately for chest penetrating wounds. In the stable patient, however, a CT scan can help localize hematomas adjacent to great vessels. The use of IV contrast helps further evaluate these structures and may demonstrate a vascular defect or false aneurysm. The major role of CT scans is as a screen for great vessel injury. Arteriograms are most helpful in identifying major intrathoracic vascular injuries within hematomas. Contrast swallows using Gastrografin may be performed on stable patients to evaluate the integrity of the esophagus. Endoscopy is sometimes used in hemodynamically stable patients with penetrating wounds of the chest or lower neck.

Emergency Department Care and Disposition

Initial management consists of attention to the ABCs of initial resuscitation. Early **endotracheal intubation** should be performed in patients with penetrating injuries to the thoracic inlet to avoid the problems associated with expanding hematomas distorting the airway. The patient in severe shock (systolic BP < 60 mm Hg) should have **immediate surgery,** along with aggressive fluid resuscitation and control of major bleeding sites. If the systolic BP is 60 to 88 mm Hg, 2 to 3 l of crystalloid should be given rapidly. If the patient remains hypotensive, then immediate surgery is required. Emergency thoracotomy is required if the patient loses vital signs in the ED. Indications for thoracotomy in the stable patient are based on chest-tube output (Table 150-3) and other clinical indicators. Bullets that enter great vessels can embolize to distant sites, and should be sought with multiple x-rays or fluoroscopy.

BLUNT TRAUMA TO THE GREAT VESSELS OF THE CHEST

Clinical Features and Diagnosis and Differential

Eighty to ninety percent of patients with injury to great vessels from blunt trauma to the chest die at the scene, and 50% of those who reach the hospital succumb within 24 h. Ninety percent of patients who arrive at the hospital alive have an injury at the isthmus of the aorta (between the left subclavian and ligamentum arteriosum). Other common sites of injury are the innominate or left subclavian artery at their origins or a subclavian artery over the first rib.

A high index of suspicion is required to diagnose traumatic rupture of the aorta. This injury can occur even when no external signs of trauma exist. This injury, therefore, should be suspected in any patient with a high-speed deceleration mechanism of injury. These patients

TABLE 150-4. Chest Radiographic Findings Associated with Traumatic Rupture of the Aorta

Superior mediastinal widening (>8.0–8.5 cm)
Deviation of esophagus or trachea at T4
Obscuration of aortic knob or descending aorta
Obliteration of the aortopulmonary window
Obscuration of medial aspects of left upper lobe
Widening of the paravertebral stripe
Fracture of 1st or 2nd rib
Apical cap

complain primarily of their associated symptoms. Retrosternal or interscapular pain, often described as a tearing sensation may be the only initial indication. Dysphagia, stridor, dyspnea, and hoarseness are reported less often.

Patients with aortic injury may show a difference in BP between the upper and lower extremities, a difference in BP between the upper extremities, or a harsh systolic murmur across the precordium or in the interscapular area. Findings associated with traumatic rupture of the aorta on plain chest x-ray are seen in Table 150-4. The most frequent radiologic finding is mediastinal widening. Many unnecessary angiograms are performed because of technically poor chest x-rays that make the mediastinum appear wide. The best chest x-ray is an upright PA chest x-ray taken from 72″. The most accurate radiographic sign of traumatic aortic rupture is deviation of the esophagus more than 1 to 2 cm to the right of the spinous process of T4. To see this, an NG tube should be inserted prior to obtaining the chest x-ray. Up to one-third of patients with traumatic aortic rupture will have a normal chest x-ray initially.

Transesophageal ultrasound is a highly sensitive diagnostic modality to evaluate for traumatic aortic rupture. It can be used at bedside at the same time as the resuscitation and yields results that are at least as good as aortography. It visualizes the aortic isthmus and descending aorta very well, and defines the pericardial cavity, cardiac valves, pulmonary veins, and regional wall motion. The utility of transesophageal ultrasound on visualizing the ascending aorta is unknown.

Contrast-enhanced CT scans of the chest have been recommended as a tool to screen for traumatic aortic rupture. The presence of a mediastinal hematoma is an indication for aortography. The use of MRI in selected patients may be particularly good for diagnosing dissecting aneurysms. Aortography is the best way to diagnose aortic rupture.

Injury to the ascending aorta usually results in immediate death. These injuries tend to occur within the pericardium and result in cardiac tamponade. With an associated valvular injury, there is a murmur of aortic insufficiency. Chest x-ray shows a widened superior mediastinum, with or without obscuring the aortic knob. The aortogram shows a pseudoaneurysm.

Injuries to the innominate artery are associated with rib fractures, flail chest, hemopneumothorax, fractured extremities, head injuries, facial fractures, and abdominal injuries. The diagnosis is difficult because there are no characteristic physical findings except for some decrease in the right radial or brachial pulse. Findings on chest x-ray are similar to those found with traumatic rupture of the aorta (see Table 150-4), except the mediastinal hematoma is usually higher.

Subclavian artery injuries are most often caused by fractures to the first rib or clavicle. Absence of a radial pulse on the affected side is the most important sign. A pulsatile mass or bruit at the base of the neck is suggestive of this injury. Associated injury to the brachial plexus is common, and complete neurologic evaluation of the upper extremity on the involved side is indicated. Chest x-ray may show a widened superior mediastinum without obscuring the aortic knob. Management is immediate operative repair.

Emergency Department Care and Disposition

Management of the patient with suspected traumatic aortic rupture requires attention to the ABCs, keeping the systolic BP below 120 mm Hg, and avoidance of valsalva maneuvers. Sedatives, analgesics, vasodilators, and beta-adrenergic blockers may be required to control the patient's BP. Insertion of an NG tube is important, but it must be done with extreme care to avoid the patient gagging. Emergency thoracotomy is the accepted standard of treatment. Delayed repair may be more appropriate in patients who are at high operative risk or when surgical conditions are not optimal.

ESOPHAGEAL AND THORACIC DUCT INJURIES

Injuries to these structures are rare. If an esophageal injury is suspected, an esophogram should be performed. Most radiologists recommend use of Gastrografin because it causes less of an inflammatory reaction than barium. The false-negative rate with this contrast agent, however, is as high as 25%. Flexible esophagoscopy also can be performed, but it carries a false negative rate of 20%. Thoracic-duct injuries result in a chylothorax in the right hemithorax.

For further reading in *Emergency Medicine: A Comprehensive Study Guide*, 4th edition, see Chapter 218, Thoracic Trauma, by Robert F. Wilson.

The primary goal in the evaluation of abdominal trauma is to promptly recognize conditions that require immediate surgical exploration. A prolonged exam to pinpoint specific injuries is potentially detrimental to the patient. The most critical mistake is to delay surgical intervention when it is needed.

Clinical Features and Diagnosis of Specific Organ Injuries

The evaluation of the patient with abdominal trauma must be performed in the context of the patient's entire clinical picture.

Hollow organs Hollow viscus rupture may result from sudden compressen by a seat belt, and should be suspected when lap belt bruises or abrasions are identified. Injuries to these organs usually result in symptoms of peritonitis. Diagnostic peritoneal lavage (DPL) and water-soluble contrast studies are helpful in diagnosing these injuries.

Stomach The stomach is generally resistant to blunt trauma. A distended stomach, however, increases the likelihood of injury. Nasogastric tube (NGT) lavage of heme-positive contents is an insensitive diagnostic technique, so contrast studies are required to confirm diagnosis.

Duodenum The retroperitoneal position of the duodenum makes the diagnosis of this injury difficult. Signs and symptoms are often slow to develop; when present, they indicate significant injury. Duodenal injuries may range in severity from an intramural hematoma to an extensive crush or laceration. The definitive test for evaluating duodenal injury is a contrast study showing extravasation.

Small bowel Small-bowel injuries are most frequently the result of penetrating trauma. However, a deceleration injury can cause a bucket-handle tear of the mesentery or a blowout injury of the antimesenteric border. In most cases, injury to the small bowel will result in early peritoneal irritation from spillage of bowel contents causing significant symptoms. DPL and CT scan are useful in confirming clinical suspicions.

Colon Large-bowel injuries may lead to excessive contamination if surgical intervention is delayed. CT scanning with rectal contrast is an excellent method to detect this injury. A Gastrografin enema with fluoroscopy remains the optimal test for evaluating colonic perforation.

Rectum Since the rectum is an extraperitoneal organ, physical exam findings may be subtle. Careful rectal palpation should be performed to detect evidence of bony penetration when there is an associated pelvic fracture, and stool should be tested for blood. Overwhelming sepsis may rapidly develop when rectal injury is associated with an open pelvic fracture. Preoperatively, broad-spectrum antibiotic coverage is indicated.

Gallbladder and biliary ducts These injuries are rare. It is suspected when DPL fluid is positive for bile.

Solid organs Injury to the solid organs causes morbidity and mortality, primarily as a result of acute blood loss. The spleen is the most frequently injured organ in blunt abdominal trauma and is commonly associated with other intra-abdominal injuries. The liver also is commonly injured in both blunt and penetrating injuries. Tachycardia, hypotension, and acute abdominal tenderness are the primary physical exam findings. Kehr's sign, representing referred left shoulder pain, is a classic finding in splenic rupture. Lower left-rib fractures should heighten clinical suspicion for splenic injury. CT scan remains the optimal diagnostic tool in the hemodynamically stable patient. If the patient is unstable, a positive DPL mandates surgical exploration.

Pancreas Pancreatic injury is most common with penetrating trauma but also occurs after a severe crush injury. The classic case is a blow to the midepigastrium from a steering wheel or the handlebar of a bicycle. CT scan is helpful in diagnosis.

Kidney Renal parenchymal injury usually results in hematuria. Most renal injuries can be managed nonoperatively, but accurate diagnosis is essential for monitoring. IVP and CT scanning are useful diagnostic tests. Indications for surgery include evidence of continuing blood loss, laceration through Gerota's fascia, or loss of function. (A more detailed discussion of genitourinary tract trauma can be found in Chap. 153.)

Diaphragm Diaphragm injuries are insidious. Often there is no herniation, and the only finding is blurring of the diaphragm or an effusion. With herniation of abdominal contents into the thoracic cavity, diagnosis is clear. Diagnosis most often is on the left, and it is frequently made with contrast studies, chest x-ray, CT scan, or DPL.

Abdominal wall With high-velocity penetrating injuries to the abdominal wall, there is high incidence of associated intra-abdominal visceral injuries, which calls for exploratory laparotomy. When a patient presents to the ED with an obvious gunshot wound to the abdomen, DPL should never be performed, as it will only delay transport to the OR. If organ evisceration is present, it should be covered with a moist, sterile dressing prior to surgery.

Vascular structures Both abdominal arterial and venous injuries are potentially life-threatening secondary to acute hemorrhage. If a patient is hypovolemic and unresponsive to massive fluid resuscitation, ED thoracotomy for aortic crossclamping to gain proximal control may be life-saving before to taking the patient to the OR.

Adjunctive Diagnostic Tests

Plain Radiographs

Chest radiograph is valuable in checking for abdominal contents in the thoracic cavity and for evidence of free air under the diaphragm. An AP pelvis radiograph is important in identifying injuries that can produce significant blood loss and that can be associated with intra-abdominal visceral injury.

Diagnostic Peritoneal Lavage (DPL)

This remains an excellent test for evaluating abdominal trauma. Advantages include sensitivity, availability, and the relative speed with which it can be performed. Disadvantages include potential for iatrogenic injury, misapplication for evaluation of retroperitoneal injuries, lack of specificity, and higher incidence of false-positive exams.

In blunt trauma, indications for DPL include patients: (1) too hemodynamically unstable to leave the ED for CT scanning; (2) with a physical exam unreliable secondary to drug intoxication, head injury, or spinal cord injury; (3) with unexplained hypotension.

In penetrating trauma, DPL should be performed when it is not clear that exploratory laparotomy should be performed. DPL is useful in evaluating patients with stab wounds if local wound exploration indicates that superficial muscle fascia has been violated. Also, it may be useful in confirming a negative physical exam when tangential wounds or wounds of the lower chest are involved.

The DPL is considered positive if more than 5 cc of gross blood is aspirated immediately, the RBC count is $> 100,000$ cells/μL, the white blood cell count is > 500 cells/μL, bile is present, or vegetable matter is present. The only absolute contraindication to DPL is when surgical management is clearly indicated, and DPL will delay patient transport to the OR. Relative contraindications include patients with advanced hepatic dysfunction, severe coagulopathies, previous abdominal surgeries, and gravid uterus.

In the evaluation of the trauma patient with hematuria who potentially has genitourinary injuries, a cystogram and IVP prior to DPL are helpful. These tests may negate the need for DPL if bladder rupture is identified.

Computed Tomography (CT)

The abdominal CT scan has greater specificity than DPL and has become the initial diagnostic test of choice at many trauma centers. Oral and IV contrast material should be given to provide optimal resolution. Advantages of CT include its ability to precisely locate intra-abdominal lesions preoperatively, to evaluate the retroperitoneum, to identify injuries that may be managed nonoperatively, and noninvasiveness. Reports conflict as to the sensitivity of the test, and there are multiple reports of missed surgical lesions. It is important to emphasize that neither DPL or CT is perfect, and both tests should be used in conjunction with the overall clinical picture and sound clinical judgment.

Ultrasonography

Recent literature has demonstrated that an ultrasound exam of the abdomen performed by ED physicians or surgeons can be helpful in accurately identifying the presence of free intraperitoneal fluid in trauma patients. Ultrasonography provides an accurate, rapid, noninvasive, and portable method for evaluating blunt abdominal trauma.

Arteriography

Evaluation of major vessel injuries can be best accomplished by arteriography. In pelvic fractures, for example, bleeding sites can be located and controlled by embolization. An aortogram remains a valuable test in evaluating thoracic aortic injury.

Emergency Department Care and Disposition

The patient sustaining abdominal trauma should be evaluated and resuscitated in a systematic manner as outlined in Chapter 144. In a multiple trauma patient, all potential and actual injuries need to be prioritized. A head, cardiac, pulmonary, or great vessel injury may take precedence over an abdominal injury. Table 151-1 lists indications for exploratory laparotomy.

TABLE 151-1. Indications for Exploratory Celiotomy

Abdominal trauma and hemodynamic instability
Abdominal wall disruption with evisceration
Clinical findings of peritoneal irritation
Free air in abdomen on x-ray
Retroperitoneal air on x-ray
Ruptured urinary bladder (intraperitoneal)
Positive peritoneal tap or lavage
Rectal perforation
Surgically correctable lesions suggested by CT scan

For further reading in *Emergency Medicine: A Comprehensive Study Guide*, 4th edition, see Chapter 219, Abdominal Trauma, by Arthur L. Ney, Jeremy Hollerman, and Robert C. Andersen.

PENETRATING TRAUMA TO THE POSTERIOR ABDOMEN

Penetrating trauma to the posterior abdomen is a distinct subcategory of penetrating torso trauma. The organs most commonly injured by penetrating trauma to this area include the liver, kidney, colon, duodenum and pancreas. Diagnosis of these injuries, however, may be difficult because of the apparent absence of physical findings.

Clinical Features

The importance of obtaining a complete history and performing a thorough physical exam must be emphasized. Mechanism of injury, description of the wounding object and time elapsed since injury are important to the evaluation. Both the chest and abdomen must be evaluated. Specific organ injuries are covered in the chapters on abdominal trauma (Chap. 151) and genitourinary tract trauma (Chap. 153).

Diagnosis and Differential

The diagnosis of specific organ injuries is often dependent on exploratory laparotomy. In the hemodynamically stable patient with no obvious visceral injury, however, adjunctive diagnostic tests, such as wound exploration, diagnostic peritoneal lavage (DPL), and computed tomography (CT) may be useful. Wound exploration should generally be reserved for superficial stab wounds with low probability of visceral injury. Sterile technique, adequate anesthesia, good exposure, and hemostasis are key. Exploration of injuries that extend through fascia or muscle is not recommended. DPL is highly accurate for detecting intraperitoneal injuries, but poor in detecting retroperitoneal injuries. DPL is indicated when injury to the diaphragm or hollow viscus is suspected. CT scanning can be accurate in detecting solid viscus intraperitoneal injuries and retroperitoneal injuries. Oral and IV contrast are necessary for an optimal study.

Emergency Department Care and Disposition

All patients with penetrating trauma should be evaluated according to a routine regimen. Initial resuscitation should follow the ABCs, as outlined in Chapter 144. Two large-bore IVs, supplemental oxygen, cardiac monitoring and nasogastric and Foley catheters should be placed. A baseline CBC, crossmatch, urinalysis, rectal examination, and chest x-ray should be performed on all patients. Trauma-team involvement or early surgical consultation should be obtained. Exploratory laparotomy is indicated for patients with hemodynamic instability, evisceration, peritonitis, intraperitoneal free air, transabdominal missile path and other gunshot wounds except superficial tangential wounds. Selective management, such as evaluating gross hematuria by CT scanning or diagnosing diaphragmatic injury by DPL, is more appropriately applied in stable patients with stab wounds. Appropriate patient management is directed by the findings. All patients should be hospitalized, with the exception of patients with clearly defined superficial tangential wounds.

If Standard Treatment Fails

Any change in the condition of the patient requires re-evaluation. Retroperitoneal and diaphragmatic injuries may be difficult to diagnose, and missile paths are often unpredictable. An ED thoracotomy with crossclamping of the aorta may be indicated in the significantly unstable patient.

PENETRATING BUTTOCK INJURIES

Penetrating trauma to the buttock has the potential to injure multiple organ systems, including gastrointestinal (GI), genitourinary (GU), and neurological systems. Significant morbidity and mortality may occur if such injuries are missed.

Clinical Features

The clinical features will vary, depending on which organ system has been injured. Blood within the rectum signifies distal colon or rectal injuries. GU trauma can present with hematuria and scrotal or penile hematomas. Vascular injuries should be suspected when an enlarging hematoma, bruit, or change in peripheral pulses is present. Neurologic injuries will present with paresthesias, sensory loss, or motor weakness.

Diagnosis and Differential

Routine proctosigmoidoscopy will identify rectal and sigmoid colon injuries. GU injuries should be investigated by retrograde urethrogram and cystogram. Routine pelvic x-rays will reveal bony injury and suggest possible missile path. CT scan of the pelvis may reveal colon, urinary tact, or vascular injury. Angiography may be indicated in the evaluation of suspected vascular injury.

Emergency Department Care and Disposition

Initial resuscitation should follow the ABCs. Two large bore IVs, oxygen, cardiac monitoring, and an NG tube should be placed. If urethral injury is suspected, a Foley catheter should *not* be placed. Baseline lab evaluation should include a CBC, type and crossmatch, urinalysis, and careful rectal examination. Hemodynamic instability, peritonitis, or blood within the GI tract are indications for operative therapy. Significant vascular or nerve injuries (sciatic or femoral nerves) usually require early operative intervention. Trauma-team evaluation or early surgical consultation should be obtained. All patients should be admitted for further evaluation and monitoring.

If Standard Treatment Fails

Penetrating buttock injuries can injure several different organ systems. The associated visceral injuries are often extraperitoneal and have subtle or minimal physical findings. A thorough, systematic evaluation is required to identify these injuries early.

For further reading in *Emergency Medicine: A Comprehensive Study Guide*, 4th edition, see Chapter 220, Penetrating Trauma to the Posterior Abdomen and Buttock, by Mark D. Odland and Arthur L. Ney.

Greg Mears

In the multiple trauma patient, the management of life-threatening injuries takes precedence over urologic injury, and the diagnostic evaluation of genitourinary trauma can be delayed. Early diagnosis and management of urologic injuries, however, are important for the restoration of normal urinary function.

Clinical Features

A careful examination of the perineum is important in evaluating for potential urologic trauma. Any blood or lacerations should be documented. A rectal exam should be performed to document the position of the prostate, rectal tone, and the presence of blood in the rectum. Evaluation of the scrotum includes noting the presence of hematomas, ecchymoses, lacerations, and testicular disruption. The penis should be examined and any blood at the meatus noted. In females, the labia should be inspected for lacerations. A bimanual vaginal exam should be done to detect bleeding. The presence of blood in the vagina requires a speculum examination. X-ray evaluation of the pelvis is necessary to document any pelvic fracture.

RENAL INJURY

A renal injury is the most frequent form of genitourinary trauma. Penetrating renal injuries associated with gunshot wounds require surgical exploration. Stab wounds to the flank may be evaluated by CT scan, but stab wounds to the abdomen often require surgical exploration. Blunt renal injuries are evaluated radiographically. Considerable force is required to cause significant renal injury. Renal injury is associated with fractured ribs, vertebral transverse process fractures, flank bruises or hematomas, and hematuria.

Renal Contusion

Renal contusion accounts for 92% of renal injures. A renal contusion is a relatively minor renal injury associated with renal parenchymal ecchymosis, minor lacerations, and subcapsular hematomas with an intact renal capsule. The IVP is usually normal, and the CT scan may reveal edema and microextravasation of contrast. Treatment is supportive, and serial vital signs, hemotocrits, and urine specimens should be performed. Gross hematuria requires bedrest until it resolves. Renal contusions usually resolve without complications.

Renal Laceration

Renal laceration accounts for approximately 5% of renal injuries. Radiographic studies demonstrate disruption of the renal outline, a perirenal hematoma, and possibly extravasation of contrast adjacent to the kidney. Almost all minor cortical lacerations heal without sequelae with conservative management. Major lacerations involving the medulla or collecting system may develop complications despite a stable hemodynamic condition. Surgery is indicated for persistent retroperitoneal bleeding associated with hemodynamic instability. Surgery also may be indicated in stable patients with extensive urinary extravasation, large devitalized renal fragments, and renal pedicle injures.

Renal Rupture

Renal rupture accounts for 1% of renal injuries. A large expanding hematoma leads to a clinically unstable patient with persistent bleeding. Radiographic studies reveal multiple lacerations, devitalized kidney fragments, and extravasation of contrast. Surgery is indicated.

Renal Pedicle Injury

Renal pedicle injuries include lacerations and thrombosis of the renal artery, vein, and their branches. These injuries account for 2% of renal injuries. High-velocity deceleration injuries and penetrating trauma are typical mechanisms of injury. In blunt trauma, the most common renal pedicle injury is thrombosis of the renal artery. With renal artery occlusion or disruption, IVP shows nonfunction, arteriogram reveals arterial contusion or bleeding, and CT scan demonstrates a nonenhanced kidney. Renal-vein thrombosis results in delayed renal function and parenchymal swelling in the absence of ureteral obstruction. Within the first 12 h, surgical repair is possible, but nephrectomy is often required.

Renal Pelvis Rupture

Renal pelvis rupture results in extravasation of urine into the perirenal space and along the psoas muscle. This injury is rare and is often associated with congenital renal anomalies. IVP reveals a normally functioning kidney with extravasation of contrast and nonvisualization of the ureter. When diagnosis is delayed, the patient develops high fever and increasing abdominal pain as the extravasation of urine filters into the retroperitoneal space. A retrograde pyelogram confirms the diagnosis. Surgical repair is required.

URETERAL INJURIES

Ureteral injuries are the rarest of all GU injuries from external trauma. Blunt trauma can produce a rupture at or just below the ureteropelvic junction. Penetrating injuries can produce a contusion or rupture of the ureter. Blast effects from gunshot wounds may cause microvascular thrombosis and delayed ureteral necrosis or fistula formation. Surgical repair is required.

BLADDER INJURIES

Bladder injuries are the second most common injury to the genitourinary tract and usually are associated with blunt trauma and pelvic fractures. Pelvic hematomas often displace the bladder and can serve as a marker on plain radiographs for pelvic injury.

Bladder Contusion

Bladder contusion is associated with hematuria secondary to bruising of the bladder wall. Cystogram demonstrates an intact bladder outline. Management is conservative.

Intraperitoneal Bladder Rupture

Intraperitoneal bladder rupture is usually secondary to a burst injury of a full bladder. Cystogram demonstrates intraperitoneal extravasation of contrast into the peritoneal cavity. Surgical repair is required.

Extraperitoneal Bladder Rupture

Cystogram demonstrates extravasation of contrast into the retroperitoneal space with extraperitoneal bladder rupture. Treatment consists of urethral-catheter drainage alone for 10 to 14 days.

URETHRAL INJURIES

Male Urethral Injuries

Urethral injuries in males occur in the posterior (prostatomembranous) and in the anterior (bulbous and penile) urethra. Posterior injuries result from pelvic fractures. A perineal hematoma and highriding, detached prostate on rectal exam are associated with complete posterior urethral disruption. Anterior injuries result from direct trauma to the urethra (fall-astride injuries, straddle injury, kick) and instrumentation, and are associated with a penile fracture. A butterfly perineal hematoma is often noted.

With anterior urethral contusions, there is blood at the external meatus, but the retrograde urethrogram is normal. Treatment is conservative with or without a urethral catheter. Anterior urethral lacerations are confirmed by contrast extravasation associated with the retrograde urethrogram. Partial lacerations are managed by an indwelling catheter placed coaxially over a guidewire under fluoroscopic control or with a suprapubic cystostomy. Complete lacerations are diagnosed when no contrast passes proximal to the injury with the urethrogram. Surgical repair is required for complete lacerations.

Partial posterior urethral lacerations are managed with a urethral catheter placed coaxially over a guidewire under fluoroscopic control or with a suprapubic catheter. Complete posterior disruptions can be managed with primary realignment with a catheter or with a suprapubic cystostomy. Complications include stricture, impotence, and incontinence.

The Full Bladder Dilemma

ED physicians in nontrauma centers may be faced with a patient with a urethral injury precluding catheterization but with a full urinary bladder. A large-bore central venous catheter may be inserted into the bladder suprapubically with the Seldinger technique. The needle should be inserted 2 finger-breadths above the pubic symphysis, and urine should be aspirated. The catheter should be threaded enough to coil within the lumen of bladder. A small amount of contrast dye should be injected into the bladder, and an x-ray should be obtained to confirm placement.

Female Urethral Injuries

Female urethral injuries should be suspected in extensive pelvic fractures; 80% of urethral injuries in women present with vaginal bleeding. Surgical repair of the injury is required with a urethral catheter in place. Complications of a delayed or missed diagnosis include labial edema, necrotizing fasciitis, and sepsis.

GENITAL INJURIES

Testicular and Scrotal Injuries

A direct blow to the testis, impinging it on the symphysis pubis, is the primary cause of blunt testicular injury. Blunt injuries are either contusions or ruptures. Rarely the testicle can be traumatically dislocated into the inguinal canal. With testicular contusion or rupture, a hematoma or hematocele appears as a large, blue, tender scrotal mass. Penetrating injuries to the testicle require surgical exploration. Doppler studies are useful to define testicular injury. Early exploration of blunt testicular injury, with the evacuation of blood clots and repair of testicular rupture, is preferable to conservative management.

Injuries to the Penis

Vacuum and Sharp Wounds

Vacuum-cleaner injuries and blade injuries are usually self-inflicted. Vacuum-cleaner injuries cause extensive damage to the glans penis and some loss of the urethra. Surgical debridement and reconstruction are often required. Blade injuries range from superficial lacerations to complete amputation. Penile amputation is managed by reimplantation (if ischemia time is less than 18 h) or local repair.

Penile rupture When an erect penis impacts forcibly on a hard object (sexual partner's pubis or the floor) traumatic rupture can occur. A cracking sound is heard, followed by pain, immediate detumescence, rapid swelling, discoloration, and distension. Urethral injures may be associated with the rupture. Immediate surgical evacuation of the blood clot and repair are required.

Penile denuding Loss of penile skin by avulsion injury or burns is managed by split-thickness skin grafting. The avulsed skin should not be reapplied.

Zipper injury Zipper injury to the penis is caused when penile skin is trapped in the trouser zipper. Mineral oil and lidocaine infiltration are useful in freeing the penile skin. Otherwise, wire-cutting or bone-cutting pliers are used to divide the median bar of the zipper, causing the zipper to fall apart.

Contusions Contusions to the perineum or penis result from straddle or toilet seat injuries. Treatment is conservative, with cold packs, rest, and elevation. If the patient is unable to void, a catheter may be required.

Diagnosis and Differential

First the clinician must suspect the diagnosis of a GU injury in any patient with a mechanism of injury that could produce trauma to the abdomen or pelvis. Second, supplementary imaging studies along with a urinalysis will help identify the location of an injury. In adult blunt-trauma patients with only microscopic hematuria, the diagnostic yield of a significant urologic injury is extremely low. Radiographic evaluation is required in adult blunt trauma patients with gross hematuria or with microscopic hematuria and shock, or significant nongenitourinary injuries. Adult penetrating trauma patients require radiographic studies regardless of the amount of hematuria. Pediatric trauma patients require radiographic evaluation with any degree of hematuria. All studies should be performed in a caudal to cephalad direction (retrograde urethrogram, cystogram, IV pyelogram).

When blood is found at the urethral meatus, a retrograde urethrogram with contrast solution determines the integrity of the urethra before any instrumentation. This will prevent the conversion of a partial urethral laceration into a complete transection. If the prostate gland is displaced on rectal exam, a urethrogram is not required, since it is obvious the urethra is transected. Thirty cc of contrast solution is injected into the urethral meatus with a syringe or a Foley catheter 1 to 2 cm into the urethra. An oblique radiograph is then taken to visualize the urethra.

A cystogram is required to evaluate the urinary bladder in the presence of a pelvic ring fracture or gross hematuria. Contrast solution, 400–500 cc in adults and 5 cc/kg in children is instilled into the bladder through the urethral catheter under gravity. After an AP film is obtained, the bladder is emptied, and another AP film is obtained.

An intravenous pyelogram (IVP) is seldom indicated in the ED setting. It has been replaced with CT scanning. CT yields more information, has fewer false-positive studies, and has fewer associated contrast-related risks.

Emergency Department Care and Disposition

After standard evaluation of the multiple trauma patient and identification of the urologic injuries, the urologic consultant should be contacted. Urologic injuries are typically not life-threatening, and urologic evaluation should not interfere with aggressive trauma resuscitation. Radiographic studies (retrograde urethrogram, cystogram, IVP, or CT scan) indicated should be performed in conjunction with the overall trauma management of the patient.

For further reading in *Emergency Medicine: A Comprehensive Study Guide*, 4th edition, see Chapter 221, Trauma to the Genitourinary Tract, by Joe Y. Lee and Alexander S. Cass.

154 | Early Management of Fractures and Dislocations

Michael P. Kefer

A delay in diagnosis of several orthopaedic emergencies can increase the chance of significant complications or poor functional outcome.

Clinical Features

Knowing the precise mechanism of injury or listening carefully to the patient's symptoms is important to diagnosing fracture or dislocation. Pain may be referred to an area distant from the injury (e.g., hip injury presenting as knee pain). If implications of the history are not appreciated, specific x-ray views needed may never be ordered.

The physical exam includes: (1) inspection for deformity, edema, or discoloration; (2) assessment of active and passive range of motion of joints proximal and distal to the injury; (3) palpation for tenderness or deformity and (4) assessment of neurovascular status distal to the injury. Careful palpation can prevent missing a crucial diagnosis due to referred pain. Document neurovascular status early, before performing reduction maneuvers.

Radiologic evaluation is based on the history and physical, not simply on where the patient reports pain. X-ray of all long bone fractures should include the joints proximal and distal to the fracture to evaluate for coexistent injury. Children may need comparison x-ray views of the opposite extremity to differentiate fracture lines from normal growth plates. A negative x-ray does not exclude a fracture. This commonly occurs with scaphoid, radial head, or metatarsal shaft fractures. The ED diagnosis is often clinical and is not confirmed until 7–10 days after the injury, when enough bone resorption has occurred at the fracture site to detect a lucency on x-ray.

An accurate description of the fracture to the consultant is crucial and should include the following details:

1. Open versus closed.
2. Location—Mid-shaft, junction of proximal and middle or middle and distal third, or distance from bone end. Intra-articular involvement with disruption of joint surface may require surgery. Anatomic bony reference points should be used, when applicable (e.g., humerus fracture just above the condyles is described as supracondylar, as opposed to distal humerus).
3. Orientation of fracture line—Transverse, spiral, oblique, comminuted (shattered), segmental (single large segment of free floating bone) and, in children, greenstick or torus.
4. Displacement—Describe the amount and direction the distal fragment is offset from the proximal fragment.

5. Separation—Degree two fragments have been pulled apart. Unlike displacement, alignment is maintained.
6. Shortening—Reduction in bone length due to impaction or overriding fragments.
7. Angulation—Angle formed by the fracture segments. Describe the degree and direction of deviation of the distal fragment.
8. Rotational deformity—Degree the distal fragment is twisted on the axis of the normal bone. It is usually detected by physical exam and not seen on x-ray.

Fractures in children that involve the epiphyseal (growth) plate may result in disturbance of bone growth. These are described by the Salter–Harris classification (Figure 154-1). The prognosis is progressively worse with increasing classification number. Salter 1 (separation of the epiphysis) and 5 (compression of epiphysis) are often not detected by x-ray and diagnosis is based on finding swelling and tenderness in the region of the physis.

Emergency Department Care and Disposition

Control swelling with application of cold packs and elevation. Administer analgesics as necessary. Remove any objects that may constrict the injury as swelling progresses such as rings or watches. Keep the patient NPO if anesthesia will be required.

Prompt reduction of fracture deformity with steady, longitudinal traction is indicated to: (1) alleviate pain; (2) relieve tension on associated neurovascular structures; (3) minimize the risk of converting a closed fracture to an open fracture when a sharp, bony fragment tents overlying skin and (4) restore circulation to a pulseless distal extremity. Whether the procedure is performed by the ED physician or the orthopaedist depends on practice environment. Of the above indications, however, distal vascular compromise is the most time-critical. Postreduction films should be obtained to confirm proper anatomic repositioning.

Open fractures are treated immediately with prophylactic antibiotics to prevent osteomyelitis. A common regimen is a first-generation cephalosporin and an aminoglycoside. Irrigation and debridement in the OR is indicated.

Immobilize the fracture or relocated joint. Fiberglass or plaster splinting material is commonly used. The chemical reaction that causes the material to set is an exothermic reaction that begins upon contact with water. The amount of heat liberated is directly proportional to the setting process, which, in turn, is directly proportional to the temperature of the water. Severe burns, therefore, can result from the splinting material, as the peak temperature to the skin is the sum of the water temperature plus the heat released by exothermic reaction. The use of water slightly warmer than room temperature is a safe practice. Padding is necessary under the splint to prevent pressure sores and irritation. Use an adequate

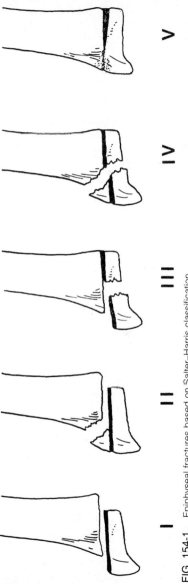

FIG. 154-1. Epiphyseal fractures based on Salter–Harris classification.

length to immobilize the injury. Splints for mid-shaft fractures should be long enough to immobilize the joint above and below the fracture.

Crutches are prescribed for the patient who has a lower extremity injury that requires nonweightbearing. Ideal crutch height is one hand width below the axilla. The pressure of the crutch pads is borne by the sides of the thorax, not the axilla, to avoid injury to the brachial plexus. Walkers and canes are appropriate for partial weightbearing conditions, they may be alternatives for patients too weak to use crutches.

The patient who is discharged home is instructed to keep the injured extremity elevated above heart level and to seek immediate re-evaluation if increased swelling, cyanosis, pain, or decreased sensation develops.

For further reading in *Emergency Medicine: A Comprehensive Study Guide*, 4th edition, see Chapter 223, Early Management of Fractures and Dislocations, by Jeffrey S. Menkes.

Michael P. Kefer

General Principles

The key concept is preservation of function by proper splinting followed by early mobilization: (1) Padded aluminum splints adequately immobilize flexion/extension movement as occurs at DIP and PIP; (2) Plaster or fiberglass is required to control rotary motion, as occurs at MCP and wrist; (3) open fracture or open joint injury is treated in the operating room; immediate IV antibiotics are indicated; (4) fractures or dislocations that compromise neurovascular function or overlying skin require urgent reduction; (5) significant crush, artery, or nerve injury requires emergent referral to a hand surgeon.

Tendon Injuries

Knowing the hand position at the time of injury predicts where, along its course, a tendon is injured. Extensor tendon repair can often be performed by the ED physician in the ED. Flexor tendon repair should be performed by a hand surgeon. Followup and rehabilitation of all tendon injuries are necessary.

Mallet Finger

This injury results from a disruption of the extensor tendon mechanism at the base of the distal phalanx. Treatment is a dorsal extension splint immobilizing the DIP. If it is associated with avulsion fracture involving more than one third of the DIP articular surface, open reduction and internal fixation are recommended.

Boutonniere Deformity

This injury results from an injury at the dorsal surface of the PIP that disrupts the extensor hood apparatus. Lateral bands of the extensor mechanism become flexors of PIP and hyperextensors of DIP. An extensor hood injury is easily missed on ED presentation. Re-exam after 7 days is indicated.

Collateral Ligaments and Volar Plate

They form a U-shaped hood around the lateral and volar aspects of the IP and MCP joints. MCP collateral ligaments are taut in flexion and lax in extension. To preserve maximum function, therefore, the MCP is immobilized at 50° to 90° flexion. Abduction and adduction stress is applied to assess collateral ligament stability; hyperextension stress will assess volar plate stability. IP partial sprains are treated by buddy tape splinting. IP complete disruptions are treated by gutter splint with 15° to 20° flexion. MCP partial sprains are treated by aluminum splint with 50° to 90° flexion. MCP complete disruptions are treated by gutter splint with 50° to 90° flexion.

Gamekeeper's Thumb

This injury results from forced radial abduction at the MCP with injury to the ulnar collateral ligament of the thumb and is the most critical of the collateral ligament injuries, since it affects pincer function. A partial tear is diagnosed when abduction stress causes the joint to open up to 20° more relative to the uninvolved side. A complete tear is diagnosed when abduction stress causes the joint to open greater than 20° more relative to the uninvolved side. Treatment is thumb spica for partial disruption, and surgical repair for complete disruption.

IP JOINT DISLOCATIONS

Dorsal dislocation

This injury is relatively common. A radiograph is indicated to distinguish dislocation from fracture–dislocation. Reduction is performed under digital-block anesthesia. The dislocated phalanx is distracted, slightly hyperextended, then repositioned. Collateral ligament damage should then be assessed and splinted accordingly.

Volar Dislocation

This is an uncommon injury. It results in boutonniere deformity from extensor mechanism injury. An x-ray may only reveal dorsal-chip fracture if spontaneously reduced. Early hand-surgeon consultation is indicated.

MCP Joint Dislocation

This injury is often unreducible due to volar-plate entrapment. Splinting and referral for surgical reduction is indicated.

Nerve Injuries

Neurapraxia results from nerve contusion. Complete nerve disruption of a major nerve or digital nerve proximal to the PIP should be repaired by a hand surgeon.

Volkmann's Contracture

This injury results from a constrictive dressing, severe fracture, or crush injury to the forearm, causing compartment syndrome from inadequate circulation. A high index of suspicion is critical, as irreversible loss of hand function can occur within 6 h.

WRIST FRACTURES

Scaphoid Fracture

This is the most common carpal fracture. The patient is tender in the anatomic snuff box. The wrist x-ray is often negative, so the diagnosis is based on physical findings. Treatment of the patient with snuff-box tenderness is thumb spica splint and referral. Without proper treatment, there is risk of avascular necrosis of the scaphoid bone.

Dorsal Chip Fracture

The triquetrum is the most commonly involved carpal bone. The patient is tender dorsally over the ulnar aspect of the wrist. The wrist x-ray is often negative, so diagnosis is based on physical findings. Treatment of the patient with tenderness, as described, is volar splint with 10° wrist extension and referral to a hand surgeon.

Lunate Fracture

This is the most important of the carpal fractures since it occupies two thirds of the articular surface of the radius. There is risk of avascular necrosis. The patient feels tenderness over the lunate fossa (distal to the rim of the radius at the base of the third metacarpal). Wrist x-ray is often negative, so diagnosis is based on physical exam findings. Treatment of patient with tenderness, as described, is thumb spica splint and referral.

Colles' and Smith's Fractures

These fractures involve the distal radius at the metaphysis. With a Colles fracture, the distal radius is dorsally displaced, causing a dinner-fork deformity. With a Smith fracture, the distal radius is volarly displaced. Treatment is hematoma block, placing the hand in a finger trap, and closed reduction.

WRIST DISLOCATIONS

Scapholunate Dissociation

This is a commonly missed diagnosis among ED physicians. The patient presents with wrist tenderness that may be localized to the scapholunate joint. The AP view on the wrist x-ray demonstrates a space between the scaphoid and lunate that is ≥3 mm. Early hand-surgeon referral for repair of the ligamentous ruptures is indicated.

Lunate and Perilunate Dislocations

The most common carpal bone dislocations are lunate and perilunate. Lateral, oblique, and AP wrist x-rays reveal the dislocation, as the normal alignment of the radius-lunate-capitate is lost. With a lunate dislocation, the lunate dislocates anterior to the radius, but the remainder of the carpus aligns with the radius. With a perilunate dislocation, the lunate remains aligned with the radius, but the remainder of the carpus is dislocated, usually dorsal to the lunate. Usually there is concomitant fracture of the scaphoid, and the proximal portion of the scaphoid remains with the lunate, and the distal portion dislocates with the carpus. Prompt referral to a hand surgeon for closed reduction or surgical repair is indicated.

HAND FRACTURES

Distal Phalanx

A tuft fracture is the most common. If associated with subungual hematoma, drainage is recommended. Transverse fractures with displacement are always associated with nail-bed laceration, which requires repair. Avulsion fracture of base results in a mallet finger.

Middle and Proximal Phalanx Fractures

This diagnosis is often suspected if the fingertips of the closed hand do not point to the same spot on the wrist, and the plane of the nail bed of the involved digit is not aligned with others. Treatment of nondisplaced fractures is gutter splint in position of function and referral. Treatment of displaced fractures usually requires surgical intervention. Rotational malalignment is a common problem and requires correction.

Metacarpal Fracture

A fourth or fifth metacarpal neck fracture, the boxer's fracture, is the most common metacarpal fracture. Angulation of 30° in the ring finger and 50° in the 5th finger can be tolerated but, ideally, angulation > 20° should be reduced. Treatment is gutter splint and referral. Second and third metacarpal fractures causing any angulation should be reduced. Treatment is gutter splint and referral. First metacarpal base fracture with intra-articular involvement, Bennett's fracture, requires consultation for surgical reduction.

Nail bed Injury

Injuries to the nail bed may result in significant deformity of the nail with associated morbidity. Significant fracture of the nail or subungual hematoma > 50% of the nail bed are indications for exploration of the nail bed. Treatment is nail removal and repair of the nail bed with

6-0 or 7-0 absorbable suture. The nail is cleaned and debrided and replaced in the nail fold as a splint.

For further reading in *Emergency Medicine: A Comprehensive Study Guide*, 4th edition, see Chapter 224, Injuries to the Wrist and Hand, by Robert R. Simon and David Slobodkin.

Stephen W. Meldon

ELBOW DISLOCATION

Although the elbow is one of the most stable joints in the body, dislocations of the elbow are commonly seen. They are usually posterior and usually result from a fall onto an outstretched hand.

Clinical Features

Clinically the patient presents with elbow in 45° of flexion. The olecranon is prominent posteriorly, however, this may be obscured by significant swelling. Neurovascular complications occur in 8% to 21% of patients, with brachial-artery and ulnar-nerve injuries most common.

Diagnosis and Differential

Elbow deformity may resemble a displaced supracondylar fracture, but the diagnosis of elbow dislocation is easily confirmed radiographically. On the lateral view, both the ulna and radius are displaced posteriorly. In the anteroposterior view, the ulna and radius have a normal relationship but may be displaced medially or laterally. Any associated fractures should be noted.

Emergency Department Care and Disposition

Appropriate treatment of elbow dislocations requires adequate reduction and recognition of neurovascular complications, associated fractures, and postreduction instability.

1. Carefully evaluate for neurovascular compromise by assessing brachial and radial pulses, and ulnar, radial, and median nerves. Document any associated fractures.
2. **Reduction**—After adequate sedation, reduction is accomplished by gentle traction on the wrist and forearm. An assistant applies countertraction on the arm. Distal traction is applied while any medial or lateral displacement is corrected with the other hand. Downward pressure on the proximal forearm will help disengage the coronoid process from the olecranon fossa. Distal traction is continued, and the elbow is flexed. A palpable *clunk* is noted with successful reduction.
3. After reduction, re-examine neurovascular status and obtain postreduction films. If full, smooth, passive range of motion is not possible after reduction, the postreduction radiograph should be examined for medial epicondyle entrapment.
4. Immobilization by a long-arm posterior splint, with the elbow in 90° of flexion, is appropriate. Cylinder casts should not be placed because of the risk of significant subsequent edema.
5. Orthopaedic followup should be arranged. Patients with instability in extension require immediate referral.

SUBLUXATION OF THE RADIAL HEAD (NURSEMAID'S ELBOW)

Subluxation of the radial head is common in young children, with peak age being between 1 and 4 y. The mechanism of injury is sudden traction on the hand while the elbow is extended, but history is not always obtained.

Clinical Features

Clinically the child appears comfortable but does not use the injured arm, which is held in slight flexion and pronation. Supination is painful and any effort to move the arm is resisted. There is no associated deformity or swelling, and the neurovascular exam is normal.

Diagnosis and Differential

A child not using an arm that is flexed and pronated, without signs of trauma, probably has a radial-head subluxation. Radiographs are unnecessary unless another diagnosis is being considered.

Emergency Department Care and Disposition

1. **Reduction** is carried out by firmly placing the thumb over the radial head, while the other hand is placed on the wrist. The forearm is supinated and the elbow is flexed. Successful reduction is shown by a palpable click and subsequent use of the affected arm.
2. Immobilization is not required. For recurrent subluxations, however, the patient's arm should be immobilized in a sling and the patient given orthopaedic referral.

If Standard Treatment Fails

If the above is not successful, reduction may be tried with radial head pressure, supination, and elbow extension. If reduction is not successful, radiographs should be obtained.

ELBOW FRACTURES

Intercondylar fractures are common in adults, and any distal humerus fracture in an adult should be assumed initially to be intercondylar. Supracondylar fractures occur most commonly in children. Ninety-five percent of these extra-articular fractures are displaced posteriorly.

Clinical Features

Intercondylar and supracondylar elbow fractures typically present with significant swelling, tenderness, and decreased range of motion. Intercondylar fractures occur from a force directed against the elbow, whereas most supracondylar fractures result from an extension force. Both can be associated with severe soft-tissue injury. Associated neurovascular injuries are common with supracondylar fractures. The anterior interosseus nerve, a motor branch of the median nerve, is particularly prone to injury. Evaluation of this nerve is performed by testing for flexion of the thumb interphalangeal and index finger distal interphalangeal joints. Acute vascular injuries present with decreased or absent radial pulse and are most frequently due to transient vasospasm.

Diagnosis and Differential

An anteroposterior and lateral radiograph of the elbow should be obtained. Careful evaluation for a fracture line separating the condyles from each other and the humerus, which distinguishes intercondylar fractures, should be made. The amount of displacement, rotation, and comminution of the fragments should be noted. In supracondylar fractures, the AP radiograph usually reveals a transverse fracture line, while the lateral view will show an oblique fracture line and displacement of the distal fragment proximally and posteriorly. The lateral radiograph may also reveal a posterior and anterior fat-pad sign. In some nondisplaced fractures, the fracture line may not be visible and the fat pad sign may be the only evidence of injury.

Emergency Department Care and Disposition

1. Carefully evaluate for neurovascular compromise.
2. Splint immobilization and orthopaedic referral is appropriate for nondisplaced fractures.
3. Displaced fractures and those with neurovascular compromise require immediate orthopaedic consultation. Supracondylar fractures are often treated by closed reduction followed by pin fixation, whereas displaced intercondylar fractures are usually treated with open reduction and internal fixation. Patients with displaced fractures or severe swelling should be admitted for neurovascular observation.

If Standard Treatment Fails

Evidence of Volkmann's ischemia may accompany supracondylar fractures that present with absent radial pulse. Signs of impending ischemia include refusal to open the affected hand, pain with passive extension of the fingers, and forearm tenderness. Volkmann's ischemia is an indication for fasciotomy or brachial artery exploration.

FOREARM FRACTURES

Fractures of both the radius and ulna occur most often from significant trauma, such as a motor vehicle accident or fall from a height. Isolated fractures of the ulna (nightstick fracture) often result from direct blows to the forearm. Radius fractures are produced by falls on the outstretched hand or by direct blows.

Clinical Features

Fractures of both bones results in swelling, tenderness, and deformity of the forearm. Open fractures are not uncommon. Isolated fractures of the ulna or radius present with swelling and tenderness over the fracture site. Fracture of the proximal ulnar shaft with radial head dislocation—a Monteggia fracture–dislocation—causes considerable pain and swelling at the elbow. A distal radial shaft fracture with associated distal radioulnar joint dislocation—Galeazzi's fracture—will present with localized tenderness and swelling over the distal radius and wrist.

Diagnosis and Differential

Fractures of the radius and ulna are easily diagnosed on an AP and lateral radiograph of the forearm. Displacement, angulation, and longitudinal alignment are easily evaluated. Any rotational malalignment should be noted. Clues to rotational deformity include a sudden change in the bone's width at the fracture site and a change in the normal orientation of the various bony prominences of the radius or ulna. Isolated ulnar fractures are considered displaced if there is $>10°$ angulation or $>50\%$ displacement. In a Monteggia fracture, the proximal ulnar fracture is clearly visible, but the radial head dislocation may be overlooked. As a rule, the radial head normally aligns with the capitellum in all radiographic views of the elbow. The distal radioulnar joint dislocation seen with a Galeazzi's fracture may also be subtle. On the lateral view, the ulna will be displaced dorsally, whereas the AP view may show only a slightly increased radioulnar joint space.

Emergency Department Care and Disposition

1. Assess for neurovascular complications and evidence of an open fracture.
2. Immobilize the extremity and obtain an AP and lateral radiograph. The entire forearm, including elbow and wrist, should be viewed. Evaluate for displacement, alignment, angulation, and associated dislocation.

Nondisplaced isolated fractures may be immobilized in a long arm cast and given orthopaedic referral. However, most of these injuries will have significant displacement and require orthopaedic consultation and management. Closed reduction is often adequate for both bone fractures in children. Open reduction and internal fixation is usually required for displaced fractures in adults and for Monteggia and Galeazzi's fracture–dislocations.

If Standard Treatment Fails

A potential complication of these injuries is compartment syndrome. The presence of a palpable pulse does not exclude this diagnosis. Direct measurements of compartment pressures is recommended. Treatment may require fasciotomy.

For further reading in *Emergency Medicine: A Comprehensive Study Guide*, 4th edition, see Chapter 225, Injuries to the Elbow, Forearm and Wrist, by Dennis T. Uehara and Harold Chin.

Stephen W. Meldon

CLAVICLE AND SCAPULA

Clavicle fractures and acromioclavicular (AC) joint injuries are common. Clavicle fractures account for approximately one half of significant shoulder girdle injuries and is the most common fracture seen in children. Although much less common, injuries to the sternoclavicular (SC) joint and scapula are important because of the association with other significant injuries.

Clinical Features

Both clavicle fractures and AC joint injuries result from direct trauma, such as falls onto the shoulder. Clavicle fractures typically present with swelling, deformity, and localized tenderness. AC joint injuries are usually clinically obvious with tenderness and deformity of the AC joint. In both cases, the supported arm is slumped inward and downward. Sprains of the SC joint present with localized pain and swelling. Anterior dislocations of this joint result in a prominent medial clavicle that appears anterior to the sternum, whereas posterior dislocations are less visible and palpable and may result in impingement on superior mediastinal structures. Scapular fractures present with localized tenderness over the scapula and the affected extremity held in adduction. They usually result from significant trauma, such as motor-vehicle crashes or falls.

Diagnosis and Differential

Routine clavicle radiographs will usually reveal clavicle fractures occuring in the middle third of the clavicle in 80%, distal third in 15%, and medial third in 5%. AC radiographs help determine the severity of AC injury and any associated fracture. Type-I AC injuries have normal radiographs. Type-II injuries result in a 25 to 50% elevation of the distal clavicle above the acromium, and type-III injuries show 100% dislocation of the AC joint and coracoclavicular space widening. The diagnosis of SC joint dislocations, which are usually anterior, is suggested clinically. CT imaging is indicated, as plain radiographs may not be diagnostic. The differential diagnosis of sternoclavicular sprains should include septic arthritis, especially in IV drug users. Fractures of the scapula can be diagnosed with radiographs of the AP shoulder with axillary and scapular views. Associated injuries to the thoracic cage, lung, and shoulder occur in 80% of patients with scapular fractures.

Emergency Department Care and Disposition

1. Carefully evaluate for neurovascular compromise. Examine for associated injuries, especially with SC dislocations and scapular fractures.

2. Simple **immobilization** with a sling is acceptable for most clavicle fractures, scapular fractures, and AC joint injuries. Figure-of-eight clavicle brace is acceptable for displaced clavicle fractures and SC dislocations.
3. Immobilization, ice, analgesics, and early range of motion exercises are appropriate components of conservative treatment. Orthopaedic followup should be arranged.
4. Orthopaedic consult is indicated for SC dislocations, displaced distal clavicle fractures, articular or complex scapular fractures, and unusual, complicated AC joint injuries.

If Standard Treatment Fails

Anterior SC dislocations may require open reduction. Although conservative treatment is usually successful, operative intervention may be indicated for complex injuries of the clavicle, AC joint, and scapula. Posterior SC dislocation may be associated with significant intrathoracic injuries.

GLENOHUMERAL JOINT AND ROTATOR CUFF INJURIES

Dislocation of the glenohumeral joint is the most common major joint dislocation. Anterior dislocations occur in 98% of cases; rotator cuff tears may accompany this injury.

Clinical Features

Glenohumeral joint dislocation is usually suspected clinically. The most common mechanism of injury is a fall onto an extended, abducted arm. The patient typically is in severe discomfort and resists abduction and internal rotation of the affected arm. The shoulder lacks the normal rounded contour, and the humeral head can be palpated anteriorly and inferiorly. Associated axillary nerve injuries present with decreased sensation over the deltoid muscle. The rare inferior dislocation (luxatio erecta) will present with the affected arm fully abducted, elbow flexed, and hand held above the patient's head. Rotator cuff tears will demonstrate tenderness on the greater tuberosity, decreased range of motion, and weakness with abduction and external rotation.

Diagnosis and Differential

Anteroposterior and lateral scapular (Y view) or axillary radiographs should be obtained before reduction. The Y view or axillary radiograph will indicate the uncommon posterior dislocation. Associated bony injuries, such as glenoid rim fractures and compression fractures of the humeral head (Hill–Sachs lesion) should be noted. Associated rotator-cuff tears are often missed. It should be suspected in patients over 40 years old, in luxatio erecta dislocations, and in patients who are unable to externally rotate or abduct the arm after a glenohumeral dislocation. Diagnosis may require an arthrogram, arthroscopy, or MRI.

Emergency Department Care and Disposition

Many reduction techniques have been described. The use of conscious sedation is recommended, but any technique may be attempted without medication if performed slowly and atraumatically.

1. Assess and document neurovascular status and any associated bony injury.
2. Modified Hippocratic technique—This method uses **traction–countertraction.** The patient is supine with the arm abducted. A sheet is placed across the thorax of the patient and tied around the waist of the assistant. The physician gradually applies traction while the assistant provides countertraction. Gentle internal and external rotation may aid reduction. A sheet placed around the patient's flexed forearm and the physician's waist may help with traction.
3. **Milch technique**—With the patient supine, the physician slowly abducts and externally rotates the arm to the overhead position. With the elbow fully extended, traction is applied.
4. **External rotation technique**—With the patient supine and the elbow at 90 flexion, the arm is slowly externally rotated. No traction is applied. This technique must be performed slowly and gently. Reduction is often subtle and occurs prior to reaching the coronal plane.
5. After reduction, reassess neurovascular status and obtain postreduction radiographs. A shoulder immobilizer or and swathe should be applied and orthopaedic followup arranged.

If Standard Treatment Fails

Conscious sedation with a short-acting benzodiazepine (e.g., versed, 0.1 mg/kg, max of 2.5 mg IV) and an opiate analgesic (e.g., morphine, 0.1 mg/kg IV) may be necessary for successful reduction. Alternatively, a different technique (e.g., Stimson, or scapular, manipulation) may be attempted. Orthopaedic consultation is recommended for glenohumeral dislocation complicated by humeral fractures or glenoid rim impaction, since open reduction may be necessary.

HUMERUS FRACTURES

Fractures of the proximal humerus are relatively common injuries typically seen in elderly osteoporotic patients after falls onto outstretched hands. In contrast, humerus shaft fractures occur in younger patients following either direct or indirect trauma.

Clinical Features

Patients with proximal humerus fractures usually present with pain, swelling, and tenderness around the shoulder. Crepitus and ecchymoses may be present. Neurovascular injuries may occur and are suggested by paresthesia, pulselessness, or expanding hematoma. Humeral-shaft fractures result in localized pain, swelling, and tenderness. Shortening of the upper extremity may occur with displaced fractures. Associated radial-nerve injury is common and will be manifested by wrist drop and decreased sensation over the dorsal first web space. The humerus is also a common site for pathological fractures.

Diagnosis and Differential

Radiographs consisting of anteroposterior and lateral shoulder and axillary views will diagnose most proximal humerus fractures. The Neer Classification is based on the relationship of the proximal humerus segments (greater and lesser tuberosities, anatomic or surgical neck) and the number of fragments significantly displaced (2-part, 3-part, or 4-part). Over 80% of proximal fractures have no significant displacement or angulation and are classified as 1-part fractures. The diagnosis of humeral shaft fractures is usually obvious on anteroposterior and lateral radiographs of the humerus.

Emergency Department Care and Disposition

ED management of humerus injuries is relatively straightforward.

1. Assess and document neurovascular status. This is particularly important in complex proximal humerus and humeral shaft fractures.
2. **Immobilization**—A sling and swathe or collar and cuff should be used for simple (1-part) proximal humerus fractures. Humeral shaft fractures can be immobilized by a sugar-tong splint or hanging cast. Alternatively, a simple sling and swathe is often adequate.
3. Immobilization, ice, analgesia, and orthopaedic referral are indicated for simple fractures. Early range of motion exercises are important in simple proximal humerus fractures.
4. Orthopaedic consultation is indicated for multipart proximal humerus fractures, significantly displaced or angulated fractures, open fractures, and any fracture with neurovascular complications.

If Standard Treatment Fails

Closed reduction, intra-operative treatment, or a combination of the two may be necessary in multipart proximal, and some midshaft humeral, fractures. Radial-nerve palsy may persist after the initial injury or closed reduction of a humeral shaft fracture. Return of nerve function will usually occur without operative intervention. Lastly, patients with fractures of the anatomic neck of the humerus should be warned about the risk of ischemic necrosis of the humeral head.

For further reading in *Emergency Medicine: A Comprehensive Study Guide*, 4th edition, see Chapter 226, Injuries to the Shoulder Complex and Humerus, by Dennis T. Uehara and John P. Rudzinski.

Although pelvic fractures constitute only 3% of all bony fractures, they are associated with a high morbidity and mortality. Large forces are required to fracture the pelvis, and concomitant abdominal, thoracic, and head injuries are common. The vascularity of the pelvic bones and proximity of pelvic vessels are responsible for large blood losses. The proximity of the urinary tract, genitals, rectum, and intestines mandate thorough evaluation of these organ systems in patients with pelvic fractures. Avulsion fractures of the pelvic bones are relatively stable fractures that occur secondary to forceful contraction of muscles attached to the pelvis. Hip fractures are common in elderly patients with osteoporosis and may occur spontaneously. Hip and femur fractures or dislocations also can occur in young, healthy patients after trauma.

PELVIS FRACTURES

Clinical Features

Pelvis fractures should be suspected whenever there is trauma to the torso or a fall from height. Pain, crepitus, or instability on palpation of the pelvis suggests a fracture. Hematoma over the inguinal ligament or perineum should increase suspicion. Hypotension may be secondary to abdominal or thoracic injuries or acute blood loss from disrupted pelvic bones or vessels.

Diagnosis and Differential

Radiographs confirm suspected pelvic fractures. The AP pelvic radiograph is the most useful; additional views include oblique hemi-pelvis and inlet (to evaluate anterior–posterior displacement) and outlet views (to evaluate superior–inferior displacement). CT scan provides more detailed information. Many classifications for pelvic fractures exist; the Young system is helpful because fractures are classified based on mechanism and directional forces (Table 158-1). Four main patterns (suggested by the alignment of pubic rami fractures, pubic symphysis diastasis, SI joint displacement) have been identified: lateral compression (LC), AP compression (APC), vertical shear (VS), and combination (CM). Complications often correlate with, and can be anticipated by, the fracture pattern.

Emergency Department Care and Disposition

Major complications include blood loss from hemorrhage; nerve root, urinary tract, gynecologic, and rectal injuries; and diaphragmatic rupture. Late complications include sepsis, venous and pulmonary thrombo-

TABLE 158-1. Injury Classification Keys According to the Young System

Category	Distinguishing Characteristics
LC	Transverse fracture of pubic rami, ipsilateral or contralateral to posterior injury I—Sacral compression on side of impact II—Crescent (iliac wing) fracture on side of impact III—LC I or LC-II injury on side of impact; contralateral openbook (APC) injury
APC	Symphyseal diastasis and/or longitudinal rami fractures I—*Slight* widening of pubic symphysis and/or anterior SI joint; stretched but intact anterior SI, sacrotuberous, and sacrospinous ligaments; intact posterior SI ligaments II—Widened anterior SI joint; disrupted anterior SI, sacrotuberous, and sacrospinous ligaments; intact posterior SI ligaments III—Complete SI joint disruption with lateral displacement; disrupted anterior SI, sacrotuberous, and sacrospinous ligaments; disrupted posterior SI ligaments
VS	Symphyseal diastasis or vertical displacement anteriorly and posteriorly, usually through the SI joint, occasionally through the iliac wing and/or sacrum
CM	Combination of other injury patterns, LC/VS being the most common

embolism, and infertility. Careful attention to life-threatening injuries is paramount in the multiply injured patient. Foley catheter should not be placed if urethral injury is suspected (perineal hematoma, blood at the urethral meatus, high-riding prostate on rectal exam) until a retrograde urethrogram is performed. Rectal examination (and bimanual pelvic examination in women) should be performed to evaluate for rectal and gynecologic injuries. If blood is found on pelvic exam, a speculum exam should be done to evaluate for vaginal lacerations (which may occur with anterior pelvic fractures). Vaginal lacerations mandate operative debridement, irrigation, and IV antibiotics. Rectal injuries are treated with irrigation, diverting colostomy, and antibiotics.

Hypotension is treated with early liberal use of **blood products** and pelvic stabilization to prevent further blood loss. MAST trousers may be used to stabilize pelvic fragments, but are contraindicated if diaphragmatic rupture is suspected. Early external fixation decreases complications such as ARDS and should be considered if there is evidence of continued blood loss with disruption of the posterior elements. **Angiography for embolization** of pelvic vessels is another option for continued major blood losses, but intra-abdominal solid organ injuries and other sources of blood loss should be considered. If DPL is performed, a supraumbilical approach should be taken to avoid disruption of pelvic hematoma.

STABLE PELVIC AVULSION FRACTURES

Avulsion fractures involve a single bone, which is avulsed during forceful muscular contraction. Diagnosis is based on physical exam and confirmed radiographically. Avulsion fractures are usually stable, heal well, and are treated symptomatically.

Clinical Features

Avulsion fracture of the anterior superior iliac spine (ASIS) occurs when forceful contraction of the Sartorius muscle causes separation of the ASIS. Symptoms include localized swelling and pain with thigh flexion and abduction. Avulsion fractures of the anterior inferior iliac spine (AIIS) occurs after forceful contraction of the rectus femoris muscle. Symptoms include groin pain and inability to flex at the hip. Radiograph reveals downward displacement of the inferior iliac spine. Avulsion of the ischial tuberosity occurs in patients under age 20 to 25 (whose apophysis have not yet united) when the hamstring forcefully contracts (as in jumping). Pain is present on sitting and thigh flexion. There is tenderness on palpation of the tuberosity on rectal examination.

Stable Fractures Involving a Single Pelvic Bone

Fracture of a single ischial bone or pubic ramus can occur in the elderly from a fall with direct trauma. A lateral film of the hip is necessary to rule out a hip fracture. The ischial bodies can be injured by a direct fall on the buttocks. Iliac wing (Duverney) fractures (from direct trauma) present with pain and swelling over the iliac wing. Intra-abdominal injuries may be coexistent. Sacral fractures may occur when large anteroposterior forces are applied to the pelvis. They may be difficult to diagnose on radiograph; subtle irregularity, buckling, or malalignment of the sacral foramina are suggestive, and the lateral view may show displacement. A bimanual rectal examination, (one finger in the rectum, and a hand on the sacrum) may reveal crepitus. Coccygeal fractures are caused by a fall in a sitting position. The diagnosis is made clinically by rectal examination which reveal crepitus. Treatment is symptomatic, with a soft doughnut cushion for sitting, ice, and analgesics.

HIP FRACTURES

Clinical Features

Hip fractures are common in elderly patients with osteoporosis. The affected leg is classically foreshortened and externally rotated. Morbidity is high, related to the premorbid conditions. Complications include infection, venous thromboembolism, avascular necrosis, and nonunion.

Diagnosis and Differential

The position of the extremity, ecchymoses, deformity, and range of motion should be evaluated. Heel percussion may elicit pain. PA, lateral, and frog-leg views will evaluate the femur and acetabulum. Hip fractures are classified as intracapsular (femoral head and neck) or extracapsular (intertrochanteric, subtrochanteric). Intracapsular fractures may compromise blood supply to the femoral head, secondary to damage of capsular vessels.

Femoral head fractures are most commonly associated with hip dislocations. Femoral neck fractures are common in elderly patients with osteoporosis. Pain radiates to the groin and inner thigh. The leg is foreshortened and held in external rotation. Radiographs may reveal fracture, but may be normal with stress fractures.

Emergency Department Care and Disposition

Nondisplaced neck fractures are treated with pin fixation; displaced fractures are treated with open reduction or prosthesis placement. A stress fracture should be suspected if there is significant pain without radiologic abnormality. They are treated conservatively with bone scan in 1 to 2 days, or followup radiograph in 10 to 14 days.

Intertrochanteric fractures occur in the elderly after a fall with rotational forces. The leg is foreshortened and externally rotated. Treatment includes nonemergent operative fixation.

Subtrochanteric fractures may be seen in elderly osteoporotic patients and young patients after major trauma. Symptoms include pain, deformity, and swelling. Immobilization with a traction apparatus is recommended, with eventual operative fixation.

Greater trochanter fractures may occur in adults (true fracture) or children (avulsion of the apophysis). Pain is present on abduction and extension. Treatment is controversial, and may include conservative treatment or operative fixation (based on patient's age and displacement of fragments).

Lesser trochanter avulsions are most common in young athletes, after avulsion of the iliopsoas muscle. Pain is present during flexion and internal rotation. If there is more than 2 cm of displacement, operative fixation with screws is recommended.

HIP DISLOCATIONS

Hip dislocations are most often the result of massive forces during trauma. The majority (90%) are posterior and 10% are anterior. Both types are treated with early closed reduction (less than 6 h) in order to decrease the incidence of avascular necrosis.

Clinical Features and Emergency Department Care

Posterior dislocations occur when a posterior force is applied to the flexed knee and may coexist with acetabular fractures. The leg is foreshortened, internally rotated, and adducted. AP, lateral, and oblique x-ray views will evaluate the status of the acetabulum and the femoral head. Treatment includes early closed reduction, with analgesics and muscle relaxants, using the Allis maneuver (hip flexion to 90°, then internal and external rotation) or the Stimson maneuver (patient prone, with the leg hanging over the edge of stretcher, and application of gentle traction). Anterior dislocations occur during forced abduction. The leg is held in abduction and external rotation. Treatment includes early closed reduction with strong, in-line traction, and flexing and externally rotating the leg, with abduction, once the femoral head clears the acetabulum.

FEMORAL SHAFT FRACTURES

Femoral shaft fractures occur commonly in young patients during motor vehicle crashes, falls, or occupational accidents. The femur has a rich vascular supply and is surrounded by soft tissue, which can accommodate 1 l or more of blood, contributing to blood loss and clinical shock. Distal neurovascular status should be thoroughly evaluated. Diagnosis is confirmed radiographically. Treatment involves immediate immobilization with Hare or Sager traction or a Thomas splint. Definitive repair is by operative fixation, or traction in children.

PEDIATRIC DISORDERS OF THE CHILD WITH A LIMP

The child who presents with a limp should be carefully evaluated for septic arthritis, transient toxic synovitis, Legg–Calvé–Perthes disease, slipped capital femoral epiphysis, and congenital hip dislocations.

Clinical Features and Emergency Department Care

Septic arthritis—Septic arthritis is most common in children under age 4, and commonly presents with a limp or refusal to ambulate. The hip joint becomes infected by hematogenous spread or local extension. The most common organisms are *S. Aureus, H. Influenza* (less common since the HIB vaccine), and group B *Streptococcus* (in neonates). The child may appear toxic, irritable, and febrile, but the symptoms may be nonspecific in younger children. The leg is classically held in abduction, flexion, and external rotation. Exam reveals pain on hip movement. Laboratory tests usually reveal an increased WBC and sedimentation rate, and blood cultures are positive in 50% of cases. Definitive diagnosis is based on hip aspiration (under fluoroscopy). Treatment mandates hospitalization, **IV antibiotics,** and **operative irrigation.**

Transient synovitis—Transient synovitis may be difficult to distinguish from a septic hip and is most common in children aged 18 mo to 12 y, with a peak in 5- to 6-y olds. The cause is unknown but may be related to antecedent viral illness. Onset of symptoms is generally gradual and the child appears less toxic. If the child is febrile with an elevated WBC and sedimentation rate, a septic hip should be ruled out by aspiration. The illness is self limited (3–5 days), and treatment is supportive (rest, ibuprofen).

Legg–Calvé–Perthes disease—Legg-Calvé-Perthes disease is an idiopathic avascular necrosis of the femoral head, found more commonly in boys aged 5 to 9. Examination reveals decreased range of motion; tests are normal. Radiographic findings (best seen on lateral view) may include necrosis, fragmentation, and resorption, but may be normal early in the disease process. Bone scan is more sensitive. Patients should be referred to an orthopaedist.

Slipped capital femoral epiphysis—This is a disease of unknown etiology, most common in children aged 10 to 16, which may occur bilaterally. It also occurs more commonly in obese and long, slender, rapidly growing adolescents. Symptoms are usually gradual in onset, with groin pain during activity, which may refer to the knee. AP and lateral radiographs may reveal a posteriorly displaced epiphyseal plate that may be normal initially. Treatment includes nonweight bearing activity, and orthopaedic referral for traction or operative fixation.

For further reading in *Emergency Medicine: A Comprehensive Study Guide*, 4th edition, see Chapter 227, Trauma to the Pelvis, Hip, and Femur, by Joseph F. Waeckerle and Mark T. Steele.

Judith Linden

Knee injuries are most often the result of ligamentous and cartilage injuries, but may include bony fractures and dislocations. Leg injuries include tibia and fibula fractures. Injury may be caused by direct blow or torquing forces. Tibia fractures have a high complication rate because they are often open and may have concomitant extensive soft tissue injury.

KNEE INJURIES

Patellar Fractures

Fractures of the patella occur most often from a direct blow or from a fall on a flexed knee but may also be caused by forceful contraction of the quadriceps muscle. Symptoms include swelling and pain over the patella, occasionally with palpable defect. Orthopaedic consultation in the ED is recommended. Treatment depends on the type of fracture: Nondisplaced transverse fractures are treated with knee immobilization, crutches, and partial weightbearing for 6 wks. Displaced transverse fractures are treated with reduction (often requiring open internal-wire fixation) and cylindrical cast. Comminuted fractures are treated operatively, with small-fragment removal and suturing of the quadriceps and patellar tendons.

Patellar Dislocations

Patellar dislocations are most common in women, where the patella is usually displaced laterally over the lateral condyle, often with disruption of the medial knee-joint capsule. Reduction is achieved by hyperextending the knee and flexing at the hip while sliding the patella back in place. Radiographs will rule out fracture. The apprehension test may be used to diagnose recurrent dislocations—attempted lateral displacement of the patella of an extended leg causes reflex contraction of the quadriceps muscle and an apprehensive facial expression in anticipation of pain. Initial dislocations are immobilized in extension. Recurrent, superior, and medial dislocations should be referred to an orthopaedic surgeon.

Patellar Tendonitis

Jumper's knee occurs most commonly in runners and basketball and volleyball players. Pain localizes to the patellar tendon and increases when standing from a sitting position and running up hills. Treatment includes ice, NSAIDs, and quadriceps-strengthening exercises. Steroid injections increase the risk of rupture and should be avoided.

Chondromalacia Patellae

This is common in young, active women. Symptoms include anterior knee pain, which increases on stair climbing and rising from a sitting position. Malalignment of the patella on the femur causes excessive stress on the lateral cartilage and degenerative changes. Diagnosis may be made by the patellar compression test. The patellar compression test is considered positive when compression of the patella distally in the trochlear groove of the extended knee and contracted quadriceps causes pain and a grinding sensation under the examiner's hand. Treatment includes rest, NSAIDs, and quadriceps-strengthening exercises.

Femoral Condyle Fractures

Condyle fractures are most often caused by direct trauma from a fall or a blow to the distal femur. Signs and symptoms include pain, swelling, and deformity, occasionally with rotation and shortening. Neurovascular status distally should be evaluated. Sensation in the web space between the first and second toe (deep peroneal nerve) should be tested. The ipsilateral hip and quadriceps apparatus should be fully evaluated. Orthopaedic consultation for treatment is mandatory. Fractures are treated with immobilization, traction, or intraoperative fixation, depending on the type of fracture.

Tibial Spine Injuries

These injuries often indicate cruciate ligament avulsions and are caused by anterior or posterior forces applied to the flexed knee. The patient is unable to fully extend the knee due to hemorrhagic joint effusion. A positive Lachman's test is present. Incomplete or nondisplaced fractures are treated with knee immobilization in full extension. Complete, displaced fractures are treated with operative reduction. Tibial tuberosity avulsions are caused by sudden force applied to the flexed knee while the quadriceps muscle is contracted, causing avulsion of the tibial tuberosity where the quadriceps mechanism attaches. Treatment of nondisplaced avulsions include immobilization; displaced or large avulsions are treated operatively.

Tibial Plateau Fractures

These fractures occur most commonly at the lateral plateau and are caused by a direct blow or axial loading, which forces the femoral condyles onto the tibia. Symptoms include pain and swelling of the knee and decreased range of motion. Radiographs may demonstrate a fracture or a joint effusion with a fat/fluid level. Tomograms or CT scan are helpful to further evaluate the fracture. Treatment for nondepressed fractures is a long leg cast and nonweightbearing activity. Depressed fractures are treated with operative elevation of the fragments.

Knee Dislocations

These occur when large forces cause disruption of multiple ligamentous supports of the knee. A very unstable knee on exam is suggestive of a spontaneously reduced dislocation. A high degree of suspicion should be maintained, as there is a high incidence of popliteal artery and peroneal nerve injury. Arteriogram is mandatory if pulses or ankle/brachial index are decreased and should be considered (but is controversial) if normal pulses are present. Orthopaedic consultation is mandatory if a dislocation is suspected, even if the knee has been spontaneously reduced.

Ligamentous and Meniscal Injuries

These injuries present with knee pain and effusion. Hemarthroses are common with ligamentous and meniscal injuries, but they may be absent if the joint capsule is completely disrupted. Ligamentous injuries include anterior, posterior, medial collateral, and lateral collateral tears. The integrity of the lateral collateral ligament is tested by applying a varus (lateral) force with the leg flexed at 30°, and medial collateral tested by valgus (medial) force. The injured side should be compared to the uninjured side. A laxity of greater than 1 cm with no firm endpoint suggests a complete tear, whereas laxity with an endpoint suggests a partial tear. If the laxity remains after testing is repeated with the leg in full extension, a more severe injury (including the cruciate ligaments) is suspected. Anterior cruciate tears are common, presenting with a large joint effusion and pain, and may include a medial meniscus tear. Posterior cruciate tears are rarer and often involve large posterior forces applied to the lower leg. A drawer sign may be elicited (laxity of greater than 6 mm when anterior/posterior forces are applied to the lower leg, which is flexed to 90°), but is not sensitive. The Lachman and pivot-shift tests are more sensitive for diagnosing ACL tears. MRI can assist in further defining the injury. Ligament injuries are treated with knee immobilization, crutches, and analgesics. Orthopaedic referral, although not emergent, is recommended.

Meniscal injuries are commonly associated with ligamentous tears. Symptoms include painful locking of the knee, a popping or clicking sensation, and the knee giving out. Exam may reveal atrophy of the ipsilateral thigh. Orthopaedic consultation is recommended. A locked knee should be unlocked by sitting the patient at the edge of the stretcher with the knee flexed to 90°. The ED physician should apply traction with internal and external rotation of the leg to unlock the joint.

KNEE INJURIES IN CHILDREN

Bony fractures are much more common than ligamentous knee injuries in children, since the ligaments are much stronger than the epiphyses.

Meniscal injuries and dislocations may occur but are rare. The opposite knee may be radiographed for comparison. Common epiphysial injuries include the distal femoral epiphysis, proximal tibial epiphysis, and tibial tubercle injuries. Osgood–Schlatter disease (epiphysial aseptic necrosis of the tibial tubercle) may be confused with tibial tubercle avulsion fractures, but it usually presents in adolescents with a vague history of pain, especially with range of motion against resistance. Treatment for Osgood–Schlatter disease is symptomatic, and the prognosis is good. Osteochondral fractures may occur infrequently at the femoral condyles or patella. The patient describes an acute injury with a pop or a snap. Treatment includes surgical removal of the fragment.

LEG INJURIES

Tibia Fractures

Symptoms include localized pain, crepitus, and soft-tissue swelling. Overlying lacerations may indicate open fracture. Complete evaluation and documentation of neurologic status (sensation and motor) and vascular status (pulses at the dorsalis pedis and anterior tibial artery) are crucial. Clinically obvious fractures should be splinted before radiographs. PA and lateral radiographs of the tibia and fibula should be obtained, including ankle and knee. If vascular compromise is present, emergent reduction should be performed prior to obtaining radiographs in order to re-establish circulation. Soft tissue injuries require debridement and meticulous wound care to prevent infection.

Fibular Fractures

Fractures most commonly involve the distal fibula at the ankle, but isolated fibular shaft fractures may occur from direct or indirect trauma. Stress fractures (commonly at the distal third) may be difficult to diagnose on x-ray, but can be confirmed by bone scan. Treatment may include a short leg walking cast and crutches for patient comfort, and commonly does not require immobilization.

Compartment Syndrome

One of the most common serious complications of lower extremity fractures is compartment syndrome (see chap. 166). Early recognition is crucial, because irreversible damage occurs within 4 to 6 h. Common causes of compartment syndrome include bony fractures, burns, electrical injuries, snake bites, prolonged immobilization (in drug intoxication), and hypo- or hyperthermia. Cardinal signs and symptoms include the five *P*'s: *P*ain (out of proportion to injury), *p*aresthesia and abnormal two-point sensation and light touch, *p*allor, *p*ulselessness (a late sign), and *p*aralysis. Pulses and capillary refill are initially normal; pain on passive stretch and paresthesia are the most sensitive sign. If suspected, compartment pressures should be measured and orthopaedic consultation obtained.

For further reading in *Emergency Medicine: A Comprehensive Study Guide*, 4th edition, see Chapter 228, Knee Injuries; and Chapter 229, Leg Injuries, by Joseph F. Waeckerle and Mark T. Steele.

The ankle bears as much weight per unit area as any other joint in the body. Its anatomic design and weightbearing function predispose it to a wide variety of injuries.

LIGAMENTOUS INJURIES

Clinical Features

A careful history of the mechanism of injury is essential in evaluation. Position of the foot at the time of injury, direction of the stresses, noises that were heard with the event such as popping, time to onset of pain and swelling, and amount of disability are all important to note. Previous injury to the ankle is important to document. Approximately 75% of all ankle injuries are sprains; over 80% involve the anterior talofibular ligament.

Ligamentous injuries are classified into 1st, 2nd, and 3rd-degree sprains. A 1st-degree sprain is stretching or microscopic tearing of a ligament associated with local tenderness, minimal swelling, and the ability to still bear weight. X-rays of the ankle are normal.

A 2nd-degree sprain is defined as a severe stretching and partial tearing of a ligament, causing marked tenderness, moderate edema, mild ecchymosis, and moderate pain with weight bearing. Standard x-rays will be normal, but stress views will be abnormal.

A 3rd-degree sprain is due to complete rupture of ligaments. The patient will have marked tenderness, swelling, ecchymosis, and often deformity. The patient will be unable to bear weight. Standard x-rays will be abnormal.

Diagnosis and Differential

A partial exam should be done on the patient prior to x-ray evaluation. Neurovascular status should be evaluated for compromise and should be documented. In the absence of gross deformity, local swelling and the loss or prominence of anatomic landmarks should be noted. Ecchymosis may be present with a sprain or fracture. The area of maximal tenderness and presence of any crepitance should be located. Both malleoli, the proximal fibula, and the fifth metatarsal should be palpated for tenderness.

Stability of all ligaments should be addressed in the physical exam. The anterior drawer maneuver is performed by grasping the calcaneus with the finger and thumb behind the malleoli, and with the opposite hand stabilizing the extreme distal tibia and fibula. Applying a forward anterior force to the calcaneus will stress the lateral ligaments. If movement is greater than 3 mm, the test is abnormal. There are many false-

855

positive and false-negative results to this test. Talar tilt or movement of the talus in the ankle mortise gives an indication of the more posterior lateral ligaments. Comparison with the uninjured ankle may be helpful with each of these tests.

Emergency Department Care and Disposition

First-degree sprains are treated with compression dressings, elevation, ice, and immobilization. The decision for nonweightbearing or partial weightbearing is an individual one. Plaster or synthetic splints or ankle braces may be used. In an athlete with a 1st-degree sprain, full athletic activity should not be resumed until the person can sprint without limping, run figure-of-eight full speed without pain, and cut at right angles off the affected foot without pain. Orthopaedic consultation should be obtained for followup and because 2nd- and 3rd-degree sprains can be managed in multiple ways.

ANKLE FRACTURE

Clinical Features

Standard x-rays will reveal fractures of the ankle. Ligamentous avulsions will usually cause transverse malleolar fractures or small chip or pull-off fractures of the tip of the malleolus. Ligamentous injuries are usually present with any fracture. The type of fracture produced by an injury depends on the position of the foot at the time of injury and the direction of the deforming force.

Diagnosis and Differential

A partial exam should be performed prior to x-ray evaluation. It is important to note that an avulsion fracture at the base of the 5th metatarsal is one of the most commonly missed fractures.

Emergency Department Care and Disposition

The goal in the treatment of all ankle injuries is to restore anatomic position. This is achieved through immobilization or surgery. Orthopaedic consultation is required for any ankle fracture. Ice, elevation, pain control, and immobilization are standard treatment measures with any fracture. Dislocations of the ankle are usually associated with malleolar fractures, and about 50% are open fracture–dislocations. Dislocations should be emergently relocated with gentle in-line traction. Open injuries require surgical debridement. A high incidence of avascular necrosis is noted following ankle dislocations.

Ankle Contusion

Direct trauma can produce contusion of the soft tissues or periosteum with swelling, discoloration, and point tenderness. X-ray evaluation may be normal or demonstrate a cortical defect. Treatment consists of ice, elevation, compression dressings, rest, and analgesics.

Tenosynovitis

Tenosynovitis is usually secondary to direct trauma or overuse of the involved tendon. Tenderness, swelling, and crepitance with movement of the tendon are usually noted. X-rays are negative, and treatment consists of ice, elevation, and rest. Partial immobilization and anti-inflammatory medication may be necessary. Corticosteroid injections should never be given due to the risk of tendon rupture.

Achilles Tendon Rupture

Achilles tendon rupture most often occurs secondary to indirect mechanisms resulting in forceful dorsiflexion of the ankle. Initiating a sprint, slipping on a stair or ladder, direct trauma, or a fall from a height may produce this injury. Rupture typically involves middle-aged men and the left Achilles tendon more often than the right.

Clinical Features

Sudden pain, an audible snap, and subsequent difficulty stepping off on the foot is typically noted. Swelling of the distal calf and a palpable defect in the tendon proximal to the calcaneus are also usually noted. A negative Thompson's test, performed by squeezing the calf, may demonstrate an absent or markedly diminished plantarflexion of the foot. X-rays are normal.

Emergency Department Care and Disposition

Treatment includes orthopaedic consultation and splinting with a posterior splint. The patient should remain nonweightbearing and elevate the extremity. Therapy consists of long leg cast immobilization or surgical repair.

Subluxing Peroneal Tendons

Subluxing peroneal tendons are uncommon entities that can be acute or chronic. This injury has been most commonly associated with skiing but can occur in various athletic endeavors, such as ice skating, soccer, and basketball. The patient often notes a snap or pop sound at the time of injury, as the peroneal tendons sublux from posterior to anterior over the lateral malleolus.

Clinical Features and Emergency Department Care

Symptoms include localized pain, swelling, and ecchymosis over the posterior aspect of the lateral malleolus. Spontaneous reduction has usually occurred prior to evaluation. The subluxation can be reproduced by having the patient dorsiflex and evert the foot against resistance. Inversion ankle sprains are included in the differential. A small piece of bone is avulsed from the posterior aspect of the lateral malleolus in 15% to 50% of cases on x-ray. Orthopaedic consultation should be obtained, since treatment may be conservative or surgical.

Ankle Injuries in Children

In adolescents over 15 or 16 years old, epiphyseal plates are closing, so injuries follow the typical adult pattern noted above. In children, the ligamentous injuries are rare, because the ligaments are stronger than the bone. This causes fractures to occur at epiphyseal plates. These fractures are described by the Salter–Harris classification. Salter–Harris types I and II are often difficult to diagnose on x-ray. Injuries should be treated conservatively with close followup or orthopaedic consultation. Complications can involve disturbance of the growth plate, resulting in angular deformities and leg-length changes.

For further reading in *Emergency Medicine: A Comprehensive Study Guide,* 4th edition, see Chapter 230, Ankle Injuries, by Joseph F. Waeckerle and Mark T. Steele.

Greg Mears

CALCANEAL FRACTURES

Clinical Features

The calcaneus is the largest and most frequently fractured tarsal bone. Injury usually is the result of a compression mechanism secondary to a fall from a height. Ten percent of all calcaneal fractures are associated with lumbar compression injuries, and 26% with other extremity injuries.

Diagnosis and Differential

The symptoms and signs associated with calcaneal fractures are swelling, pain, and ecchymosis at the fracture site. Often the fracture site will be exquisitely tender locally, with decreased range of motion. The patient may be unable to bear weight. The patient must be examined closely for injuries associated with calcaneal fractures, including back, pelvic, hip, and knee injuries. Special radiographic views of the calcaneus or CT may be needed to define the fracture.

Emergency Department Care and Disposition

A thorough physical exam to rule out associated injures must be performed. The treatment of calcaneal fractures consists of immobilization of the foot using a posterior splint. Elevation and ice may be used to control the swelling. Pain control should be provided based on the overall evaluation of the patient. Early orthopaedic consultation should be obtained since hospitalization may be required.

TALUS FRACTURES

Clinical Features

Talus fractures are the second most common foot fracture. Dislocation of the talus is often associated with the fracture. The mechanism of injury that produces a talus fracture or dislocation is usually hyperextension. Avascular necrosis of the talus can occur.

Diagnosis and Differential

The patient complains of intense pain and is unable to bear weight. Localized swelling, discoloration, and tenderness to palpation are noted. Documentation of the neurovascular status of the foot should be done initially. Routine radiographs of the foot are diagnostic.

Emergency Department Care and Disposition

The treatment of a talus fracture is dependent on the extent of the fracture. Simple, nondisplaced minor chips or avulsion fractures require immobilization, ice, elevation, pain control, and followup. Fractures of the neck and body of the talus may be difficult to treat, especially if there is dislocation. These fracture dislocations are often treated operatively. Orthopaedic consultation should be obtained on all talus fractures.

MIDFOOT FRACTURES

Clinical Features

Fractures of the midfoot are rare but, if they occur, they may involve multiple fractures. This area of the foot includes the five tarsal bones, their articulating surfaces, and the ligamentous support. Subluxation or dislocation is common. The navicular bone is the most commonly fractured bone in the foot.

Diagnosis and Differential

Signs and symptoms of a fracture include pain, swelling, and tenderness over the involved area. Standard radiographic views of the foot are diagnostic.

Emergency Department Care and Disposition

The treatment of a midfoot fracture is ice, elevation, pain control, and immobilization, if there is no displacement. Orthopaedic consultation should be obtained and, if displacement of the fracture is noted, operative repair may be required.

TARSAL–METATARSAL INJURIES

Clinical Features

The tarsal–metatarsal joint is referred to as Lisfranc's joint; injuries to this area are uncommon. The mechanism of injury is usually an axial load applied directly to the heel, with the foot fixed to the ground in severe hyperextension of the forefoot on the midfoot, causing dorsal dislocation. A fracture at the base of the second metatarsal is almost pathognomonic for this injury.

Diagnosis and Differential

The signs and symptoms of a tarsal–metatarsal fracture or dislocation include pain, swelling, discoloration, loss of range of motion, loss of weightbearing and possibly, some paresthesia in the midfoot. Standard radiographs of the foot are diagnostic.

Emergency Department Care and Disposition

Neurovascular status of the extremity should be documented. All tarsal–metatarsal fractures or dislocations require early orthopaedic consultation. Treatment is difficult using closed reduction methods, so open reduction is often required with internal fixation.

METATARSAL FRACTURES

Clinical Features

Mechanisms of injury producing metatarsal fractures include direct trauma, crush injuries, or an indirect force such as a twisting-type injury. Frequently, more than one metatarsal is fractured. Fractures are described as being in the neck or shaft of the metatarsal. A fracture at the base of the 5th metatarsal is the most common. A transverse fracture through the base of the 5th metatarsal is called a Jones fracture. A pull-off or avulsion fracture at the base of the 5th metatarsal is called a *ballet dancer's fracture*. Stress fractures typically involve the 2nd and 3rd metatarsal proximal to the head. These fractures are usually insidious and may not appear on a radiograph for 2 to 3 wks.

Diagnosis and Differential

Fractures of the metatarsals are associated with local tenderness. The patient may bear weight uncomfortably. Fifth metatarsal fractures are often confused with lateral ankle injuries, so it is important visualize the base of the 5th metatarsal on routine ankle radiographs. Routine radiographs of the foot are diagnostic except with stress fractures. Stress fractures often require a repeat radiograph in 2 to 3 wks, or a bone scan to delineate the fracture site. Fractures at the base of the 5th metatarsal can be confused with a secondary growth center apophysis.

Emergency Department Care and Disposition

Metatarsal fractures are treated with ice, elevation, pain medication, and immobilization by splinting. Orthopaedic consultation should be obtained. Casting is usually required for metatarsal fractures other than the 5th. Fractures at the base of the 5th metatarsal can be treated with a postoperative or fracture shoe and crutches. Stress fractures require rest and immobilization.

PHALANGEAL INJURIES

Clinical Features

Injuries to the phalanx are common and usually result from direct trauma.

Diagnosis and Differential

Pain, swelling, and discomfort when wearing shoes and walking are common features. In some instances, when dislocation or subluxation has occurred, obvious deformity results. Routine radiographs of the foot are diagnostic.

Emergency Department Care and Disposition

Treatment consists of reduction of the subluxation or dislocation and reduction of the fracture to its most anatomic position. Ice, elevation, and immobilization are required. Digital block is useful prior to manipulation of any fracture or dislocation. Immobilization can be accomplished through dynamic splinting (buddy taping), a postoperative shoe or if necessary, with a walking boot cast. Unstable phalangeal fractures require early orthopaedic referral for possible internal fixation. Open phalangeal fractures demand adequate tissue treatment and early referral or close followup. Prophylactic antibiotics should be used with open fractures.

PLANTAR FASCIITIS

Clinical Features

Plantar fasciitis is the most common cause of heel pain. Inflammation and degeneration of the plantar fascia at the calcaneal tuberosity is noted.

Diagnosis and Differential

A history of increased running activity and improper footwear is often noted. Pain is described as burning in nature and gradual in onset along the medial aspect of the calcaneus. Pain is usually worse with weightbearing, stairclimbing, or standing on toes. X-rays of the foot may reveal a heel spur. The differential includes calcaneal stress fracture and tarsal tunnel syndrome.

Emergency Department Care and Disposition

Treatment consists of rest, ice, elevation, NSAIDs, and padded heel cups. In recalcitrant cases, local injection of corticosteroids may be helpful, but multiple injections of corticosteroids have been associated with rupture of the plantar fascia.

TARSAL TUNNEL SYNDROME

Clinical Features

Tarsal tunnel syndrome is an entrapment neuropathy of the posterior tibial nerve (comparable to the carpal tunnel syndrome in the wrist).

This fixed space is prone to allow compression of the nerve when any condition causing inflammation and swelling of the area occurs. Fractures, dislocations, gout, and rheumatoid arthritis can result in this syndrome.

Diagnosis and Differential

Pain is located at the medial malleolus with radiation to the heel and sole of the foot. Nocturnal pain is common and pain may be increased with walking or dorsiflexion of the foot. Paresthesias, dysethesias, and hypoesthesias may occur. A loss of two-point discrimination over the plantar aspect of the foot and toes is often noted. Tapping over the nerve (Tinel sign) may reproduce the pain.

Emergency Department Care and Disposition

Rest, NSAIDs, and well-fitting shoes are all part of the initial treatment. Referral for orthotic devices to improve biomechanics may be necessary. Local corticosteroid injections also may be helpful. If no improvement is noted with conservative measures, surgical release of the flexor retinaculum is indicated.

For further reading in *Emergency Medicine: A Comprehensive Study Guide*, 4th edition, see Chapter 231, Foot Injuries, by Joseph F. Waeckerle and Mark T. Steele.

21 | MUSCULAR, LIGAMENTOUS, AND RHEUMATIC DISORDERS

Cervical, Thoracic, and Lumbar Pain Syndromes

Charles J. Havel, Jr.

The list of potential causes of cervical, thoracic, and lumbar pain is long and includes trauma, infection, neoplasms, and inflammatory processes. As in many other conditions, diagnosis will often be achieved with a thorough history and physical exam and the appropriate use of adjunct testing, particularly imaging modalities. Attention in the ED must be paid to identifying causes of permanent disability and life-threatening entities.

Clinical Features

Patients with neck pain will often have associated complaints of stiffness and limited range of motion. They will also routinely present with an identifiable inciting or provocative maneuver or position that can be reproduced. Localized neck tenderness may or may not be present. Radiation of the pain, particularly in a dermatomal pattern, should suggest a radiculopathy. Pain may be accompanied by a variety of neurogenic symptoms and signs, such as muscle weakness or hypertonicity, reflex changes, and sensory abnormalities.

Pain from the thoracic spine is less common than either cervical or lumbar pain syndromes. Localized pain and tenderness may or may not be present. Radicular pain is common and may be associated with chest or abdominal pain. If long tract signs are present, e.g., hyperreflexia, Babinski's sign, or urinary incontinence, then intrinsic or extrinsic spinal cord pathology must be suspected.

Lumbosacral pain carries a long differential diagnosis including diseases of structures remote from the spine itself. An important goal of evaluation, therefore, is the distinction between musculoskeletal versus neurogenic versus more remote causes of pain. Localized bony pain and percussion tenderness points to musculoskeletal disease; radicular pain is common, particularly with musculoskeletal and neurologic processes. A neurologic deficit can be associated with either spinal or extraspinal pathology. It is important to note the presence or absence of systemic symptoms and signs; these in association with an abnormal abdominal, neurologic, or rectal exam strongly suggest an extraspinal cause of pain, including potentially life-threatening conditions.

Diagnosis and Differential

The mainstay of the diagnostic process is a thorough history and physical exam. The patient's age, medical history, and review of systems can be helpful in prioritizing differential diagnosis. Other specific factors of importance include any history of trauma and the mechanism of injury, the character and distribution of pain, any identifiable exacerbating or abating positions, and the presence or absence of neurogenic or systemic symptoms. With trauma, the initial physical exam will often be restricted to identifying areas of bony tenderness, crepitus, or step-off, and noting any neurologic deficit. Positive findings mandate the need for radiographic imaging before further spine evaluation and manipulation. For hemodynamically unstable patients, a more focused examination is also done to identify neurologic deficit and other abnormal findings (e.g., a pulsatile abdominal mass) whereas resuscitation and other evaluations are begun. Otherwise, in stable patients with atraumatic pain syndromes, the examination can be completed before considering imaging or other lab testing.

For suspected cervical lesions, range of motion testing, spine compression, and distraction techniques to reproduce pain and radicular symptoms, assessments of distal upper extremity pulses, and thorough neurologic exam are important diagnostic procedures. If imaging is required, a minimum of a three-view cervical spine plain film series should be ordered, with oblique views or flexion–extension views added selectively. CT scan or MRI is useful in the workup for patients with suspected radiculopathy or myelopathy.

The differential diagnosis in neck pain begins with vertebral fracture, especially in the setting of trauma, to be confirmed by plain film or CT imaging. In the absence of fracture, cervical soft-tissue injury, colloquially known as *whiplash* and, more accurately, as acceleration flexion–extension neck injury, is common. These injuries may be accompanied by a host of nonspecific symptoms, such as dizziness, dysesthesias, tinnitus, dysphagia, and spatial instability, but without focal neurologic deficits. Patients with radiculopathy will have neck pain associated with radiation of pain in a dermatomal pattern, with or without demonstrable sensory changes or muscle weakness in the appropriate distribution (Table 162-1). Neck pain with long tract signs signifies a myelopathy, upper extremity hyperreflexia with Hoffman's reflex indicating a lesion above C5, lower extremity hyperreflexia, upgoing great toe, and sphincter changes, suggesting cervical stenosis or epidural metastasis. Acute cervical disk herniation may present with a radiculopathy or myelopathy; radicular symptoms in these patients will often be worsened in extension and lateral flexion and relieved with flexion and distraction. X-rays may be negative even with large herniations, prompting the need for MRI or myelography to confirm the diagnosis. Chronic degenerative disk disease may continue on to cervical spondylosis and subsequently to spinal stenosis, producing a spectrum of symptoms from simple pain and stiffness to myelopathy. Neck pain with reproducible scalp pain on palpation at the occipital notch is diagnostic of occipital neuralgia. Conditions causing thoracic pain include fractures resulting from direct trauma and hyperflexion injuries. In the elderly, especially females, pathologic fractures may also occur-

TABLE 162-1. Symptoms and Signs of Cervical Radiculopathy

Disk Space	Cervical Root	Pain Complaint	Sensory Change	Motor Weakness	Altered Reflex
C1–2	C1–2	Neck, scalp	Scalp	None	None
C4–5	C5	Neck, shoulder, upper arm	Shoulder, thumb	Spinati, deltoid, biceps	Biceps reflex
C5–6	C6	Neck, shoulder, upper medial scapular area, proximal forearm, thumb	Thumb and index finger, lateral forearm	Deltoid, biceps, pronator teres, wrist extensors	Biceps and brachioradialis reflexes
C6–7	C7	Neck, posterior arm, dorsum and proximal forearm, chest, medial third of scapula, middle finger	Middle finger, forearm	Triceps, pronator teres	Triceps reflex
C7–T1	C8	Neck, posterior arm, medial proximal forearm, medial inferior scapular border, medial hand, ring and little fingers	Ring and little fingers	Triceps, flexor carpi ulnaris, hand intrinsic muscles	Triceps reflex

with minimal or no trauma; those due to osteoporosis are generally stable, whereas those due to metastatic lesions may present with myelopathy and long tract signs. CT, MRI, or myelography is needed to distinguish between relatively rare thoracic disk herniation and neoplasm. Localized thoracic pain and tenderness are characteristic of acute facet syndrome. Osteoarthritis can cause radicular pain and localized stiffness, and progress to thoracic spinal stenosis. Herpes zoster neuralgia presents with acute thoracic radiculopathy, often before the appearance of the characteristic vesicular skin eruption. Diabetic radiculopathy may have an abdominal pain component as well; electromyography (EMG) is useful for diagnosis.

The physical exam of patients with lumbar pain must include spinal, neurologic, abdominal, vascular, and lower extremity evaluation. Pelvic and rectal examinations are often valuable as well. Lumbosacral X-rays should be ordered in the setting of trauma and in the elderly, but otherwise are not prerequisite. Additional lab testing, and imaging studies such as ultrasound and CT scans, are indicated in the evaluation of patients with low back pain, other systemic symptoms, and abnormal visceral or vascular physical findings.

Spinal causes of lumbar pain include a spectrum of degenerative spinal processes, inflammatory sacroiliitis, and compression fractures. Acute disk herniation can reveal itself by pain alone or accompanied by radiculopathy (Table 162-2) or myelopathy; epidural hematoma, abscess, and neoplasm all have a similar neurologic picture. Pain exacerbated by ambulation is typical of both peripheral vascular disease and spinal stenosis and may require arteriography, CT scan, or MRI for definitive diagnosis. Lumbar pain may be a manifestation of visceral pathology; pyelonephritis and other renal disease, peptic ulcer disease, pancreatic disease, diverticulitis, pelvic disease, abdominal aortic aneurysm, and others fall into this category.

TABLE 162-2. Symptoms and Signs of Lumbar Radiculopathy

Disk Space	Lumbar Root	Pain Complaint	Sensory Change	Motor Weakness	Altered Reflex
L2–3	L3	Medial thigh, knee	Medial thigh, knee	Hip flexors	None
L3–4	L4	Medial lower leg	Medial lower leg	Quadriceps	Knee jerk
L4–5	L5	Anterior tibia, great toe	Medial foot	Extensor hallicus longus	Biceps femoris
L5–S1	S1	Calf, little toe	Lateral foot	Foot plantar flexors	Achilles

Emergency Department Care and Disposition

Patients sustaining significant trauma with or without a neurologic deficit and those with significant life or limb-threatening conditions must be aggressively evaluated, resuscitated, and consultation obtained for inpatient care, as appropriate. Patients with intractable pain, evidence of progression of neurologic deficit, or myelopathy are candidates for initiation of treatment in the ED and hospital admission. The majority of patients, however, can be managed as outpatients; the primary goal being pain relief with **anti-inflammatory medications** and analgesics (muscle relaxants are of questionable value), relative rest, cold or heat applications, and other supportive measures. Close followup is advisable to monitor for the appearance or progression of neurologic deficits.

If Standard Treatment Fails

As suggested above, a failure of outpatient care (e.g., progression of deficits or intractable pain) requires hospital admission and further evaluation and more intensive treatment. For chronic pain management, tricyclic antidepressant and anticonvulsant medications have been used with good success. Other adjunctive measures include diathermy, traction, and other rehabilitative interventions. The vast majority of pain syndromes do not require surgical intervention, but failure of more conservative treatment may prompt consideration of this option in selected cases.

For further reading in *Emergency Medicine: A Comprehensive Study Guide*, 4th edition, see Chapters 232, Neck Pain; and Chapter 233, Thoracic and Lumbar Pain Syndromes, by Myron M. LaBan.

Charles J. Havel, Jr.

Shoulder pain is a common musculoskeletal complaint, representing both acute and chronic conditions. The origin of pain may be either pathology intrinsic to the shoulder joint or to extrinsic disorders causing referred pain.

Clinical Features

The pain of musculoskeletal shoulder pathology is often described by patients as an aching sensation, particularly in the setting of a more chronic process. It may be exacerbated by specific motions, and this history is helpful in making a specific diagnosis. Associated with certain conditions may be decreased range of motion, crepitus, weakness, or muscular atrophy. Any systemic symptoms, such as shortness of breath, fever, or pain radiating from the chest or abdomen, should raise suspicion for extrinsic and potentially life-threatening problems.

Diagnosis and Differential

The primary diagnostic maneuver is thorough history and physical exam. Exam of the shoulder joint should include range of motion and muscle strength testing, palpation for local tenderness or other abnormality, and identification of any neurovascular deficit. Specific tests for impingement and individual tests of rotator cuff muscle function are often helpful in intrinsic disease. Plain radiographic studies of the shoulder joint are rarely diagnostic but may be helpful to rule out bony abnormalities in selected patients or to evaluate for abnormal calcifications. In patients in whom extrinsic causes of shoulder pain are suspected, further diagnostic testing may be indicated, such as lab studies, additional x-rays, and EKG.

Differential diagnosis includes a variety of intrinsic musculoskeletal disorders. Impingement syndrome is a painful overuse condition characterized by positive findings with impingement testing and relief of pain with anesthetic injection of the subacromial space. Both subacromial bursitis and rotator cuff tendinitis are associated with impingement. Subacromial bursitis is generally seen in patients less than 25 years old and presents with positive impingement tests and tenderness at the lateral proximal humerus or in the subacromial space. Rotator cuff tendinitis occurs primarily in the 25- to 40-age group and is distinguished by tenderness of the rotator cuff with mild to moderate muscular weakness. In more chronic disease, crepitus, decreased range of motion, and osteophyte formation visible on x-ray also may be apparent. Rotator cuff tears occur primarily in people over 40 and are associated with muscular weakness (especially with abduction and external rotation) and cuff tenderness. Ninety percent will be chronic tears with a history of minimal or no trauma; in severe disease, muscular atrophy may be present. Acute tears may occur in patients of any age and result from significant force, producing a tearing sensation with immediate pain and disability. Abnormal calcifications on x-ray in a clinical setting of painful shoulder with rotator cuff tenderness and often crepitus suggest calcific tendinitis. Osteoarthritis is characteristically associated with degenerative disease in other joints (primary) or previous fracture or other underlying disorder (secondary). The hallmark of adhesive capsulitis is significantly painful and limited range of motion, often but not always associated with a period of immobilization. Radiographs should be done to rule out posterior glenohumeral dislocation.

A number of extrinsic conditions should also be considered as causes of shoulder pain. Degenerative disease of the cervical spine, brachial plexus disorders, and suprascapular nerve compression are neurologic processes that should be sought in patient evaluation. Vascular pathology, notably axillary artery thrombosis, may also cause shoulder pain. Lastly, acute cardiac, pulmonary, and abdominal pathology may cause pain referred to the shoulder, and the clinician must remain alert to this possibility.

Emergency Department Care and Disposition

For intrinsic disease, the primary goals of ED care are to reduce pain and inflammation and prevent progression of disease. For most conditions, this translates to relative **rest** of the joint helped by use of a sling (full immobilization is not suggested), **NSAIDS,** further analgesics as needed, and cold packs. Joint space injection with glucocorticoids should be used judiciously, because of potentially deleterious effects on soft tissues—such as tendon rupture with direct injection. Do not exceed recommended limitation of three injections into a single area. In calcific tendinitis and where calcifications can be localized, these can be needled with an 18-gauge needle. For all intrinsic disorders, followup with a primary care physician with expertise in joint disease or orthopedic referral is suggested within 7 to 14 days.

In extrinsic disease, the treatment and referral pattern will be diagnosis dependent. Neurologic problems will require analgesia and anti-inflammatory medications and may require neurology or neurosurgical followup. Vascular causes of shoulder pain must be carefully evaluated and, with axillary artery thrombosis, immediate consultation is required to initiate thrombolysis. Treatment of other extrinsic conditions depends on the specific diagnosis and will entail immediate consultation with other specialists or subspecialists.

If Standard Treatment Fails

Failure of therapy should immediately cause reassessment of the initial diagnosis. Of particular concern is the misdiagnosis of extrinsic causes of shoulder pain, especially potentially life-threatening etiologies (e.g., cardiac ischemia). A thorough history and physical exam, a high index of suspicion for extrinsic disease, and prompt patient referral for followup will help greatly in guarding against treatment failures.

For further reading in *Emergency Medicine: A Comprehensive Study Guide*, 4th edition, see Chapter 234, Shoulder Pain, by D. Monte Hunter.

Overuse injuries are caused by repetitive, stressful forces applied to tendons and muscles. Acute pain from inflammation and chronic degenerative changes at the tendon insertion are characteristic. Treatment generally includes rest, cold compresses, and NSAIDs.

CARPAL TUNNEL SYNDROME

CTS occurs when repetitive wrist flexion (typing, craftwork, assembly-line work, instrument playing) causes irritation, inflammation, and compression of the median nerve as it passes between the flexor retinaculum and the common flexor sheath at the volar wrist. Conditions that increase edema, such as pregnancy and hypothyroidism, may contribute. Symptoms include pain and paresthesia in the index, middle, and radial aspects of the ring finger, and often are worse on awakening (caused by wrist flexion while sleeping). The aching sensation may radiate up the forearm to the elbow. Diagnosis is suggested by a positive Tinel's sign (tapping on the volar aspect of the wrist) and Phalen's sign (hyperflexion of the wrist for 1 min), which reproduce the paresthesia's. There may be atrophy of thenar muscles in advanced cases. Treatment includes rest from the repetitive motion, a cockup wrist splint, and NSAIDs. Referral to a hand specialist for steroid injections or surgery is appropriate if symptoms persist.

ULNAR NEURITIS (GUYON'S CANAL SYNDROME, CUBITAL TUNNEL SYNDROME)

Caused by repetitive stretching and friction (cycling, pitching, playing tennis), symptoms include numbness and weakness in the 4th and 5th fingers (if involving Guyon's canal at the wrist) or medial elbow pain (if involving the cubital tunnel at the elbow). Diagnosis is confirmed when tapping on the ulnar nerve reproduces symptoms. Diagnosis of cubital tunnel syndrome is confirmed when hyperflexing the elbow for 1 min reproduces symptoms (pain over dorso-ulnar hand). Froment's sign may be positive due to ulnar innervation of the adductor pollicis muscle, causing weak thumb abduction. Diagnosis of Guyon's canal syndrome is confirmed if there is numbness of the 4th and 5th fingers, without Froment's sign or dorsal hand symptoms. Treatment includes rest, wrist splinting (Guyon's canal), NSAIDs, steroid injection, and surgical decompression in refractory cases.

DeQUERVAIN'S TENOSYNOVITIS

This occurs when repetitive activity (assembly-line work, weeding, laundry) causes inflammation of the abductor pollicis longis and extensor pollicis brevis tendons. Patients present with pain from the radial styloid to the thumb IP joint. Diagnosis is confirmed by a positive Finkelstein's test (pain on forced ulnar deviation of the fisted thumb). Treatment includes rest, a thumb spica splint, and NSAIDs.

LATERAL (TENNIS ELBOW) AND MEDIAL (GOLFER'S ELBOW) EPICONDYLITIS

These conditions occur with manual labor, sports, or spontaneously. Lateral epicondylitis is commonly caused by racquet sports (a faulty backhand). Medial epicondylitis may be caused by repetitive motions in golfing, pitching, and racquet sports. Symptoms of lateral epicondylitis include pain at the insertion of distal arm extensors at the lateral epicondyle/radial head; pain is increased on pronation of the forearm and dorsiflexion of the wrist against resistance (lifting a chair). Medial epicondylitis presents with pain at the insertion of distal arm flexors at the medial epicondyle; pain is increased on pronation and wrist flexion against resistance. Patients also may complain of ulnar neuritis. Treatment includes rest, NSAIDs, and gradual resumption of sport after 6 wks. Utilizing supination in picking up objects may help in lateral epicondylitis. Orthopaedic referral is helpful.

GROIN STRAIN

Activities that involve sudden acceleration or directional changes may cause groin strain. Symptoms include pain during hip adduction and flexion against resistance. Exam elicits tenderness on palpation of the thigh adductors. Differential diagnosis includes inguinal hernia, testicular pathology, renal colic, bladder injury, pelvic stress fractures, and avulsion fractures. Radiographs of the pelvis are recommended (especially in adolescents) to rule out pelvic avulsion fractures. Treatment includes rest, cold compresses, NSAIDs, gentle stretching exercises once pain decreases, and orthopaedic referral for persistent pain.

ILIOTIBIAL BAND SYNDROME

This is most common in football players, military recruits, cyclists, dancers, and runners. Long stride and downhill running increase the pain, as friction against the lateral femoral condyle increases. Symptoms include lateral knee pain which increases as the foot strikes ground. Diagnosis is aided by the Renne test and the Noble test. The Renne test is performed when the patient stands on the affected leg and flexes until pain occurs at about 30°. The Noble compression test elicits pain on palpation of lateral femoral condyle while the patient lies supine and extends the knee from flexion (at 30°). Treatment includes rest, NSAIDs, ice, stretching of the band, and a gradual increase in activity over 6 wks. Orthopaedic referral is appropriate in refractory cases (for steroid injection and gait analysis).

POPLITEUS TENDONITIS

Caused by excessive downhill running, symptoms include lateral knee pain radiating deeply to the knee. Exam reveals pain on palpation of the posterolateral knee while the knee is flexed with the ankle crossing over the other knee. Treatment includes avoidance of downhill running, ice, NSAIDs, and resumption of activity when the pain decreases.

ANTERIOR TIBIAL STRAIN (ATS), MEDIAL TIBIAL STRESS SYNDROME (MTSS), AND TIBIAL STRESS FRACTURES

These conditions, commonly called *shin splints*, are a group of overuse syndromes that present with pain over the tibia. ATS is common in new runners, and MTSS is more common in experienced runners, from hyperpronation. Tibial stress fractures are caused by an increase in activity. The pain of ATS and MTSS typically occur after activity. In ATS pain is typically along the anterolateral border of the proximal two-thirds of the tibia and anteromedial at the distal third. In MTSS pain is localized to the medial border of the distal third of the tibia. Tibial stress fractures present with pain that begins during activity and tenderness on palpation of the tibial bone. X-ray may reveal periosteal reaction, but bone scan is more sensitive. Treatment includes avoidance of the inciting activity for 5 to 7 days, with gradually increasing activity as tolerated, ice, and NSAIDs. Stress fractures require 3 to 6 wks of rest. Gradual activity may be resumed when the patient is pain-free for 10 days. Orthopaedic referral is advised.

ACHILLES TENDONITIS

Caused by uphill running (repetitive hyperpronation) and wearing high-heeled shoes. Patients present with pain 6″ proximal to the insertion of gastrocnemius and soleus muscles at the heel. There is tenderness on palpation of the Achilles tendon. Treatment includes 1 to 2 days of immobilization, low heel lifts, and flexibility stretching. Steroid injections are not recommended as they predispose to tendon rupture. NSAIDs also are not recommended, as they may lead to premature resumption of activity.

For further reading in *Emergency Medicine: A Comprehensive Study Guide*, 4th edition, see Chapter 235, Overuse Syndromes, by Beverly Timerding and D. Monte Hunter.

Muscle injuries are the most commonly reported sports-related injury, usually occurring when excessive stretching forces are applied. The musculotendinous junction is vulnerable to injury, and therefore the most common site of rupture. Muscles at highest risk for rupture are those that cross two joints (biceps, hamstrings, quadriceps, and gastrocnemius). All muscle ruptures are treated with ice, elevation, and analgesics in order to decrease swelling and pain.

GASTROCNEMIUS/SOLEUS MUSCLE (ACHILLES TENDON) RUPTURE

This is most common in middleaged, intermittent athletes. It occurs with foot dorsiflexion while extending the knee and pushing off. There is often a delay in seeking treatment, and up to 25% of Achilles tendon ruptures are missed on first exam due to minimal symptoms. Symptoms include a popping noise or sensation of being struck in the heel, progressive pain, edema, and the inability to stand on tiptoes. Diagnosis is facilitated by Thompsen's Test (squeezing the calf while in prone position should cause plantar flexion of the foot; if not present, the test is positive and suggests tendon rupture). A defect may be palpable proximal to the insertion of the Achilles tendon at the heel. Orthopaedic consultation is recommended. The lower leg is casted in equinus position for at least 6 wks of nonweight bearing, and then protected weightbearing for 6 wks. Surgical repair is an option, especially in competitive athletes.

BICEPS RUPTURE

Most common in the 4th to 6th decades, biceps rupture is rare in young athletes. Steroids (oral or injectable) increase the risk. Almost all (97%) biceps ruptures involve the proximal musculotendinous unit. Symptoms include anterior shoulder pain and occasionally an auditory pop during muscle contraction against resistance (lifting heavy object). There is pain and swelling over the bicipital groove (proximal) or antecubital fossa (distal). There is an asymmetric biceps muscle bulge on arm flexion, which is not present on the unaffected arm. Radiographs are often negative but are recommended to rule out avulsion fractures. Treatment includes a sling with early mobilization. Orthopaedic consultation is recommended to plan treatment (surgical repair is an option).

TRICEPS RUPTURE

Triceps rupture is most frequent in young males who present with localized pain at the triceps and difficulty extending the elbow. The mechanism is often a fall on an outstretched arm, but it may occur spontaneously or after a direct blow. There is palpable defect proximal to the olecranon, with localized tenderness and swelling at the distal triceps. Radiographs may reveal avulsion fracture of the olecranon. Treatment includes sling immobilization and orthopaedic consultation for possible surgical repair.

QUADRICEPS RUPTURE

Quadriceps rupture is most common after a direct blow to the thigh. Symptoms include swelling and pain on leg extension. Exam reveals swelling and tenderness at the anterior midthigh. The ability to extend the leg is maintained, although with pain. There is usually no palpable muscular defect secondary to hematoma formation. Radiographs are necessary only if a femur fracture is suspected. Treatment includes knee immobilization in full extension with nonweightbearing and crutches. Heat therapy after 48 h aids hematoma resolution. Early mobilization is recommended. Orthopaedic consultation is suggested for high-performance athletes, since surgical repair may be considered.

QUADRICEPS TENDON RUPTURE

This injury is most common in elderly people after sudden contraction of the quadriceps (landing after a jump). Symptoms include sharp pain at the proximal knee on ambulating. If the tear is complete, the patient will be unable to extend the leg from knee flexion, although the ability to straight-leg raise may be maintained (due to an intact retinaculum). There may be a palpable defect, with tenderness and swelling at the suprapatellar region, and the patella may migrate distally (patella Baja). Radiographs will rule out a patellar or femoral avulsion fracture. The differential includes patellar fracture or tendon rupture, tendonitis, and muscle strain. The treatment for a complete tear is surgical repair. Partial tears are treated similarly to quadriceps muscle tears.

PATELLAR TENDON RUPTURE

Most common in young athletes with a history of tendonitis, this injury occurs after violent quadriceps contraction. Symptoms include pain inferior to the patella. On exam, there is a defect inferior to the patella, with the inability to extend the knee. The patella may be high riding (*patella alta*). Radiographs will rule out patellar fractures or avulsions. Differential includes patella tendonitis or strain, avulsion of tibial tuberosity, and quadriceps tendon rupture. Treatment includes orthopaedic consultation, possible admission for repair, knee immobilization, and crutches.

HAMSTRING RUPTURE AND STRAINS

Hamstring injuries are the most common thigh injuries. They occur during repetitive high-velocity activity and are associated with inadequate warmup, poor endurance, or exercise in cold-weather conditions. Symptoms include sudden onset of pain in the posterior thigh during activity and pain on knee flexion. Exam shows local tenderness at the posterior thigh, ecchymosis, and a palpable defect in the muscle. Radiographs will rule out avulsion fractures of the ischium if there is proximal pain. Treatment includes crutches and orthopaedic followup in 1 wk for rehabilitation. Hamstring injuries often heal slowly and recur.

For further reading in *Emergency Medicine: A Comprehensive Study Guide*, 4th edition, see Chapter 236, Muscle Ruptures, by Robert P. Petrilli and D. Monte Hunter.

Compartment syndromes are due to an increased pressure within a closed tissue space resulting in compromised blood flow through the space and subsequent tissue necrosis. Increased pressures can be caused by compression of the compartment by an outside force or by volume increase inside the compartment secondary to a hematoma or edema (see Table 166-1).

Clinical Features

Virtually any muscle invested in fascia can develop a compartment syndrome under the proper set of conditions. The upper arm has an anterior and posterior compartment. The anterior compartment contains the biceps–brachialis muscle and the ulnar, median, and radial nerves. The posterior compartment contains the triceps muscle. Compartment syndromes are extremely uncommon in the upper arm. The forearm has volar and dorsal compartments. The volar compartment contains wrist and finger extensors.

There are three gluteal compartments on the buttocks. One contains the tensor muscle of the fascia lata, another the gluteus medius and minimus, and the third the gluteus maximus. The sciatic nerve lies adjacent to the gluteus maximus and can be compressed by it.

The thigh has three compartments: anterior, medial, and posterior. The anterior compartment contains the vastus lateralis, vastus intermedius, and the vastus medialis muscles, as well as the sartorius and rectus femoris muscles. The femoral artery and nerve also traverse the anterior compartment. The medial compartment contains the adductor longus, the adductor brevis, and the adductor magnus muscles, plus the gracilis muscle. The posterior compartment contains semimembranosus, the semitendinosus, and biceps femoris muscles. The sciatic nerve also traverses the posterior compartment.

The leg has four compartments: anterior, lateral, deep posterior, and the superficial posterior. The anterior compartment is the most frequent compartment to develop this syndrome. The tibialis anterior muscle and the extensor muscles of the toes are located in this compartment, as well as the anterior tibial artery and the deep peroneal nerve. The lateral compartment—which is frequently involved with an anterior compartment syndrome—contains the peroneus longus and brevis muscles, as well as the superficial peroneal nerve. The deep posterior compartment contains the tibialis posterior muscle, the flexor digitorum longus muscle, and the flexor hallucis longus muscle. It also contains the posterior tibial artery and the tibial nerve. The superficial posterior compartment contains the gastrocnemius muscle, the soleus muscle, and the sural nerve.

TABLE 166-1. Classification of Acute Compartment Syndromes

Decreased compartment size
  Constrictive dressings and casts
  Closure of fascial defects
  Thermal injuries and frostbite
Increased compartment contents
  Primarily edematous accumulation
    Postischemic swelling
      Arterial injuries
      Arterial thrombosis or embolism
      Reconstructive vascular and bypass surgery
      Replantation
      Prolonged tourniquet time
      Arterial spasm
      Cardiac catheterization and angiography
      Ergotamine ingestion
    Prolonged immobilization with limb compression
      Drug overdose with limb compression
      General anesthesia with knee-chest position
    Thermal injuries and frostbite
    Exertion
    Venous disease
    Venomous snakebite
  Primarily hemorrhagic accumulation
    Hereditary bleeding disorders, e.g., hemophilia
    Anticoagulant therapy
    Vessel laceration
  Combination of edematous and hemorrhagic accumulation
    Fractures
      Tibia
      Forearm
      Elbow, e.g., supracondylar
      Femur
    Soft tissue injury
    Osteotomies, e.g., tibia
  Miscellaneous
    Intravenous infiltration, e.g., blood, salin
    Popliteal cyst
    Long leg brace

From Mubarak and Hargens. Used by permission.

Diagnosis and Differential

The ED physician must maintain a strong clinical suspicion for compartment syndrome in patients at risk. The history, including mechanism of injury, is very important since many patients at risk for this syndrome are severely ill or injured and cannot verbally relate if they are experiencing pain. Awake patients will virtually always say they are experiencing severe and constant pain over the involved compartment (Table 166-2). Palpation of the compartment will elicit pain. Active contraction

TABLE 166-2. Symptomatology of Acute Compartment Syndromes

UPPER EXTREMITY	
Upper arm	
Anterior compartment	Pain on active and passive flexion and extension of the elbow
	Hypesthesia in the distribution of the median, ulnar, and radial nerves
Posterior compartment	Pain on active and passive flexion and extension of the elbow
	Hypesthesia over the dorsum of the hand
Forearm	
Volar compartment	Pain on active and passive flexion and extension of the fingers
	Hypesthesia over the palm of the hand
Dorsal compartment	Pain on active and passive flexion and extension of the fingers
Hand	
Thenar and hypothenar compartments	Pain on thumb and little finger opposition
Interosseous compartments	Pain on abduction and adduction of the fingers
LOWER EXTREMITY	
Gluteal compartments	Pain on active and passive flexion and extension of the hip
	Sciatic nerve paresthesias
Thigh compartments	Pain on active and passive flexion and extension of the knee
	Sciatic nerve paresthesias with posterior compartment involvement
Leg	
Anterior compartment	Pain on active and passive dorsiflexion and plantar flexion of the foot
	Hypesthesia of the first web space
Lateral compartment	Pain on active and passive eversion and inversion of the foot
	Hypesthesia of the first web space
Superficial posterior compartment	Pain on active and passive plantar flexion and dorsiflexion of the foot
	Hypesthesia of the lateral foot
Deep posterior compartment	Pain on dorsiflexing the toes and everting the foot
	Hypesthesia of the plantar surface of the foot

of the involved muscles will increase the pain, as will passive stretching of the muscles. Hypoesthesia resulting from compromise of nerves traversing the involved compartment appears later than muscle weakness and pain.

Compartment syndromes are commonly associated with fractures and penetrating wounds. Prompt surgical consultation should be obtained. Diagnosis of compartment syndrome can only be confirmed by compartment pressure measurement. Ideally, orthopedic or surgical consultation should be obtained for this procedure. Compartment pressures of 20 mmHg or greater are considered serious and potentially damaging.

Emergency Department Care and Disposition

Treatment of compartment syndromes consists of initial stabilization, elevation, ice to the injured area, and **compartment pressure measurement** by an ED physician experienced in the procedure or by surgical consultation. Treatment is based on the measured compartment pressures. Compartment pressures greater than 20 mmHg can be damaging if they persist for hours and require **hospital admission** or surgical consultation. Pressures between 15 and 20 mmHg are problematic, and the patient should have followup in 12 to 24 h for re-evaluation and remeasurement if there is not clinical improvement. Pressures of 30 to 40 mmHg are generally considered grounds for **emergency fasciotomy.**

For further reading in *Emergency Medicine: A Comprehensive Study Guide*, 4th edition, see Chapter 237, Compartment Syndrome, by Ernest Ruiz.

Michael P. Kefer

Life-threatening complications are rare in rheumatology. However, certain manifestations require prompt intervention to prevent increased mortality and serious morbidity.

RHEUMATIC EMERGENCIES ASSOCIATED WITH RISK OF MORTALITY

Respiratory System

Death may result from airway obstruction, respiratory muscle failure, or pulmonary tissue involvement.

Airway Obstruction

Relapsing polychondritis begins with abrupt onset of pain, redness, and swelling of the ears or nose. The tracheobronchial cartilage is involved in approximately 50% of cases. Hoarseness and throat tenderness over cartilage is noted. Repeated attacks can lead to airway collapse. Treatment of an exacerbation is high-dose steroids and admission for observation.

Rheumatoid arthritis may involve the cricoarytenoid joints causing pain with speaking, hoarseness, or stridor. The joints may fix in a closed position mandating emergency tracheostomy.

Respiratory Muscle Failure

Dermatomyositis and *polymyositis* may lead to respiratory failure from respiratory muscle involvement in poorly controlled disease.

Pulmonary Tissue Involvement

Pulmonary hemorrhage complicates Goodpasture's disease, systemic lupus erythematosus, Wegener's granulomatosis, and other vasculitic conditions. *Pulmonary fibrosis* complicates ankylosing spondylitis, scleroderma, and other conditions. *Pleural effusion* complicates rheumatoid arthritis and systemic lupus erythematosus.

The Heart

Many rheumatologic conditions involve the heart.

Pericarditis occurs in rheumatoid arthritis and systemic lupus erythematosus.

Myocardial infarction may occur from coronary artery involvement in Kawasaki's disease or polyarteritis nodosa.

Pancarditis is noted in acute rheumatic fever.

Valvular heart disease is noted in ankylosing spondylitis, relapsing polychondritis, and rheumatic fever. Further, involvement may extend into the conduction system.

Adrenal glands Glucocorticoids are used often in the treatment of many rheumatic conditions. Any acute condition that prevents the patient's steroid requirement from being met, such as vomiting or acute illness or injury that increase the physiologic requirements, may result in adrenal insufficiency. The patient should receive stress-dose steroid therapy.

RHEUMATIC PRESENTATIONS ASSOCIATED WITH RISK OF MORBIDITY

Cervical Spine and Spinal Cord

Patients with rheumatologic involvement of the C-spine may be at high risk for serious C-spine or spinal cord injury from otherwise trivial trauma. This includes manipulation during endotracheal intubation if extreme caution is not exercised. Ligamentous destruction of the transverse ligament of C-2, with resultant symptoms of cord compression, may complicate rheumatoid arthritis. C-spine inflexibility from ankylosing spondylitis predisposes to injury out of proportion to mechanism. Anterior spinal artery syndrome may result from rheumatologic conditions causing vasculitis, aortic dissection, or embolism.

The Eye

Rheumatologic involvement ranges from mild irritation to complete blindness.

Temporal arteritis is a cause of sudden blindness and should be considered in any patient older than 50 who presents with new onset headache, visual changes, or jaw or tongue claudication. Lab investigation reveals an elevated Westergren sedimentation rate (> 50 mm/ h), anemia, and elevated alkaline phosphatase. Treatment consists of prednisone 60 mg/day and is initiated immediately, based on clinical and laboratory findings. Treatment is not delayed for definitive diagnosis which requires temporal artery biopsy. Biopsy however, must be obtained within the 1st week of treatment to be accurate.

Dry eyes and dry mouth from Sjogren's syndrome may occur alone or coexist with many rheumatologic conditions.

Episcleritis is a self-limiting, painless injection of the episcleral vessels. It is in the differential diagnosis of the red eye in patients with rheumatoid arthritis.

Scleritis, also seen in patients with rheumatoid arthritis, presents with marked ocular tenderness. The eye has a purple discoloration. The potential for visual impairment and scleral rupture mandate emergent ophthalmologic consult and high dose steroids.

Kidney

Renal insult is common in rheumatologic conditions and is due either to the primary disease process, the drugs used to treat the disease, or both.

Nephritis is a common complication of systemic lupus erythematosus and systemic vasculitis. Renal dysfunction from malignant hypertension occurs with scleroderma.

Nephrotic syndrome in patients with systemic lupus erythematosus predisposes to renal vein thrombosis.

Renal insufficiency from prostaglandin inhibition by NSAIDs is more frequent in the elderly. It also may result from rhabdomyolysis in the patient with florid myositis.

Joint

Synovial fluid analysis is important in accurate diagnosis of articular problems. Fluid is sent for a gram-stain, culture, cell count, and crystal analysis, and evaluated for turbidity and mucin clot. Fluid may be categorized as normal, noninflammatory, or inflammatory (Table 167-1).

Traumatic arthritis with a hemarthrosis causes swelling within minutes of an injury. A sprain causes swelling over hours.

Septic arthritis is a medical emergency as the inflammatory response can destroy a joint within h. Pain may develop over h. On initial exam, effusions may be scant. Both active and passive range of motion will be resisted secondary to pain. A previously diseased or injured joint is more prone than a normal joint so flare of a single joint, in a patient with rheumatoid arthritis or gout, for example, may represent infection.

Staph, strep, and H. flu are the most common causes of septic arthritis. The patient presents with typical symptoms. Gonococcus causes a migratory arthritis and tenosynovitis followed by a septic arthritis. Vesiculopustular lesions, especially on the fingers, are an important clue. Synovial fluid cultures are often negative. Cultures of the throat, urethra, cervix, and rectum before antibiotics increase the yield of the organism. Mycoplasma and ureaplasma occur in immunosuppressed patients. Tuberculous and fungal arthritides may smolder for months before diagnosis is made. A synovial biopsy is required to identify the organism.

Osteomyelitis adjacent to a joint may elicit a sympathetic effusion that is sterile with a low cell count.

Lyme disease is characterized by a migratory arthritis in the second phase of the disease and a chronic arthritis, especially of the knee, in the third phase.

Gout and *pseudogout* are crystal induced arthritides that occur mainly in middleaged and elderly adults. Arthrocentesis is required to make the initial diagnosis. Gout classically involves the MTP of the great toe but commonly involves any extremity joint. Microscopic examination

TABLE 167-1. Examination of Synovial Fluid

	Normal	Noninflammatory	Inflammatory	Hemarthrosis
Gross appearance	Transparent, clear	Transparent, yellow	Cloudy, yellow	Bloody
String sign	Normal	Normal	Diminished or absent	Approaches peripheral
WBC/mm³	<200	<200	>2000	
PMNs	<25%	<25%	>50%	
Culture	Negative	Negative	>50% positive	Negative
Crystals	Negative	Negative	±Positive	Negative
Associated conditions		Osteoarthritis, trauma, neuropathic arthritis, SLE, hypertrophic osteoarthritis, rheumatic fever	Septic arthritis, crystal arthritis, seronegative spondyloarthritis, RA, SLE, polymyositis, acute rheumatic fever, Lyme disease	See Table 238-6 (in Emergency Medicine: A Comprehensive Study Guide)

under polarized light reveals negatively birefringent, needle-shaped urate crystals. A uric acid level does not aid in the diagnosis, as it is typically low to normal during an acute exacerbation.

Pseudogout also commonly involves extremity joints. Microscopic exam under polarized light reveals positively birefringent, rhomboid-shaped calcium pyrophosphate crystals. Treatment of gout and pseudogout is the same. NSAIDs are effective such as indomethacin (50 mg PO tid). An alternate is colchicine (0.6 mg PO q h) until pain relief or GI side-effects occur. IV colchicine is also available. When a suspected attack of gout or pseudogout is unresponsive to treatment, one should suspect other causes, such as septic arthritis, and evaluate with repeat arthrocentesis.

Baker's cyst classically occurs in patients with rheumatoid arthritis. It is formed when inflammatory joint fluid dissects into the popliteal space. Rupture of the cyst mimics a DVT. Three features distinguishing this condition from DVT are: (1) swelling spares the foot; (2) crescent sign is present where blood layers below the medial malleolus around the ankle ligaments and tendons, forming a purple crescent; (3) history of sudden decline in size of effusion or popliteal fullness. An arthrogram is diagnostic (ultrasound may be). Treatment consists of arthrocentesis and steroid injection.

Septic bursitis is associated with a puncture wound or overlying cellulitis. WBC counts are only 10% of those seen in septic arthritis. Treatment requires drainage; the needle should be tunneled subcutaneously 1 to 2 cm to the bursa to minimize the risk of a chronic fistula.

Avascular necrosis most commonly affects the femoral head and manifests as progressive focal bone pain that worsens with weightbearing. X-ray findings lag behind symptom onset by about 2 wks. MRI will detect the condition earlier.

For further reading in *Emergency Medicine: A Comprehensive Study Guide*, 4th edition, see Chapter 238, Musculoskeletal Disorders in Adults, by Mary Chester Morgan.

Infectious and NonInfectious
Inflammatory Conditions
of the Hand

Michael P. Kefer

As with traumatic injuries to the hand, rest and elevation are the main-stays of treatment for nontraumatic conditions to decrease inflammation, avoid secondary injury, and prevent spread of any existing infection. The optimal position of the hand for splinting is the position of function: wrist—15° extension; MCP—50° to 90° flexion; PIP—10° to 15° flexion; DIP—10° to 15° flexion.

Noninfectious Conditions

Tendonitis and tenosynovitis These conditions are usually due to over-use. Treatment usually consists of immobilization and NSAIDs. Nonin-fectious synovitis also may be treated by injection of deposteroids. Triamcinolone (40 mg/ml) mixed with 0.5% bupivacaine is injected into the synovial sheath.

Trigger finger This is a tenosynovitis of the flexor sheaths of the digits and may result in stenosing of the tendon sheath. Impingement and snap release of the tendon occurs as the finger is extended from a flexed position. Steroid injection may be effective treatment for early stages. Definitive treatment is surgery.

Dupuytren's contracture This condition, resulting from fibrous changes in the subcutaneous tissues of the palm, may lead to tethering and joint contractures. Referral to a hand surgeon is indicated.

Infectious Conditions

The most common organism causing hand infection is *Staph aureus*. Infections from animal bite wounds may be infected with *Pasteurella multocida*, and human bite wounds with *Eichenella corrodens*. Ab-scesses always require surgical drainage.

In treating wounds of the hand, jet irrigation is the optimal method of cleansing the wound. Prophylactic antibiotics are indicated in acute open hand injuries. A cephalosporin or a penicillinase-resistant penicil-lin is a good choice. Erythromycin or clindamycin is an alternate for penicillin-allergic patients.

Felon This is an infection of the pulp space of the fingertip. Pain results from a buildup of pus in the fibrous septae of the finger pad. Treatment consists of drainage by the lateral approach to protect the neurovascular bundle. An incision begins 5 mm distal to the DIP crease and continues just palmar to and parallel with the paronychium folds, stopping distally at the tip of the distal phalangeal tuft. The incision should be deep enough to extend across the entire finger pad to divide the septae at the bony insertions. Unless there is a pointing abscess, the radial aspect of the index and long finger, and the ulnar aspect of the thumb and small finger, should be avoided. Pack the wound loosely. Splint the finger and wrist in the position of function. Check the wound in 24 and 48 h. Then pull the packing and begin warm soaks.

Paronychia This is an infection of the lateral nail fold. Treatment of a small paronychia consists of inserting a #11 blade into the nail fold parallel to the nail to drain the abscess. In an advanced infection, or when pus is seen beneath the nail, the corner of the paronychium should be incised and the nail fold lifted. A portion of the nail may have to be removed and a wick placed for adequate drainage. Avoid injury to the nail bed. Check the wound and replace the wick in 24 h. After 48 h, pull the wick and begin warm soaks.

Herpetic whitlow This is a viral infection of the fingertip involving intracutaneous vesicles. Clinically, it may present similar to a felon. Treatment is to prevent autoinoculation and transmission by covering with a dry dressing.

Pyogenic flexor tenosynovitis This is most commonly caused by skin organisms and *Pseudomonas*. Clinically, four cardinal signs are: (1) tenderness over the flexor tendon sheath; (2) symmetric swelling of the finger; (3) pain with passive extension; and (4) flexed position of the involved digit. ED care is splinting, elevation, IV antibiotics, and emergent surgical consult.

Web space infection This occurs after penetrating injury to the web space. Clinically, dorsal and volar swelling of the web space with separation of the digits is noted. ED care is splinting, elevation, IV antibiotics, and emergent surgical consult.

Midpalmar space infection This occurs from spread of a flexor tenosynovitis or penetrating wound to the palm causing infection of the radial or ulnar bursa of the hand. ED care is splinting, elevation, IV antibiotics, and emergent surgical consult.

Human bite wound This condition, a clenched fist injury to the MCP, results from punching an opponent in the mouth and hitting the teeth. Risk of infection spreading along the extensor tendons is high. The most common organisms are mouth flora: α- and ß-hemolytic strep, *S. aureus, E. corrodens*, and *Neisseria* species. Appropriate antibiotic coverage includes penicillin and a penicillinase-resistant penicillin effective against staph. Erythromycin or clindamycin are alternatives for penicillin-allergic patients. Wounds penetrating the skin should be explored and irrigated in the operating room and allowed to heal by secondary intention. When inspecting for extensor tendon injury, remember to consider the position of the hand at the time of injury. Extensor tendon repair should be delayed 5 days or until the wound is clean.

For further reading in *Emergency Medicine: A Comprehensive Study Guide*, 4th edition, see Chapter 239, Infectious and NonInfectious Inflammatory States of the Hand, by Robert R. Simon and David Slobodkin.

Chronic foot problems often present to the ED for initial diagnosis and management. Advanced age, poverty, and female gender are associated with an increased risk.

TINEA PEDIS

Clinical Features

Tinea Pedis is estimated to affect 10% of the population. The most common form of infection is interdigital, usually between the fourth and fifth toes. The interspaces appear white, macerated, and soggy. The infected areas are pruritic and may become painful. Some types of organisms may infect the entire foot or produce vesicular lesions.

Diagnosis and Differential

Diagnosis of tinea pedis is made clinically since fungal cultures usually have a very low yield. Juvenile plantar dermatosis may be confused with tinea. Affected children have dry, cracked, red scaly patches on the toe pads and anterior planter surface of the feet with sparing of the interdigital spaces. Treatment consists of lubrication and occlusion. Contact dermatitis also may mimic tinea. It typically involves only the dorsum of the foot with well-demarcated red patches that may contain tiny vesicles. Psoriasis presents with thick scaly lesions that spare the interdigital areas and affects the heel. Erythrasma is a low-grade chronic infection that may involve the interdigital areas but is also typically present in the groin and axilla. These lesions will fluoresce bright coral red under a Wood's lamp.

Emergency Department Care and Disposition

Due to interactive bacterial infections and other factors, the ideal medication for tinea must be antifungal, antibacterial, anti-inflammatory, and have a local drying effect. The imidazole group of **antifungals** (miconazole, clotrimazole, econazole, ketoconazole, oxiconazole, and sulcomazole) meet these criteria and also cover Candida. Creams and solutions are most appropriate. Ointments hold the active ingredient in place longer but should not be used on oozing or moist lesions. Sprays are effective. It is important to stress proper hygiene including daily foot cleaning, drying, and changes in socks and footwear. High-risk patients should not walk barefoot.

ONYCHOMYCOSIS

Clinical Features

Fungal infections of the nail plate can lead to severe disturbances in nail growth. The affected toenails may appear opaque, discolored, and hyperkeratotic. The infection can spread to the surrounding skin. Autoavulsion and traumatic avulsion of the involved toenail is common.

Emergency Department Care and Disposition

Treatment is difficult due to the poor absorption of topical antifungals. If less than one half of the nail is involved, an empiric trial of imidazole antifungals should be done. Repeated debridement of the nail is necessary so the patient should be referred for continued care. Surgical or chemical removal of the nail may be required. Even with optimal care, recurrence is high.

ONCHOCRYPTOSIS (INGROWN TOENAIL)

Clinical Features

Ingrown toenails occur when a segment of the nail plate penetrates the nail sulcus and subcutaneous tissue. This is most commonly due to curvature of the nail plate and is often associated with external trauma or self-treatment. Inflammation, swelling, and infection of the medial or lateral aspect of the toenail are present. The great toe is most commonly affected. In patients with underlying diabetes or arterial insufficiency, cellulitis, ulceration, and necrosis may lead to amputation if diagnosis and treatment is delayed.

Emergency Department Care and Disposition

If infection is not present, simple elevation of the nail with a wisp of cotton between the nail plate and the skin, daily foot soaks, and avoidance of pressure on the area are usually sufficient treatment. A small corner of the offending nail including the embedded portion also may be removed after a digital block. If granulation or infection is present, **partial removal of the nail** is indicated under a digital block. Using a nail splitter or scissors, the nail is cut parallel to the toe, including the portion under the cuticle. The affected cut portion is then removed by grasping and pulling with a hemostat. The nail groove is then debrided. The nail plate may be cauterized by clinicians experienced in this procedure. A nonadherent gauze and antibiotic ointment should be placed on the wound, and the wound should be checked in 24 to 48 h.

PUNCTURE WOUND

Clinical Features

Features depend on the penetrating material, footwear at the time, time of injury, and overall health of the patient. Typically, the location is on the plantar surface of the foot.

Emergency Department Care and Disposition

The wound must be examined for removal of any foreign body and potential joint involvement. Plain radiographs are helpful, but CT, MRI, and ultrasonography also may be needed for further evaluation. Fluoroscopy may aid in removal of foreign bodies. After a foreign body has been removed or excluded, the wound should be cleaned, irrigated and, if necessary, closed. **Antibiotics** are indicated for infected wounds. Pseudomonal coverage should be used in wounds which have penetrated through sneakers. Recurrent infection, deep-tissue tenderness, and increased soft tissue swelling raise the possibility of a retained foreign body and deep-tissue infection. Specialty referral and possible admission is indicated.

FOOT ULCERS

Clinical Features

Foot ulcers are typically either ischemic or neuropathic. Ischemic ulcers present with a cool foot, dependent rubor, pallor on elevation, atrophic shiny skin, and diminished pulses. Neuropathic ulcers occur as a result of loss of sensation. Ulcers then result from localized ischemia associated with ill-fitting shoes, foreign bodies, abnormal bony prominences, or the daily stresses of walking. Neuropathic ulcers are typically well-circumscribed with a surrounding white callus-like material. If no vascular disease is present, the foot will have a normal temperature, color, and pulse, but defects in touch, pressure, and proprioception are noted.

Emergency Department Care and Disposition

An infected ulcer requires debridement and complete pressure relief. Wet-to-dry dressings are not a substitute for debridement. Antibiotics and, often, admission are warranted for the treatment of infected ulcers. Cultures of drainage material should be obtained. Broad-spectrum antibiotic coverage include clindamycin along with an aminoglycoside, cefoxitin, ticarcillin disodium, or clavulanate potassium. Cellulitis or signs of deep-tissue infection require admission. Abscesses should be incised and drained. X-rays should be considered to assess for osteomyelitis, subcutaneous gas, foreign body, and Charcot foot.

For further reading in *Emergency Medicine: A Comprehensive Study Guide*, 4th edition, see Chapter 240, Soft Tissue Problems of the Foot, by Frantz Melio.

Dexter L. Morris

Psychiatric disorders are classified according to the Diagnostic and Statistical Manual of Mental Disorders (DSM-IV), which has three major axes (categories) from which to chose a diagnosis. Brief descriptions of the clinical features of the major illnesses are provided below.

PSYCHIATRIC SYNDROMES (AXIS I DISORDERS)

Dementia

The main feature of dementia is a decrease in cognitive functioning. This can occur in several areas, including, memory, abstract thinking, judgment, and personality. These functions can be assessed by a mental status examination and history from the family. Memory disturbance is usually the earliest sign to appear. Anxiety and depression may accompany early dementia. Onset of dementia is usually gradual.

Delirium

Delirium is also characterized by global impairment in cognitive function but has several additional features. Patients with delirium have clouding of consciousness, decreased awareness and altered alertness, including sensory misperception, drowsiness, and stupor. Onset of delirium is usually acute, and intensity can fluctuate widely.

SUBSTANCE-INDUCED DISORDERS

Defined as impairment of judgment, perception, attention, emotional or psychomotor control that accompanies a recent exposure to an exogenous substance, a patient with induced substance-abuse disorder should not have other features of delirium or hallucinosis. Repeated episodes result in a diagnosis of a substance-abuse disorder. Withdrawal is a term used for withdrawal symptoms that are mild and without signs of delirium.

SCHIZOPHRENIA AND OTHER PSYCHOTIC DISORDERS

These disorders are marked by delusions (fixed false beliefs not shared by others of similar cultural backgrounds) and hallucinations. One of the most serious health problems in the world, patients with psychosis take up a significant portion of health-care resources.

Schizophrenia

The features of schizophrenia are: (1) deterioration in functioning; (2) the presence of hallucinations, delusions, disorganized speech, or catatonic behavior for at least 1 mo; and (3) the absence of a mood disorder. The disease usually manifests in late adolescence or early adulthood and a prodromal period of decreased functioning usually precedes the active psychotic features. Antipsychotic medications usually help the active symptoms but may not affect the level of function of the patient as much. Schizophrenics commonly present or are brought to the ED after stopping or running out of their medications. A schizophreniform disorder is similar to schizophrenia, but the symptoms have not been present long enough (6 mo) to confirm diagnosis.

Brief Psychotic Disorder

This is a psychosis which lasts less than two wks and is generally precipitated by a traumatic experience such as death of a loved one or a life-threatening situation.

Delusional Disorder

Persistent nonbizarre delusions are the hallmark of this disorder that distinguish it from schizophrenia. Patients usually are functional and outwardly normal appearing.

MOOD DISORDERS

Mood or affective disorders are the most prevalent psychiatric disorders and affect 10% to 15% of the general population during their lifetimes. They tend to be episodic with periods of remission and normal function.

Major Depression

The features of this disorder include a persistent dysphoric mood and loss of interest in usual activities lasting for at least 2 wks. Feelings of self-reproach, worthlessness, anhedonia, and recurrent thoughts of death or suicide are common. Vegetative symptoms are also present and include loss of appetite, sleep disturbances, fatigue, and inability to concentrate. The illness is more common in women, persons with a family history of depression or suicide and people with medical or other psychiatric illnesses.

Bipolar Disorder

Mania is the main characteristic of this disorder, formerly termed manic-depressive illness. Manics are expansive, energetic, elated, but quickly become argumentative, hostile, or sarcastic if their plans are thwarted. Other signs include decreased need for sleep, rapid speech, and racing thoughts. Poor judgment in monetary or sexual matters may lead to problems that prompt treatment. Manics often have grandiose ideas and lack insight into their surroundings, thus consultation with family or friends is important. Patients also have periods of depression. The disorder has no sex preference and has onset in the 3rd or 4th decades. Depressive episodes are more common than manic ones and suicide and drug abuse is common.

Dysthymic Disorder

This is a chronic and less severe form of depression. A depressed mood must be present more days than not for at least 2 years. Patients have a lifelong gloomy outlook but remain functional.

ANXIETY DISORDERS

Panic Disorder

Recurrent panic attacks are the hallmark of this disorder. These attacks consist of a sudden surge of anxiety, along with autonomic signs including palpitations, tachycardia, shortness of breath, chest tightness, dizziness, and sweating. Patients often present to the ED with these symptoms. Careful history, including questions about domestic violence and sexual abuse is indicated.

Generalized Anxiety Disorders

These patients have constant anxiety rather than panic attacks. They may have some of the autonomic symptoms of those patients with panic disorder.

Phobic Disorders

These are anxiety disorders associated with specific exposures, such as heights, social occasions, etc. The symptoms are similar to panic disorders.

SOMATOFORM DISORDERS

This is a group of disorders in which patients have particular complaints for which no physical cause can be found. When the complaint is specific, such as paralysis, it is called a conversion disorder. Less specific complaints are classified as somatization disorders. Reassuring the patient that there is no major physical problem and referring them for further care is appropriate.

PERSONALITY DISORDERS

Individuals with personality disorders have difficulty perceiving, relating to, and reacting to their environment and interpersonal relations. They are often easy to recognize, manipulative, but very frustrating to treat in the ED. It is important to establish firm limits on their behavior and focus on the chief complaint.

For further reading in *Emergency Medicine: A Comprehensive Study Guide*, 4th edition, see Chapter 241, Behavioral Disorders: Clinical Features, by Stephen C. Olsen and Douglas A. Rund.

171 | Behavioral Disorders: Emergency Assessment and Stabilization

Burton Bentley II

INITIAL EVALUATION

A thorough medical–psychiatric history and physical exam are the most effective tools for the ED evaluation of behavioral disorders. An immediate goal is to attempt to distinguish organic from functional disorders. Since few functional disturbances begin abruptly, a sudden onset of a major change in behavior, mood, or thought is most likely to result from an organic cause. The following life-threatening conditions may result in abrupt behavior disturbances and must be systematically ruled out:

1. Central nervous system infection (meningitis or encephalitis)
2. Intoxication
3. Alcohol or drug withdrawal
4. Hypoglycemia
5. Hypertensive encephalopathy
6. Hypoxia
7. Intracranial hemorrhage
8. Poisoning
9. Head trauma
10. Seizure
11. Acute organ system failure

For the severely impaired patient, third-party accounts may be the only reliable source of historical information. The changed behavior is an excellent starting point for inquiry, and it should always be evaluated relative to the patient's previous level of functioning. In addition to the standard questions asked during the history of present illness, evaluation of the behaviorally disturbed patient should include the following data:

1. Thorough review of systems, focusing on neurologic symptoms (e.g., confusion, recently impaired speech, headaches).
2. Description of previous and recent highest level of functioning.
3. Previous psychiatric illness and treatment.
4. History of substance abuse, prescribed drugs, and over-the-counter medication usage.
5. Exposure to occupational hazards or toxins (e.g., heavy metals, organic solvents).
6. Identity of stressors in the patient's environment that may provoke or accentuate disturbed behavior.

MENTAL STATUS EXAMINATION

Important components of the mental status examination include assessment of affect, orientation, language, memory, thought content, perceptual abnormalities, and judgment. Impaired language performance, including difficulty with speech, reading, writing, and word finding may indicate a neurologic disorder. The patient's affect should be evaluated for sadness, euphoria, or anxiety. This observation may help to distinguish between psychiatric illness induced by affective disorders versus true organic dementia. The experience of hallucinations should also be reviewed; visual hallucinations favor organic etiologies, whereas auditory hallucinations are often functional. Lastly, the clock-face test may be useful. To perform this test, the physician draws a circle and asks the patient to fill in the numbers and hands to form the face of a clock. The inability to perform this task suggests organic disease.

PHYSICAL AND LABORATORY EVALUATIONS

The physical exam should identify problems that may have caused or impacted up the behavioral disorder. Also, it should uncover medical problems that require special care or that may be inappropriate for management in a psychiatric-hospital setting.

A thorough neurologic examination is essential and should include a search for focal neurologic deficits, such as apraxia, agnosia, right–left disorientation, aphasia, asymmetric reflexes, and paresis.

Many medical illnesses cause both acute behavioral disturbances and a change in vital signs. Abnormal vital signs must never be dismissed as being secondary only to the behavioral disturbance itself. For example:

1. Bradycardia may be secondary to: hypothyroidism, Stokes–Adams syndrome, elevated intracranial pressure, cholinergic poisoning.
2. Tachycardia may be secondary to hyperthyroidism, infection, heart failure, pulmonary embolism, alcohol withdrawal, anticholinergic or sympathomimetic poisoning.
3. Fever may be secondary to thyroid storm, vasculitis, alcohol withdrawal, sedative–hypnotic withdrawal, infection.
4. Hypothermia may be secondary to sepsis, hypoendocrine status, CNS dysfunction, alcohol intoxication.
5. Hypotension may be secondary to shock, Addison's disease, hypothyroidism, medication side effect.
6. Hypertension may be secondary to hypertensive encephalopathy, stimulant abuse.
7. Tachypnea may be secondary to metabolic acidosis, pulmonary embolism, cardiac failure, fever.

SUICIDE

Suicide attempts are made by roughly 1% of the population and regardless of how trivial the attempt may seem, the action must be taken seriously. Medical problems must be addressed efficiently, and the suicide risk should be assessed.

Schizophrenia, substance abuse, and depression are psychiatric diagnoses that place patients at a relatively high suicide risk. Personality or adjustment disorders are frequent diagnoses in people who attempt suicide, although they have a lower risk of completion. Violent suicide attempts (e.g., shooting, hanging) are considered high risk for a future attempt. In general, the risk of a successful suicide increases with advancing age. Other factors that contribute to suicide risk include male gender, divorced or widowed marital status, unemployment, poor health, prior suicide attempts, history of poor achievement, and social isolation.

During the clinical interview, patients who display hopelessness, helplessness, exhaustion, overwhelming depression, or clear suicidal intent obviously remain at high risk; immediate psychiatric consultation and hospitalization is required. Patients at lower suicide risk often show remorse or embarrassment about the attempt, and the action may have been taken during a period of transient anger. Patients who refuse to provide any information about the event must be considered to be at high risk. Patient disposition can also be aided by considering the lethality of the attempt and the likelihood of rescue. For example, the patient who attempts to hang himself while alone at home is at much greater risk than the patient who takes a few pills in front of friends.

High-risk patients with strong suicidal intent require immediate psychiatric hospitalization. Moderate-risk patients are those who have a positive response to initial intervention and favorable social support. They are judged not to be in immediate danger and may often be treated right away in the outpatient setting. This determination is made in concert with a psychiatric consultant and requires the support of family or friends. Low-risk patients often present following suicide threats or minor attempts that occur in the context of a clearly definable external crisis. Provided they have a responsive and available social support system, they may be managed as outpatients once immediate followup has been arranged. Any patient whose suicide risk cannot be determined must be evaluated by a psychiatric consultant and considered for hospitalization.

Physical and Chemical Restraint

In order to protect patients from harming themselves and others, violent behavior demands immediate physical restraint. This action should only be undertaken by trained personnel such as hospital security teams or local police. An initial show of force may be sufficient to induce the patient to accept physical or chemical restraint without further resistance. This approach usually requires five team members with each one assigned to a limb, and the leader controlling the head. All restrained patients should be disrobed, gowned, and searched for weapons.

Chemical restraint is indicated for those patients whose behavior remains dangerously uncontrolled despite adequate physical restraint.

Lorazepam (Ativan) is often considered to be the agent of choice for control of the agitated patient. It has rapid onset of action, a wide therapeutic index, and may be given orally, IV, or IM. Typical starting doses of lorazepam are 1 to 2 mg IM or 1 mg IV, repeated every 30 min, as necessary. Respiratory depression may occur and can be treated with flumazenil (Romazicon). **Haloperidol** (Haldol) and **droperidol** (Inapsine) are neuroleptic tranquilizers that may be used as single-line agents or to augment the effect of lorazepam. They are particularly good for patients whose agitation has psychotic features. The dose of haloperidol may be titrated, starting at 2.5 to 5 mg IM Droperidol's onset of action is rapid by both the IV and IM routes, and is usually started at 2.5 to 5 mg via either route. Hypotension from either agent usually responds to crystalloid infusion.

Potentially violent behavior requires a nonthreatening attitude by the physician and staff while an adequate backup force is summoned. This force should be clearly visible, and the patient must be informed that certain types of unacceptable behavior will result in restraint. The physician should avoid excessive eye contact, maintain a somewhat submissive posture, and stand in a location that neither threatens the patient nor blocks his own retreat from the room. Potentially violent situations may be defused by allowing the patient to ventilate feelings verbally while the physician makes neutral comments and sets limits on behavior.

The decision to release a patient from restraints should be made jointly by medical and nursing personnel on the basis of the patient's behavior and not as a result of bargains or threats. Restraints are then released in steps, over time.

For further reading in *Emergency Medicine: A Comprehensive Study Guide*, 4th edition, see Chapter 242, Emergency Assessment and Stabilization of Psychiatric Patients, by Jeffery C. Hutzler and Douglas Rund.

There are five major classes of psychotropic medications with which the emergency physician should be familiar: antipsychotics, anxiolytics, sedatives, antidepressants, and lithium.

ANTIPSYCHOTICS (NEUROLEPTICS)

Indications and Guidelines

In the ED, neuroleptics are used to control both psychotic and nonpsychotic agitation. Prior dystonic reactions, pregnancy, and a history of neuroleptic malignant syndrome are relative contraindications to usage. High-potency antipsychotics such as haloperidol (Haldol) and fluphenazine (Prolixin) have relatively few anticholinergic side-effects and are generally safe. Management of acute psychotic agitation often combines one of these agents with a benzodiazepine. A typical regimen might include 5 mg of IM haloperidol and 1 mg of IM lorazepam (Ativan), with dosing repeated as necessary.

Side-Effects

Acute dystonic reactions are the most common neuroleptic side-effect. Spasms may involve the neck (torticollis), muscles of mastication (trismus), back (opisthotonos), eyes (oculogyric crisis), or larynx (laryngospasm). Treatment with 1 to 2 mg of benztropine, IV or IM, or 25 to 50 mg of diphenhydramine, IV or IM, rapidly abolishes the dystonia. Dystonia may recur despite discontinuance of the neuroleptic, so prophylactic medication is required. Effective regimens include 1 mg of oral benztropine or 25 mg of oral diphenhydramine given 3 to 4 times daily for several days.

Akathisia is a syndrome of motor restlessness mainly characterized by the patient's inability to keep the lower extremities still. It may begin days to weeks after neuroleptics are started and is often misdiagnosed as anxiety or increasing psychosis, which may then prompt a detrimental increase in the patient's medication. Treatment may consist of decreasing the neuroleptic dosage, adding benztropine, or discontinuing the medication entirely.

Antipsychotic-induced Parkinsonism syndrome is common in elderly patients within the 1st month of treatment. Patients may display any or all of the classic Parkinsonian features, including bradykinesia, resting tremor, cogwheel rigidity, shuffling gait, masked facies, or drooling. Reduction in the neuroleptic dosage and addition of benztropine is usually effective.

Anticholinergic effects range from sedation to delirium, and may include dry mouth, blurred vision with mydriasis, urinary retention, or ileus. Symptomatic improvement is usually seen with discontinuation of the neuroleptic and supportive care. Life-threatening anticholinergic symptoms may be temporized with careful administration of 1 to 2 mg of IV physostigmine.

Cardiovascular side effects result from α-adrenergic blockade and include orthostatic hypotension and decreased myocardial inotropy. IV fluids, norepinephrine (Levophed), or metaraminol (Aramine) may be required.

Neuroleptic malignant syndrome (NMS) is an idiosyncratic reaction manifested by rigidity, fever, autonomic instability, and confusion. NMS is a true medical emergency with a mortality of 20%. Treatment includes ICU admission, discontinuation of the neuroleptic, avoidance of anticholinergics, and meticulous supportive care of cardiorespiratory function.

Clozapine and Risperidone

Clozapine (Clozaril) is a unique antipsychotic medication that has no extrapyramidal side-effects, although it may rarely cause NMS. It is still strongly anticholinergic, lowers the seizure threshold, and may produce sedation and hypotension. The predominant adverse reaction is agranulocytosis, requiring consultation with a hematologist. Risperidone (Risperdal) is a newer antipsychotic that also causes fewer extrapyramidal symptoms, especially at low doses. Agranulocytosis does not occur, and side-effects are mild, including constipation, insomnia, and anxiety. Seizures occur in 0.3% of patients.

ANXIOLYTICS

Indications and Guidelines

Short-term anxiolysis may be beneficial for the anxious, agitated patient during a psychosocial crisis or acute panic reaction. Nonpsychiatric uses include sedation and muscle relaxation during procedures, seizure control, and treatment of alcohol and sedative withdrawal. Benzodiazepines are effective anxiolytics with a high therapeutic index. The short-acting benzodiazepines, which are most useful in the ED, include lorazepam (Ativan), oxazepam (Serax), and alprazolam (Xanax); alprazolam is the drug of choice for acute anxiety disorders and panic attack. Only lorazepam (Ativan) and midazolam (Versed) have reliable intramuscular absorption and may be given by this route. All benzodiazepines require careful dosage titration; higher dosages may be required in patients with a history of alcohol or sedative/hypnotic abuse, and lower dosages are used in patients with hepatic disease or debilitation.

Side-Effects

Sedation and ataxia are the most common side-effects and are managed by dosage reduction and restriction of hazardous activities. Paradoxical responses of insomnia and agitation require discontinuation of the medication. Benzodiazepines are respiratory depressants, and extreme caution must be exercised if they are given to intoxicated or hypercarbic patients.

HETEROCYCLIC ANTIDEPRESSANTS (HCAs)

HCAs are used to treat a number of psychiatric and nonpsychiatric entities including major depression, panic disorder, obsessive–compulsive disorder, enuresis, and chronic pain syndromes.

MONOAMINE OXIDASE INHIBITORS (MAOIs)

MAOIs are useful in the treatment of atypical major depressive episodes. Only two agents, phenelzine (Nardil) and tranylcypromine (Parnate) are commonly used in the United States. ED initiation of therapy with these agents is not recommended.

SELECTIVE SEROTONIN REUPTAKE INHIBITORS (SSRIs)

SSRIs are the most widely prescribed antidepressants in the United States, and include fluoxetine (Prozac), sertraline (Zoloft), and paroxetine (Paxil).

LITHIUM

Lithium is indicated for the treatment of several major depressive disorders, including bipolar disorder. The long latency of action precludes its use as an emergency psychotropic medication.

For further discussion on the toxicologic effects and treatment of heterocyclic antidepressants, MAOIs, SSRIs, and lithium, see Chapter 92, Psychopharmacologic Agents, by Keith Mausner.

For further reading in *Emergency Medicine: A Comprehensive Study Guide*, 4th edition, see Chapter 243, Psychotropic Medications, by Kathy Shy.

Dexter L. Morris

Eating disorders affect 5% to 10% of young women, with anorexia more common at ages 13 to 14 and 17 to 18, and bulimia at ages 17 to 25. These disorders can cause death, as well as medical and social disability.

Clinical Features

Anorexia is suggested by the refusal to maintain normal body weight, intense fear of becoming obese, the perception of being obese even though underweight, and the absence of at least 3 consecutive expected menstrual cycles. Bulimia is suggested by 2 episodes of binge eating per week for 3 mo, self-induced vomiting, use of laxatives, strict dieting or fasting to prevent weight gain, and overconcern with body shape and weight.

Eating disorder patients can present with several serious medical problems. Binge eating can produce acute gastric distention and pancreatitis (10% mortality rate). Starvation can lead to hypoglycemia (which can also be fatal) and changes in respiratory muscles. Cardiovascular changes include arrhythmias and cardiomyopathy, as well as secondary problems due to electrolyte abnormalities. Other medical problems include pretibial edema, peripheral neuropathy, stress fractures, and osteoporosis. Young diabetics with frequent hospitalizations may have underlying eating disorders.

Emergency Department Diagnosis, Care and Disposition

In addition to a careful history and physical exam, testing for electrolyte and cardiac abnormalities is indicated. Toxicology for diuretics or stool samples for phenolphthalein (laxative) may be useful. Patients with severe metabolic derangements should have slow correction with IV fluids and parenteral nutrition. Fluid overload should be avoided. Psychiatric consult should be obtained and consideration for admission given if the weight loss is severe, significant depression is evident, or the patient is unsafe to return to an outside environment. Some medications, such as antidepressants, have been found to be useful, but such decisions should be left to the psychiatrist. ED physicians should remember that although these disorders may seem benign, they do cause death.

For further reading in *Emergency Medicine: A Comprehensive Study Guide*, 4th edition, see Chapter 244, Anorexia Nervosa and Bulimia Nervosa, by Alexander H. Sackeyfio and Susan J. Gottlieb.

174 | Panic Disorder

C. Crawford Mechem

Panic disorder is a subcategory of anxiety disorders, characterized by a variety of autonomic symptoms, at times associated with altered states of mind such as depersonalization or derealization. Panic disorder is more common in young women, and the illness tends to prevail through midlife.

Clinical Features

The early phase of panic disorder is characterized by brief episodes that terminate in less than 10 min. During the attack the patient is overwhelmed by anxiety, with associated tachycardia, tachypnea, dyspnea, chest tightness, weakness, and dizziness. Once the first attack has occurred, it is likely to be followed by recurrent attacks, all usually of 10-min duration. Recurrent attacks can lead to agoraphobia, secondary depression, and an increased risk of suicide.

Diagnosis and Differential

Careful history and physical exam should rule out significant physical illnesses, including acute myocardial infarction, hypoglycemia, hyperthyroidism, pheochromocytoma, complex partial seizures, mitral valve prolapse, alcohol and drug withdrawal, excessive caffeine use, drug abuse, and sleep disorders. Lab findings associated with panic disorder have been identified in recent years, but their usefulness is limited to research at this time.

Emergency Department Care and Disposition

Treatment is divided into drug and behavior therapy. Traditional psychotherapy is usually ineffective. For patients willing to take medication, **imipramine** (10 to 25 mg), may be given at night as a starting dose, up to 150 mg/d. Alcohol and caffeine should be avoided. Anticholinergic side-effects, hypotension, and sedation may be seen. SSRIs, such as fluoxetine, sertraline, and clomipramine have been shown to be effective. These agents are likely to cause initial drug-induced anxiety, however, and should be used with caution. **Alprazolam** (1 to 2 mg/d), will rapidly relieve panic symptoms in mildly affected patients. This drug should be discontinued gradually because of the risk of withdrawal symptoms. Clonidine can be effective during the first 4 wks of treatment, but tachyphylaxis may develop. Desipramine is not associated with tolerance and is generally considered safe for long-term use.

Many communities now have specialty clinics and support groups. Patients should be guided into one of these programs. Careful listening, explanation, and reassurance frequently bring about a positive thera-peutic response.

For further reading in *Emergency Medicine: A Comprehensive Study Guide*, 4th edition, see Chapter 245, Panic Disorder, by Suck Won Kim.

Conversion Reactions

Dexter L. Morris

Conversion reactions are rare, more common in women, and usually present during adolescence or early adulthood.

Clinical Features

Conversion reactions usually present as a single symptom with sudden onset. It is by definition associated with a specific stressful event. Classic symptoms of conversion reactions include paralysis, aphonia, seizures, coordination disturbances, blindness, other visual disturbances, anesthesia, and paresthesia. Less commonly, vomiting and autonomic disturbances can be seen.

Diagnosis and Differential

Conversion reaction is a diagnosis of exclusion. Careful history and physical exam are paramount, both for ruling out significant pathology and for understanding the underlying stress. Appropriate lab and ancillary studies should be ordered to rule out possible organic disease. Tests for true neurologic deficit, such as dropping the hand over the face or the Hoover test can be useful. The ED physician should keep in mind that some diseases (SLE, MS, polymyositis, and Lyme disease) have insidious onset with nonspecific symptoms that can be mistaken for a conversion reaction.

Emergency Department Care and Disposition

The patient should be reassured that no serious medical problem is present and that symptoms will resolve. Confronting the patient is not helpful. Referral to both medical and psychiatric resources is helpful for patient reassurance, stress management, and close followup.

For further reading in *Emergency Medicine: A Comprehensive Study Guide*, 4th edition, see Chapter 246, Conversion Reactions, by Gregory P. Moore and Kenneth C. Jackimczyk.

PEDIATRIC ABUSE

The spectrum of pediatric abuse includes child neglect, physical abuse, sexual abuse, and Munchausen syndrome by proxy. The physical stigmata of such abuse may be characteristic or subtle. Recognition of abuse is aided by knowledge of normal child development.

Clinical Features

Child neglect in early infancy results in the syndrome of failure to thrive (FTT). Overall, physical care and hygiene are frequently poor. FTT infants have very little subcutaneous tissue, prominent appearing ribs, and loose skin over the buttocks. Muscle tone is usually increased. Distinct behavioral characteristics include wariness, poor eye contact, difficult consolability, and even irritability, with interpersonal interaction. Children over the age of 2 to 3 with emotional neglect are termed psychosocial dwarfs. These children manifest the classic triad of short stature; bizarre, voracious appetite; and a disturbed home environment. They are frequently hyperactive and have delayed speech.

The spectrum of injuries in physical abuse is wide; however, certain clinical features should be suggestive. Multiple areas of ecchymoses, especially over the lower back, buttock, thighs, cheeks, ear pinnae, ankles, or wrists, and bruises of uniform but unusual shape (secondary to belts or cords) should arouse suspicion. Scald burns caused by immersion in hot water do not show a splash configuration but rather involve an entire hand or foot (glove and stocking pattern) or the buttocks and genitalia. Skeletal injuries often present with unexplained swelling of an extremity or refusal to walk or use the affected extremity. Head injuries may be manifested by subgaleal hematomas, bruising around the eyes or ears, or mental status changes. Intracranial hemorrhage with associated retinal hemorrhages may result from vigorous shaking of an infant. Injuries to the abdomen are equally serious. Symptoms include recurrent vomiting, abdominal pain and tenderness, and diffuse distension. Lastly, abused children are often submissive and compliant, do not resist painful medical procedures, and may be overly affectionate to the medical staff.

The clinical features of sexual abuse are also varied. GU symptoms, including vaginal discharge or bleeding and urinary tract infections, and behavioral disorders such as sexually oriented behavior, encopresis, regression, and nightmares, are common. Genital and perianal injury may result in abrasions, hematomas, fissures, or scarring.

Munchausen syndrome by proxy (MSBP) is a relatively uncommon form of child abuse in which a parent induces or fabricates an illness in a child. Typically reported symptoms include bleeding, seizures, apnea, diarrhea, vomiting, and fever. MSBP should be a consideration in children with medically perplexing cases and extensive previous workups.

Diagnosis and Differential

The diagnosis of child abuse should be suggested by an inconsistent history and the previously mentioned clinical features. Be highly suspicious when evaluating children for GU complaints or serious trauma. Weight, length, and head circumference should be measured in FTT infants. The body-mass index (BMI = weight [Kg]/height [m^2]) may be less than 5%. Weight gain after hospital admission is considered to be the sine qua non of environmental FTT. Children with suspected physical abuse should be evaluated with a complete blood cell count, including platelets, coagulation studies, and a skeletal survey. Inflicted injuries are suggested by spiral fractures of a long bone, metaphyseal chip fractures, multiple fractures at different stages of healing, and unusual fracture sites such as ribs, lateral clavicle, and scapula. Infants and children with suspected intracranial or intra-abdominal trauma should be elevated with CT scan. Rarely, pathological conditions such as leukemia or aplastic anemia, and osteogenesis imperfecta can mimic physical abuse. The diagnosis of sexual abuse can often be confirmed by careful inspection of the genital and perianal areas. The hymenal orifice should be measured and any hymenal notches (concavities) should be noted. Anal tone should be assessed. Children seen immediately after an assault should be evaluated for the presence of forensic evidence, such as semen. Swabs of the vagina, rectum, and oral cavity should be performed. These areas should also be cultured for gonorrhea. A vaginal culture for chlamydia should be included. Rapid antigen assays for chlamydia are unreliable in prepubescent children. It is important to remember that the absence of physical findings does not preclude abuse.

Emergency Department Care and Disposition

Medical management of pediatric abuse should be guided by physical findings and nature of injury. A full social service assessment should be obtained. Infants with significant environmental FTT and MSBP should be admitted. Victims of physical abuse frequently require admission. Reporting of suspected cases of abuse is mandatory, and a verbal report should be made to the police department or child protection agency. A suspicion of child sexual abuse also mandates such reporting. Although it is likely that the child may be removed from the home, a followup appointment for culture results and a referral for psychological counseling should be arranged.

ELDER ABUSE

Elder abuse continues to be under-recognized and under-reported. Current estimates indicate that elder abuse affects nearly 10% of the elderly population.

Clinical Features

Most elderly victims of abuse live with the perpetrator. The abuser is often dependent on the victim for housing and financial or emotional support. Alzheimer disease and other dementias are associated with greater risk for physical abuse. Patients with dependency needs (immobility, hygiene assistance) are more often victims of elder neglect. Other important historical features include presence of caretaker mental illness or drug or alcohol abuse; family history of violence; patient isolation; and recent stressful life events for the caretaker. The physical exam should note signs or symptoms of poor personal hygiene, inappropriate or soiled clothing, dehydration, malnutrition, and decubiti. Specific injuries suggestive of abuse include unexplained fractures, lacerations, or ecchymoses; injuries to the head or face; and unusual burns. In addition, certain interactions between the patient and caretaker are suggestive of abuse. These include patient fear; conflicting accounts of the injury or illness; an indifferent or angry attitude; inordinate concern with the cost of treatment; and caretaker denial to let the patient interact privately with the medical staff.

Diagnosis and Differential

Diagnosis of elder abuse should be considered in the differential diagnosis when evaluating the patient with frequent falls, failure to thrive, dementia, and dehydration or malnutrition. Diagnosis can be made in most cases by simple direct questioning regarding abusive relationships and careful physical exam.

Emergency Department Care and Disposition

Management of elder abuse involves both specific treatment for the injuries or illnesses detected and immediate intervention. Social services consultation and adult protective services involvement should be obtained in cases of proven or strongly suspected elder abuse. Elderly patients with medical problems requiring hospital admission should be admitted to the appropriate medical service. Patients who do not medically require admission may need to be admitted for protective placement if they cannot be safely discharged. If indicated, caregivers should be provided with intervention options such as home health services, Meals on Wheels, transportation, and medical and mental health services.

For further reading in *Emergency Medicine: A Comprehensive Study Guide*, 4th edition, see Chapter 250, Child Abuse and Neglect, by Carol Berkowitz; and Chapter 253, Abuse in the Elderly and Impaired, by Ellen Tallaferro and Patricia R. Salber.

177 | Male and Female Sexual Assault

Stephen W. Meldon

Sexual assault accounts for 6% of reported crimes. One study revealed that 1 in 8 women have been victims of rape, and it is estimated that only 1 in 4 cases are reported. Male sexual assault is similarly under-recognized and under-reported and has an estimated incidence of 2% to 4% of reported rapes.

Clinical Features

A brief, tactfully obtained history should include the following components: Who—assailant known, number of attackers? What happened—other physical assaults, injuries? When—time since assault? Where—where did penetration occur; vaginal, oral, rectal? Douching, showering, teeth brushing, or changing of clothing—any of these activities should be noted. Important past medical history to document includes last menstrual period, birth control method, time of last intercourse, and allergies. The physical exam should document bruises, lacerations, or other visible trauma. A pelvic examination may reveal vaginal discharge or genital lacerations or abrasions. Application of toluidine blue stain to the posterior fourchette may reveal small, subtle vulvar lacerations, which will appear as a linear blue stain. Careful oral or rectal examinations should be performed with attention to ecchymoses, lacerations, or fissures, if oral or rectal penetration has occurred. The male rape examination should entail the same history-taking as noted above. The physical exam should search for abrasions to the abdomen or anterior chest and submissive injuries, such as facial and head trauma. The anal area should be inspected for signs of trauma such as abrasions, lacerations, or fissures.

Diagnosis and Differential

Rape is a legal determination, not a medical diagnosis. The legal definition contains three elements: carnal knowledge, nonconsent, and compulsion or fear of harm. Because of the legal considerations, careful documentation and sample collection is important. Preprinted diagrams can aid in accurate representation of injuries. A prepackaged rape kit with equipment and directions on sample collection should be used. If no kit is available, smears from the vagina and cervix are made, labeled, and air dried. A wet mount from the same areas should be microscopically inspected for sperm. A vaginal aspirate using 5 to 10 mL of normal saline should be tested for acid phosphatase. Premoistened rectal or buccal swabs for sperm should be collected. A Wood's lamp will cause semen to fluoresce and may aid in sperm collection. If sodomy has occurred, rectal swabs should be taken, slides made, labeled, and air dried. A rectal aspirate using 10 mL of normal saline should be examined for sperm.

Emergency Department Care and Disposition

Treatment of the rape victim includes management of any injuries, such as laceration repair and tetanus prophylaxis, counseling, and pregnancy and sexually transmitted disease (STD) prophylaxis. Although the risk of pregnancy is very low, women rape victims should be offered pregnancy prophylaxis. Currently accepted therapy is **Ovral** (norgestrel and ethynyl estradiol) 2 tablets initially, and 2 tablets 12 h later. A negative pregnancy test should be documented prior to providing this regimen. Prophylaxis must be initiated within 72 h of the sexual assault to be effective. **STD prophylaxis** for gonorrhea and chlamydia should also be given. Current recommendations include Ceftriaxone (125 mg IM) or Ciprofloxacin (500 mg po) once, followed by Doxycycline (100 mg po BID for 7d) or Azithromycin (1 g po) once. In addition, a baseline VDRL should be obtained. **HIV testing** and counseling should be discussed with the patient, with the understanding that the risk of transmission is very low, prophylaxis with AZT has not been shown to prevent HIV transmission, and HIV testing is needed every 3 mo for a minimum of 6 mo. Indications for admission are related to the nature of injuries sustained. Only 1% to 2% of patients require hospitalization. Counseling should be available 24 h a day; often the counselor can assess and prepare the patient for exam prior to physician assessment. If counseling is not immediately available, followup with a local mental health or rape counseling center should be provided. A followup medical appointment in 7 to 14 days is appropriate. If the patient wishes to prosecute, it is the physician's added responsibility to provide police with corroborative medical evidence.

For further reading in *Emergency Medicine: A Comprehensive Study Guide*, 4th edition, see Chapter 251, Male and Female Sexual Assault, by Marion Hoelzer.

INDEX

Page numbers followed by the letters *f* and *t* indicate figures and tables respectively.